ERYTHROCYTE STRUCTURE AND FUNCTION

PROGRESS IN CLINICAL AND BIOLOGICAL RESEARCH

Volume 1: **ERYTHROCYTE STRUCTURE AND FUNCTION**
George J. Brewer, *Editor*

Volume 2: **PREVENTABILITY OF PERINATAL INJURY**
Karlis Adamsons and Howard A. Fox, *Editors*

Volume 3: **INFECTIONS OF THE FETUS AND THE NEWBORN INFANT**
Saul Krugman and Anne A. Gershon, *Editors*

Volume 4: **CONFLICTS IN CHILDHOOD CANCER**
Lucius F. Sinks and John O. Godden, *Editors*

ERYTHROCYTE STRUCTURE AND FUNCTION

Proceedings of the Third International Conference on Red Cell Metabolism and Function held at the University of Michigan, Ann Arbor, October 16–19, 1974.

Editor, George J. Brewer
Department of Human Genetics and Medicine
(Simpson Memorial Institute)
University of Michigan
Ann Arbor, Michigan

Alan R. Liss, Inc. • New York, N. Y. • 1975

Address all inquiries to the publisher:

Alan R. Liss, Inc.
150 Fifth Avenue
New York, New York 10011

Printed in the United States

Library of Congress Cataloging in Publication Data

International Conference on Red Cell Metabolism and
Function, 3d, University of Michigan, 1974.
Erythrocyte structure and function.

(Progress in clinical and biological research; 1)
Includes bibliographies.
1. Erythrocytes – Congresses.
2. Erythrocyte disorders – Congresses.
3. Sickle cell anemia – Congresses.
I. Brewer, George J., 1930 – II. Title. III. Series.
RC641.7.S5157 1974 612'111 75–999
ISBN 0-8451-0001-7

We gratefully acknowledge the generous support of:

Meyer Laboratories Incorporated
1900 West Commercial Boulevard
Fort Lauderdale, Florida 33309

Allen H. Meyers Foundation Incorporated
P. O. Box B
Tecumseh, Michigan 49286

Dow Chemical U.S.A.
Midland, Michigan 48640

PREFACE

Research on the red cell and red cell-related areas have continued at an exciting rate in the two and one-half year period since the Second International Conference on Red Cell Metabolism and Function. On October 16-19, 1974, crystallographers, chemists, biochemists, biophysicists, membrane physiologists, geneticists, anthropologists, hematologists, and physicians from many medical disciplines met in the Towsley Center for Continuing Medical Education at the University of Michigan in Ann Arbor to present new data on red cell-related topics. The meeting was dedicated to Dr. Shigeki Minakami, Chairman of the Department of Biochemistry, Kyushu University School of Medicine, Fukuoka, Japan, in recognition of his many fine contributions to red cell work, in particular to the understanding of the control of red cell glycolysis.

One of the most fascinating aspects of the total picture of red cell research is the beginning integration of the various structural and functional components of the cell into a system. For instance, in sickle cell anemia it appears that the polymerization of deoxyhemoglobin S is only the initiating step in a sequence of reactions which leads to irreversible sickling. Subsequent steps involve the structure of the red cell membrane and metabolic components in the cell and within the membrane which lead to an irreversibly sickled cell. Another area illustrative of the many emerging interactions is the area of oxidation. Numerous interactions occur between hemoglobin, the red cell membrane, red cell metabolism, and red cell systems designed to protect the cell against damage such as oxidation. Aspects of these interactions continually emerged from papers and discussions during the meeting. In addition to the more traditional areas, the Conference focussed on the molecular biology of the globin genes, red cell membranes, the fluorocarbon blood substitutes, trace metals and their blood cell effects, and biological oxidation.

The program got off to its usual strong start with a paper from M.F. Perutz, Nobel Laureate, on the nature of haem-haem interaction. Dr. Perutz illustrated his presentation with a beautiful filmstrip which showed the nature of the globin chain movement and interaction with DPG during oxygenation and deoxygenation. Other interesting papers were presented on various aspects of hemoglobin, such as the effect of salt bridges, NMR studies, a hemoglobin variant with an elongated β chain, and hemoglobin-zinc interaction. Research on the globin genes was reviewed, and a paper utilizing this system, which suggests a structural gene deletion for hydrops fetalis, was also presented. Red blood cell metabolism was considered, as usual, from many viewpoints, including the roles of pH, DPG, pyruvate kinase, and of cyclic nucleotide-membrane protein interaction. Papers on malaria, an inherited red cell cation defect, actylcholinesterase in autoimmune hemolytic anemia, and methemoglobin reduction were also presented. As with the first and second conferences a session was devoted to sickle cell hemoglobin and sickle cell anemia. Basic research areas such as the surface activity of Hb S and the allosteric properties of sickle cell hemoglobin were covered. Clinically oriented papers included factors predisposing to vascular occlusions, and approaches to treatment including in vitro carbamylation and the use of oral zinc therapy. Studies of carbamyl phosphate in animals, the potential of procaine and related drugs as antisickling agents, and the use of an animal model for testing the effects of new antisickling agents were presented.

An entire session was devoted to progress in understanding cell membranes, and papers included the effects of hormones, biophysical studies, crystallographic studies, studies of phosphorylation, and determinants of membrane elasticity. Exciting new developments in the use of fluorocarbons as blood substitutes were the topics of two papers. Animals can be kept alive after a complete exchange transfusion and also can be kept alive while breathing liquid fluorocarbons. The important developments in this field have obvious application in many important hematologic areas. A session on trace metals included the role of zinc in man, the role of selenium in glutathione peroxidase, studies of magnesium in alcohol-induced sideroblastic anemias, and the relationship of copper to the biosynthesis of heme.

Perhaps one of the most exciting new areas is the biological oxidation area because of new findings regarding superoxide and related radicals. Papers on hydrogen peroxide toxicity in erythrocytes, on the role of superoxide in G6PD-type hemolysis, superoxide in inflammation, and superoxide in the bactericidal actions of granulocytes were presented.

This volume contains the proceedings of this third conference. It includes the formal papers and much of the formal discussion after the papers. As with the previous two conferences, it represents a compilation of the present state of the art and the status of current thinking in the various areas discussed above.

The editor would like to point out that without the help of a great many people this conference could not have occurred. In particular, a great debt of gratitude is owed to Ms. Nellie Gill for her able work in all phases of the conference and publication of the volume. I also owe much gratitude to my wife, Lucia Feitler Brewer, who again worked very hard on all aspects of conference organization thereby assuring whatever success we obtained. I wish to thank Dr. Fred J. Oelshlegel, Jr., Dr. John W. Eaton, and Dr. Lorna Grindlay Moore, Ms. Nancy Noble, and Mr. Eric Schoomaker for serving as an ad hoc advisory committee for program development and also for much additional sage counsel. Thanks are also due to Mr. Tom Gilroy, Ms. Anita Schoomaker, Dr. Walter Kruckeberg, Mr. Barry Sander, Ms. Virginia Crews, and Mr. Conrad Knutsen for their assistance. The staff of post-graduate medicine, in particular Mr. Jack Burmeister, Ms. Janet Johnson, Mr. Robert Richards, and Dr. Roland Hiss were quite helpful. Ms. Barbara Warnick and Ms. Kathleen Hosner (and Ms. Nellie Gill) deserve a great deal of credit for whatever success we have achieved in publishing the discussion. Financial support from Meyer Laboratories, Inc., Fort Lauderdale, Florida, Allen H. Meyers Foundation, Inc., Tecumseh,

Michigan, and Dow Chemical U.S.A., Midland, Michigan, made the conference possible.

THE EDITOR

October 24, 1974

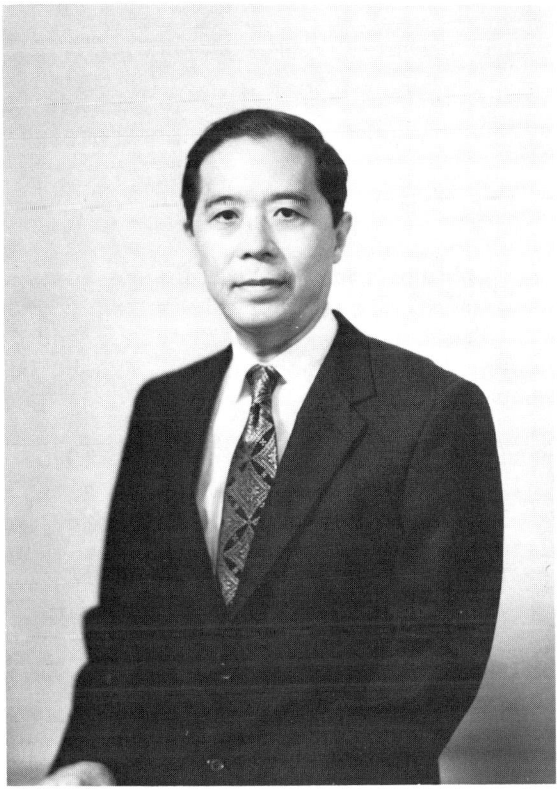

DEDICATION

OF THE THIRD INTERNATIONAL CONFERENCE ON

RED CELL METABOLISM AND FUNCTION TO

DR. SHIGEKI MINAKAMI

KYUSHU UNIVERSITY SCHOOL OF MEDICINE

FUKUOKA, JAPAN

It is a privilege and great pleasure for me, on behalf of Dr. George Brewer, Conference Chairman, to dedicate this meeting to Dr. Shigeki Minakami, Professor and Chairman of the Second Department of Biochemistry, Kyushu University School of Medicine.

Dr. Minakami was born on January 10, 1930, in Tokyo. He received his M.D. from the Tokyo University Faculty of Medicine in 1953. After completing his internship, he became a graduate student in Dr. Haruhisa Yoshikawa's Department of Physiological Chemistry and Nutrition of Tokyo University Faculty of Medicine in 1954. Thus at the early age of 24 he began a long and most productive association with Professor Yoshikawa, whom he greatly admires as a scientist and as his teacher.

Dr. Minakami was appointed an instructor in 1958 and was awarded the degree of Doctor of Medical Sciences (Ph.D.) in 1959. He came to the United States as a Fulbright Scholar in 1960, working first under Dr. T.P. Singer at the Edsel Ford Institute in Detroit and then under Dr. B. Chance at the Johnson Research Foundation in Philadelphia. He returned to Tokyo in 1962 and was promoted to associate professor in 1964. In July, 1967, he accepted his current position of Professor and Chairman of the newly formed Second Department of Biochemistry, Kyushu University School of Medicine in Fukuoka. Kyushu University is the third oldest university in Japan, after Tokyo and Kyoto. Dr. Minakami is currently a councilor of the Japanese Biochemical Society and is on the editorial board of the Journal of Biochemistry. He has an impressive bibliography of some 81 publications, all in English except for one.

Aside from his work in red cell metabolism to which I shall turn in a moment, Dr. Minakami has contributed significantly in several fields. Early in his career, he purified cytochrome c from baker's yeast, elucidated its properties, and in collaboration with Drs. K. Titani, H. Ishikura, and K. Takahashi, studied the catalytic activity of cytochrome c modified in various ways by chemical or enzymatic treatment. He worked on heme synthesis with Drs. Y. Yoneyama and Y. Sugita, discovering in liver mitochondria ferrochelatase, the enzyme responsible for the last step of heme synthesis. In an important series of five papers in the Journal of Biological Chemistry, he and his colleagues described the isolation and properties of the NADH dehydrogenase of the respiratory chain.

But it is for his contributions in the area of red cell metabolism and function that we particularly wish to honor him here today. His accomplishments are especially impressive when one realizes the difficult research conditions in Japan at the time. In a landmark series of papers beginning in 1965 on studies on erythrocyte glycolysis, Dr. Minakami, Dr. Yoshikawa, and associates described the complete analysis of glycolytic intermediates and nucleotides in human erythrocytes, studied systematically the effect of pH, then demonstrated the importance of phosphofructokinase as a controlling step, showed the value of calculating intracellular free energy changes in understanding glycolysis, examined the effect of inorganic phosphate on glycolysis, and stressed the importance of the application of the "cross over" theorem in the study of red cell glycolysis. These classical studies have established Minakami and Yoshikawa as familiar names among red cell investigators throughout the world.

Certain additional studies performed in collaboration

with his colleagues deserve mention; with Dr. H. Ohyama he determined changes in glycolytic intermediates during maturation of rabbit reticulocytes and also during storage of ACD blood; with Dr. M. Oguchi he crystallized glyceraldehyde-3-phosphate dehydrogenase from human red cells; with Dr. T. Saito he reported on the control of red cell glycolysis by ATP and NAD levels; with Dr. T. Asakura he published in 1966 that the 2,3-diphosphoglycerate (DPG) level together with the overall glycolytic rate increased when red cells were incubated anaerobically and extended previous work on the pH dependency of the DPG content in red cells. They also studied the metabolism of polyols, especially that of xylitol in erythrocytes, and showed that xylitol could be utilized as a substrate for methemoglobin reduction in red cells.

More recently, with his younger colleagues, Drs. N. Hamasaki, A. Tomoda, and S. Tsuda, he has reported on the effect of oxygen tension on glycolysis, the kinetics of DPG changes in glycolysis, the correlation of DPG with arterial pH, oxygen tension, and hematocrit value, and the problem of intracellular pH of red cells in reference to regulation of glycolysis and in blood preservation.

I have purposefully mentioned the names of some of Dr. Minakami's collaborators. This I have done because Dr. Minakami, in spite of his many significant contributions, wished to have it made clear that in honoring him we were thereby honoring the many Japanese scientists who have contributed so greatly in the area of red cell metabolism and function.

Dr. Minakami, it is our pleasure to honor you with this meeting, and with the published volume which will result from this Conference.

Kouichi R. Tanaka, M.D.
Harbor General Hospital
Torrance, California

CONTENTS

PARTICIPANTS

Bernard M. Babior, New England Medical Center Hospital, Boston, Massachusetts.

Richard F. Baker, School of Medicine, University of Southern California, Los Angeles, California.

George J. Brewer, Department of Human Genetics, University of Michigan, Ann Arbor, Michigan.

H. Franklin Bunn, Peter Bent Brigham Hospital, Boston, Massachusetts.

Oswaldo Castro, Department of Medicine, Yale University, New Haven, Connecticut.

Samuel Charache, The Johns Hopkins Hospital, Baltimore, Maryland.

Leland C. Clark, Jr., Children's Hospital Research Foundation, Cincinnati, Ohio.

Gerald Cohen, Mount Sinai School of Medicine, New York, New York.

C. Lockard Conley, The Johns Hopkins Hospital, Baltimore, Maryland.

Dennis A. Diederich, University of Kansas Medical Center, Kansas City, Kansas.

Jochen Duhm, Physiologisches Institut, Universität München, München, Germany.

John W. Eaton, Department of Medicine, University of Minnesota, Minneapolis, Minnesota.

Evan A. Evans, Department of Biomedical Engineering, Duke University, Durham, North Carolina.

Robert P. Geyer, Department of Nutrition, Harvard School of Public Health, Boston, Massachusetts.

John G. Gilman, Department of Human Genetics, University of Michigan, Ann Arbor, Michigan.

Bertil E. Glader, The Children's Hospital Medical Center, Boston, Massachusetts.

Alfred C. Greenquist, Department of Clinical Pathology and Laboratory Medicine, University of California Medical Center, San Francisco, California.

John D. Hines, Cleveland Metropolitan General Hospital, Cleveland, Ohio.

Chien Ho, Department of Biophysics and Microbiology, University of Pittsburgh, Pittsburgh, Pennsylvania.

William G. Hoekstra, Department of Biochemistry, University of Wisconsin, Madison, Wisconsin.

Harry Jacob, University of Minnesota Medical School, Minneapolis, Minnesota.

Yuet W. Kan, San Francisco General Hospital, San Francisco, California.

John V. Kilmartin, MRC Laboratory of Molecular Biology, Cambridge, England.

Lorraine M. Kraus, University of Tennessee Center for the Health Sciences, Memphis, Tennessee.

Samuel Krimm, Department of Physics, University of Michigan, Ann Arbor, Michigan.

P.L. La Celle, University of Rochester, School of Medicine and Dentistry, Rochester, New York.

Rosanne M. Leipzig, Department of Human Genetics, University of Michigan, Ann Arbor, Michigan.

Joe M. McCord, Duke University Medical Center, Durham, North Carolina.

Nydia Meyers, Department of Human Genetics, University of Michigan, Ann Arbor, Michigan.

Shigeki Minakami, Department of Biochemistry, Kyushu University, Fukuoka, Japan.

Ronald L. Nagel, Albert Einstein College of Medicine, Yeshiva University, Bronx, New York.

Fred J. Oelshlegel, Jr., Department of Human Genetics, University of Michigan, Ann Arbor, Michigan.

James M. Orten, Department of Biochemistry and Graduate Affairs, Wayne State University School of Medicine, Detroit, Michigan.

M.F. Perutz, MRC Laboratory of Molecular Biology, Cambridge, England.

Ananda S. Prasad, Department of Medicine, Wayne State University, Detroit Michigan.

Howard Rasmussen, Department of Biochemistry, University of Pennsylvania, Philadelphia, Pennsylvania.

Luigi Rossi-Bernardi, Cattedra di Enzimologia, University of Milan, Milan, Italy.

Arthur I. Skoultchi, Department of Cell Biology, Albert Einstein College of Medicine, Yeshiva University, Bronx, New York.

Yoshika Sugita, Department of Biochemistry, Kanazawa University School of Medicine, Kanazawa, Japan.

Kouichi R. Tanaka, Harbor General Hospital, Torrance, California

REGISTRANTS

Arthur Arnone, Department of Biochemistry, University of Iowa, Iowa City, Iowa.

David Ballou, Department of Biological Chemistry, University of Michigan, Ann Arbor, Michigan.

Marion I. Barnhart, 540 E. Canfield, Detroit, Michigan.

A. Gerald Beaudoin, 23280 Manistee, Oak Park, Michigan.

Michael C. Brain, Department of Medicine, McMaster University, Hamilton, Ontario, Canada.

Robert J. Broersma, Dow Chemical Company, Midland, Michigan.

Ray K. Brown, Wayne State University School of Medicine, Detroit, Michigan.

Lawrence N. Button, Children's Hospital Medical Center, Boston, Massachusetts.

Robert T. Card, Department of Medicine, University Hospital, Saskatoon, Saskatchewan Canada.

William G. Chaney, Department of Biochemistry, Michigan State University, East Lansing, Michigan.

Lyubica Dabich, Simpson Memorial Institute, University of Michigan, Ann Arbor, Michigan.

R. Ben Dawson, Division of Hematology, School of Medicine, University of Maryland, Baltimore, Maryland.

Louis DeFilippi, Department of Biological Chemistry, University of Michigan, Ann Arbor, Michigan.

Thomas F. Deuel, Department of Medicine, The University of Chicago, Chicago, Illinois.

Stephen H. Embury, Stanford University School of Medicine, Division of Hematology, Stanford, California.

James Fee, Biophysics Research Division, University of Michigan, Ann Arbor, Michigan.

Ellis A. Fuller, 4910 Crofton Road, Louisville, Kentucky.

Leslie Wo-Mei Fung, University of Pittsburgh, Pittsburgh, Pennsylvania.

Thomas G. Gabuzda, Lankenau Hospital, Philadelphia, Pennsylvania.

Gary Geller, University of Minnesota, Minneapolis, Minnesota.

Ronald O. Gilcher, Central Blood Bank of Pittsburgh, Pittsburgh, Pennsylvania.

Victor Ginsberg, 6 Hickory Hill, Roslyn Estates, New York.

Harry L. Greene, Peter Bent Brigham Hospital, Boston, Massachusetts.

Roy Greenwell, Meyer Laboratories, Inc., Fort Lauderdale, Florida.

William Hasey, Meyer Laboratories, Inc., Fort Lauderdale, Florida.

A.B. Henderson, 9041 Dexter, Blvd., Detroit, Michigan.

John Hercules, National Institutes of Health, Sickle Cell Disease Branch, Bethesda, Maryland.

Donald E. Hultquist, Department of Biological Chemistry, University of Michigan, Ann Arbor, Michigan.

Robert Hsu, University of Chicago, Chicago, Illinois.

Rudolph E. Jackson, National Institutes of Health, Sickle Cell Disease Branch, Bethesda, Maryland.

Michael E. Johnson, Biophysics Department, University of Pittsburgh, Pittsburgh, Pennsylvania.

Patricia Kelly, Simpson Memorial Institutes, University of Michigan, Ann Arbor, Michigan.

Yeong Wook Kim, Department of Physics, Wayne State University, Detroit, Michigan.

Walter Kruckeberg, Department of Human Genetics, University of Michigan, Ann Arbor, Michigan.

Martha Ludwig, Biophysics Research Division, University of Michigan, Ann Arbor, Michigan.

Jeanne Lusher, Children's Hospital of Michigan, Detroit, Michigan.

M. David MacFarlane, Meyer Laboratories, Inc., Fort Lauderdale, Florida.

Jeannine A. Majde, Office of Naval Research, 536 S. Clark, Chicago, Illinois.

Michael K. McCormack, Dight Institute for Human Genetics, University of Minnesota, Minneapolis, Minnesota.

Thomas D. Miale, Department of Pediatrics, University of Florida College of Medicine, Gainesville, Florida.

Denis R. Miller, Cornell Medical Center, New York Hospital, New York, New York.

Harry J. Miller, 2500 Ridge Avenue, Evanston, Illinois.

Hiroshi Mizukami, Department of Biology, Wayne State University, Detroit, Michigan.

Makio Murayama, National Institutes of Health, Bethesda, Maryland.

Peter J. O'Brien, Department of Biological Chemistry, University of Michigan, Ann Arbor, Michigan

S. Ogawa, Bell Laboratories, 600 Mountain Avenue, Murray Hill, New Jersey.

Eugene P. Orringer, Department of Medicine, University of North Carolina School of Medicine, Chapel Hill, North Carolina.

Judith L. Page, Chemical Biology Research, Dow Chemical Company, Midland, Michigan.

David Petering, Department of Chemistry, University of Wisconsin, Milwaukee, Wisconsin.

P.H. Pinkerton, Sunnybrook Medical Centre, Toronto, Ontario Canada.

Y. Ravindranath, Children's Hospital of Michigan, Detroit, Michigan.

Robert E. Reed, Veterans Administration Hospital, Ann Arbor, Michigan.

James W. Reid, 633 Lord Dunmore Drive, Virginia Beach, Virginia.

Ronald A. Rohe, E.J. Meyer Memorial Hospital, Buffalo, New York.

Zelda B. Rose, Institute for Cancer Research, Philadelphia, Pennsylvania.

Richard L. Roth, 64 Sheldon Trail, New Haven, Connecticut.

J.M. Salhany, Department of Biophysics, Bell Telephone Laboratories, Murray Hill, New Jersey.

Jerome S. Schultz, Department of Chemical Engineering, University of Michigan, Ann Arbor, Michigan.

J. Gerald Scott, Toronto General Hospital, Toronto, Canada.

Nicole Simard-Duquesne, Ayerst Research Laboratories, Montreal, Quebec, Canada.

James B. Stamatoff, Physics Department, University of Michigan, Ann Arbor, Michigan.

Ivan J. Stern, Travenol Laboratories, Morton Grove, Illinois.

William J. Stith, Fenwal Laboratories, Division of Travenol Laboratories, Round Lake, Illinois.

Kenneth A. Stoutenborough, Simpson Memorial Institute, University of Michigan, Ann Arbor, Michigan.

Abraham Sumoza, Mayo Clinic, Rochester, Minnesota.

Basil Tatsis, L.I. Jewish-Hillside Medical Center, Queens Hospital Affiliation, Jamaica, New York.

Garson H. Tishkoff, American Red Cross, 1800 E. Grand River Avenue, Lansing, Michigan.

R.C. Trueworthy, Department of Pediatrics, University of Kansas Medical Center, Kansas City, Kansas.

Vernon L. Verhoef, Department of Biochemistry, Michigan State University, East Lansing, Michigan.

May Votaw, Simpson Memorial Institute, University of Michigan, Ann Arbor, Michigan.

Davorin Vugrincic, Simpson Memorial Institute, University of Michigan, Ann Arbor, Michigan.

Charles H. Wallas, Blood Bank, University of Kansas Medical Center, Kansas City, Kansas.

Y.M. Wang, Department of Pediatrics, M.D. Anderson Hospital and Tumor Institute, The University of Texas System Cancer Center, Houston, Texas.

Karen Wiechelman, Department of Biophysics and Microbiology, University of Pittsburgh, Pittsburgh, Pennsylvania.

Robert D. Woodson, 1300 University Avenue, Madison, Wisconsin.

Raymond L. Woosley, Meyer Laboratories, Inc., Fort Lauderdale, Florida.

Robert Zand, Department of Biological Chemistry, Institute of Science and Technology, University of Michigan, Ann Arbor, Michigan.

HEMOGLOBIN STRUCTURE AND FUNCTION

Chairman: M. F. Perutz

HAEMOGLOBIN BEHAVES AS AN ALLOSTERIC PROTEIN

M.F. Perutz

MRC Laboratory of Molecular Biology,
Cambridge, England.

On the basis of the allosteric theory of Monod, Wyman and Changeux (1965) haem-haem interaction and the Bohr effect should be due to a reversible transition between two, or at least two, alternative structures; one, the tense (T) structure having a low oxygen affinity and the other relaxed (R) structure a high one. These two structures should differ by the distribution and/or energy of the bonds between the four subunits and therefore also by the conformational constraints imposed upon them. The theory predicts that the shape of the curve is determined by only two experimentally verifiable parameters $L = [T]/[R]$, i.e. the concentration ratio of the tense and relaxed structures in the absence of oxygen; and $c = k_R/k_T$, the ratio of the dissociation constants of oxygen from the subunits in the R or T states, assuming them to be equal for the α and β subunits.

Figure 1 is a diagrammatic representation of the allosteric model. The left diagram shows a tense structure in which the four subunits are held together by four clamps against the pressure exercised by four springs. The haem pockets are too narrow to admit oxygen easily. When oxygen nevertheless combines, the structure becomes progressively more strained, until the clamps give way, the haem pockets of all four subunits expand simultaneously (no matter

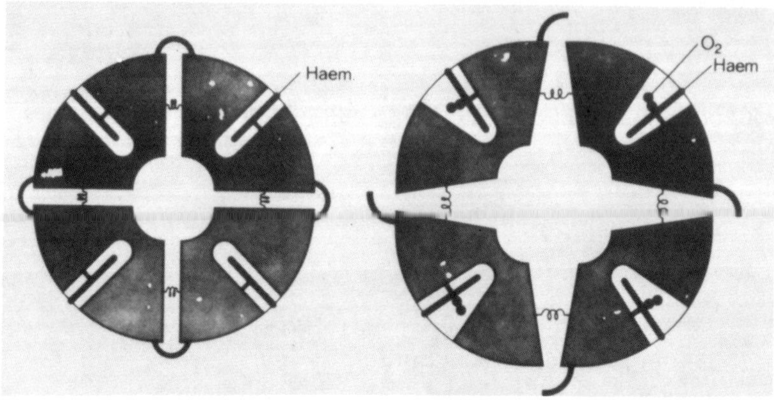

Fig 1. Diagrammatic representation of allosteric transition of haemoglobin between tense and relaxed states.

whether they contain oxygen or not) and the structure assumes the relaxed state pictured on the right. This transition can happen at any stage of the reaction.

X-ray analysis did indeed reveal two alternative structures, deoxy- and oxyhaemoglobin, and showed evidence for the deoxy structure being constrained by bonds between the subunits which are absent in the oxy structure (Muirhead and Greer, 1970; Bolton and Perutz, 1970; Perutz, 1970). These bonds take the form of salt bridges between charged groups as pictured in figure 2. Most of the polar groups which form the salt bridges have pK's well above or below the physiological range of pH, but a few contain histidines or α-amino groups with pK's between 6.5 and 8.0, so that they are strengthened by a drop, and weakened by a rise, of pH (acid pH increases the fraction of histidines and α-amino groups carrying positive charges). Consequently acid pH tightens the bonds between the subunits in the deoxy structure, but may have little or no effect on the stability of the oxy structure. 2,3-diphosphoglycerate (DPG) is pictured as an additional clamp held fast by four salt bridges between the β chains (actually there are seven). It too should add to the stability of the deoxy structure but leave the oxy structure unaffected (in fact it does have a very low affinity for the oxy structure).

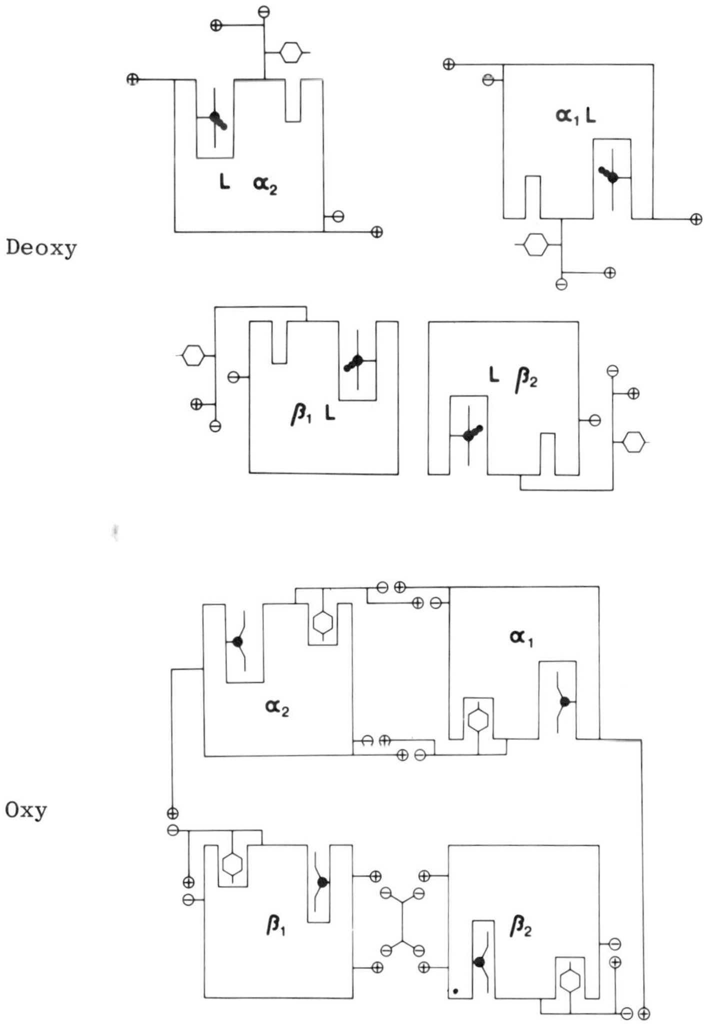

Fig 2. Top: deoxyhaemoglobin with all salt bridges intact and DPG clamped between the β subunits. Note the iron out of the plane of the porphyrin and the narrow haem pockets in the β chains. Bottom: oxyhaemoglobin with all salt bridges broken, DPG dissociated, planar haems and wider haem pockets in the β subunits (Perutz, 1970).

PROPERTIES PREDICTED BY ALLOSTERIC THEORY

What predictions can we make about the properties of haemoglobin on the basis of the allosteric theory and the experimentally determined stereochemistry of the two alternative structures?

1. In the absence of a change of quaternary structure there should be no haem-haem interaction. If all the molecules remain in the oxy or R structure the Bohr effect should also be absent, but if they remain in the deoxy or T structure, there may be a Bohr effect if rupture of the salt bridges is directly linked with oxygen uptake.

2. The two structures should be in dynamic equilibrium in solution.

3. The free energy of haem-haem interaction should be a function of the number and strength of the salt bridges that must be broken in the transition from the T to the R structure. Near physiological pH it should therefore rise with increasing concentration of DPG and $[H^+]$.

4. The allosteric constant L and Hill's constant n should be related by a bell-shaped curve (Rubin and Changeux, 1966; Edelstein, 1971).

EXPERIMENTAL EVIDENCE

Evidence for 1. There are many examples of the inhibition of haem-haem interaction in haemoglobin derivatives or mutants which remain in the R state in the absence of oxygen (NES-desArg haemoglobin (Kilmartin and Hewitt, 1971): desArg haemoglobin at high pH; BME haemoglobin* (Simon, 1967); haemoglobin Kempsey (Perutz *et al*, 1974a).

---

* In BME haemoglobin cysteine 93β and histidine 97β are joined by the bifunctional reagent Bismaleimidomethylether which shifts the allosteric equilibrium towards R. NES stands for N-ethylsuccinamide on SH93β.

In every case which has been investigated haem-haem interaction can be restored by the addition of organic phosphates, showing that these haemoglobins are capable of regaining it if their allosteric equilibrium is shifted sufficiently towards the T state. The oxygen equilibrium curves of these haemoglobins coincide with the asymptote K_4 for normal human haemoglobin (see accompanying paper by Kilmartin et al).

Inhibition of haem-haem interaction in the T state has been demonstrated in haemoglobin Kansas, but not convincingly since the heterogeneity between the α and β chains is too large to restore interaction, either by stripping the haemoglobin of phosphates or by raising the pH. However, the valency hybrid haemoglobin Milwaukee (Val E11β→Glu) does show haem-haem interaction when stripped of phosphates; this is inhibited by DPG which prevents the transition to the R state (Udem, Ranney, Bunn and Pisciotta, 1970). In both haemoglobins Kansas and Milwaukee the oxygen equilibrium curves in the T state coincide with K_1 for normal haemoglobin (see accompanying paper by Kilmartin et al).

Evidence for 2. The existence of a dynamic equilibrium in solution can be demonstrated in three modified haemoglobins in which some of the residues forming salt bridges which stabilize the deoxy structure have been either removed or blocked: desArg 141α; desTyr 145-His 146β and BME haemoglobin. In each case the deoxy derivative of horse crystallizes in the R and that of human in the T form. In horse the R structure is the less soluble, but in human the T structure. Consequently, when the two structures are in dynamic equilibrium in a saturated solution, the less soluble one crystallizes out.

Evidence for 3. The dependence of the free energy of haem-haem interaction on pH and DPG is demonstrated by Kilmartin in the accompanying paper and by Tyuma et al (1973).

Evidence for 4. The predicted bell-shaped relation between L and n was first demonstrated tentatively for normal haemoglobin under various conditions and for two mutant haemoglobins by Edelstein. However, the values of n do not all lie on the same bell-shaped curve unless the intrinsic oxygen affinities in the R and T states are the same for all derivatives, which is not always true. To overcome this difficulty Kilmartin measured the oxygen affinities of the free α and β chains of many derivatives and mutants with abnormal oxygen affinities; Baldwin (1974) then made $k_R = (k_\alpha \times k_\beta)^{\frac{1}{2}}$ and expressed the observed mean oxygen affinities $k_m(p_{50})$ relative to k_R. Using Rubin and Changeux's equations this allowed her to plot the observed values of n against L. They did fall on a set of bell-shaped curves, rather than a single one, which is consistent with the very different values of c found by Kilmartin in different derivatives and mutants (figure 3).

STABLE AND UNSTABLE INTERMEDIATE STRUCTURES

A central feature of the allosteric theory is the concept of symmetry, that is to say the ligand affinities of the subunits in any one quaternary structure should be independent of the state of ligation of the other subunits; this is a restatement of condition 1 and has been confirmed experimentally. However, the theory does not postulate the existence of only two alternative quaternary structures but of "at least two", and the often made references to it as a "two state model" are a misrepresentation. The X-ray evidence shows that in the transition between the R and T quaternary structures most of the movement occurs at the $\alpha_1\beta_2$ contact which is dovetailed so that two relative positions of the α_1 and β_2 subunits are more stable than all others. I therefore argued that intermediates in the reaction with oxygen are likely to have either the T or R quaternary structure, but cautioned that in view of the high speed of the reaction with oxygen the occurrence of unstable intermediate quaternary structures could not be excluded (Perutz, 1970).

Valency hybrids are regarded as good models for intermediates as they can be made to have one pair of haems in a high, and another in a low, spin state similar to deoxy- and oxyhaemoglobin. In X-ray studies the best model so far has

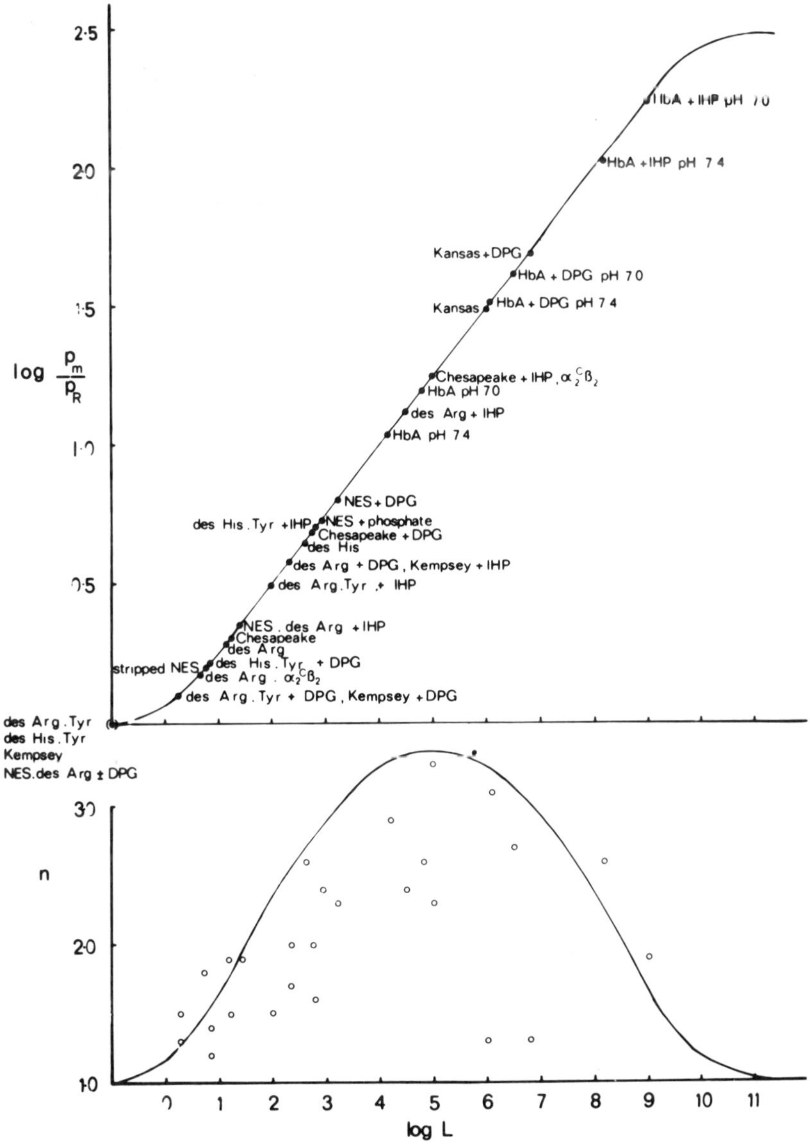

Fig 3. Dependence of the mean oxygen affinity k_m/k_R and of Hill's constant n on the allosteric constant L. (Reproduced by permission of Baldwin, 1974).

been haemoglobin Milwaukee where the haems in the β chains are locked in a ferric high spin structure and bias the allosteric equilibrium towards the T state. Results showed that $\alpha_2^{deoxy}\beta_2^{+Mil}$ has the T structure and $\alpha_2^{CO}\beta_2^{+Mil}$ the R structure, indicating that these are the only two stable quaternary structures accessible to the system (Perutz, Pulsinelli and Ranney, 1972). Cyanomet hybrids have one pair of haems locked in a ferric low spin state which biases the allosteric equilibrium strongly towards the R state. They have not yet been crystallized but NMR spectra indicate that $\alpha_2^{+CN}\beta_2^{deoxy}$ in "stripped" solutions has the R structure but in solutions containing phosphates (inorganic or organic) the T structure. $\alpha_2^{deoxy}\beta_2^{+CN}$ maintain the R structure even in the presence of inorganic phosphate or DPG, but inositolhexaphosphate (IHP) switches it to the T structure (Ogawa and Shulman, 1972). When the ferrous chains have combined with oxygen, both hybrids have the R structure. So the X-ray and NMR evidence indicates that stable intermediates have either one or the other quaternary structure. However, there is kinetic evidence in favour of short-lived intermediates with ligand affinities intermediate between those of the R and T structures (Gibson, 1973); spectroscopic evidence indicates that IHP can combine with ferrous and ferric low spin compounds and somehow modify the R structure (Perutz et al, 1974c; Adams and Schuster, 1974); the absorption spectrum of the modified oxy structure is related to that of the kinetic intermediate seen by Gibson and may be indicative of an intermediate quaternary structure unstable in the absence of IHP*. Furthermore, a major change in the quaternary structure of oxyhaemoglobin occurs on going below pH 6.0, and this transition may be the cause of the acid Bohr effect (Perutz, 1954 and 1970); a minor change occurs near pH 7.0 which may be related to the small pH dependence of the fourth Adair constant observed by Imai and Yonetani (1974).

---

* Gibson (1973) reported a heterogeneity in the velocities of combination with oxygen which he attributed to differences between the α and β chains, but on the basis of my spectroscopic results I suspect that his kinetic heterogeneity is in fact between the R structure and an intermediate.

REGULATION OF ALLOSTERIC EQUILIBRIUM BY HAEM LIGANDS

How does the uptake of ligands by the haem regulate the allosteric equilibrium? One can envisage two effects. A direct steric one by the ligand itself, as pictured in figure 1, and an indirect one by ligand altering the structure of the haem complex. The X-ray evidence shows a marked widening of the haem pocket on combination of ligand with the β subunits, but an only just detectable one in the α subunits. It also shows a marked change in the structure of the haem complex in both subunits. This change consists of a movement of the iron atom and of the haem-linked histidine (F8) relative to the plane of the porphyrin ring (figure 4 and Table 1) and is caused by an electronic transition in the iron atom on going from the five-coordinated high spin deoxyhaemoglobin to the six-coordinated low spin oxyhaemoglobin. The transition shortens the bonds between the iron atom and its surrounding

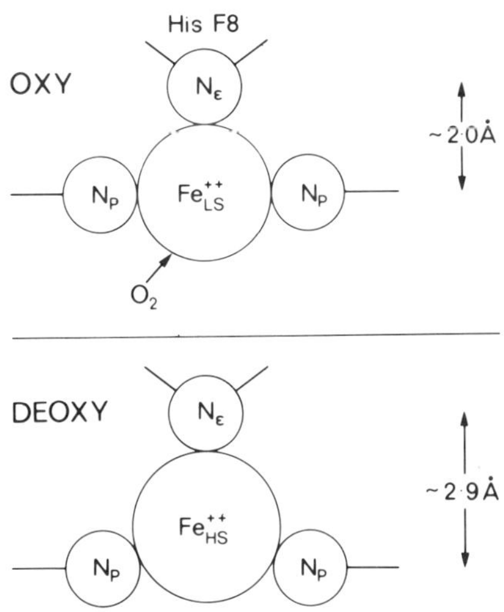

Fig 4. Position of iron and N_{ε} of histidine F8 relative to the plane of the porphyrin in oxy- and deoxyhaemoglobin.

TABLE 1

MOVEMENTS IN THE HAEM-POCKET ON TRANSITION FROM DEOXY TO METHAEMOGLOBIN

	From centre of porphyrin to		Deoxy	Met	Δ Deoxy - Met
			Å	Å	Å
	N_ε His F8	α	2.7	2.1	+0.6
		β	2.8	2.2	+0.6
$C_{\gamma 1}$	Val E11	α	6.7	6.7	0
		β	5.1	6.4	-1.3

The movement of the N_ε His F8 relative to the centre of the porphyrin ring is due to the shortening of the Fe-N bond distances on going from the high spin ferrous five-coordinated deoxy to the high spin ferric six-coordinated aquomet structure. On transition to the low spin ferrous six-coordinated oxy structure the movement probably amounts to 0.9 Å.

$C_{\gamma 1}$ of valine E11 obstructs the ligand binding site in the deoxy structure and moves out of the way on transition to the liganded oxy or met form. It responds directly to the steric effect of the ligand. (The changes in distances were calculated by Dr Elizabeth Heidner from the real space refined coordinates of horse deoxy- and methaemoglobin determined by A.D. McLachlan.)

nitrogen atoms (Hoard, 1968; Perutz, 1970). Both direct and indirect steric effects of ligation therefore play a part in regulating the allosteric equilibrium. In view of the recent controversies (Hoffmann, Spilburg and Petering, 1971; Hoard and Scheidt, 1973) it is worth pointing out that I stated this explicitly in the summary as well as the text of my 1970 paper in Nature. Another statement in that summary has given rise to misunderstanding, even though I amplified it in the text and in subsequent papers. This says that the structural changes in the subunits are triggered by the movement of the iron relative to the porphyrin, which is indeed true for the oxygenation reaction of normal haemoglobin; however, it is made clear in the text that the more important and generally valid parameter is the distance of the proximal histidine from the plane of the porphyrin ring. So if I had to write the summary today, I would say that reaction with ligand alters the allosteric equilibrium between the two alternative stable quaternary structures of mammalian haemoglobin by changing the distance of the proximal histidine from the plane of the porphyrin ring and by the direct steric effect of the ligand on the β subunits.

What evidence, other than structural, is there to support this hypothesis?

1. pH dependence of the cooperativity of the oxidation of deoxy- to methaemoglobin. In the reaction of haemoglobin with oxygen, the free energy of haem-haem interaction rises slightly with falling pH (Imai and Yonetani, 1974) while in the oxidation reaction it rises steeply with rising pH (Antonini et al, 1964; Kilmartin, 1973). This seems curious at first sight, since both oxy- and methaemoglobin have the same quaternary structure. In the oxygenation reaction the distance moved by the proximal histidine relative to the plane of the porphyrin is independent of pH and the small rise of the free energy of haem-haem interaction with falling pH occurs because $[H^+]$ strengthens the salt bridges between the subunits in the T structure. In the oxidation reaction, on the other hand, the distance moved by the histidine relative to the porphyrin is pH-dependent. At acid pH, the transition is between two high

spin structures involving a movement of the proximal histidine relative to the plane of the porphyrin ring by only ∿0.6 Å, while at alkaline pH the transition is between a high and a low spin structure involving a movement by ∿0.9 Å; thus the bigger movement raises the free energy of haem-haem interaction which corresponds to a lowering of the allosteric constant c. The detailed mechanism is discussed by Perutz et al 1974b.

2. Cobalt haemoglobin exhibits haem-haem interaction even though the divalent cobalt ion remains formally in the low spin state in both oxy- and deoxyhaemoglobin (Hoffmann, Spilburg and Petering, 1971). However, electron spin resonance has shown that in oxyhaemoglobin a large fraction of the electron density of the single unpaired electron is transferred to the oxygen, so that the cobalt becomes effectively trivalent. X-ray studies of model compounds have shown that the transfer of the unpaired electron from the metal to the oxygen shortens the bond from the cobalt to the proximal histidine as well as moving the cobalt slightly nearer to the plane of the porphyrin ring (Hoard and Scheidt, 1973). As a result the proximal histidine would move relative to the plane of the porphyrin by only about one third of the distance in iron haemoglobin (Hoard and Scheidt 1973). The free energy of haem-haem interaction is correspondingly diminished to about one third of its value in iron haemoglobin (Woodruff, Spiro and Yonetani, 1974).

3. Valency hybrids. I have already mentioned the valency hybrids in which one pair of subunits can be either high or low spin ferric. The distance from the plane of the porphyrin to the N_ε of the proximal histidine (D_{pN}) is at least 0.3 Å longer in high than in low spin derivatives, and both contain ligands in the sixth coordination position. It is possible, therefore, to examine the influence on the allosteric equilibrium of changes in D_{pN} without gain or loss of ligand at the ferric haems.

The results of spectroscopic and ligand equilibrium studies show a bias of the allosteric equilibrium of valency hybrids towards the T structure when the ferric iron is high spin and towards the R structure when it is low spin (Perutz et al, 1974c; Szabo and Karplus, in press).

4. Effect of inositolhexaphosphate (IHP). This organic phosphate binds to the same site as DPG (Arnone and Perutz, 1974) and biases the allosteric equilibrium strongly towards the T state. It switches the two high spin ferric derivatives aquo- and fluoro-methaemoglobin to a structure which has a similar SH reactivity and UV absorption and circular dichroism as deoxyhaemoglobin, but does not switch the two low spin derivatives cyano- and azide-methaemoglobin to that structure, showing that the shorter D_{pN} distance in the low spin derivatives opposes the action of IHP (Perutz et al, 1974b).

5. If it were possible to construct a system in which the metal-nitrogen bonds remained unaltered on ligand binding, so that one could isolate the direct from the indirect effects of ligation, such a system would also be found to bind ligand cooperatively. However, in practice the metal-nitrogen bonds will always be longer in a five-coordinated transition metal complex than in the corresponding six-coordinated one, so that one observes varying combinations of the two effects.

CHANGES OF TERTIARY AND QUATERNARY STRUCTURE ON LIGAND BINDING

Monod et al (1965) assumed all the subunits in the quaternary T state to be in the unreactive form, and those in the R structure to be in the reactive form. In their paper they related identical affinities with identical structures but they envisaged the possibility that this assumption might prove too simple and this is indeed the case. In fact, the haemoglobin subunits change their tertiary structure in response both to ligand binding and to the change of quaternary structure. The change in tertiary structure in response to ligand binding may be regarded as an example of induced fit in response to a change in conformation of the coenzyme (the haem) on reacting with the substrate (oxygen) as predicted by Koshland (1958). However, it is important to realise that even though the subunits change their tertiary structure sequentially in response to ligand binding, there is no evidence that this change in tertiary structure affects the ligand affinities or the electronic and NMR spectra of the neighbouring subunits, unless there is a change of quaternary structure. Functionally, therefore, haemoglobin behaves strictly according to the allosteric model of Monod *et al* (1965) rather than the sequential one of Koshland *et al* (1966).

EFFECT OF CHANGES IN QUATERNARY STRUCTURE OF THE GLOBIN UPON THE HAEM

In recent years my own studies have been directed towards the effect of the change in quaternary structure on the state of the haem. The results indicate that the interaction between the haem and the globin is a reciprocal one, as indeed it must be on elementary principles of action and reaction, so that changes in quaternary structure of the globin in turn alter the tension at the haems. Our recent results confirm this idea and suggest that haem-haem interaction works in the following way. Starting with fully oxygenated haemoglobin in the R state, loss of oxygen from one or more subunits would change the quaternary structure to the T state. The resulting tension at the haems and narrowing of the haem pocket in the β subunits would lower the oxygen affinity and facilitate the release of the remaining oxygen. Starting with fully deoxygenated haemoglobin in the T state, uptake of oxygen by some of the subunits would change the quaternary structure to the R state, thereby releasing the tension on the haems, opening out the haem pockets in the β subunits, and speeding full oxygenation. In summary, haem-haem interaction is coupled to a change of tension at the haem, transmitted by a change of quaternary structure of the globin (Perutz, 1972; Hopfield, 1973; Perutz *et al*, 1974c).

REFERENCES

Adams, M.L. & Schuster, T. (1974). Phosphate-dependent spectroscopic changes in liganded haemoglobin. Biochem. Biophys.Res.Comm. 58, 525.

Antonini, E., Wyman, J., Brunori, M., Taylor, J.F., Rossi-Fanelli, A. & Caputo, A. (1964). Studies on the oxidation-reduction potentials of heme proteins. I. Human haemoglobin. J.Biol.Chem. 239, 907.

Arnone, A. & Perutz, M.F. (1974). Structure of inositol-hexaphosphate human haemoglobin complex. Nature, 249, 34.

Baldwin, J.M. (1974). Structure and function of haemoglobin. Progress in Biophys. and Mol.Biol. In press.

Bolton, W. & Perutz, M.F. (1970). Three-dimensional Fourier synthesis of horse deoxyhaemoglobin at 2.8 Å resolution. Nature, 228, 551.

Edelstein, S.J. (1971). Extensions of the allosteric model for haemoglobin. Nature, 230, 224.

Gibson, Q.H. (1973). The contribution of the α and β chains to the kinetics of oxygen binding to and dissociation from hemoglobin. Proc.Nat.Acad.Sci.US, 70, 1.

Hoard, J.L. (1968). Some aspects of heme stereochemistry. In: Structural Chemistry and Molecular Biology (Ed A. Rich and N. Davidson). Freeman : San Francisco.

Hoard, J.L. & Scheidt, W.R. (1973). Stereochemical trigger for initiating cooperative interaction of the subunits during the oxygenation of cobaltohemoglobin. Proc.Nat. Acad.Sci.US, 70, 3919.

Hoffmann, B.M., Spilburg, C.A. & Petering, D.H. (1971). Coboglobins: Cobalt substitution and the nature of the prosthetic group - apoprotein interaction in hemoglobin and myoglobin. Cold Spring Harb.Symp.Quant.Biol. 36, 343.

Hopfield, J.J. (1973). Relation between structure, cooperativity and spectra in a model of hemoglobin action. J.Mol.Biol. 77, 207.

Imai, K. & Yonetani, T. (1974). pH dependence of the Adair constants of human hemoglobin: non-uniform contribution of successive oxygen bindings to the alkaline Bohr effect. J.Biol.Chem. in press.

Kilmartin, J.V. (1973). The interaction of inositolhexaphosphate with methaemoglobin. Biochem.J. 133, 725.

Kilmartin, J.V. & Hewitt, J.A. (1971). The effect of removal of C-terminal residues on cooperative interactions in hemoglobin. Cold Spring Harb.Symp.Quant.Biol. 36, 311.

Koshland, D.E. (1958). Application of a theory of enzyme specificity to protein synthesis. Proc.Nat.Acad.Sci.US, 44, 98.

Koshland, D.E., Némethy, G. & Filmer, D. (1966). Comparison of experimental binding data and theoretical models in proteins containing subunits. Biochemistry, 5, 365.

Monod, J., Wyman, J. & Changeux, J.P. (1965). On the nature of allosteric transitions: a plausible model. J.Mol.Biol. 12, 88.

Muirhead, H. & Greer, J. Three-dimensional Fourier synthesis of human deoxyhaemoglobin at 3.5 Å resolution. Nature, 228, 516.

Ogawa, S. & Shulman, R.G. (1972). High resolution nuclear magnetic resonance spectra of hemoglobin. III. The half-ligated state and allosteric interactions. J.Mol.Biol. 70, 315.

Perutz, M.F. (1954). The structure of haemoglobin. III. Direct determination of the molecular transform. Proc.Roy. Soc. A.225, 264.

Perutz, M.F. (1970). Stereochemistry of cooperative effects in haemoglobin. Nature, 228, 726.

Perutz, M.F (1972). Nature of haem-haem interaction. Nature, 337, 495.

Perutz, M.F., Pulsinelli, P.D. & Ranney, H.M. (1972). Structure and subunit interaction of haemoglobin M Milwaukee. Nature New Biol. 237, 259.

Perutz, M.F., Ladner, J.E., Simon, S.R. & Ho, C. (1974a). Influence of globin structure on the state of the heme. I. Human deoxyhaemoglobin. Biochemistry, 13, 2163.

Perutz, M.F., Fersht, A.R., Simon, S.R. & Roberts, G.C.K. (1974b). Influence of globin structure on the state of the heme. II. Allosteric transitions in methaemoglobin. Biochemistry, 13, 2174.

Perutz, M.F., Heidner, E.J., Ladner, J.E., Beetlestone, J.G. Ho, C. & Slade, E.F. (1974c). Influence of globin structure on the state of the heme. III. Changes in heme spectra accompanying allosteric transitions in methaemoglobin and their implications for heme-heme interaction. Biochemistry, 13, 2187.

Rubin, M.M. & Changeux, J.P. (1966). On the nature of allosteric transitions: implications of non-exclusive ligand binding. J.Mol.Biol. 21, 265.

Simon, S.R. (1967). Ph.D. thesis. Rockefeller University, New York.

Szabo, A. & Karplus, M. In press.

Tyuma, I., Imai, K. & Shimizu, K. (1973). Analysis of the oxygen equilibrium of haemoglobin and control mechanism of organic phosphates. Biochemistry, 12, 1491.

Udem, L., Ranney, H.M., Bunn, H.F. & Pisciotta, A. (1970). Some observations on hemoglobin $M_{Milwaukee-1}$. J.Mol.Biol. 48, 489.

Woodruff, W.H., Spiro, T.G. & Yonetani, T. (1974). Resonance Raman spectra of cobalt-substituted hemoglobin: cooperativity and displacement of the cobalt atom upon oxygenation. Proc.Nat.Acad.Sci.US. 71, 1065.

FUNCTIONAL ROLE OF THE SALT BRIDGES IN HEMOGLOBIN

J.V. Kilmartin, K. Imai* and R.T. Jones

MRC Laboratory of Molecular Biology,
Cambridge, England.
* MRC Abnormal Haemoglobin Unit, Cambridge,
England.

The allosteric theory of Monod et al (1965) explains the cooperativity of multi-subunit proteins by proposing that the subunits can associate in two different quaternary structures in equilibrium with each other. These quaternary structures differ in their intersubunit contacts which constrain the subunits to have different affinities for ligands. A subunit in the T, or tense, structure has low affinity for the ligand and a subunit in the R, or relaxed, structure has high affinity. Binding ligand to the protein shifts the equilibrium towards the R structure. High cooperativity is only observed when there is a complete transition between T and R during ligation. The model uses two parameters. L, the allosteric constant, is the equilibrium constant between T and R in their unliganded forms; c is the ratio of ligand affinities of subunits in the R and T structures.

When this theory is applied to hemoglobin (Perutz, 1970) the T structure corresponds to the deoxyhemoglobin quaternary structure (Muirhead and Greer, 1970; Bolton and Perutz, 1970). The subunits are constrained by various bonds including salt bridges that oppose the entry of ligand and cause low oxygen affinity. The R structure corresponds to the oxyhemoglobin quaternary structure (Perutz et al, 1968) where the constraints are broken so that the hemoglobin subunits revert to their naturally high oxygen affinity similar to that of the isolated α and β chains (Antonini et al, 1965). Because the affinities of the α and β chains in both R and T structures are likely to be different, the parameter c must be replaced by three parameters c_α, c_β, and γ, where $c_\alpha = K^R_\alpha/K^T_\alpha$, $C_\beta = K^R_\beta/K^T_\beta$ and $\gamma = K^R_\alpha/K^R_\beta$ (Ogata and McConnell, 1972; Szabo and Karplus, 1972; Baldwin, 1974). This modification of the model has five parameters: L, K^R_α, K^T_α, K^R_β and K^T_β whereas all hemoglobin equilibrium curves can be described by four parameters, the Adair constants (Adair, 1925). Hence it is not possible to obtain the allosteric parameters from one equilibrium curve without making additional assumptions. Despite these disadvantages the allosteric theory provides a highly attractive explanation for the functional properties of hemoglobin because its parameters have been given a firm structural basis. Thus changes in functional properties resulting from modifications of the structure can usually be readily understood in terms of the modification having altered one of the parameters (Morimoto et al, 1971).

FUNCTIONAL PROPERTIES OF THE R AND T STRUCTURES

One absolute prediction of the allosteric theory is that high cooperativity can only be observed on a complete transition from the T to R states during ligation. Thus in a highly cooperative hemoglobin the bottom extreme end of the equilibrium curve (plotted as a Hill plot, see figure 1) will correspond to oxygenation of the T structure only and the top extreme end the oxygenation of the R structure only. The slope of the Hill plot will be unity at these two extreme ends or asymptotes of the equilibrium curve, and the positions of the asymptotes correspond to the oxygen affinities of the R and T structures.

Previously, the measurement of the positions of these asymptotes required the time-consuming gasometric techniques developed by Roughton et al (1955). However, the introduction of a modified spectrophotometric technique by Imai et al (1970) has enormously facilitated these

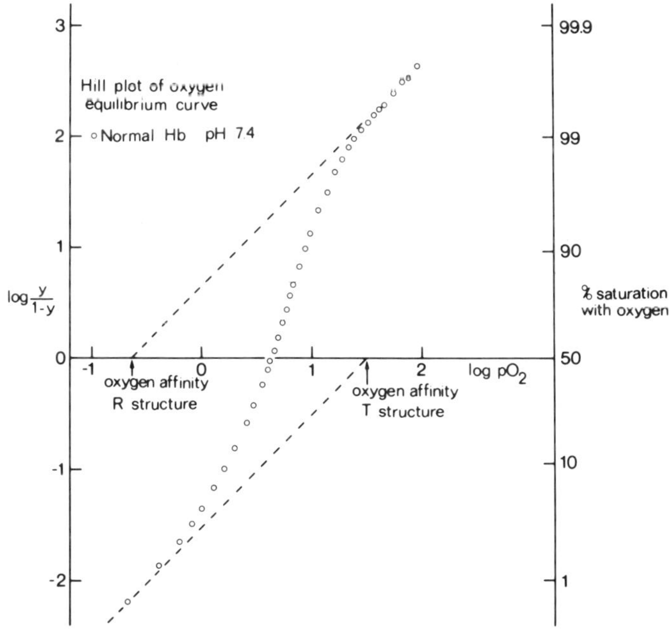

Fig 1. Hill plot of oxygen equilibrium curve of human hemoglobin (1 mg/mℓ) in 0.05 bis-tris, 0.1 M $C\ell^-$ pH 7.4 at $25^{o}C$ showing the positions of the two asymptotes. y is the fractional saturation with oxygen.

measurements and in addition requires only small amounts of sample.

Figure 1 shows a Hill plot of the data for normal hemoglobin at pH 7.4 with the positions of the two asymptotes corresponding to the affinities of the R and T structures. It can be seen that data around 1% saturation and between 99 and 99.9% saturation is needed to fix the positions of the asymptotes, hence the presence of impurities with high or low oxygen affinity in amounts as low as 0.5% of the total hemoglobin must be excluded. Kilmartin et al (1974b) chromatographed mixtures of oxy- and deoxyhemoglobin which would have removed these components if they were present and found no change in the positions of the asymptotes, hence these accurately reflect the affinities of the R and T structures of normal hemoglobin.

If a modified hemoglobin has a highly stable R or T structure then the allosteric theory predicts that this hemoglobin should have a non-cooperative equilibrium curve corresponding to the top or bottom asymptote. Des-(Arg 141α, His 146β) hemoglobin (Kilmartin and Hewitt, 1971) lacks the salt bridges involving residues His 146β and Arg 141α which stabilise the deoxy or T quaternary structure and consequently has a relatively stable R structure so that it would remain in this structure even when unliganded. This was confirmed when the deoxy form of this modified hemoglobin crystallized in a form closely related to the oxy or R quaternary structure (Perutz and Ten Eyck, 1971). In contrast, hemoglobin Kansas in the presence of inositolhexaphosphate (IHP) remains in the T structure even when liganded as shown by NMR studies (Ogawa et al, 1972). IHP is an organic phosphate which binds strongly to the deoxy or T quaternary structure thereby stabilising it (Benesch et al, 1968). The inherently high stability of the T structure of hemoglobin Kansas was confirmed when ligation of crystals of deoxy Kansas with CO failed to break them up in contrast to the behaviour of normal deoxyhemoglobin crystals (N.L. Anderson, unpublished results).

The equilibrium curves of these two hemoglobins are shown, together with the curve for normal hemoglobin, in figure 2.

It is clear that the equilibrium curves for these hemoglobins are close to the asymptotes of the curve for normal hemoglobin. The slight difference in the case of des-(Arg 141α, His 146β) hemoglobin is probably due to alterations in K_α^R and K_β^R caused by the modifications (Kilmartin et al, 1974a). Similarly, in hemoglobin Kansas the mutation or bound IHP could change K_β^T or K_α^T thus giving a slightly different bottom asymptote from that of normal hemoglobin.

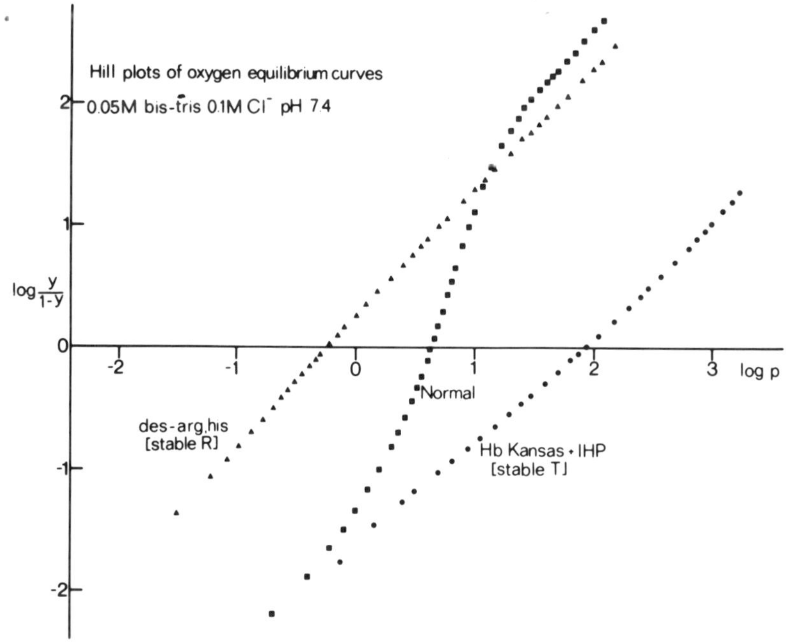

Fig 2. Hill plots of oxygen equilibrium curves of des-(Arg 141α, His 146β) hemoglobin (▲ - ▲), normal hemoglobin (■ - ■) and hemoglobin Kansas + 1 mM IHP (● - ●). Conditions as in figure 1. The data for hemoglobin Kansas were taken at 10°C because of the low affinity of this hemoglobin. The position of the curve was adjusted along the log pO_2 axis until the curves for normal hemoglobin at 10°C and 25°C coincided.

RELEASE OF BOHR PROTONS DURING LIGATION

In an extensive study of the effect of pH on the oxygen equilibrium curve Imai and Yonetani (1974) have shown that the position of the bottom asymptote is pH dependent while that of the top asymptote is pH independent. Equilibrium curves of normal hemoglobin at pH 7.4 and 9.1 are shown in figure 3. This result confirms the earlier less extensive data of Roughton (1963) on sheep hemoglobin by the more laborious gasometric methods. In cooperative hemoglobins the pH dependence of the position of the bottom asymptote, which

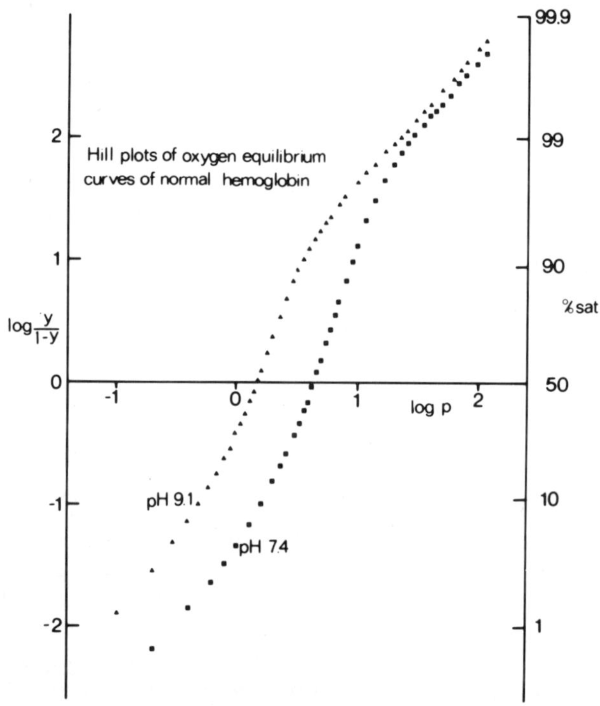

Fig 3. Hill plots of oxygen equilibrium curves of normal hemoglobin (1 mg/mℓ) in 0.05 M bis-tris, 0.1 M $C\ell^-$ pH 7.4 (■ - ■) and 0.05 M tris, 0.1 M $C\ell^-$ pH 9.1 (▲ - ▲) at 25°C.

is a direct measure of the oxygen affinity of the T structure, means that protons affect the oxygen affinity of the T structure. From the theory of linkage (Wyman, 1964) the converse of this must be true so that oxygenation of the T structure must change the affinity of groups in the protein for protons, that is, change their pK values. The groups in the protein with neutral pK values which are changed between deoxy and fully oxygenated hemoglobin are the Bohr groups. The simplest interpretation of the pH dependence of the bottom asymptote is that ligation of the T structure breaks these same Bohr group salt bridges: thus the Bohr effect or release of protons is linked to tertiary structure changes in the T structure. The change in the position of the bottom asymptote in figure 3 is closely similar to the change in log p_{50} which means that when the hemoglobin molecule is in the T state most of the Bohr protons associated with one subunit are released on its ligation. This is confirmed by the finding that hemoglobin Kansas in the presence of IHP still has a substantial Bohr effect (Kilmartin, Ogawa and Shulman, unpublished results).

The pH independence of the position of the top asymptote, measuring the oxygen affinity of the R structure in cooperative hemoglobins means that R structure hemoglobins should have no Bohr effect. This is confirmed by the absence of a Bohr effect in des-(Arg 141α, His 146β) hemoglobin and des-(Arg 141α, Tyr 140α) hemoglobin (Kilmartin *et al*, 1974a), the latter hemoglobin still having the major alkaline Bohr group His 146β present. Thus the R structure is unable to form its Bohr group salt bridges. Hence during ligation the release of protons from subunits not yet ligated will be linked to the change in quaternary structure from T to R.

EFFECT OF REMOVAL OF SALT BRIDGES ON THE OXYGEN EQUILIBRIUM CURVE

If the Bohr groups are involved in the pH dependence of the position of the bottom asymptote then their removal should displace this asymptote relative to that of normal hemoglobin.

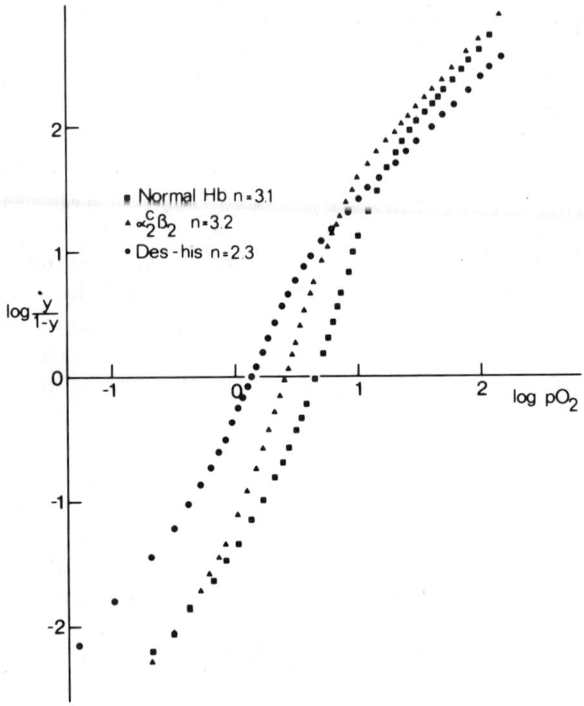

Fig 4. Hill plots of oxygen equilibrium curves of normal hemoglobin (■ - ■), hemoglobin specifically modified by carbamylation on the α chain α-amino group $\alpha_2^c\beta_2$ (▲ - ▲) and des-(His 146β) hemoglobin (● - ●). Conditions as in figure 1.

Figure 4 shows the oxygen equilibrium curves of hemoglobin lacking two Bohr group salt bridges. In $\alpha_2^c\beta_2$, the α-amino group of the α chain has been specifically modified with cyanate (Kilmartin et al, 1973a) to block the salt bridge between this group and the C-terminal carboxyl group of Arg 141α (Perutz, 1970). This group is responsible for a minor part of the alkaline Bohr effect, about 20% (Kilmartin et al, 1973b). It is clear from figure 4 that the asymptotes of $\alpha_2^c\beta_2$ are practically unchanged from normal hemoglobin hence this salt bridge does not contribute to the lowering of the oxygen affinity of the T structure.

The increase in oxygen affinity at 50% saturation is due to the general destabilization of the T structure, that is a change in the allosteric parameter L, caused by the modification.

Removal of His 146β by carboxypeptidase B digestion of isolated β chains (Kilmartin and Wootton, 1970; Kilmartin et al, 1974a) followed by recombination with α chains gives des-(His 146β) hemoglobin in which two salt bridges between His 146β and Asp 94β, and Lys 40α and the α-carboxyl of His 146β have been removed. The equilibrium curve is shown in figure 4. Clearly the bottom asymptote is substantially shifted, showing that the absence of His 146β raises the oxygen affinity of the T structure. Part of this shift may be due to the presence of a small amount of R structure in the absence of ligand since the cooperativity of this hemoglobin is reduced. The top asymptote has also been lowered by removal of His 146β. This is probably because K_β^R is changed in this hemoglobin as a consequence of the lowered oxygen affinity of the isolated des-(His 146β) chains (Kilmartin et al, 1974a).

The C-terminal carboxyl group of Arg 141α actually forms a salt bridge with two groups, the α chain α-amino group as described above and Lys 127α (Muirhead and Greer, 1970; Perutz, 1970). The contribution of the salt bridge involving Lys 127α can be assessed by specifically blocking the C-terminal carboxyl of Arg 141α. This has been done by reaction with hydrazine to make hydrazide-hemoglobin in the following way. Trypsin can catalyse the removal of a hydrazide from the α-carboxyl group of lysine or arginine:

$$-CONHNH_2 + H_2O \rightleftharpoons -COOH + NH_2NH_2 \qquad (1)$$

The equilibrium constant of this reaction (Fersht and Requena, 1971; Fastrez and Fersht, 1973) is such that in high concentrations of hydrazine the hydrolysis is reversed and trypsin will catalyse the formation of the hydrazide. Accordingly CO-hemoglobin (10 mg/mℓ) was incubated with trypsin (1 mg/mℓ) and 2 M hydrazine at pH 6.5 at 4°C for 48 hours. Chromatography on CM-cellulose gave two peaks, one of which was normal hemoglobin. The other was further purified from normal hemoglobin by preparative isoelectric focussing and was characterised as hemoglobin specifically modified on the α chain C-terminal carboxyl group by hydrazine. The preparation of this hemoglobin will be described in detail later, its characterization is described briefly below:

(i) digestion with carboxypeptidase B failed to release Arg 141α, whereas digestion with carboxypeptidase A released both His 146β and Tyr 145β.

(ii) in the absence of hydrazine trypsin should catalyse the hydrolysis of the hydrazide in equation (1). Treatment of hydrazide hemoglobin with trypsin in the absence of hydrazine releases 1.0 mole of hydrazine per αβ dimer and changes the isoelectric point of the hemoglobin so that it is now identical to normal hemoglobin on isoelectric focussing. Digestion of this trypsin-treated hemoglobin with carboxypeptidase B now released 1.0 mole of arginine per αβ dimer.

(iii) treatment of des-(Arg 141α) hemoglobin with trypsin and 2 M hydrazine gave no changes in isoelectric point on isoelectric focussing, showing that the change in isoelectric point found on treating normal hemoglobin with trypsin and 2 M hydrazine is due to a reaction with Arg 141α.

(iv) SDS electrophoresis in 15% gels (Weber and Osborn, 1969) showed that trypsin had not cleaved at any part of the chains of hydrazide hemoglobin.

The oxygen equilibrium curve of both hydrazide hemoglobin and trypsin-treated hydrazide hemoglobin are shown in figure 5.

The trypsin-treated hydrazide hemoglobin is identical to normal hemoglobin. The hydrazide hemoglobin has an unchanged top asymptote showing that no changes have occurred in the R structure of this hemoglobin. The oxygen affinity at half saturation is greater than that for $\alpha_2^c\beta_2$

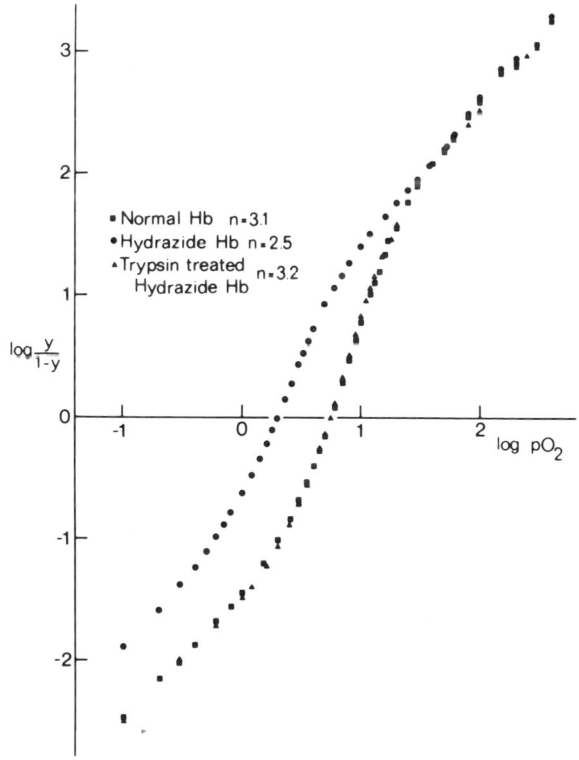

Fig 5. Hill plots of oxygen equilibrium curves of normal hemoglobin (■ - ■), hydrazide hemoglobin (● - ●) and trypsin-treated hydrazide hemoglobin (▲ - ▲). Conditions as for figure 1.

because an additional salt bridge between Lys 127α and the α-carboxyl of Arg 141α has been broken in hydrazide hemoglobin. This salt bridge must contribute substantially to the lowering of the oxygen affinity of the T structure since the bottom asymptote is shifted considerably in hydrazide hemoglobin but not in $\alpha_2^{\S}\beta_2$ (figure 4). However, as explained earlier for des-(His 146β) hemoglobin, part of this shift may be due to the presence of a small fraction of the R structure in the absence of oxygen because the Hill's constant n is lowered in this hemoglobin.

Finally, the Bohr effect of hydrazide hemoglobin was measured by direct proton titration. At pH 7.4, 0.38 protons/heme were released on oxygenation compared with a value of 0.53 protons/heme for normal hemoglobin. The reduction is due to the inability of the α chain α-amino group to form its salt bridge with the α-carboxyl of Arg 141α, and is the same reduction as found in $\alpha_2^c\beta_2$ (Kilmartin *et al* 1973a).

In conclusion, these results show that the salt bridges between His 146β and Asp 94β, Lys 40α and the α-carboxyl of His 146β, and between Lys 127α and the α-carboxyl of Arg 141α contribute to the lowering of the oxygen affinity of the T structure. The salt bridge between the α-amino of Val 1α and the α-carboxyl of Arg 141α does not. None of these salt bridges contribute significantly to the properties of the R structure.

Acknowledgement

JVK thanks Professor B.S. Hartley for drawing his attention to the potentialities of the trypsin hydrazine system as a synthetic method.

REFERENCES

Adair, G.S. (1925). The hemoglobin system. VI The oxygen dissociation curve of hemoglobin. J.Biol.Chem. 63, 529-545.

Antonini, E., Bucci, E., Fronticelli, C., Wyman, J. and Rossi-Fanelli, A. (1965). The properties and interactions of the isolated α and β chains of human haemoglobin. III. Observations on the equilibria and kinetics of the reactions with gases. J.Mol.Biol. 12, 375-384.

Baldwin, J.M. (1974). Structure and function of haemoglobin. Progress in Biophysics and Molecular Biology. In press.

Benesch, R., Benesch, R.E. and Yu, C.I. (1968). Reciprocal binding of oxygen and diphosphoglycerate by human hemoglobin. Proc.Nat.Acad.Sci.USA, 59, 526-532.

Bolton, W. and Perutz, M.F. (1970). Three dimensional Fourier synthesis of horse deoxyhaemoglobin at 2.8 Å resolution. Nature, 228, 551-552.

Fastrez, J. and Fersht, A.R. (1973). Demonstration of the acyl-enzyme mechanism for the hydrolysis of peptides and anilides by chymotrypsin. Biochemistry, 12, 2025-2034.

Fersht, A.R. and Requena, Y. (1971). Free energies of hydrolysis of amides and peptides in aqueous solution at 25°. J.Amer.Chem.Soc. 93, 3499-3504.

Imai, K., Morimoto, H., Kotani, M., Watari, H., Hirata, W. and Kuroda, M. (1970). Studies on the function of abnormal hemoglobins. I. An improved method for automatic measurement of the oxygen equilibrium curve of hemoglobin. Biochim.Biophys.Acta, 200, 189-196.

Imai, K. and Yonetani, T. (1974). pH dependence of the Adair constants of human hemoglobin: non-uniform contribution of successive oxygen bindings to the alkaline Bohr effect. J.Biol.Chem. In press.

Kilmartin, J.V. and Wootton, J.F. (1970). Inhibition of Bohr effect after removal of C-terminal histidines from haemoglobin β chains. Nature, 228, 766-767.

Kilmartin, J.V. and Hewitt, J.A. (1971). The effect of removal of C-terminal residues on cooperative interations in hemoglobin. Cold Spring Harb.Symp.Quant.Biol. 36, 311-314.

Kilmartin, J.V., Fogg, J., Luzzana, M. and Rossi-Bernardi, L. (1973a). Role of the α-amino groups of the α and β chains of human hemoglobin in oxygen-linked binding of carbon dioxide. J.Biol.Chem. 248, 7039-7043.

Kilmartin, J.V., Breen, J.J., Roberts, G.C.K. and Ho, C. (1973b). Direct measurement of the pK values of an alkaline Bohr group in human hemoglobin. Proc.Nat.Acad.Sci.USA, 70, 1246-1249.

Kilmartin, J.V., Hewitt, J.A. and Wootton, J.F. (1974a). Alteration of the functional properties associated with the change in quaternary structure in unliganded hemoglobin. J.Mol.Biol. Submitted.

Kilmartin, J.V., Imai, K. and Jones, R.T. (1974b). In preparation.

Monod, J., Wyman, J. and Changeux, J.P. (1965). On the nature of allosteric transitions: a plausible model. J.Mol.Biol. 12, 88-118.

Morimoto, H., Lehmann, H. and Perutz, M.F. (1971). Molecular pathology of human haemoglobin: stereochemical interpretation of abnormal oxygen affinities. Nature, 232, 408-413.

Muirhead, H. and Greer, J. (1970). Three-dimensional Fourier synthesis of human deoxyhemoglobin at 3.5 Å resolution. Nature, 228, 516-519.

Ogata, R.T. and McConnell, H.M. (1972). Mechanism of cooperative oxygen binding to hemoglobin. Proc.Nat.Acad. Sci.USA, 69, 335-339.

Ogawa, S., Mayer, A. and Shulman, R.G. (1972). High resolution proton magnetic resonance study of the two quaternary states in fully ligated hemoglobin Kansas. Biochem.Biophys.Res.Comm. 49, 1485-1491.

Perutz, M.F. (1970). Stereochemistry of cooperative effects in haemoglobin. Haem-haem interaction and the problem of allostery. The Bohr effect and combination with organic phosphates. Nature, 228, 726-739.

Perutz, M.F., Muirhead, H., Cox, J.M. and Goaman, L.C.G. (1968). Three-dimensional Fourier synthesis of horse oxyhaemoglobin at 2.8 Å resolution. II. The atomic model. Nature, 219, 131-139.

Perutz, M.F. and Ten Eyck, L.F. (1971). Stereochemistry of cooperative effects in haemoglobin. Cold Spring Harb.Symp. Quant.Biol. 36, 295-310.

Roughton, F.J.W. (1963). The accurate determination of the oxygen-hemoglobin equilibrium in dilute solutions of sheep hemoglobin. Clin.Chem. 9, 682-709.

Roughton, F.J.W., Otis, A.B. and Lyster, R.L.J. (1955). The determination of the individual equilibrium constants of the four intermediate reactions between oxygen and sheep haemoglobin. Proc.Roy.Soc.(Lond). B.144, 29-54.

Szabo, A. and Karplus, M. (1972). A mathematical model for structure-function relations in hemoglobin. J.Mol.Biol. 72, 163-197.

Weber, K. and Osborn, M. (1969). The reliability of molecular weight determinations by dodecylsulphate-polyacrylamide gel electrophoresis. J.Biol.Chem. 244, 4406-4412.

Wyman, J. (1964). Linked functions and reciprocal effects in hemoglobin: a second look. Adv.Protein Chem. 19, 223-286.

DISCUSSION
(of both Dr. Perutz's and Dr. Kilmartin's Papers)

Dr. Salhany: I'd like to address a question to Dr. Kilmartin. It's not clear to me just how you rule out the possibility that the effect that you see in the bottom of the equilibrium curves is not due to the alternation of the R-T equilibrium by these modifications.

Dr. Kilmartin: I think if the Hill's constant is high, which it is in most of these modified hemoglobins, they all have values around 2.5, then I think you can be reasonably sure that you're looking mainly at the T structure at the bottom of the curve. I would agree with you that when the Hill's constant goes down to 2, then you're going to get a significant R contribution at the bottom.

Dr. Salhany: Perhaps this is too technical a question, but how much difference in K_T (binding constant to the T state) do you estimate there is from these modifications?

Dr. Kilmartin: This is very difficult to evaluate because we should really allow for changes in both the α and β chain affinities in the T structure as well as for changes in the allosteric constant L. All that we can say so far is that the changes in the bottom part of the equilibrium curve cannot be explained solely on the basis of a change in the allosteric constant L, so the affinity of the T structure must change.

Dr. Ogawa: Dr. Kilmartin, in your measurements, about how much dependence do you have on wave length? Dr. Sugita suggested that in the deoxy Soret spectra region there is a difference between α and β; the α chain changes from chain to tetramer, but the β chain does not. If the wave length dependence is very little, it means that α and β are very equivalent in functional properties.

Dr. Kilmartin: We have not measured the wavelength dependence of our equilibrium curves because in their initial report of the method Imai *et al*. measured a large number of wave lengths and found very little difference. It seems to me that the kinetic work of Gibson et al. has shown that most of the spectral difference between the α and β chains occurs at around the isosbestic points and not at the wave lengths around 560 nm where the oxygen equilibrium curves are measured.

Dr. Ogawa: What is the relative ratio of the extinction between the ferrous side and the ferric side?

Dr. Kilmartin: The change would be something like an eighth or a ninth as much.

Dr. Ogawa: Eighty percent?

Dr. Kilmartin: No, I'm saying one-eighth, about 15% of the change in OD. I think if you measure around the isosbestic points, then you'll pick up such changes. But, I think when you're measuring at 560, you're way off this. In the original work that Imai did, equilibrium curves were measured at a large range of wave lengths so they couldn't see very much difference between them. I must confess that in these studies we only measured at a single wave length, but I've no reason to think that it would be any different.

Dr. Ogawa: No, the difference between α and β in deoxy Soret may be large. In your measurements, say 15% in the extinction.

Dr. Kilmartin: Under these conditions in the Milwaukee, where I think the changes will be much less, you're getting two separate spectral changes occurring. I'm sure if you did a kinetic experiment you'd see an enormous change, an enormous factor for the wave length.

Dr. Ogawa: In the early part of curve, if you had very little wave length dependence, that would mean that α and β chains are equivalent.

Dr. Kilmartin: Yes, but it depends on where you measure it.

Dr. Ogawa: Yes, I know. That's what I'm saying about dependence.

Dr. Kilmartin: Yes, I think at 560 you will, but I'm saying that if you measure around an isosbestic point you should possibly pick up something happening there if your data is good enough, but the difficulty is that the change in OD is so small, and the equilibrium curve takes such a long time that any slight drift in the spectrophotometer would completely invalidate the results.

Dr. Ogawa: Yes, I see. Thank you.

Dr. Sugita: I measured the different spectra between the isolated chains and the reconstituted hemoglobin. I prepared the isolated chain which had the protoheme in the α chain and the metaheme in the β chain and took the different spectra. And I found that hyperchromicity in the Soret region appeared at the wave lengths of the protoheme. When we changed the heme, vice versa, the wave lengths of the peak in the Soret region corresponded to that of the heme in the α chain. It's very complicated; but anyway, the absorption in the α chain increased when it is incorporated into tetramer.

Dr. Petering: Dr. Perutz, in analyzing the Bohr effect, can you fit that to a Monod model? Presumably when you break the salt bridges which appear to be pH dependent and change the position of that equilibrium, you're fooling around with the parameter L in the Monod model. Now, if I recall right, it seems to me that if you change L, you're going to change the shape of the curve; and one of the peculiar things about hemoglobin is that as you change the pH, the oxygenation curve is essentially invariant in shape...

Dr. Perutz: No! That is a well-worn fallacy which Imai, Kilmartin and Jones's results have dispelled. Roughton showed many years ago that the shape of the oxygen equilibrium curve is pH-dependent. That is to say, the first Adair constant is pH dependent as Imai and Yonotani have shown; it is much higher at acid than at alkaline pH; consequently the free energy of heme interaction rises with falling pH. I think Imai himself has misunderstood the Monod model and my salt bridge model when he published a paper in PNAS saying that you need a three stage model to account for the pH dependence of the equilibrium curve.

The crystallographic results suggest (though this is not yet proved) that a rise in pH from 6.5 to 9 does not lead to a different deoxy structure, but that the same structure persists with some of the salt bridges opened. The effect of a rise of pH, therefore, consists merely in a gradual loosening of some of the clamps which constrain the deoxy or T structure. We must regard protein structures as somewhat soft, so that the opening of one of the clamps would loosen the structure, thereby reducing the tension of the hemes and raising their oxygen affinity. Once you introduce a three-state model, you should really introduce a 500-state model, because there are so many salt bridges which you can open and close and you can put in DPG and release it; you can strip the hemoglobin free of phosphate or even of chloride; removal of any of these anions changes the lower part of the oxygen equilibrium curve, because it changes the number and kinds of constraints in the T structure, but the T structure always remains much the same.

Dr. Salhany: I'd like to ask a question of Dr. Kilmartin relevant to the point of whether the change in the bottom part of the curve is due to the allosteric equilibrium versus the c values; if it is the latter, then does that mean that you have a change in the tertiary structure of the subunit or subunits that are being affected, either by changing pH or by the chemically modified hemoglobins that you are using? And is it possible to localize by your different chemically modified hemoglobins specific chain heterogeneity so that you can demonstrate tertiary changes in either the α or the β chains?

Dr. Kilmartin: Well, I think that there obviously must be tertiary changes occurring. But if the affinity of one structure is lowered by a particular group, then when you either break the salt bridge of that group or remove it, there must be some sort of change occurring which makes the affinity of that structure higher after the bridge is broken or the residue is removed. If this happens, then there must be a change in the optical spectrum of that particular chain, but I suspect that these changes are going to be pretty small. If you do a kinetic experiment I'm sure that you can pick something out, but for an equilibrium experiment, I just don't think you have much chance, because it just takes too long.

Dr. Dawson: This is a conceptual question for you, Dr. Perutz. Can you decide from looking at your models which chain a β chain is going to take with it when it rotates? What I'm asking is, when the alpha, beta dimers move apart, or change to allow DPG to fit in, are they moving according to the dimers that we know from chemical separations and are there certain salt bridges that are stronger between a particular β chain and one of the α chains than between the β chain and the other α chain?

Dr. Perutz: The $alpha_1$-$beta_1$ dimer behaves almost but not quite as a rigid unit but the two subunits are not linked by salt bonds, these interactions do not change much when the quaternary structure changes.

Dr. Dawson: Those, then would be stronger forces...?

Dr. Perutz: Yes, yes, the forces that hold one $alpha_1$-$beta_1$ dimer together are much stronger than those that link two such dimers to form a tetramer, as evidenced by the very low dissociation constant of the dimer to produce free α and β chains from the alpha beta dimer.

Dr. Dawson: That answers my question.

RECENT NMR STUDIES ON QUATERNARY STRUCTURAL TRANSITIONS IN HUMAN HEMOGLOBINS

Chien Ho, Leslie W.-M. Fung, Karen J. Wiechelman,
Greta Pifat, and Michael E. Johnson

Department of Biophysics and Microbiology
University of Pittsburgh,
Pittsburgh, Pennsylvania 15260

ABSTRACT

High-resolution proton nuclear magnetic resonance (NMR) spectroscopy at 250 MHz has been used to investigate structural and functional properties of human normal and abnormal hemoglobins upon ligand binding. Organic phosphates have been shown not only to induce different ligand affinities between the α and β chains but also to induce quaternary structural changes especially in those mutant hemoglobins having amino acid substitutions in the $\alpha_1\beta_2$ subunit contacts. The hemoglobin-ligand reactions are found to be hemoglobin, ligand, organic phosphate, and pH specific. NMR spectra of human hemoglobins in water reveal several exchangeable proton resonances which are indicators of the quaternary structures of both the liganded and unliganded molecules. By comparing the spectra of normal adult hemoglobin with those of $\alpha_1\beta_2$ mutants as well as with several chemically modified hemoglobins, we have found that the resonance at ∿ -9.4 ppm from H_2O at 30^oC is due to the hydrogen bond between β99(G1)Asp and α42(C7)Tyr in the $\alpha_1\beta_2$ subunit interface and is characteristic of the deoxy quaternary structure. A resonance at ∿ -5.8 ppm from H_2O which is characteristic of the oxy conformation appears to originate from the hydrogen bond between α94(G1)Asp and β102(G4)Asn in the $\alpha_1\beta_2$ subunit interface. Two resonances (at -8.2 and -7.3 ppm) which remain *invariant in the two quaternary structures could come from the exchangeable protons in the* $\alpha_1\beta_1$ *subunit interface. The relationships of these results to the molecular mechanism of the cooperative oxygenation of hemoglobin will be discussed.*

INTRODUCTION

The hemoglobin (Hb) molecule is perhaps the best studied protein in terms of its structure and function. In spite of extensive efforts that have been devoted to this molecule, the detailed molecular mechanism for the cooperative oxygenation process is not yet understood. X-Ray diffraction studies have provided valuable information about the structural differences between deoxy- and methemoglobin in the crystalline state (Perutz, 1970; Perutz and Ten Eyck, 1971). So far, very little information is available on the sequence and nature of structural changes in the hemoglobin molecule during the oxygenation process. Hence, we need to have a number of structural probes to monitor the changes in the tertiary and quaternary structures during the oxygenation process and to relate these changes to the mode of action of the hemoglobin molecule.

High-resolution proton nuclear magnetic resonance (NMR) spectroscopy has been used to investigate the structure-function relationships in hemoglobins. It has provided detailed and in some cases unique information about the heme environment or the tertiary structure around the heme groups (Davis *et al.*, 1969; Davis *et al.*, 1971; Ogawa and Shulman, 1972; Lindstrom *et al.*, 1972; Lindstrom and Ho, 1973; Ho *et al.*, 1973), the functional properties of individual hemes in the hemoglobin molecule (Lindstrom *et al.*, 1971; Lindstrom and Ho, 1972; Lindstrom *et al.*, 1973; Johnson and Ho, 1974; Wiechelman *et al.*, 1974), the subunit interactions (Davis *et al.*, 1971; Ho *et al.*, 1973; Perutz *et al.*, 1974a; Wiechelman *et al.*, 1974; Fung and Ho, 1974), and the acid-base properties of a Bohr group (Greenfield and Williams, 1972; Kilmartin *et al.*, 1973).

In this communication, we wish to report our recent 250 MHz proton NMR studies on the quaternary structural transitions in hemoglobins.

MATERIALS AND METHODS

Human adult hemoglobin (Hb A) was prepared from fresh whole blood samples obtained from the local blood bank by the standard procedure used in this laboratory (Lindstrom and Ho, 1972). Mutant hemoglobins Chesapeake, Mälmo, Kempsey, Yakima, and M Milwaukee were isolated and purified from individual heterozygous hemolysates by standard methods with either DEAE-Sephadex or Bio-Rex 70 column chromatography (Davis *et al.*, 1971; Lindstrom *et al.*, 1972; Lindstrom *et al.*, 1973; Perutz *et al.*, 1974a). Hemoglobins Des-Arg, NES-Des-Arg, and Des-His were prepared from Hb A according to the procedures of Kilmartin and Hewitt (1971). The hemoglobin samples were made phosphate-free by passing through a Sephadex G-25 column using as buffer 0.01M Tris-HCl with 0.1M NaCl at pH 7.45 (Berman *et al.*, 1971). The samples were buffered at the desired pH by adding appropriate amounts of stock buffers. Calculated amounts of 2,3-diphosphoglycerate (DPG) or inositol hexaphosphate (IHP) were added to the hemoglobin samples when required. For some studies, the hemoglobin samples were exchanged with D_2O so as to suppress the intense proton signal from water in aqueous samples. The reported pH values were the direct pH readings obtained from a Radiometer Model 4 or Model 26 pH meter equipped with a Beckman Model 39030 frit junction combination electrode. The pD values of the samples in D_2O were obtained by adding 0.4 pH units to the pH readings (Glasoe and Long, 1960). Samples for NMR studies were prepared by the usual methods used in this laboratory (Lindstrom and Ho, 1972). Hb Chesapeake, Hb Yakima, and Hb Kempsey in IHP were found to be unstable when O_2 was added and significant amounts of methemoglobins were formed. NMR experiments were carried out in the presence of the methemoglobin reductase system of Hayashi *et al.* (1973). The presence of this reductase system was found not to interfere with our NMR results. The sample concentration was 8-16 gm % hemoglobin.

Proton NMR spectra at 250 MHz were obtained from the MPC-HF 250 MHz superconducting spectrometer, interfaced with a Sigma 5 computer (Dadok *et al.*, 1970). The signal-to-noise ratio was enchanced by the NMR correlation technique (Dadok and Sprecher, 1974). Proton chemical shifts were referenced with respect to the water signal, which was 4.75 ppm downfield from the proton resonance of 2,2-dimethyl-2-silapentane-5-sulfonate (DSS) at 30°C, the ambient temperature of the probe. Chemical shifts downfield from the proton resonance of water were assigned negative values with ± 0.2 ppm accuracy.

RESULTS

Figure 1 shows the hyperfine shifted proton resonances of deoxyhemoglobins A, Chesapeake (FG4α92 Arg→Leu), Yakima (G1β99 Asp→His), and Kempsey (G1β99 Asp→Asn). These resonances arise from the hyperfine interactions between the unpaired electrons in the ferrous atoms of the heme groups and the protons on the porphyrin rings and/or the amino acid protons positioned sufficiently close to the heme groups. They have been shown to be very sensitive to the heme environment and to the heme-globin interactions (Davis *et al.*, 1971; Ogawa and Shulman, 1972; Ho *et al.*, 1973). By comparing the spectrum of Hb A with those of appropriate mutant hemoglobins, we have assigned the resonance at ∿ -18 ppm to protons from the β chain and the resonances at ∿ -12 and ∿ -8 ppm are due to proton groups from the α chains of Hb A (Davis *et al.*, 1971; Lindstrom *et al.*, 1972). These hyperfine shifted resonances return to their normal diamagnetic resonance positions when the hemoglobin molecule becomes diamagnetic by combining with ligands, such as oxygen or carbon monoxide. The hyperfine shifted proton resonances of deoxyhemoglobins Chesapeake, Yakima, and Kempsey are different from one another and also differ from those of deoxy Hb A as first reported by Davis *et al.* (1971). The addition of inositol hexaphosphate to these three mutants can alter the chemical shift and line shape of their hyperfine shifted resonances to those similar to deoxy Hb A.

Figures 2 and 3 summarize the results on the functional properties of α and β chains in Hb A, Hb Chesapeake, Hb Yakima, and Hb Kempsey. Since hyperfine shifted proton

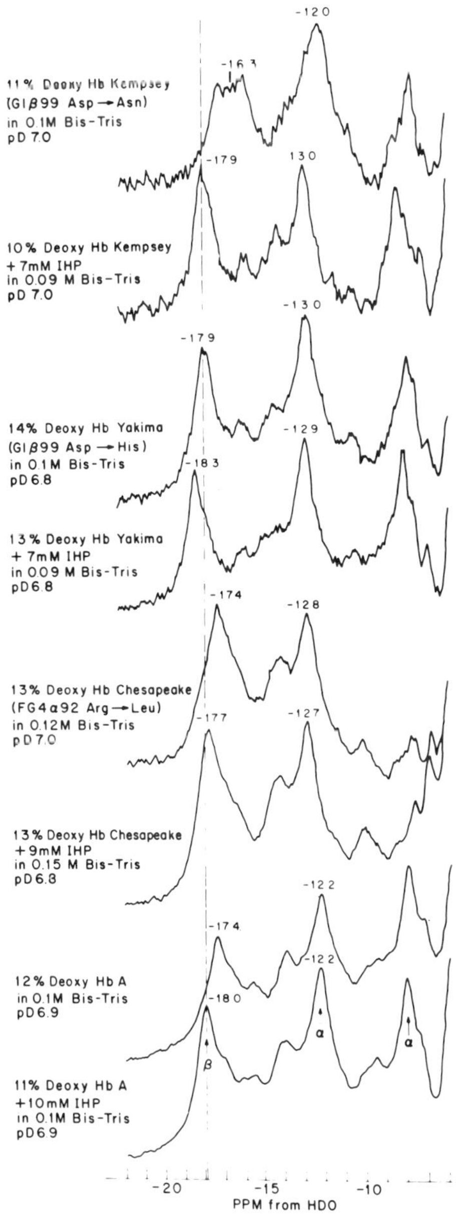

Fig.1. 250 MHz NMR Spectra of 12% Hemoglobins in H_2O and 0.1M Bis Tris at pH 6.6 and 30^0 C. Ho, Fung, Wiechelman, Pifat, and Johnson, "Recent NMR Studies on Quaternary Structural Transitions in Human Hemoglobins.

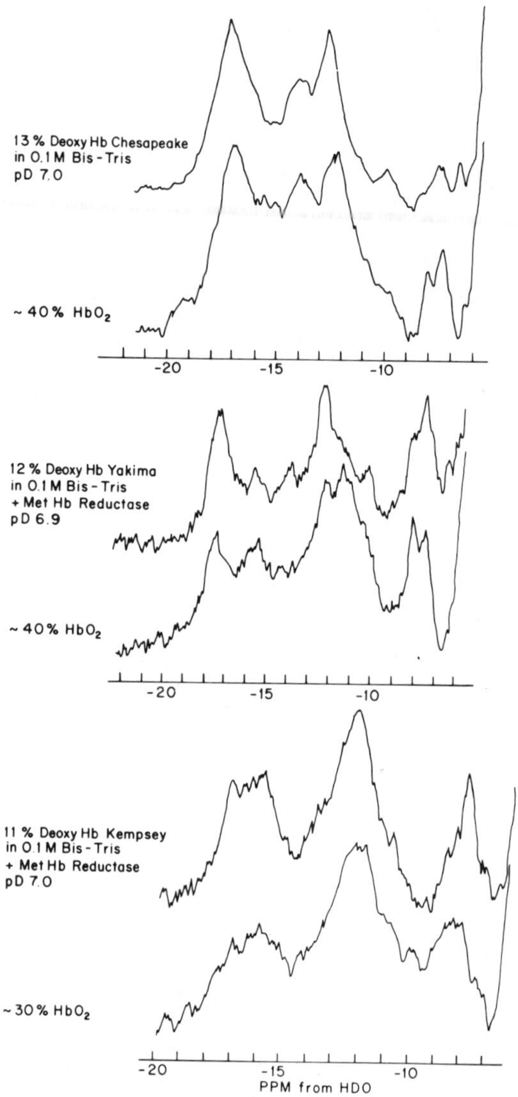

Fig.2. 250 MH_Z NMR Spectra of α_1 β_2 Hb Mutants on Oxygenation at 30^0 C. Ho, Fung, Wiechelman, Pifat, and Johnson, "Recent NMR Studies on Quaternary Structural Transitions in Human Hemoglobins.

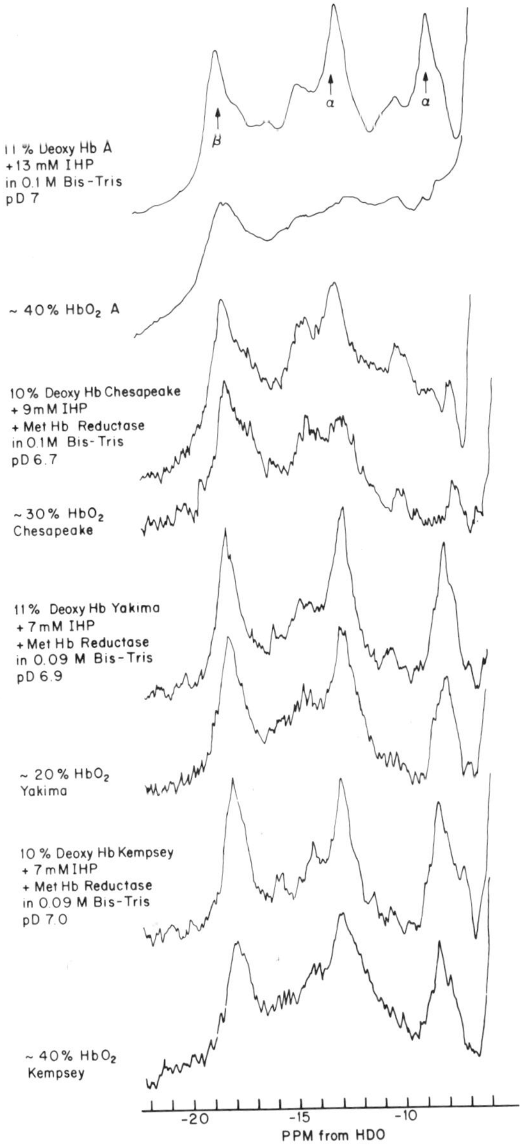

Fig. 3. 250 MH_Z NMR Spectra of HbA and α1 β2 Mutants on Oxygenation in the Presence of IHP at 30° C. Ho, Fung, Wiechelman Pifat, and Johnson, "Recent NMR Studies on Quaternary Structural Transitions in Human Hemoglobins.

resonances only occur in deoxyhemoglobins and some of them have been assigned to specific proton groups in α and β chains (Davis *et al.*, 1971; Lindstrom *et al.*, 1972; Johnson and Ho, 1974), the measurement of the intensity ratios of the α resonance (at ∿ -12 ppm) and the β resonance (at ∿ -18 ppm) as a function of ligand saturation provides a unique way to determine the functional properties of α and β chains in hemoglobins. Figure 2 shows the oxygen saturation studies of Hb Chesapeake, Hb Yakima, and Hb Kempsey in 0.1M Bis-Tris buffer at pD 7 and at 30°C. In the case of Hb Chesapeake, the intensity ratios of the α-heme resonance (at ∿ -12 ppm) and the β-heme resonance (at ∿ -17 ppm) remain constant on oxygenation suggesting that oxygen molecules bind to the α and β chains of this mutant with no preference (Wiechelman *et al.*, 1974). On the other hand, the intensity of the β-heme resonance decreases much more rapidly than that of the α-heme resonance (at ∿ -12 ppm) in Hb Yakima and Hb Kempsey suggesting that the β chains in these two mutants have a higher affinity for O_2 than the α chains. Figure 3 shows the oxygen saturation studies of Hb A, Hb Chesapeake, Hb Yakima, and Hb Kempsey in 0.1M Bis-Tris buffer plus IHP at pD ∿ 7 and at 30°C. For Hb A in the presence of IHP, oxygen exhibits almost exclusive binding to the α chains (Johnson and Ho, 1974). In the case of Hb Chesapeake in the presence of IHP, the intensity ratios of the α- to β-heme resonances decrease on oxygenation suggesting that O_2 binds to the α chains in preference to the β chains (Wiechelman *et al.*, 1974). IHP also has a profound effect on the functional properties of Hb Yakima and Hb Kempsey. In the presence of IHP, the intensity ratios of the α- to β-heme resonances remain constant on oxygenation suggesting that O_2 binds to the α and β chains of these two mutants at random.

Figure 4 gives the downfield proton NMR spectra of oxy, carbonmonoxy, and deoxy Hb A at pH 6.6 in H_2O and at 30°C. In the deoxy Hb A spectrum, the three prominent hyperfine shifted proton resonances (at -17.6, -12.1, and -8.0 ppm from H_2O) remain the same in H_2O as in D_2O (Figures 1 and 4). Additional resonances at about -9.4, -6.4, and -5.2 ppm as well as the two resonances at -8.3 and -7.6 ppm from H_2O

Fig.4. 250 MH_Z Proton NMR Spectra 15% Hb A in H_2O an 0.1 Bis Tris at pH 6.6 and 30^0 C. Ho, Fung, Wiechelman, Pifat, and Johnson, "Recent NMR Studies on Quaternary Structural Transitions in Human Hemoglobins."

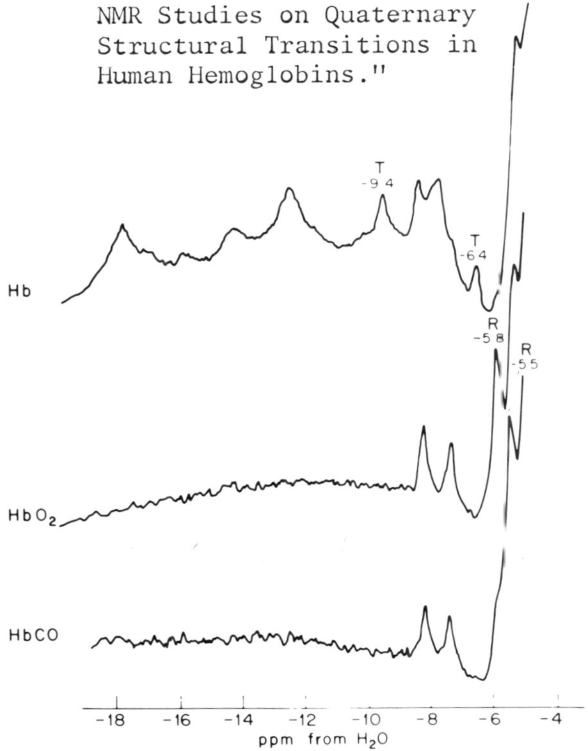

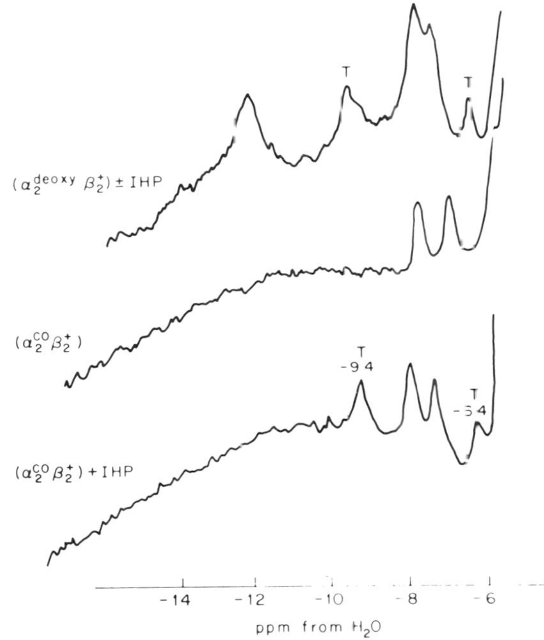

Fig. 5.250 MH_Z Proton NMR Spectra of 15% Hb M Milwaukee in H_2O and 0.1M Bis Tris at pH 6.6 and 30^0 C. Ho, Fung, Wiechelman, Pifat, and Johnson, "Recent NMR Studies on Quaternary Structural Transistions in Human Hemo-globins.

which are superimposed upon the -8 ppm hyperfine shifted resonance, are from the hydrogen bonded NH and/or OH protons of the hemoglobin molecule (Fung and Ho, 1974). In the spectra of both oxy and carbonmonoxy samples, the -9.4 and -6.4 ppm resonances are absent; instead, new resonances appear at -5.8 and -5.5 ppm respectively (Figure 4). Figure 5 shows the effect of IHP on Hb M Milwaukee (E11β67 Val→Glu), a natural valency hybrid with the β hemes in the ferric state. The -9.4 and -6.4 ppm resonances which are present in the deoxy spectrum disappear in the spectrum of HbCO M Milwaukee, but when IHP is added to the sample these two resonances reappear due to the conversion from oxy to deoxy quaternary structure (Perutz *et al.*, 1972; Fung, Pisciotta, and Ho, unpublished results). The exchangeable resonances at -9.4, -6.4, and -5.8 ppm, can be used as quaternary structural probes.

There are no observable differences in the exchangeable proton resonances among Hb A, Hb Des-Arg(α141), Hb Des-His-(β146), and Hb Chesapeake in the deoxy form and IHP has no effect on the exchangeable proton resonances of these hemoglobins (Fung and Ho, 1974). Figure 6 shows the deoxy spectra of hemoglobins NES-Des-Arg, Yakima, Kempsey as well as Hb A in the presence and absence of IHP in H_2O at pH 6.6 and at 30°C. The exchangeable proton resonances of these modified hemoglobins are significantly different from those of deoxy Hb A. The resonances at -9.4 and -6.4 ppm are missing in deoxy Hb NES-Des-Arg, but reappear upon the addition of IHP to the sample. The resonance at -9.4 ppm in the spectra of deoxy Hb Yakima and Hb Kempsey is missing even in the presence of IHP, and the resonance at -6.4 ppm is shifted slightly upfield (∿ 0.2 ppm) in these two mutants. It should be noted that the resonance at -5.8 ppm (characteristic of the oxy conformation) shows up in the deoxy spectrum of Hb Yakima in the presence of IHP at -5.9 ppm but not in those of deoxy Hb NES-Des-Arg and Hb Kempsey.

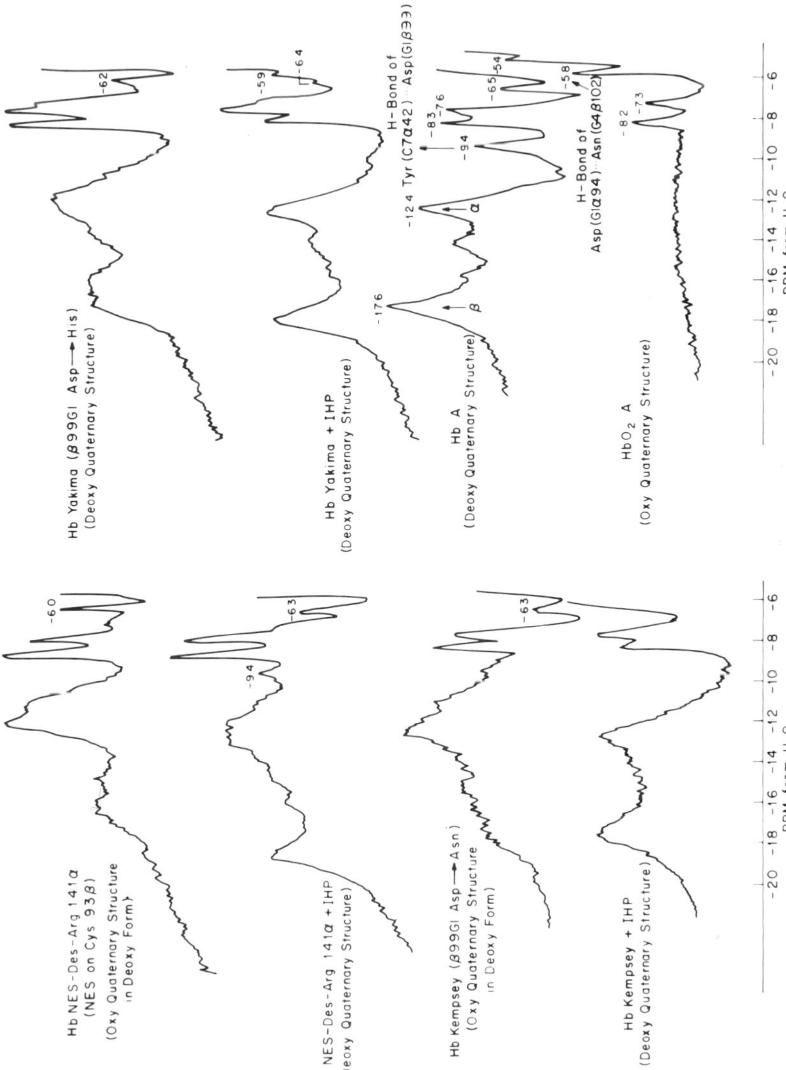

Fig.6. 250 MHz NMR Spectra of 12% Hemoglobins in H_2O and 0.1M Bis Tris at pH 6.6 and 30^0 C. Ho, Fung, Wiechelman, Pifat, and Johnson, "Recent NMR Studies on Quaternary Transitions in Human Hemoglobins."

DISCUSSION

Structural Changes in the $\alpha_1\beta_2$ Subunit Interface

The mutant hemoglobins Chesapeake, Yakima, and Kempsey have single amino acid substitutions in the $\alpha_1\beta_2$ subunit interface (Perutz and Lehmann, 1968). These single amino acid mutations result in a decrease in the cooperativity of the hemoglobin and an increase in their oxygen affinity. The hyperfine shifted proton resonances of deoxyhemoglobins Chesapeake, Yakima, and Kempsey clearly show that a mutation in the $\alpha_1\beta_2$ subunit interface alters the heme environment of both the mutated chain and also that of the normal chain (Figure 1). It is possible that in the oxygenation of Hb A, the reverse process could occur, i.e., tertiary structural changes in the vicinity of one heme could influence the structure of other hemes by altering the tertiary structure of the amino acid residues in the $\alpha_1\beta_2$ subunit interface. This region of the molecule is known to undergo significant structural changes in going from the deoxy to oxy conformation (Perutz, 1970; Perutz and Ten Eyck, 1971). We have suggested that this is one way in which conformational changes of those amino acid residues near the heme groups can be transmitted to the $\alpha_1\beta_2$ subunit interface and on to the neighboring heme groups (Davis *et al.*, 1971; Ho *et al.*, 1973). In other words, we believe that tertiary structural changes induced in the heme groups by the binding of ligands can alter the $\alpha_1\beta_2$ subunit interactions and can in this manner facilitate the quaternary structural transition during the cooperative oxygenation of hemoglobin.

Both hemoglobins Chesapeake and Yakima are known to assume both oxy and deoxy quaternary structures (or R type and T type structures). Our NMR results indicate that each of the mutant hemoglobins has its own characteristic quaternary structures which differ from those of Hb A. The functional properties of these hemoglobins along with our NMR results suggest that the mutant hemoglobins may assume a characteristic quaternary structure which may resemble "intermediate" structures occurring in the Hb A structural transition on ligand binding. The addition of IHP to each of these mutants results in hyperfine shifted spectra similar to those of Hb A suggesting that IHP can affect quaternary structural transitions in these mutants. This finding is in agreement with oxygen equilibrium measurements which show that addition of IHP to deoxy hemoglobins Chesapeake (Imai, 1974) and Kempsey (Gibson *et al.*, 1974) results in an increase in the cooperativity as measured by the Hill coefficient and a decrease in the oxygen affinity of these mutants.

Functional Properties of α and β Chains in Hemoglobins

The hyperfine shifted proton resonances have been used to monitor the ligand binding properties of α and β chains in the hemoglobin molecule (Davis *et al.*, 1971; Lindstrom *et al.*, 1971; Lindstrom and Ho, 1972; Ho *et al.*, 1973; Johnson and Ho, 1974; Wiechelman *et al.*, 1974). Figures 2 and 3 summarize our studies on the binding of O_2 to Hb A, Hb Chesapeake, Hb Yakima, and Hb Kempsey in the presence and absence of IHP. Johnson and Ho (1974) reported that in the absence of organic phosphate, O_2 binds to the α and β chains of Hb A with little preference and that in the presence of IHP, O_2 exhibits almost exclusive binding to the α chains (Figure 3). More recently, Wiechelman *et al.* (1974) reported that in the absence of IHP, oxygen binds to the α and β hemes of Hb Chesapeake essentially at random (Figure 2) and that in the presence of IHP, oxygen binds to the α chains of Hb Chesapeake in preference to the β chains (Figure 3). In the cases of Hb Yakima and Hb Kempsey in 0.1M Bis-Tris buffer at pD 7, oxygen binds to the β hemes in preference to the α hemes (Figure 2). On the other hand, in the presence of IHP oxygen binds to the α and β hemes of these two mutants essentially at random (Figure 3). For a detailed discussion on the functional properties of the α and β chains in hemoglobins as a function of organic phosphate, ligand, and pH, refer to Lindstrom *et al.* (1971), Lindstrom and Ho (1972), Ho *et al.* (1973), Lindstrom *et al.* (1973), Breen *et al.* (1974), Johnson and Ho (1974), and Wiechelman *et al.* (1974). These results suggest that the hemoglobin-ligand reactions are hemoglobin, ligand, organic phosphate, and pH specific.

Quaternary Structural Probes

Most of the proton NMR spectra of proteins were obtained by exchanging proteins with D_2O so as to suppress the intense proton signal of H_2O in aqueous samples. This experimental procedure which makes proton NMR spectra of proteins more readily obtainable sacrifices the signal from the NH and/or OH exchangeable protons. Some of these exchangeable proton resonances can provide valuable information about the hydrogen bonds in proteins. Recently, with the development of high-frequency NMR spectrometers, proton NMR spectra of proteins in H_2O can be obtained (Glickson *et al.*, 1969; Patel *et al.*, 1970; Ogawa *et al.*, 1972; Ho *et al.*, 1973; Mayer *et al.*, 1973; Breen *et al.*, 1974; Ogawa *et al.*, 1974).

The identification of the proton resonances at -9.4, -8.2, -7.3, -6.4, -5.8, and -5.5 ppm from H_2O as exchangeable proton resonances is based on two types of experiments. One is the conventional method of comparing the proton NMR spectra of samples in H_2O with those in D_2O and the second method is by the use of the double resonance technique (for details, refer to Fung and Ho, 1974). The -9.4 and -6.4 ppm resonances in Figure 4 are associated with some specific hydrogen-bonded protons in the deoxyhemoglobin molecule, whereas the -5.8 ppm (or -5.5 ppm in HbCO) resonance is associated with a specific hydrogen bond in the oxy quaternary structure. This conclusion is supported by the NMR results of Hb M Milwaukee (Figure 5). NMR and other studies have shown that the addition of IHP can convert the fully ligated Hb M Milwaukee which has an oxy quaternary structure to a deoxy conformation (Perutz *et al.*, 1972; Perutz *et al.*, 1974b; Fung, Pisciotta, and Ho, unpublished results). As shown in Figure 5, the T structure indicators, the -9.4 and -6.4 ppm resonances reappear in the spectrum when IHP is added to Hb M Milwaukee saturated with carbon monoxide. In conclusion, the -9.4 ppm and -6.4 ppm resonances are probes of the deoxy quaternary structure and the -5.8 ppm resonance is characteristic of the oxy conformation. Ogawa and co-workers have shown that the proton resonance at -9.4 ppm (or ∿ -14 ppm from DSS) can be used as a quaternary structural probe in the hemoglobin molecule (Ogawa *et al.*, 1972; Mayer *et al.*, 1973; Ogawa *et al.*, 1974); however, they did not specify the origin of the exchangeable resonances.

We have investigated the origin of these exchangeable proton resonances. In deoxyhemoglobins Yakima and Kempsey, even in the presence of IHP, the -9.4 ppm resonance is absent, clearly indicating that this resonance is related to the β99 aspartic acid, which is replaced by histidine in Hb Yakima and by asparagine in Hb Kempsey. Hence, we have assigned this resonance to the proton in the hydrogen bond between the phenolic hydroxyl of Tyr at C7α42 and the carboxyl of Asp at G1β99 in the $\alpha_1\beta_2$ subunit interface of the deoxy quaternary structure. This intersubunit hydrogen bond is one of the most characteristic features of the deoxy conformation in the hemoglobin molecule (Perutz, 1970; Perutz and Ten Eyck, 1971). X-Ray diffraction studies of Hb Yakima at 3.5 Å resolution have shown that deoxy Hb Yakima is isomorphous with deoxy Hb A, but the important $\alpha_1\beta_2$ subunit hydrogen bond between α42 and β99 is missing; instead a new hydrogen bond is formed between Asp at G1α94 and Asn at G4β102 (Pulsinelli, 1973). This hydrogen bond is normally found only in the oxy conformation of Hb A (Perutz and Ten Eyck, 1971). Crystals of deoxy Hb Kempsey are found to be isomorphous with those of oxy Hb A (Perutz *et al.*, 1974a). The same hydrogen bond which is not found in deoxy Hb Yakima is also missing in deoxy Hb Kempsey (Figure 6). Our NMR studies indicate that deoxy Hb Yakima and Hb Kempsey have their heme environments as well as $\alpha_1\beta_2$ subunit interfaces altered as revealed by the hyperfine shifted proton resonances, but these resonances can be converted to those similar to Hb A upon the addition of IHP (Figure 1). The hydrogen bond between Tyr at α42 and Asp at β99 cannot be formed in deoxy Hb Yakima and Hb Kempsey even in the presence of IHP presumably due to the amino acid substitutions at β99. A chemically modified hemoglobin, deoxy Hb NES-Des-Arg, which has a quaternary structure similar to deoxy Hb Kempsey

(Perutz *et al.*, 1974a) has also been studied (Figure 6). In this modified hemoglobin, the -9.4 ppm resonance is missing in the deoxy form. In the presence of IHP, it reappears with somewhat reduced intensity. This finding indicates that it is possible to have deoxy Hb NES-Des-Arg in the T type structure with the formation of the crucial deoxy hydrogen bond in the presence of IHP and this finding is also consistent with the results obtained by other techniques recently reported by Perutz *et al.* (1974a). The reduced intensity of this resonance may imply that the molecules have not fully resumed the T type quaternary structure.

The -6.4 ppm resonance clearly comes from an amino acid residue which changes its conformation upon ligation. There are several amino acids that fall into this category. The penultimate tyrosines (HC2) occupy pockets between helicies F and H of both α and β chains in the deoxy form and their phenolic hydroxyls are hydrogen bonded to the carboxyls of Val at FG5 (Perutz, 1970). In the oxy form, these tyrosines are pushed out of the heme pockets and form no such hydrogen bonds. The NH proton of tryptophan at C3β37 could be another candidate for the -6.4 ppm resonance. This tryptophan is in the $\alpha_1\beta_2$ subunit interface and its conformation is sensitive to a change in the quaternary structure (Perutz and Ten Eyck, 1971). The presence of the -6.4 ppm resonance in the spectra of deoxyhemoglobins Des-Arg and Des-His with IHP eliminates the likelihood of having the salt bridges of the C-terminal histidine of the β chain (β146) and of the C-terminal arginine of the α chain (α141) as possible candidates for the origin of this resonance (Fung and Ho, 1974). Further work is needed to make a specific assignment of the resonance at -6.4 ppm.

The appearance of a resonance at -5.9 ppm in deoxy Hb Yakima in the presence and absence of IHP leads us to speculate that the -5.8 ppm resonance in HbO_2 A may come from the proton of the hydrogen bond between aspartic acid at G1α94 and asparagine at G4β102 in the $\alpha_1\beta_2$ subunit interface in the oxy conformation. According to the X-ray diffraction studies of Hb Yakima, the crucial hydrogen bond between Tyr at C7α42 and Asp at G1β99 in the $\alpha_1\beta_2$ subunit interface (in the deoxy conformation) is broken as a result of the amino acid substitution at β99 in this mutant, but a new hydrogen bond between Asp at G1α94 and Asn at G4β102, which is normally found in oxy form of Hb A, is formed (Pulsinelli, 1973). The recent proton NMR study of Hb Mälmo (FG4β97 His→Gln) in H_2O provides an indirect support for the assignment of the resonance at -5.8 ppm as due to the hydrogen bond between Asp at G1α94 and Asn at G4β102 in the oxy quaternary structure. The proton resonances in the region between -5.5 and -10 ppm from H_2O are the same for HbO_2 A and HbO_2 Mälmo (Fung, Fairbanks, and Ho, unpublished results). Thus, the -5.8 ppm resonance cannot originate from the hydrogen bond between Thr at C6α41 and His at FG4β97, which is another important hydrogen bond in the $\alpha_1\beta_2$ subunit interface characteristic of the oxy conformation (Perutz and Ten Eyck, 1971). It should be noted that the hydrogen bond in the $\alpha_1\beta_2$ subunit interface senses a slight difference in the environment between HbO_2 A and HbCO A as manifested by a 0.3 ppm difference in the chemical shift (Figure 4). The exact implication of this difference between HbO_2 A and HbCO A is not known.

The -8.2 and -7.3 ppm resonances which remain invariant in the two quaternary structures (Figures 4 and 5) could come from the exchangeable protons in the $\alpha_1\beta_1$ subunit interface. This interface undergoes only a slight change on ligation and the number of hydrogen bonds probably remains unchanged (Perutz and Ten Eyck, 1971). There is additional evidence to provide indirect support to this assignment. For example, the exchangeable proton resonances of the isolated α and β chains in the CO form are very different from those of HbCO A (Pifat, Fung, Bertoli, and Ho, unpublished results; Patel *et al.*, 1970). These results suggest that these two resonances cannot come from the intrachain hydrogen bonds in the α or β chains. Another possibility is that these two resonances could originate from tryptophans at A12 of both α and β chains which remain unchanged during the transition from deoxy to oxyhemoglobin (Perutz *et al.*, 1974a). Further work is needed to ascertain the origin of these two resonances. If they indeed come from the hydrogen bonds in the $\alpha_1\beta_1$ subunit interface, they could provide a probe to monitor the $\alpha_1\beta_1$ subunit interactions in the hemoglobin molecule during the ligand binding process.

In conclusion, our NMR studies of hemoglobins can be summarized as follows: First, we have observed the proton resonances of the hydrogen bonds in the subunit interfaces in the hemoglobin molecule and have assigned two specific resonances to the important hydrogen bonds in the $\alpha_1\beta_2$ subunit interface, one in the oxy (R type) and the other in the deoxy (T type) conformation. Second, the NMR results clearly indicate the existence of oxy (R type) and deoxy (T type) quaternary structures in the hemoglobin molecule in solution and that organic phosphate (such as inositol hexaphosphate) can alter the quaternary structural transitions in hemoglobins. Third, the amino acid substitutions in the $\alpha_1\beta_2$ subunit interface produce tertiary structural changes in the vicinity of the mutation. These changes can also be transmitted to the neighboring heme groups via the $\alpha_1\beta_2$ subunit interface. The NMR results suggest that the $\alpha_1\beta_2$ mutants may have quaternary structures which are different from those of normal adult hemoglobin under the same experimental conditions. Fourth, hemoglobin-ligand reactions are found to be hemoglobin, ligand, organic phosphate, and pH specific. Thus, our NMR results suggest that there are several features of the hemoglobin molecule that are consistent with the allosteric model proposed by Monod *et al.* (1965) and also with the sequential model proposed by Koshland *et al.* (1966). In order to understand the molecular mechanism for the cooperative oxygenation of hemoglobin, it is essential to follow structural changes in different regions of the molecule and to relate these structural changes to the functional properties of the protein. By making additional resonance assignments to specific tertiary and quaternary structures in the molecule, high-resolution NMR spectroscopy offers a distinct possibility of providing further insight into the molecular mechanism for the oxygenation of hemoglobin.

ACKNOWLEDGEMENT

We are grateful to Dr. H. F. Bunn, Dr. S. Charache, Dr. V. F. Fairbanks, Dr. J. V. Kilmartin, Dr. A. V. Pisciotta, and Dr. R. D. Koler for providing the blood samples containing mutant hemoglobins and the chemically modified hemoglobins needed for this work. This work was supported by research grants from the National Institute of Health (HL-10383, HL-15165, and RR-00292) and the National Science Foundation (GB-37096X).

REFERENCES

Berman, M., Benesch, R., and Benesch, R. E. (1971). The Removal of Organic Phosphates from Hemoglobin. *Arch. Biochem. Biophys. 145:236.*

Breen, J. J., Bertoli, D. A., Dadok, J., and Ho, C. (1974). Proton Magnetic Resonance Studies of Human Adult Hemoglobin in Water. *Biophys. Chem. 2:49.*

Dadok, J., and Sprecher, R. F. (1974). Correlation NMR Spectroscopy. *J. Magn. Resonance 13:243.*

Dadok, J., Sprecher, R. F., Bothner-By, A. A., and Link, T. (1970). Time Sharing High Resolution NMR Spectrometer with Superconducting Solenoid. *Abstracts, Section C-2 of the 11th Experimental NMR Conference, Pittsburgh, Pa.*

Davis, D. G., Charache, S., and Ho, C. (1969). Nuclear Magnetic Resonance Studies of Hemoglobins. II. Evidence for the Nonequivalence of α- and β-Chains in Azide Derivatives of Methemoglobins. *Proc. Nat. Acad. Sci. (U.S.A.) 63:1403.*

Davis, D. G., Lindstrom, T. R., Mock, N. H., Baldassare, J. J., Charache, S., Jones, R. T., and Ho, C. (1971). Nuclear Magnetic Resonance Studies of Hemoglobins. VI. Heme Proton Spectra of Human Deoxyhemoglobins and their Relevance to the Nature of Cooperative Oxygenation of Hemoglobin. *J. Mol. Biol. 60:101.*

Gibson, Q. H., Bunn, H. F., Wohl, R., Bradley, T. B., and Cooley, M. (1974). Functional Properties of Hemoglobin Kempsey. *J. Biol. Chem., in press.*

Glasoe, P. K., and Long, F. A. (1960). Use of Glass Electrodes to Measure Acidities in Deuterium Oxide. *J. Phys. Chem. 64:188.*

Glickson, J. D., McDonald, C. C., and Phillips, W. D. (1969). Assignment of Tryptophan Indole NH Proton Resonances of Lysozyme. *Biochem. Biophys. Res. Commun. 35:492.*

Greenfield, N. J., and Williams, M. N. (1972). Proton Magnetic Resonance Studies of Human Hemoglobin Histidine Titrations. *Biochim. Biophys. Acta 257:187.*

Fung, L. W.-M., and Ho, C. (1974). A Proton Nuclear Magnetic Resonance Study of Subunit Hydrogen Bonds in Human Hemoglobins: An Investigation of Quaternary Structure. *Submitted to Biochemistry for publication.*

Hayashi, A., Suzuki, T., and Shin, M. (1973). An Enzymic Reduction System for Metmyoglobin and Methemoglobin, and its Application to Functional Studies of Oxygen Carriers. *Biochim. Biophys. Acta 310:309.*

Ho, C., Lindstrom, T. R., Baldassare, J. J., and Breen, J. J. (1973). Magnetic Resonance Studies of Human Hemoglobins and their Implications to the Structure-Function Relationships in Human Normal and Abnormal Hemoglobins. *Ann. N. Y. Acad. Sci. 222:21.*

Imai, K. (1974). Hemoglobin Chesapeake (92α, Arginine→Leucine):Precise Measurements and Analysis of Oxygen Equilibrium. *J. Biol. Chem., in press.*

Johnson, M. E., and Ho, C. (1974). Effects of Ligands and Organic Phosphates on Functional Properties of Human Adult Hemoglobin. *Biochemistry 13:3653.*

Kilmartin, J. V., Breen, J. J., Roberts, G. C. K., and Ho, C. (1973). Direct Measurement of the pK Values of an Alkaline Bohr Group in Human Hemoglobin. *Proc. Nat. Acad. Sci. (U.S.A.) 70:1246.*

Kilmartin, J. V., and Hewitt, J. A. (1971). The Effect of Removal of C-terminal Residues on Cooperative Interactions in Hemoglobin. *Cold Spring Harb. Symp. Quant. Biol. 36:311.*

Koshland, D. E., Nēmethy, G., and Filmer, D. (1966). Comparison of Experimental Binding Data and Theoretical Models in Proteins Containing Subunits. *Biochemistry 5:365.*

Lindstrom, T. R., and Ho, C. (1972). Functional Nonequivalence of α and β Hemes in Human Adult Hemoglobin. *Proc. Nat. Acad. Sci. (U.S.A.) 69:1707.*

Lindstrom, T. R., and Ho, C. (1973). Effects of Anions and Ligands on the Tertiary Structure around Ligand Binding Site in Human Adult Hemoglobin. *Biochemistry 12:134.*

Lindstrom, T. R., Baldassare, J. J., Bunn, H. F., and Ho, C. (1973). Nuclear Magnetic Resonance and Spin-Label Studies of Hemoglobin Kempsey. *Biochemistry 12:4212.*

Lindstrom, T. R., Ho, C., and Pisciotta, A. V. (1972). Nuclear Magnetic Resonance Studies of Haemoglobin M Milwaukee. *Nature 237:263.*

Lindstrom, T. R., Olson, J. S., Mock, N. H., Gibson, Q. H., and Ho, C. (1971). Nuclear Magnetic Resonance Studies of Hemoglobins. VIII. Evidence for Preferential Ligand Binding to the β Chains with Deoxyhemoglobin. *Biochem. Biophys. Res. Commun. 45:22.*

Mayer, A., Ogawa, S., Shulman, R. G., and Gersonde, E. (1973). High-Resolution Proton Nuclear Magnetic Resonance Studies of the Quaternary State of Hemoglobin M Iwate. *J. Mol. Biol. 81:187.*

Monod, J., Wyman, J., and Changeux, J.-P. (1965). On the Nature of Allosteric Transitions: A Plausible Model. *J. Mol. Biol. 12:88.*

Ogawa, S., and Shulman, R. G. (1972). High Resolution Nuclear Magnetic Resonance Spectra of Hemoglobin. III. The Half-ligated State and Allosteric Interactions. *J. Mol. Biol. 70:315.*

Ogawa, S., Mayer, A., and Shulman, R. G. (1972). High Resolution Proton Magnetic Resonance Study of the Two Quaternary States in Fully Ligated Hemoglobin Kansas. *Biochem. Biophys. Res. Commun. 49:1485.*

Ogawa, S. Patel, D. J., and Simon, S. R. (1974). Proton Magnetic Resonance Study of the Switch between the Two Quaternary Structures in High-Affinity Hemoglobins in the Deoxy State. *Biochemistry 13:2001.*

Patel, D. J., Kampa, L., Shulman, R. G., Yamane, T., and Fujiwara, M. (1970). Proton NMR Studies of Hemoglobin in H_2O. *Biochem. Biophys. Res. Commun. 40:1224.*

Perutz, M. F. (1970). Stereochemistry of Cooperative Effects in Haemoglobin. *Nature 228:726.*

Perutz, M. F., and Lehmann, H. (1968). Molecular Pathology of Human Haemoglobin. *Nature 219:902.*

Perutz, M. F., and Ten Eyck, L. F. (1971). Stereochemistry of Cooperative Effects in Hemoglobin. *Cold Spring Harb. Symp. Quant. Biol. 36:295.*

Perutz, M. F., Pulsinelli, P. D., and Ranney, H. M. (1972). Structure and Subunit Interaction in Haemoglobin M Milwaukee. *Nature New Biol. 237:259.*
Perutz, M. F., Ladner, J. E., Simon, S. R., and Ho, C. (1974a). Influence of Globin Structure on the State of the Heme. I. Human Deoxyhemoglobin. *Biochemistry 13:2163.*
Perutz, M. F., Heidner, E. J., Ladner, J. E., Beetlestone, J. G., Ho, C., and Slade, E. F. (1974b). Influence of Globin Structure on the State of the Heme. III. Changes in Heme Spectra Accompanying Allosteric Transitions in Methemoglobin and their Implications for Heme-Heme Interaction. *Biochemistry 13:2187.*
Pulsinelli, P. D. (1973). Structure of Deoxyhemoglobin Yakima: A High-Affinity Mutant Form Exhibiting Oxy-like $\alpha_1\beta_2$ Subunit Interactions. *J. Mol. Biol. 74:57.*
Wiechelman, K. J., Charache, S., and Ho, C. (1974). Nuclear Magnetic Resonance Studies of Hemoglobin Chesapeake: An $\alpha_1\beta_2$ Mutant. *Biochemistry, in press.*

DISCUSSION

Dr. Perutz: I should like to ask a question and then answer it. IHP can change nitric oxide hemoglobin from the R to the T state but it can't do that to carbonmonoxy or oxyhemoglobin. The equilibrium between these two forms is governed mainly by the displacement of the proximal histidine from the plane of the porphyrin ring, i.e., by the iron-nitrogen distances which are short in oxy and carbonmonoxy hemoglobin and long in deoxyhemoglobin. Why can nitric oxide hemoglobin which is a low spin compound like oxy or CO undergo the switch? The answer is provided by some beautiful X-ray crystallographic studies by R. Scheidt on nitrosoporphyrins at Notre Dame. These show that the distance from the iron atom to the nitrogen of the proximal histidine in CO hemoglobin is estimated as 2.00 angstroms, in oxy is 2.07, but the nitric oxide is 2.18. This huge increase occurs because nitric oxide has an unpaired electron which is transferred to the iron atom on ligation and repels the nitrogen of the proximal histidine making the $Fe-N_{\varepsilon}$ bond stretchable. Consequently, IHP can switch the NO derivative to the T state while it cannot switch CO or O_2.

Dr. Salhany: Drs. S. Ogawa, R. G. Shulman and J. M. Salhany at Bell Laboratories have recently investigated the structural and functional properties of fully liganded adult hemoglobin and hemoglobin Kansas (1,2,3). The structural studies employed high resolution nuclear magnetic resonance (NMR) and ultraviolet circular dichroism (CD) techniques. The functional properties of these hemoglobins were studied by measuring the CO replacement reaction by NO. The NMR marker used to indicate the T state is the -14 ppm peak for hemoglobin in H_2O, downfield from DSS. This peak is only seen for hemoglobins which are in the deoxy quaternary structure, independent of the degree of ligation (4). The CD marker consists of the appearance of the negative peak in the spectrum at about 285 nm. Simon and Cantor (5) and Perutz et al. (6,7) have shown that the appearance of this negative CD peak indicates the transition to T, also independent of the degree of ligation.

Table 1 summarizes the recent NMR and CD measurements made by Salhany, Ogawa and Shulman (2,3). As can be seen, there is an excellent agreement between the observation of the -14 ppm NMR line and the observation of the negative CD peak at 285 nm. These results show that IHP switches adult nitrosyl hemoglobin to the fully liganded T state. Furthermore, simply binding NO to stripped hemoglobin Kansas favors the formation of the fully liganded T state.

Recently, Drs. R. W. Briehl and J. M. Salhany (8), working at the Albert Einstein College of Medicine and Bell Laboratories, have found that nitrosyl sickle cell hemoglobin + IHP (a) gels; (b) shows birefringence under the polarizing microscope, and (c) shows changes in the ultracentrifuge characteristic of polymerization (9). Since it is rather well established that polymerization of sickle cell hemoglobin stereochemically requires the deoxy quaternary structure, it would seem that the above evidence of Briehl and Salhany offers strong support for the conclusion that nitrosyl hemoglobin + IHP is in the fully liganded deoxy quaternary structure at neutral pH.

Table 1
Structural Markers for Hemoglobin

All Molecules are Fully Liganded pH 7.0	Observation of the -14 ppm NMR peak	Observation of the Negative CD Peak at 285 nm	Quaternary Structure
Stripped adult HbCO	-	-	R_4
Stripped Kansas HbCO	-	-	R_4
Adult HbCO + IHP	-	-	R_4
Stripped Adult HbNO	-	-	R_4
Stripped Kansas HbNO	+	+	T_4
Kansas HbCO + IHP	+	(+)	T_4
Adult HbNO + IHP	+	+	T_4
Kansas HbNO + IHP	(+)	(+)	T_4

This situation allowed us to test the model of Monod <u>et al</u>. (10) kinetically using the CO replacement reaction <u>by NO</u>. One earlier attempt had been made to test this model (11). NO replaces CO because of its much higher affinity. Furthermore, since NO binds with extreme rapidity and is at relatively high concentration, all of the protein molecules remain fully saturated with either CO or NO during the reaction. The rate determining step in this replacement reaction is the CO off rate. The CO off rate will be influenced by the structure of the protein during the course of the reaction as well as the point in the reaction where the structure switches.

Figure 1 shows the various kinetic results (see reference 2 for more details). Line 1 is the normalized kinetic time course for the CO off rate of stripped adult hemoglobin. As Table 1 indicates, the molecule is in the R state for both CO and NO in the complete absence of all phosphates. The time course reflects these structural measurements by showing a slow, first order rate of CO dissociation. Adult hemoglobin bound by CO starts in R and ends in T when NO replaces CO in the presence of IHP (Table 1). This explains why the reaction accelerates (Fig. 1, line 2). Stripped hemoglobin Kansas at pH 7.0

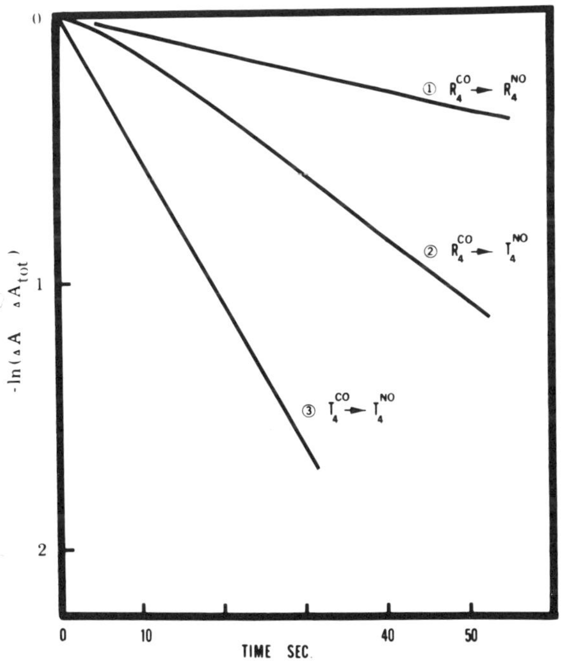

also falls in this category (Fig. 1, line 2) because with CO it is in R, but with NO it is in T (Table 1). Finally, the CO form of hemoglobin Kansas + IHP is in T to start with and remains in that structure throughout the replacement reaction according to the results of Table 1. Line 3 of Figure 1 shows that the CO off rate in this case is about an order of magnitude faster than the same rate for the molecule which remains in R throughout the reaction. The NO off rate has also been shown to reflect the quaternary transitions in nitrosyl hemoglobin presented in Table 1 (3).

These combined structural and functional changes offer strong support for the Monod model (10) as opposed to a Koshland type model (12). The importance of the present structural and kinetic findings with nitrosyl hemoglobin is not merely that this compound can switch quaternary structure, but that these structural changes cause the kinetics to change in a manner predicted by the two state model (13).

REFERENCES

1. Salhany, J. M., Ogawa, S. and Shulman, R. G. (1974). Fed. Proc. 33, 1225.
2. Salhany, J. M., Ogawa, S. and Shulman, R. G. (1974). Proc. Nat. Acad. Sci. (U.S.) 71, 3359-3361.
3. Salhany, J. M., Ogawa, S. and Shulman, R. G. (to be published).
4. Shulman, R. G., Ogawa, S., Mayer, A. and Castillo, C. L. (1973). Annals N.Y. Acad. Sci. 222, 9-19.
5. Simon, S. R. and Cantor, C. R. (1969). Proc. Nat. Acad. Sci. (U.S.) 63, 205-212.
6. Perutz, M. F., Ladner, J. E., Simon, S. R. and Ho, C. (1974). Biochemistry 13, 205-212.
7. Perutz, M. F., Fersht, A. R., Simon, S. R. and Roberts, G. C. K. (1974). Biochemistry 13, 2174-2186.
8. Briehl, R. W. and Salhany, J. M. (to be published).
9. Briehl, R. W. and Ewert, S. (1973). J. Mol. Biol. 80, 445-458.
10. Monod, J., Wyman, J. and Changeux, J. P. (1965). J.

Mol. Biol. 12, 88-118.
11. Cassoly, R., Gibson, Q. H., Ogawa, S. and Shulman, R. G. (1971). Biochem. Biophys. Res. Commun. 44, 1015-1021.
12. Koshland, D. E., Nemethy, G. and Filmer, D. (1966). Biochemistry 5, 2957.
13. Hopfield, J. J., Shulman, R. G. and Ogawa, S. (1971). J. Mol. Biol. 61, 425-443.

Dr. Salhany: One additional comment. Drs. Ogawa, Shulman, and I have done some EPR measurements on adult nitrosyl hemoglobin and IHP and stripped nitrosyl hemoglobin Kansas and the evidence in EPR seems in agreement with this view, that is that there seems to be more electron density on the iron, probably lengthening the bond to the N_{ε} of histidine.

Dr. Ogawa: I would like to ask Dr. Ho two questions. In the alpha-beta nonequivalence experiment on oxygenation of hemoglobin, does the peak intensity decrease in the alpha chain preferentially due to the kinetic broadening of the deoxy alpha peak or not? Have you measured the temperature dependence?

Dr. Ho: Yes. We have done a temperature dependence study of Hb A in a paper published in Biochemistry [3, 3653, (1974)]. This study was done in a 90 MHz NMR spectrometer and covered the range 12°C to 37°C. We don't see any line broadening at all. If the d-heme resonance intensity were a kinetic effect, you would expect significant changes in the NMR spectra. Second, also in this paper, we have done a computer simulation of the Hb NMR spectra during oxygen ligation. In this computer simulation we have used the parameters derived from the experimental spectra to generate calculated spectra. Using the α/β intensity ratios we obtained experimentally and then assuming a line broadening of 8 Hz per 1% ligation (the value observed at 250 MHz), we find that the agreement between the calculated and the observed spectral parameters is very good.

Dr. Ogawa: The second question is on the assignment of this T quaternary structure sensitive peak, the 9.4 ppm peak.

There are two possibilities for why you don't see that peak even in T in water. One is the stability of the T state, the life time of the T state possibly being too short to get reasonable line width to be observable. Second is the local structural disturbance around the proton. The local structural disturbance may facilitate the exchange rate of the proton and if that happens you have no resonance. We have been working on this peak, and on this identification, and we have tried many things. One experiment shows that it is impossible to have this proton in $\alpha_1\beta_2$ interfaces. Putting a paramagnetic spin label at the β-93, we looked for the paramagnetic broadening due to this radical. In this spin labeled hemoglobin I can see this -9.4 ppm. peak. Some years ago I went to Dr. Perutz's laboratory and put spin label in the deoxy model and estimated the position of the label. I calculated the distances from this label to the potential candidates in the $\alpha_1\beta_2$ interface. Your assigned proton is about 5 angstroms away from the spin level. I tried a couple of other spin labels just to make sure that this is not simply limited to a label. Even if we are off 5 angstroms in this distance, the magnetic broadening radius is about 15 angstroms. So it is probably very unlikely to be that proton. I also tried the other spin lebel at β-112, which is at the $\alpha_1\beta_1$ interface. All the exchangeable proton is wiped out. And if you reduce spin level in hemoglobin you can get the peak back. We have some candidates for the -9.4 ppm. peak which is tentatively assigned to histidine 122 in the chain.

Unidentified Speaker: What residue did you assign?

Dr. Ogawa: We tentatively assign it to the NH proton of histidine 122 of α chain. There is one problem here. That is the des Arg hemoblobin case in which some effect on this peak might be expected, but we can see this peak in des Arg hemoglobin as in normal hemoglobin but slightly broader. We may have to push this assignment or look for some other candidate. We need a little more work on this.

Dr. Ho: May I answer some of your questions? The first question you raised is a good one; if we have a fast exchange rate (based on the NMR time scale), we would not have seen this exchangeable proton resonance. One way to settle this question is to carry out a careful variable temperature experiment. As I have pointed out in my talk, the reappearance of the -9.4 ppm resonance in the deoxy Hb NES-Des-Arg upon the addition of IHP and not in Hb Kempsey suggests that this resonance is associated with the hydrogen bond between β99 Asp and α42 Tyr. This hydrogen bond is missing in Hb Kempsey due to the amino acid substitution at β99. Based on a number of experimental results, we know that Hb Kempsey and Hb NES-Des-Arg have similar structural and functional properties. Hence, since the two hemoglobins are very similar, it appears unlikely that the $\alpha_1\beta_2$ interface will differ sufficiently between them to allow a high enough exchange rate for Hb Kemsey to wipe out the -9.4 ppm. resonance, but still leave a sharp resonance at -9.4 ppm. Hb NES-Des-Arg. We have also labelled the β93 sulfhydryl group and examined the exchangeable resonances of this spin labelled hemoglobin. The spin label that we used is a six-membered iodoacetamide, the so-called "Ogawa" spin label. We have found no significant broadening of the -9.4 ppm resonance in the spin labelled hemoglobin. The lack of broadening at the -9.4 ppm resonance could be due to a number of factors, as for example, the orientation, mobility, etc. of the spin label. We have estimated that the distance between the nitrogen atom of the nitroxyl group of the spin label at β93 and the hydrogen atom of the hydroxyl group of α42 tyrosine is much greater than 5Å.

Dr. Ogawa: No, it's mostly dependent on dipolar...

Dr. Ho: Your previous EPR studies of this spin labelled hemoglobin suggested that the spin label at β93 has a weakly immobilized conformation in deoxy Hb A [Ogawa, McConnell, and Horwitz, Proc. Nat. Acad. Sci. 61:401 (1968)]. If the spin label is relatively mobile, it is possible that there could be a partial averaging out of the dipolar interactions. Thus, the broadening may not be as much as in the case when the spin label is rigidly pointed to a given group. Some time ago, we obtained the hyperfine shifted and ring-current shifted proton resonances of spin labelled Hb A. We have found that the β heme resonance is shifted slightly to lower field but exhibits no broadening [Davis et al., J. Mol. Biol.

60:101 (1971)] and that the ring-current shifted resonances of spin labelled HbCO A in the region of βE11 are altered but show no drastic broadening as compared to those of the unlabelled HbCO A.

Dr. Ogawa: Oh yes, we calculated that too. It is not in the range of magnetic broadening.

Dr. Ho: You don't see much broadening either?

Dr. Ogawa: You don't see any broadening.

Dr. Ho: You said that you have labelled the sulfhydryl group of β112 cysteine in the $\alpha_1\beta_1$ subunit interface. I am concerned as to whether you can reconstitute the hemoglobin molecule if you attach a spin label at β112. Have you examined the exchangeable proton resonances of Hb Des-His and Hb Des-Arg? We have found that the exchangeable proton resonances of these two modified hemoglobins are the same as those of Hb A.

Dr. Ogawa: I don't know whether this des Arg problem is due to assignment error or it doesn't matter for this arginine. This NH proton of histidine is really stabilized through the bonds with the aspartate and the arginine.

Dr. Ho: I think we can settle this later.

HEMOGLOBIN CRANSTON, AN UNSTABLE VARIANT HAVING AN ELONGATED BETA CHAIN

H. Franklin Bunn and Geoffrey J. Schmidt

Department of Medicine, Peter Bent Brigham

Hospital, Harvard Medical School, Boston, Mass.

INTRODUCTION

Structural and functional studies on human hemoglobin variants have provided valuable insights into the genetic basis of hemoglobin biosynthesis. Over 180 structurally different variants have been reported to date. Of these, the great majority are single amino acid substitutions due to a single base substitution in the corresponding triplet codon. A few of the unstable variants have been found to have deletions of one or more amino acids in sequence. Recently, abnormal hemoglobins have been encountered having elongated subunits. Hemoglobin Constant Spring is found quite frequently in association with α thalassemia. Clegg, Weatherall and Milner (1971) showed that this variant contains 31 additional residues at the C-terminus of the α chain. The chain elongation can be explained by the substitution of C for U in the termination codon (UAA) permitting the translation of the subsequent segment of mRNA. Two years ago Seid-Akhavan et al reported structural studies on hemoglobin Wayne. This α chain variant contains 5 additional residues due to a frameshift at the codon corresponding to position 139. Because of the deletion of an adenine nucleotide at this site a new sequence of amino acids is translated until a termination codon is reached. A specific base sequence at the C-terminal end of the αA chain can be deduced which is in perfect accord with the primary structures of hemoglobins A, Constant Spring and Wayne. Independent support for the structure of this portion of the α chain gene has been provided by Marotta et al (1974). They found several base sequences of synthetic human globin mRNA which match or overlap the postulated base sequences of the αA and α Constant Spring chains.

We are reporting preliminary structural studies on hemoglobin Cranston, an unstable variant having an elongated β chain probably due to a frameshift mutation.

METHODS

Blood was collected in acid-citrate dextrose. Hemolysates were analysed by isoelectric focusing on polyacrylamide gels (Drysdale, et al, 1971). Hemoglobins were isolated by chromatography on DEAE cellulose equilibrated with 0.05 M Tris-H Cl buffer, pH 8.1 and developed with a linear NaCl gradient. Globin was prepared on purified hemoglobins by precipitation in acid acetone. Alpha and beta subunits were then isolated by chromatography on CM-Cellulose in 8 M urea (Clegg et al, 1966). The purified chains were aminoethylated prior to desalting and lyophilization. Following digestion with trypsin, peptide maps were prepared on cellulose thin layer plates (Jensen et al, 1973). 1.0-1.5 mg of βchain tryptic digest was applied to 0.25 mm thick cellulose layers on glass plates (Analtech Inc., Newark, Del.). Electrophoresis was performed in a water: acetic acid:pyridine (2700:10:300) buffer, pH 6.5 at 1000V, 0°C, for three hours. Ascending chromatography was then run in water:pyridine:1-propanol:isobutyl alcohol:n-amyl alcohol (30:30:10:10:10) for four hours at room temperature. Plates were then sprayed with 0.2% ninhydrin in butanol in order to permit detection of the spots. Stains specific for arginine, tyrosine, tryptophan, histidine and sulfur containing residues were also employed for identification of specific peptides (Easley, 1965). Peptides, stained with 0.02% ninhydrin were eluted from the plates in warm 1 M acetic acid. After drying, they were hydrolyzed in constant boiling 6 N HCl, 110°C for 16 hours. Amino acid content was determined on a Durrum D-500 amino acid analyser (AAA Laboratory, Seattle, Wash.). Carboxypeptidase A was obtained from Sigma Chemical Co., and prepared as described by Ambler (Method 1).

RESULTS AND DISCUSSION

A 46 year old woman with a mild form of systemic lupus erythematosis was found to have a compensated hemolytic state: hemoglobin 13.5 g/100 ml, 8% reticulocytes. Electrophoresis of the hemolysate on cellulose acetate pH 8.6 and by gel electrofocusing revealed an abnormal component which behaved similarly to hemoglobin S. Heinz bodies were seen after the blood was incubated with 1% Crystal violet for three hours at 37°C. The patient's hemolysate formed a precipitate when incubated in 17% isopropanol (Carrell and Kay, 1972) but showed no instability when heated to 50°C in neutral phosphate or tris buffers. One of the three children of the proband had similar hematologic findings.

When the proband's hemolysate was chromatographed on DEAE-cellulose, two abnormal hemoglobin peaks were eluted between A_2 and A. Designated Cr_1 and Cr_2, these components comprised 10% and 20% of the total hemoglobin. We have been unable to show any spectral, electrophoretic or structural difference between these two abnormal hemoglobin components. Hybridization with canine hemoglobin showed that the structural abnormality resided in the β chain. A peptide map of a tryptic digest of βCr_2 is shown diagramatically in Figure 1. The fingerprint was identical to that of β-A except that βTp15 was missing and a new spot was detected that was negative for histidine and tyrosine. β-Cr_2Tp14 was shown to have the same amino acid compostion as β-ATp14. The new peptide contained equimolar amounts of serine, isoleucine, threonine and lysine. Analysis of the dansylated peptide indicated that serine is the N-terminal residue. Since these results cannot be explained by a single amino acid replacement at β Tp15, a different genetic mechanism must be involved. The total amino acid

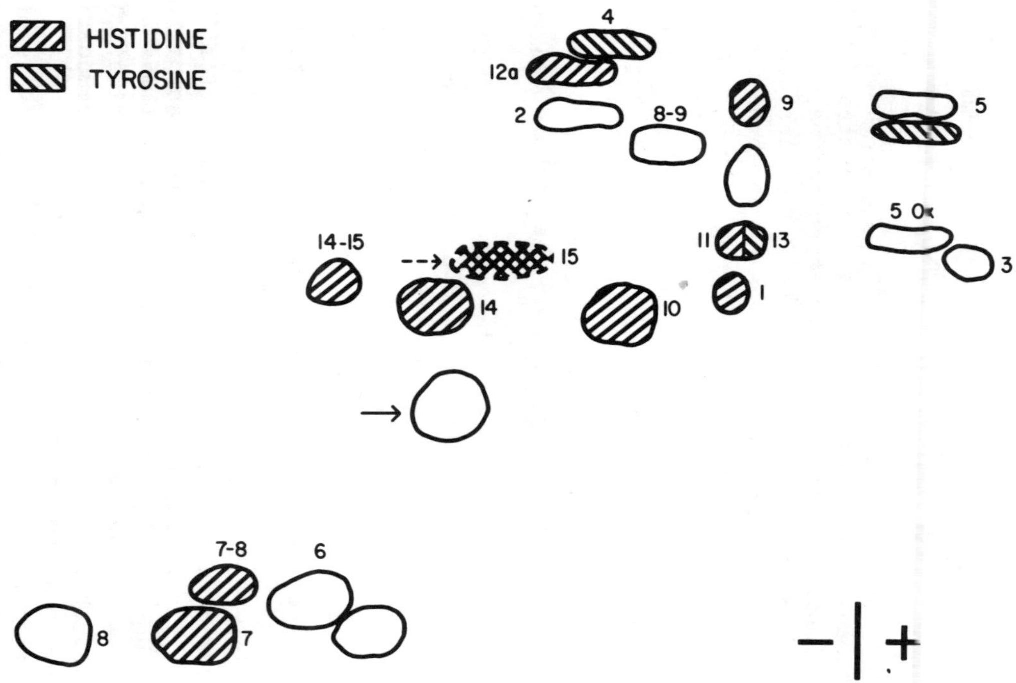

Figure 1: Diagram of β Cr_2 tryptic digest. Peptides containing histidine and tyrosine are shown. βATp15 is missing and a new peptide is seen (arrow) which does not contain either histidine or tyrosine.

compositons of β Cr_1 and Cr_2 were compared to β A following hydrolysis of the intact subunits in 6 N HCl, 110°C for 24, 48, and 96 hours. The variant β chains contained one less histidine and 0.5 less tyrosine residues, one additional aspartic acid, isoleucine, threonine and phenylalanine residues and two additional leucine and serine residues. Thus hemoglobin Cranston has an elongated β chain with a "new" sequence of amino acids beginning at β 145. It is the first adult human hemoglobin known to contain isoleucine. In order to determine the amino acid sequence at the C-terminal end of β Cranston, the intact subunit was incubated with carboxypeptidase A (enzyme:substrate 1:100, 0.01 M bis Tris buffer, pH 7.2, 37°C). In each of four experiments, up to 0.5 moles of tyrosine per mole of globin was released during the first few minutes of incubation followed by 1.0 moles of phenylalanine. Thus, about half of the βCr_1 and βCr_2 chains terminate with tyrosine. Perhaps some type of endogenous peptidase is responsible for cleaving tyrosine from the C-terminal end. More than one mole of leucine was released per mole of β Cranston, indicating the presence of two leucine residues near the C-terminus. The carboxypeptidase data and the analysis of the abnormal peptide fit best with the following sequence:

```
-Lys-Ser-(Ile-Thr)-Lys-(Leu-Asn)-Ala-Ser-Leu-Phe-Tyr-COOH
144 145  146 147  148  149 150  151 152 153 154 155
```

Hemoglobin Cranston has a very hydrophobic C-terminal tryptic peptide which we have not yet been able to isolate and identify on fingerprints. We are now using other solvent systems and proteolytic enzymes in order to isolate and analyse this fragment. At this time, the proposed structure for hemoglobin Cranston must be considered tentative.

It is likely that this variant arose because of a non-homologous crossover during meiosis. The β-chain genes can be lined up so that a crossover at position 144 (AAG) can incorporate an additional AG into the mRNA base sequence:

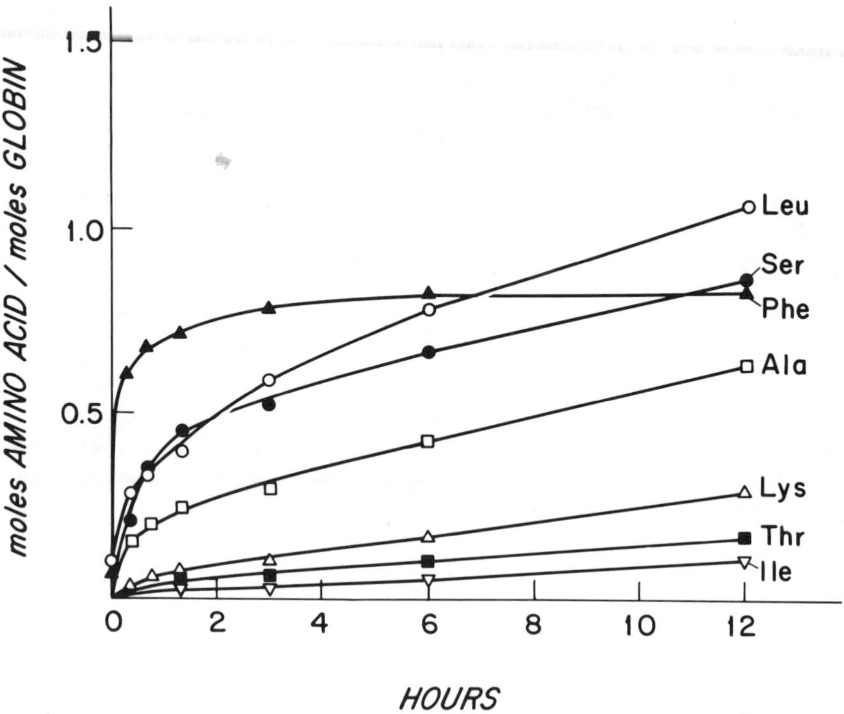

Figure 2: Digestion of βCr_2 with carboxypeptidase A. Experimental conditions are stated in the text.

	144	145	146			
	Lys	Tyr	His	Term		
βA	AAG	UAU	CAC	UAA	GCN * ...	
βA	AAG	UAU	CAC	UAA	GCN * ...	
βCr	AAG	AGU	AUC	ACU	AAG	CUN ...
	Lys	Ser	Ile	Thr	Lys	Leu ...
	144	145	146	147	148	149

The only other elongated β chain variant that has been reported to date is hemoglobin Tak (Flatz et al, 1971). It has a primary structure identical to that of β A except that it contains 10 additional residues beyond β 146 His. These are similar but not identical to the additional residues found in hemoglobin Cranston. The structure of hemolgobin Tak cannot be explained by a single base substitution at the UAA termination codon. It is difficult to deduce a precise genetic basis for the mutation in Tak because the base sequence beyond the termination codon is not yet known.

SUMMARY

A patient with compensated Heinz body hemolytic anemia was found to have an unstable hemoglobin variant with an elongated β chain. Hemoglobin Cranston has a unique amino acid sequence following β 144 lysine. The subunit contains 155 residues, nine more than β A. The presence of a segment of hydrophobic residues at the C-terminus of the β chain probably accounts for the decreased stability of the variant. The structure of hemoglobin Cranston can be explained by a crossover at position 144 wherein two nucleotide bases (AG) have been inserted into the mRNA, resulting in a frameshift.

---

* This base sequence was derived from Marotta et al (1974) and from the genetic code.

ACKNOWLEDGEMENTS

We are indebted to Mrs. D. M. and to Dr. Robert Dluhy for their continued cooperation in providing blood specimens and to Drs. Lowell Ericsson and Bernard Forget for many helpful discussions.

This work was supported by Grant HL 16927-01 and Contract NO 1-HB-42973 and by the Nehemias Gorin Foundation.

REFERENCES

Ambler, R.P. (1967). Enzymic hydrolysis with carboxypeptidases. Methods. Enzymol. 11:155.

Carrell, R.W. and Kay, R. (1972). A simple method for the detection of unstable hemoglobins. Brit. J. Haemat. 23:615.

Clegg, J.B., Naughton, M.A. and Weatherall, D.J. (1966). Abnormal human hemoglobins. Separation and characterization of the α- and β- chains by chromatography, and the determination of two new variants, Hb Chesapeake and Hb J (Bangkok). J. Mol. Biol. 19:91.

Clegg, J.B., Weatherall, D.J. and Milner, P.F. (1971). Haemoglobin Constant Spring - a chain termination mutant? Nature 234:337.

Drysdale, J.W., Righetti, P. and Bunn, H.F. (1971). The separation of human and animal hemoglobins by isoelectric focusing in polyacrylamide gel. Biochim, Biophys. Acta. 229:42.

Easley, C. (1965). Combinations of specific color reactions useful in the peptide mapping technique. Biochim. Biophys. Acta 10:386.

Flatz, G., Kinderlerer, J.L., Kilmartin, J.V. and Lehmann, H. (1971). Hemoglobin Tak: a variant with additional residues at the end of the β-chains. Lancet 1:732.

Jensen, M., Nathan, D.G. and Bunn, H.F. (1973). The reaction of cyanate with the α and β subunits in hemoglobin. Effects of oxygenation, phosphates and carbon dioxide. J. Biol. Chem. 248:8057.

Marotta, C.A., Forget, B.G., Weissman, S.M., Verma, I.M., McCaffrey, R.P. and Baltimore, D. (1974). Nucleotide sequences of human globin messenger RNA. Proc. Nat. Acad. Sci. (U.S.A.) 71:2300.

Seid-Akhavan, M., Winter, W.P., Abramson, R.K. and Rucknagel, D.L. (1972). Hemoglobin Wayne: a frameshift variant occuring in two distinct forms. Blood 40:927 (Abstact).

DISCUSSION

Dr. Charache: If you use conventional cellulose acetate electrophoresis, do the two abnormal bands show up?

Dr. Bunn: No.

Dr. Charache: So you have to use isoelectric focusing--but it does separate on DEAE columns?

Dr. Bunn: Yes, but the two column peaks don't correspond to the gel focusing peaks. The two abnormal column peaks give gel focusing patterns that are indistinguishable.

Dr. Charache: The experiment must be terribly hard, but have you tried to find out what DPG does? I mean maybe if you started partially saturated and went up?

Dr. Bunn: We tried adding DPG to hemolysates; and got varying amounts of precipitate. The data are not very clean. We really don't have a good idea as to the interaction of DPG with the variant.

Dr. Winter: Did you try playing around with hemoglobin Tak sequence to see if you could make any sense at all out of the possible nucleotide combinations?

Dr. Bunn: I believe that Fitch has suggested that Tak might be a frame shift due to the insertion of two bases at the UAA termination codon, producing additional residues following β 146 histidine. This would produce a subunit which should have the same C-terminal sequence as Cranston. We can find no precise homology even though there are a number of residues in common between Tak and hemoglobin Cranston. I know John Kilmartin was involved in the structural work on Tak. Maybe he has a comment on this.

Dr. Kilmartin: I just want to emphasize that some parts of this sequence are solid and other parts are less solid. The solid parts are residues 147 and 148, because there is a tryptic peptide: Tyr-His-Thr-Lys whose amino acid sequence was determined. The other end is solid as well; the Phe-Tyr because these residues are removed when the protein is digested with carboxypeptidase A. Unfortunately the results were somewhat ambiguous on further digestion because residue 154 was resistant. Residues 149-154 were placed after isolation of a peptide from the fingerprint of Tak. However the sequence here must remain tentative until further overlap peptides are found.

Dr. Bunn: I might add that β Cranston may have a ragged C terminal end. When we do the CPA analysis, we get some tyrosine coming off very early. Perhaps, while the hemoglobin is circulating in the patient's red cells, there is some sort of carboxy peptidase digestion of the variant subunit so that varying amounts of tyrosine are cleared

Dr. Jacob: You suggest that the alteration of β 145 and 146 with the accompanying inability to make salt bridges may lead to hemoglobin instability. Is hemoglobin stripped of its last two amino acids as with carboxypeptidase, unstable?
Dr. Bunn: I think Dr. Kilmartin can answer that. The instability of our variant is probably related to the fact that we have a very hydrophobic group at the C-terminal end of the molecule. Does anybody have any further ideas as to why we are getting this heterogeneity? We are at a loss to explain this.

Dr. Kraus: Have you looked at the amino terminal end to see if there is any blocking in one and not in the other? This might change.

Dr. Bunn: That is an interesting suggestion. The fingerprints of the two abnormal subunits are identical. We have analysed β Tpl of Cranston-2, but not Cranston-1.

HEMOGLOBIN-ZINC INTERACTION: FUNCTIONAL AND STRUCTURAL EFFECTS

John G. Gilman, Fred J. Oelshlegel, Jr., and George J. Brewer

Department of Human Genetics
University of Michigan

INTRODUCTION

During a study of zinc deficiency in patients with sickle cell anemia, Oelshlegel and colleagues (1973, 1974) found that the oxygen affinity of red cells could be increased by the addition of zinc. They showed that the binding of .4 moles of zinc per mole of hemoglobin caused the p50 to decline from 25 mm. Hg to about 19, and the value of the Hill constant n fell from 2.9 to 2.2. They also showed that zinc does not alter the Bohr effect, and that zinc does not alter hemoglobin function by interfering with diphosphoglyceric acid (DPG) binding.

The purpose of the present study was to determine the number of binding sites for zinc in hemoglobin, and if possible to find where zinc binds and how it causes its functional effects. Our strategy was to perform comparative experiments on various animal hemoglobins. By relating effects of zinc to differences in amino acid sequence among the various hemoglobins, we hoped to draw some conclusions on the nature of the zinc binding site.

MATERIALS AND METHODS

In all experiments reported here, the hemoglobin

preparation used was essentially unpurified hemolysate; in the case of human hemoglobin, and in one experiment on chicken hemoglobin, organic phosphates were removed by a method similar to that of Benesch and colleagues (1969): The hemolysate was dialyzed against the buffer appropriate to the experiment, which contained sodium chloride at a concentration .1 M or greater, at about neutral pH.

For experiments on the binding of zinc to hemoglobin, the buffer used was .02 M in bis-tris, pH 7.2, containing .1 M sodium chloride. A given amount of zinc sulfate containing radioactive zinc-65 was added to the hemolysate, which was .2 mM in tetramers. The sample was dialyzed in the cold for 22 hours against the same bis-tris buffer. After dialysis, the radioactivity and hemoglobin concentration were measured, and the amount of zinc bound to the hemoglobin was thereby determined.

For experiments on the effects of zinc on the oxygen dissociation curve of hemoglobin, the hemolysate was in a buffer used originally in earlier work on the effects of zinc on red cells (Oelshlegel and colleagues, 1974). It contained .122 M NaCl, .025 M $NaHCO_3$ and 200mg/100 ml of glucose. Hemoglobin concentration was 4.5-6 g.%. A given sample of hemoglobin was divided into several aliquots, and different amounts of zinc sulfate were added to different aliquots in such a way that the final hemoglobin concentration was the same in each case. Oxygen dissociation curves of each sample were measured at 37° using an Instrumentation Lab 317 Blood Gas Laboratory (IL 317). In general, 3 or 4 points were obtained for each sample, and the points were fitted to the Hill equation by the method of least squares to obtain values of p50 and n.

In ultracentrifuge studies, human oxyhemoglobin from which DPG had been removed by dialysis was mixed with a stock solution of triethylamine hydrochloride (TEA/HCl), pH 6.8, to the desired concentration. Hemoglobin concentration was .4%. The sample was split and a two fold ratio of zinc to hemoglobin was added to one sample, and water to the other. The two samples were placed in different cells, one of which contained a wedge window, and both samples were centrifuged simultaneously at 44770 rpm in a Beckman Spinco Model E analytical ultracentrifuge. The temperature was 20 C. Corrections to $s_{20,w}$ were made assuming that the density of the TEA/HCl was one, as noted by Edelstein and colleagues (1970), so that only viscosity corrections were made.

The human hemoglobin samples were obtained using the blood of the first author. Cow hemoglobin for one experiment on functional effects of zinc was generously provided by Dr. H. Kitchen; the cow was a Holstein, and beta chains were of type A. For the other experiment on functional effects of zinc, and for the zinc-65 binding study, blood from another cow was provided by Kappler Packing Co., Ann Arbor, Michigan; that cow was a heterozygote for beta chains of types A and B. Chicken blood was from one white Leghorn chicken.

The following is the mathematical argument by which we show that, for a system of two hemoglobins with different oxygen affinities but identical values of n, the apparent value of n for the mixture must be less than the true value of n: The Hill equation adequately defines the behavior of hemoglobin between 15% and 85% saturation with oxygen (Antonini and Brunori, 1971). In that equation, y, the fractional saturation with oxygen, is equal to $p^n/(p50^n + p^n)$, where p is the partial pressure of oxygen in the solution, and p50 is the partial pressure of oxygen such that y = .5. The parameter n is generally considered to be a measure of cooperativity of the hemoglobin, and it is empirically determined as the slope of the line obtained by plotting $\log\{y/(1-y)\}$ versus log p. Therefore, the value of n is defined as the first derivative of $\log\{y/(1-y)\}$ with respect to log p. If one assumes a solution containing an arbitrary mixture of two pure hemoglobins, both of which have identical values of the Hill constant n but different values of p50, then the following equation should adequately define the oxygen dissociation curve of the mixture, as long as the oxygen affinities of the two hemoglobins do not differ too markedly: $y = qp^n/(A^n + p^n) + (1 - q)p^n/(B^n + p^n)$, where q is the fraction of the mixture which is hemoglobin of the type with the lower value of p50, defined as A, and (1 - q) is the fraction of the mixture which is hemoglobin of the type with the higher value of p50, defined as B. Let $u = A^n + p^n$, $v = B^n + p^n$, and $z = B^n - A^n$. Then, with considerable algebraic manipulation, one can show that the apparent value of n is equal to the real value of n multiplied by the factor $(1 - \delta/D)$, where $\delta = z^2p^n(q - q^2)$, and $D = qz(uv - 2p^nu) + u^2B^n - q^2p^nz^2$. If $p < B$, then D will certainly be positive. Since, by definition, $q \leq 1$, δ is greater than or equal to zero, and it must be the case that $(1 - \delta/D) \leq 1$, so that the apparent value of n must be less than or equal to the true value, at least in a range of p between the values of p50 of the two hemoglobins.

RESULTS AND DISCUSSION

We first determined that there are two zinc binding sites per tetramer of oxyhemoglobin. Figure 1 shows the results of experiments on cow and human hemoglobin, in which the amount of zinc bound to the hemoglobin after dialysis against zinc-free buffer is plotted against the amount originally added to the hemolysate. The dotted line in this figure shows the result expected under the hypothesis that there are exactly two sites to which zinc binds stoichiometrically. Assuming that hypothesis, all zinc added, up to two zinc per tetramer, should stick to the hemoglobin and not be removable by dialysis. The actual data show that this is a close approximation. Almost all of the zinc added, up to two zinc per hemoglobin, binds to the hemoglobin; adding more than two zinc per hemoglobin leads to the binding of only a little more than two zinc.

Since this is true for both human hemoglobin, which binds DPG, and cow hemoglobin, which does not, it confirms the report by Oelshlegel and colleagues (1973) that zinc does not exert its functional effects on hemoglobin by competing with DPG binding. These results also show that zinc does not bind at either of the buried cysteines of human hemoglobin, since cow hemoglobin lacks those cysteines. Oelshlegel and colleagues (1974) had already shown that

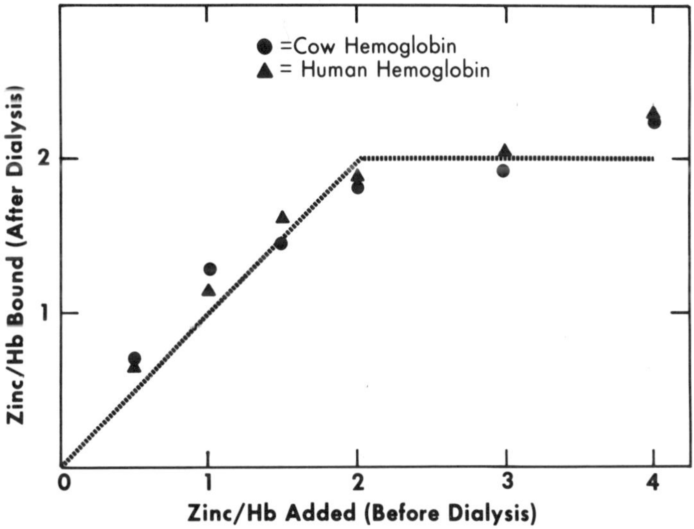

Figure 1. The amount of zinc bound per hemoglobin tetramer after dialysis as a function of the relative amount added prior to dialysis against zinc-free buffer.

blocking the free cysteines of hemoglobin does not prevent zinc binding. These results are rather surprising, because cysteine is one of the amino acids with greatest affinity for zinc.

Our next step was to determine whether these two sites in hemoglobin, to which zinc binds almost stoichiometrically, are the sites at which zinc exerts its functional effects. The binding studies made this seem likely, and the functional studies illustrated in figure 2 confirmed it. These data show that adding up to two zinc per hemoglobin caused a decrease in p50, which means that there was an increase in oxygen affinity. Adding more than two zinc per hemoglobin led to almost no change in p50. This was true for the hemoglobins of human, chicken and cow. The undialyzed hemolysate of human hemoglobin, presumably containing most of the original DPG, had a p50 of 21 without zinc and 7 with

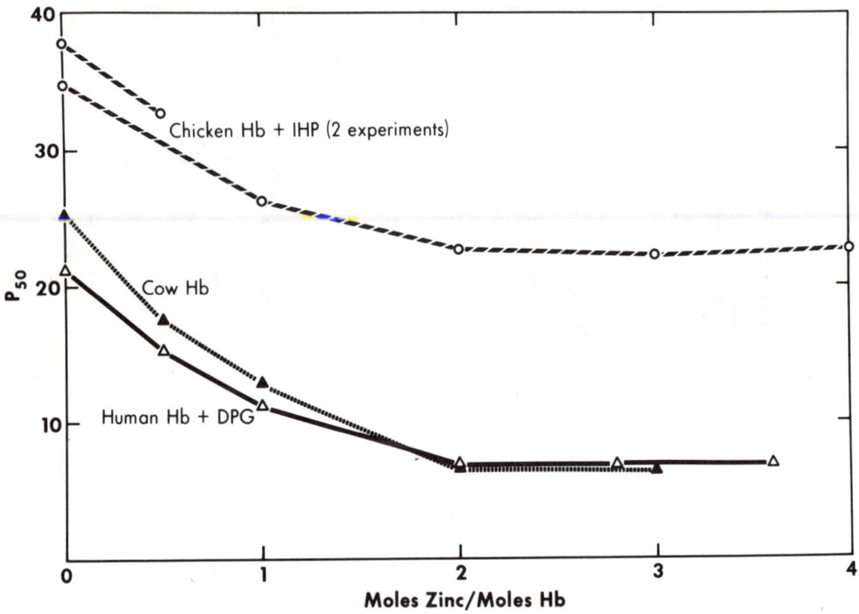

Figure 2. The effect of zinc on the oxygen affinities of several hemoglobins.

two zinc per tetramer. Undialyzed chicken hemolysate, with most of the original inositol pentaphosphate presumably present, had a p50 of 35 without zinc and 22 with two zinc added per hemoglobin tetramer. Dialyzed chicken hemolysate, to which inositol hexaphosphate (IHP) had been added in a 1:1 ratio to hemoglobin, had a p50 of 39 without zinc and 34 with .5 zinc per hemoglobin. Cow hemolysate, with neither DPG nor IHP, had a p50 of 25 without zinc and 7 with two zinc per hemoglobin.

We concluded from these studies that human, cow and chicken hemoglobins all have two zinc binding sites which lead to increased oxygen affinity when zinc is bound. Because there is considerable variability in amino acid sequence among these three hemoglobins, these results help to narrow the possible range of positions at which zinc could be binding, although the results do not specify any particular residues as being the likeliest candidates for the binding site.

It was originally reported by Oelshlegel and colleagues (1974) that zinc causes a decrease in the value of the Hill constant n of human hemoglobin--from 2.9 to 2.2 when about .4 moles of zinc were bound per hemoglobin molecule. Since n is generally considered to be a measure of cooperativity, or heme-heme interaction, this implied that zinc markedly decreases cooperativity. The data of figure 3 show that we saw a similar effect when less than two zinc were added per molecule of hemoglobin. With .5 zinc per tetramer, the value of n declined from 2.87 to 2.2. One zinc per tetramer caused n to fall further, to 2.1. However, two zinc per tetramer caused n to return almost to normal, to

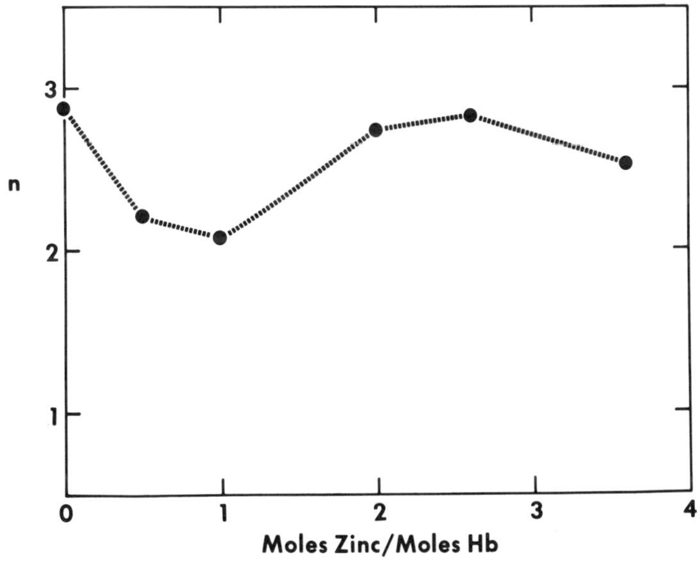

Figure 3. The effect of zinc on the Hill constant n of human hemoglobin in the presence of DPG.

2.74. With 2.8 zinc per hemoglobin, n was essentially the same as that of hemoglobin without zinc, at 2.82.

The simplest explanation for this initial fall in n and subsequent rise almost to normal is that zinc does not affect cooperativity at all. The apparent change in n could simply have been due to the fact that the measurements were performed on mixtures of hemoglobins of different oxygen affinities. For example, if one assumes that zinc binds randomly to its two binding sites in hemoglobin, mixing equimolar amounts of zinc and hemoglobin should lead to 25% of the hemoglobin having two zinc bound and high oxygen affinity, 25% having no zinc bound and low oxygen affinity, and 50% having one zinc bound and intermediate oxygen affinity. Using the Hill equation, we have shown mathematically, for a two component system, that the apparent value of n must decline (see MATERIALS AND METHODS for details). Thus, oxygen dissociation curves of a mixture of two hemoglobins with different oxygen affinities but the same degree of cooperativity will show an apparent reduction in the Hill coefficient n.

So we have concluded that zinc exerts little or no effect on cooperativity of human hemoglobin in the presence of DPG.

Figure 4, however, demonstrates that zinc can cause a decrease in the value of n, but that zinc can also cause n to increase, depending on the hemoglobin and the experimental conditions. In the case of cow hemoglobin, the value of n without zinc is about 3 and the value of n with two zinc bound is 2.6. Two independent experiments gave almost identical results. For human hemoglobin, as just discussed, the change in n with the binding of two zinc is much smaller--from 2.87 to 2.74. In the case of chicken hemoglobin in the presence of inositol pentaphosphate or inositol hexaphosphate, however, the effect of zinc was to increase the value of n. In one experiment, .5 zinc per hemoglobin increased n to 2.65 from the value 2.47 seen in the absence of zinc. In another experiment, one zinc per hemoglobin changed n to 2.51 from the value 2.30 seen without zinc, and with two zinc the value

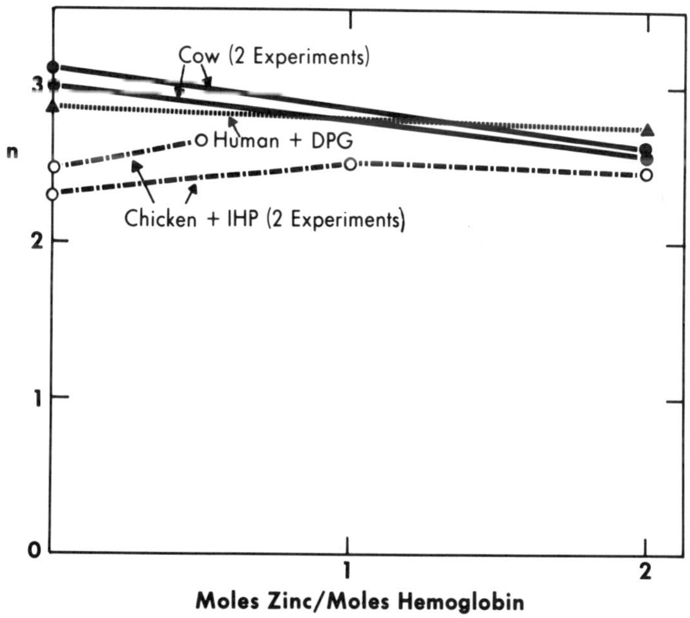

Figure 4. The effect of zinc on the Hill constant n of several hemoglobins. For cow hemoglobin and human hemoglobin + DPG, only points for 0 Zn/Hb and 2 Zn/Hb are shown.

of n was virtually the same as with one zinc--2.48.

One way of making sense of these conflicting results, that zinc decreases cooperativity in the case of cow hemoglobin but increases cooperativity of chicken hemoglobin in the presence of IHP, is to plot the value of n versus the p50 of a given hemoglobin preparation, as shown in figure 5. (The data used in figure 5 are from the same experiments as the data of figures 2 and 4.) Bunn and Guidotti (1972) have reported that "a detailed reexamination of the relationship between the value of the Hill constant, n, and . . . p50, indicates that there is a slight dependence of n on p50 for normal human hemoglobin. The value of n varies between 2.3 and 3.1 over a 50-fold variation in the value of p50." Our

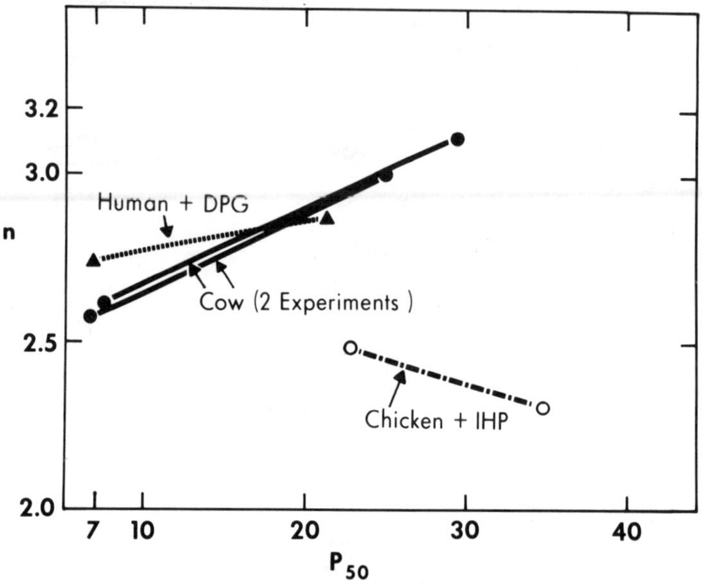

Figure 5. The value of n plotted against p50 for hemoglobins with 0 Zn/Hb and 2 Zn/Hb; the two points of a given experiment are connected by a line.

results are not directly comparable with theirs, since our experiments were performed under different experimental conditions and on animal as well as human hemoglobins. However, our results are qualitatively similar to those of Bunn and Guidotti, in that deviations of p50 from normal--which we were considering to be the p50 of normal human blood about 25 mm Hg--result in some decrease in the value of n.

The data of Figure 5 suggest, therefore, that the simplest hypothesis to explain the effect of zinc on cooperativity is that it occurs as a consequence of zinc shifting the R ↔ T equilibrium towards R, and that otherwise zinc does not cause any gross abnormality in hemoglobin structure. The data also make it improbable that zinc binds in the vicinity of the $\alpha_1\beta_2$ contact of hemoglobin, since perturbations at that contact generally lead to drastic alterations in cooperativity (Perutz and colleagues, 1968; Morimoto and colleagues, 1971).

We have some data that suggest that zinc may be perturbing hemoglobin structure in the vicinity of the other contact region between the alpha and beta chains, the $\alpha_1\beta_1$ contact. This could be occurring either through direct binding of zinc at $\alpha_1\beta_1$ or because of more indirect effects of zinc. We developed this hypothesis early in our investigations. One of the reasons for this hypothesis was the analogy between the effects of zinc on hemoglobin function and the effects of high concentrations of certain salts, namely potassium iodide (KI) and triethylamine hydrochloride (TEA/HCl). Both of these salts cause hemoglobin oxygen affinity to increase, the value of n does not change in the case of TEA/HCl, and both salts promote dissociation of hemoglobin tetramers to dimers and monomers. Tomita and colleagues (1973) showed, for KI, that an increase in the oxygen affinity of hemoglobin was apparently correlated with the ability of KI to cause some monomer formation. Current theory has it that the split from tetramer to dimer takes place at the $\alpha_1\beta_2$ contact, while the split from dimer to monomer occurs at $\alpha_1\beta_1$ (Rosemeyer and Huehns, 1967), so that the ability of KI to increase oxygen affinity of hemoglobin is associated with its ability to cleave the $\alpha_1\beta_1$ contact. Tomita and colleagues also showed that KI causes the value of n to decline, but there is no way of knowing whether this effect is real or due to molecular heterogeneity. In the case of TEA/HCl, which is more effective than KI in promoting the dissociation of hemoglobin to monomers as well as dimers, Amiconi and colleagues (1971) showed that oxygen affinity increases but that there is little change in the value of n.

By analogy with the effects of dissociating salts, we hypothesized that zinc alters the conformation of hemoglobin at the $\alpha_1\beta_1$ contact. To test this, we decided to compare the effects of salts on the dissociation of hemoglobin treated with zinc as compared with untreated hemoglobin. We felt that, if zinc were altering the conformation at the $\alpha_1\beta_1$

contact, then zinc treated hemoglobin would dissociate to a different extent than hemoglobin without zinc. What in fact we did find was that zinc causes an increased dissociation of oxyhemoglobin tetramers to dimers and monomers in the presence of potassium iodide or triethylamine hydrochloride.

Figure 6 shows the results of a study using the analytical ultracentrifuge. The experiments on the zinc treated and untreated samples were performed simultaneously in the same ultracentrifuge run. The data of figure 6 show that, at every concentration of TEA/HCl used, $s_{20,w}$ for hemoglobin treated with two zinc is lower than the value for hemoglobin without zinc. Since a smaller value of $s_{20,w}$ indicates a lower average molecular weight, figure 6 demonstrates that zinc enhances the dissociation of hemoglobin caused by TEA/HCl. At one of the concentrations shown, 2 M TEA/HCl, the value of $s_{20,w}$ for hemoglobin without zinc

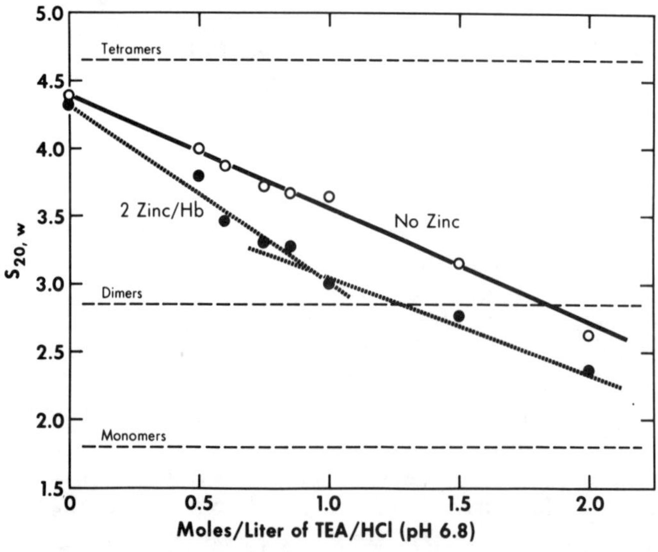

Figure 6. Ultracentrifuge study of hemoglobin treated with 2 Zn/Hb compared to hemoglobin without zinc, in the presence of triethylamine hydrochloride.

is less than that expected for dimers, showing that there must be very little tetramer left in the solution. Nevertheless, in this situation zinc still decreases $s_{20,w}$ significantly, showing that zinc must increase the dissociation of hemoglobin from dimers to monomers at this salt concentration.

We have additional independent evidence that zinc increases monomer formation in the presence of salts that cause dissociation to monomers. Using KI, one can obtain hybridization of canine and human hemoglobins, as Tomita and colleagues (1973) have shown. We have found that zinc causes a small amount of increased hybridization of canine and human hemoglobins at KI concentrations of .35 M and .45 M. Theory suggests that this means that zinc enhances monomer formation, which implies that zinc promotes splitting of the $\alpha_1\beta_1$ contact of hemoglobin.

The simplest hypothesis that explains the effects of zinc on the dissociation of hemoglobin in various salts is that zinc promotes the dissociation of hemoglobin dimers to monomers. In other words, the reaction $\alpha\beta \leftrightarrow \alpha + \beta$ is shifted to the right because of the effects of zinc. By the law of mass action, this would then imply that the tetramer to dimer equilibrium, $\alpha_2\beta_2 \leftrightarrow 2\alpha\beta$, is also shifted to the right. However, it may also be possible that zinc acts more directly to increase dissociation of tetramers to dimers.

Since we have found that zinc can enhance the tendency of hemoglobin to split at the $\alpha_1\beta_1$ contact, leading to increased monomer formation, we have been assuming that the mechanism by which zinc increases the oxygen affinity of hemoglobin may be related to its causing a structural change at the $\alpha_1\beta_1$ contact. However, we do not necessarily assume that zinc binds at the $\alpha_1\beta_1$ contact, nor do we assume that the increased dissociation to monomers that zinc can cause is itself the mechanism by which it exerts its functional effects.

We are also interested in the $\alpha_1\beta_1$ contact in terms of its possible involvement in the functional evolution of hemoglobin among the various animal species. If hemoglobin has evolved functionally, in terms of oxygen affinity, it seems likely that such changes would not have been accompanied by major alterations in cooperativity, which would be potentially deleterious. Changes at the $\alpha_1\beta_1$ contact offer the possibility of causing change in oxygen affinity while leaving cooperativity unaffected, as considerable evidence in the literature demonstrates. Besides the data just discussed concerning the effects of certain salts on hemoglobin functioning, we are aware of three human hemoglobin mutants which have altered oxygen affinity associated with perturbations involving the $\alpha_1\beta_1$ contact. These are hemoglobins Peterborough (Morimoto and colleagues, 1971) and Yoshizuka (Imamura and colleagues, 1969), with reduced oxygen affinities and normal values of n, and San Diego (Nute and colleagues, 1974), with high oxygen affinity and a reportedly low value of n. This low value of n reported for hemoglobin San Diego does not show, however, that perturbations at $\alpha_1\beta_1$ can affect cooperativity. Hemoglobin San Diego was not analyzed in pure form but as a mixture with normal human hemoglobin, which has lower oxygen affinity. The apparently decreased cooperativity may therefore be spurious and due to heterogeneity of the system.

Consequently, one must conclude that the experimental evidence shows that change involving $\alpha_1\beta_1$ can lead to altered oxygen affinity while having very little effect on cooperativity. Thus, the $\alpha_1\beta_1$ contact is one region of the hemoglobin molecule at which evolution leading to changes in oxygen affinity may have occurred. In fact, there is some evidence that this sort of evolution has actually occurred in primates. Bonaventura and colleagues (1974) found that "hemoglobin of the prosimian primate _Lemur fulvus fulvus_ is quite similar to human hemoglobin in its primary structure but is significantly different in its functional behavior. Equilibrium and kinetic studies show that the sequence differences in Lemur hemoglobin do not affect cooperativity, but do produce a decreased oxygen affinity, a decreased Bohr effect, and a decreased response to organic phosphates. The decreased effect of organic phosphates on Lemur hemoglobin may be partially accounted for by the presence of leucine at the $\beta2$ position. . . . The other functional differences cannot be readily accounted for in terms of the current stereochemical model." Their data show, however, that of 46 differences between Lemur and human hemoglobin, 7 of these differences occur at the $\alpha_1\beta_1$ contact. It seems reasonable to propose that the decreased oxygen affinity of Lemur hemoglobin could be due to changes in structure at the $\alpha_1\beta_1$ contact.

SUMMARY

We have shown that there are two binding sites for zinc in several animal hemoglobins, and that zinc binding at those sites leads to increased oxygen affinity. Zinc binding does not lead to altered cooperativity, except as might be expected due to the reported relationship between n and p50 (Bunn and Guidotti, 1972). Zinc probably alters the R $\leftrightarrow$ T equilibrium towards R, perhaps by causing structural changes at the $\alpha_1\beta_1$ contact.

ACKNOWLEDGEMENTS

The work in this paper was supported in part by NIH contract N01-HB-2-2918-B and by NIH postdoctoral fellowship F02 HL55564-01. We thank C. Knutsen for valuable technical assistance and Dr. F. Gurd (Indiana University, Bloomington, Indiana) for discussions.

REFERENCES

Amiconi, G., Antonini, E., Brunori, M., Chiancone, E., and Vecchini, P. (1971). Studies on the Relations between Molecular and Functional Properties of Hemoglobin. VIII. Equilibria and Kinetics of the Reactions of Hemoglobin with Ligands in Concentrated Solutions of Triethylamine Hydrochloride. J. Biol. Chem. 246:1883.

Antonini, E., and Brunori, M. (1971). Hemoglobin and Myoglobi in their Reactions with Ligands. American Elsevier Publishing Col, Inc., New York.

Benesch, R.E., Benesch, R., and Yu, C.I. (1969). The oxygenation of hemoglobin in the presence of 2,3-diphosphoglyerate. Effects of temperature, pH, ionic strength and hemoglobin concentration. Biochemistry 8:2567.

Bonaventura, C., Sullivan, B., and Bonaventura, J. (1974). Effects of pH and anions on functional properties of hemoglobin from Lemur fulvus fulvus. J. Biol. Chem. 249:3768.

Bunn, H.F., and Guidotti, G. (1972). Stabilizing interactions in hemoglobin. J. Biol. Chem. 247:2345.

Edelstein, S.J., Rehmar, M.J., Olson, J.S., and Gibson, Q.H. (1970). Functional aspects of the subunit association-dissociation equilibria of hemoglobin. J. Biol. Chem. 245:4372.

Imamura, T., Fujita, S., Ohta, Y., Hanada, M. (1969). Hemoglobin Yoshizuka (G10(108)β asparagine→aspartic acid): a new variant with a reduced oxygen affinity from a Japanese family. J. Clin. Invest. 48:2341.

Morimoto, H., Lehmann, H., and Pertuz, M.F. (1971). Molecular pathology of human haemoglobin: stereochemical interpretation of abnormal oxygen affinities. Nature 232:408.

Nute, P.E., Stamatoyannopoulos, G., Hermodson, M.A., and Roth, D. (1974). Hemoglobinopathic erythrocytosis due to new electrophoretically silent variant, hemoglobin San Diego (β109(G11)Val→Met). J. Clin. Invest. 53:320.

Oelshlegel, F.J., Jr., Brewer, G.J., Knutsen, C., Prasad, A.S., and Schoomaker, E.B. (1973). Effect of zinc on increasing oxygen affinity of sickle and normal red blood cells. Biochem. Biophys. Res. Commun. 53:560.

Oelshlegel, F.J., Jr., Brewer, G.J., Knutsen, C., Prasad, A.S., and Schoomaker, E.B. (1974). Studies on the interaction of zinc with human hemoglobin. Arch. Biochem. Biophys. 163:748.

Perutz, M.F., Muirhead, H., Cox, J.M., and Goaman, L.C.G. (1968). Three-dimensional Fourier synthesis of horse oxyhaemoglobin at 2.8 Å resolution: the atomic model. Nature 219:131.

Rosemeyer, M.A., and Huehns, E.R. (1967). On the mechanism of the dissociation of haemoglobin. J. Mol. Biol. 25:253.

Tomita, S., Enoki, Y., Ochiai, T., Kawase, M., and Okuda, T. (1973). Cleavage at the $\alpha_1\beta_1$ contact and its effect on the oxygen equilibrium of human haemoglobin. J. Mol. Biol. 73:261.

DISCUSSION

Dr. Ho: May I discuss the effects of zinc on hemoglobin as studied by NMR? The first slide shows the effects of zinc on the hyperfine shifted proton resonances of deoxy Hb A, on the ring-current shifted proton resonances of HbCO A, and on the exchangeable proton resonances of both oxy and deoxy Hb A. From these results, it is clear that the addition of 2-3 molar excess of zinc to deoxy Hb A at pH 7 alters only the β heme resonance and not the α heme resonances. The hyperfine shifted proton resonances of deoxy Hb A plus zinc resemble those of deoxy Hb Mälmo (FG4β97 His→Glu). We have found that zinc alters the ring-current shifted proton resonances of HbCO A which suggests that the E11 valine conformations have been altered, and in turn implies that the tertiary structure of the heme pocket in the CO form of Hb A has been affected by the addition of zinc. We have found that zinc produces no effect on the exchangeable proton resonances suggesting that it does not bind near those subunit hydrogen bonds which are characteristic of both oxy and deoxy quaternary structures as discussed in my talk. The next slide shows the effects of zinc on the aromatic proton resonances of Hb A and Hb S in the CO form. The results clearly show that zinc alters some of the histidine residues in both HbCO A and HbCO S.

You have suggested that zinc binds to the $\alpha_1\beta_1$ region of the hemoglobin molecule. Your conclusion depends on the nature of the Hb dimer, namely is it an $\alpha_1\beta_1$ or $\alpha_1\beta_2$ dimer? There is some controversy in the literature on the nature of the Hb dimer.

I would like to ask you a question. Do the two zinc binding sites on the hemoglobin molecule have the same affinity for zinc?

Dr. Gilman: I don't know.

Dr. Ho: By making a Scatchard plot of your data, you may find out whether or not the two zinc binding sites are equivalent.

Dr. Perutz: I wonder what the binding constant for zinc is?

Dr. Gilman: We know the affinity is obviously high, but we haven't measured it.

Dr. Bunn: I have three questions. Did you have an opportunity to do hybridization experiments to see if the zinc does facilitate monomer formation? In mixtures of two hemoglobins such as human and canine hybrid formation might be facilitated by the addition of zinc. Have you tried that?

Dr. Gilman: I did it in the presence of potassium iodide. In high concentrations, such as 1.0 M you get precipitation when zinc is present, but using lower concentrations like 0.35 M I could see that the presence of zinc did cause more hybrid formation.

Dr. Bunn: Are you able to prepare globin from your zinc treated hemolysate? Does the zinc remain on the globin?

Dr. Gilman: I never tried that.

Dr. Bunn: Finally, in view of the possibility that zinc binds at the $\alpha_1\beta_1$ interface, have you tested human fetal hemoglobin (hemoglobin F)?

Dr. Gilman: No. What would you suggest?

Dr. Bunn: Dr. Perutz has shown recently that the absence of a sulfhydryl group at the alpha$_1$ gamma$_1$ interface is probably the explanation for the stability of hemoglobin F to alkali. Therefore human F and A hemoglobins may interact differently with zinc.

Dr. Perutz: But Frank, Gilman showed that Zn binds to cow hemoglobin which lacks both SH groups α104 and β112.

Dr. Gilman: I can mention one interesting observation, which is that zinc decreases the rate of alkali denaturation of human and mouse hemoglobin. However, the problem with this type of experiment and the problem with the experiment using high concentrations of TEA is that I think under these conditions, more zinc may be binding than the original two. So it's not really clear in those experiments which binding sites are causing the effects whether they're the same as are involved in the functional change in hemoglobin.

Dr. Perutz: If there are no more questions, I'd like to answer one of Sam Charache's questions who asked me what do I mean by Nε.

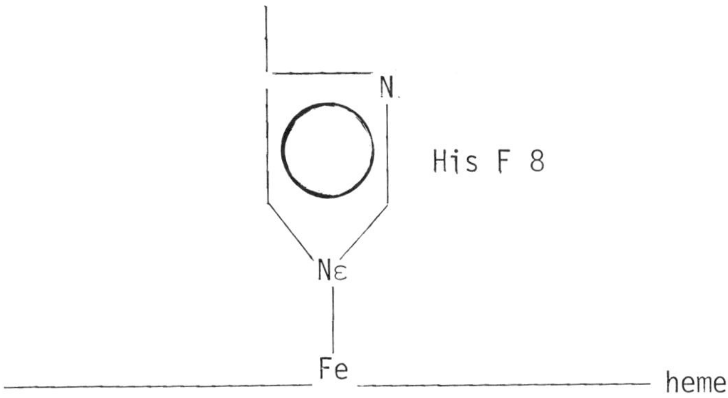

EQUILIBRIA OF HEMOGLOBINS M WITH ETHYLISOCYANIDE

Kazuko Nishikura[1], Masako Nagai[1], Yoshiki Sugita[1], Yoshimasa Yoneyama[1], Anthony V. Pisciotta[2], and Paul Heller[3]

[1]Department of Biochemistry, Kanazawa University School of Medicine, Kanazawa, Japan
[2]The Medical College of Wisconsin, Milwaukee
[3]Veterans Administration West Side Hospital and University of Illinois, Chicago

INTRODUCTION

Abnormal human hemoglobins are very useful to elucidate the role of specific amino acid residues in the ligand binding properties of hemoglobin. We have studied four kinds of Hbs M, in which the hemes of abnormal chains are usually in ferric state, to investigate the effects of amino acid substitutions located in regions close to a heme iron on cooperative ligand binding.

Oxygen equilibria of normal chains in these Hbs M have been studied and ligand binding properties very different from those of Hb A have been reported for every variant (Hayashi et al., 1966, Suzuki et al., 1966, Ranney et al., 1968, Hayashi et al., 1969, and Gersonde et al., 1973). However, there are many disagreements between the results reported previously. The reasons for the discrepancies may be the contamination of Hb A in the samples and the unstable oxidation state of normal chains in the preparations of hemoglobin M. We could obtain the purified Hb M Iwate, Hyde Park, Saskatoon and Milwaukee-I which are free from contamination of Hb A, and found the conditions for stable valency hybrid hemoglobins, in which normal chains are in ferrous state and abnormal chains in ferric state. In this paper we report the studies on equilibria of the four hemoglobins M with ethylisocyanide (EIC), which is a non-oxidizing ligand and equilibrates rapidly with hemoglobins, both in half ferric and totally reduced states.

MATERIALS AND METHODS

Hemoglobin M Iwate, M Saskatoon and M Milwaukee-I were isolated from Hb A with an Amberlite CG-50 column. Hemolysates were dialyzed against 0.05 M phosphate buffer, pH 7.0, and applied on the column previously equilibrated with the same buffer. After Hb A was washed out with the same buffer, Hb M remained on the column was eluted by a linear gradient from 0.05 M to 0.2 M phosphate buffer, pH 7.0. The hemolysate containing Hb M Hyde Park was applied on a hydroxylapatite column equilibrated with 0.05 M phosphate buffer, pH 7.0, and most of Hb A was eluted with the same buffer. Hb M Hyde Park was eluted with 0.2 M phosphate buffer, pH 7.0, concentrated by vacuum filtration, oxidized to methemoglobin by potassium ferricyanide, dialyzed against 0.015 M sodium phosphate buffer, pH 7.0, and purified by preparative electrophoresis on 15% starch gel. Purity of the hemoglobins M was examined with methemoglobin, prepared by oxidation of the sample with potassium ferricyanide, by starch gel electrophoresis.

Half ferric Hbs M, in which normal chains contain ferrous hemes and abnormal chains ferric hemes, were prepared as follows. A solution of Hb M Iwate was deoxygenated in a cell by bubbling with Q gas, and an ascorbate solution was added to give a final concentration of 5 mM. Hb M Hyde Park was treated similarly but the amount of ascorbate was a little more than the equivalent to normal chains. Ascorbate reduced the heme irons in normal chains but not those in abnormal chains of these Hbs M substituted at proximal histidine. As abnormal chains in Hb M Saskatoon and Hb M Milwaukee-I were reduced by ascorbate, these two hemoglobins were reduced totally with sodium dithionite, and then remaining dithionite was removed by Sephadex G-25. Abnormal chains were rapidly oxidized by dissolved oxygen, while oxidation of normal chains was slow. To examine the complete oxidation of abnormal chains, absorption spectra were recorded successively. Usually about 30 min after passage through a Sephadex column at room temperature, an absorption spectrum for half ferric hemoglobin was given. The concentration of ferrous heme was determined as CO binding capacity by micromanometric method of van Slyke and Plazin (1961).

Hb M in which all the hemes are in ferrous state was prepared as follows. About 3 ml of Hb M solution in a quartz cell was deoxygenated by bubbling with Q gas and added with 3 mg of sodium dithionite, except for Hb M Iwate, to reduce ferric hemes. For the reduction of Hb M Iwate 9 mg of sodium dithionite and standing overnight at room temperature were required.

Equilibria with EIC were determined spectrophotometrically essentially the same as the method described by Anderson et al. (1970).

RESULTS

The absorption spectra for half ferric hemoglobin M, except for Hb M Milwaukee-I, showed no peak at 630 nm which is due to acid met derivative of normal chains, but shoulders characteristic of abnormal chains at shorter wave lengths were observed. Hb M Milwaukee-I gives the absorption peak at 620 nm in which contributions from normal and abnormal chains are hardly distinguished. ESR spectra for purified Hb M Hyde Park and Hb M Iwate in half ferric state are shown in Fig. 1. The spectrum represents only the ferric heme iron in abnormal chains. The spectrum for Hb M Hyde Park was different from that of CO liganded, when normal α chains were deoxygenated. The results agreed well with those for Hb M Hyde Park in fresh red cells reported by Hayashi et al. (1967) and indicate that our preparation retains native properties. The ESR spectrum for half ferric Hb M Iwate shows about the same signal as that reported previously (Bemski, 1968), and did not change with

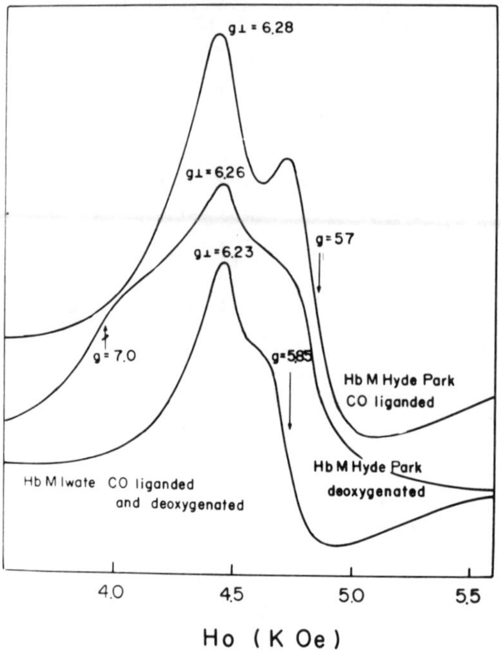

Fig. 1. ESR spectra of Hb M Hyde Park and Hb M Iwate at liquid nitrogen temperature.

the different ligand states of the normal chains.

The EIC dissociation curves of Hbs M, in which normal chains contain ferrous heme and abnormal chains ferric heme, were determined in the pH range from 6.5 to 8.0. The CO binding capacity of Hb M Iwate was 51.1% of the total heme concentration. Other three hemoglobins were used when their absorption spectra were the same as those of half ferric state which had been determined manometrically. Slow oxidation of normal chains less than 5% per 30 min did not affect the EIC equilibrium determination which took about 30 min. The value for n in Hill's equation, which is indicative of heme-heme interaction, was 1.0 for Hb M Iwate and Hb M Hyde Park at all the pHs

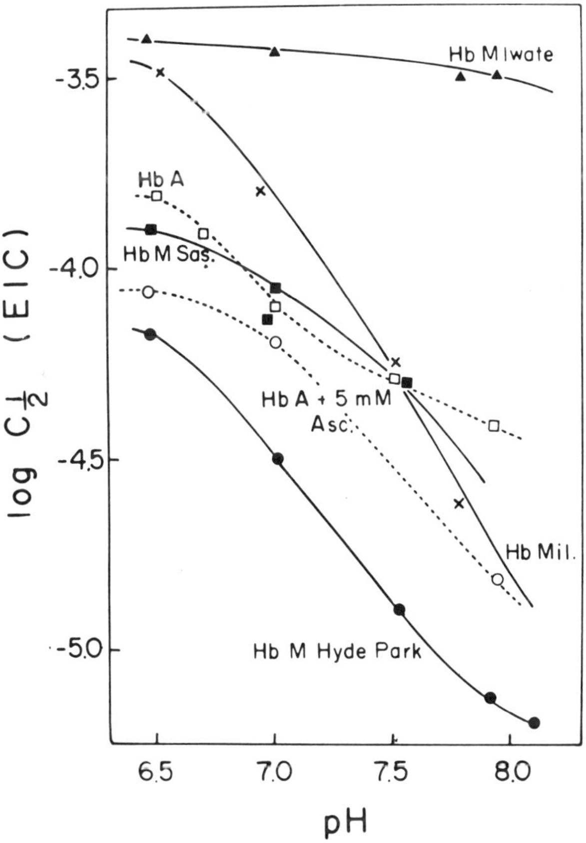

Fig. 2. Effect of pH on affinity of Hbs M for EIC in half ferric state. EIC concentrations required for half-saturation are plotted against pH.

tested. In contrast to the low value of n for the Hbs M which have substitution at proximal histidine, Hb M Milwaukee-I and Hb M Saskatoon showed the value of 1.3 for n, indicating the presence of heme-heme interaction. The effects of pH on EIC affinity are shown in Fig. 2. EIC affinity of Hb M Iwate was very low and that of Hb M Hyde Park was increased. Hb M Sas-

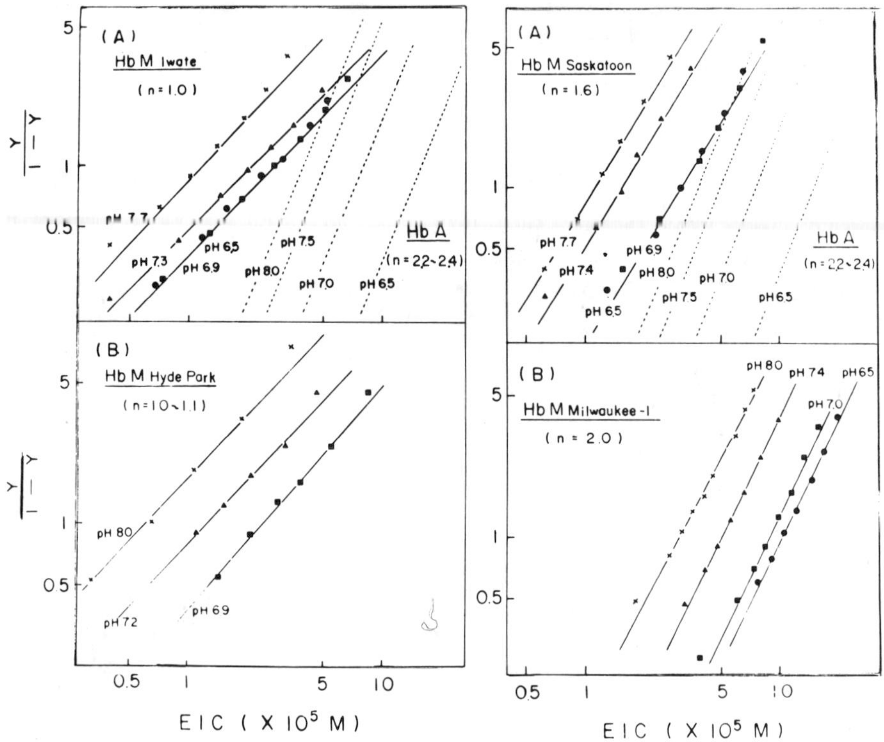

Fig. 3. EIC dissociation curves of Hbs M at different pHs in totally reduced state.

katoon showed approximately the same affinity and Bohr effect as Hb A. Hb M Milwaukee-I showed low affinity at low pH and large Bohr effect similar to the properties in oxygen binding (Hayashi et al., 1969).

EIC equilibrium curves for Hbs M in totally reduced state are shown in Fig. 3. The effect of pH on the affinity are shown in Fig. 4. The n value in EIC binding for Hb M Iwate and Hb M Hyde Park was 1.0 to 1.1, suggesting that cooperativity is lost as in the half ferric state. Hb M Saskatoon and Hb M Milwaukee-I, which have a substitution at the site of

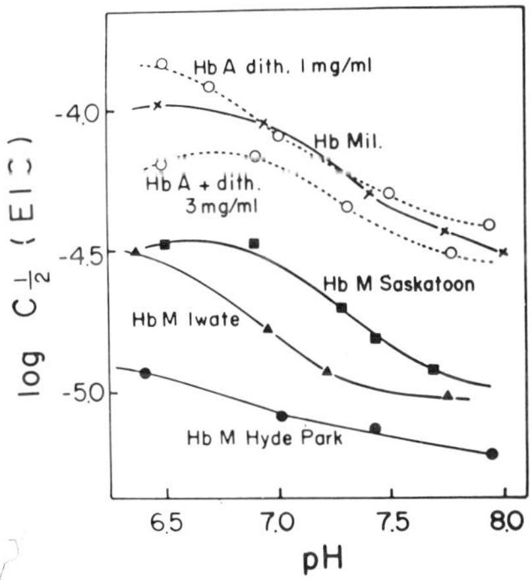

Fig. 4. Effect of pH on affinity of Hbs M for EIC in totally reduced state. EIC concentration required for half saturation are plotted against pH.

distal histidine, showed considerably high n values, namely 1.6 and 2.0, respectively, which are greater than those in the half ferric state. Bohr effect of Hb M Hyde Park was smaller than that of Hb A, and other three Hbs M showed normal magnitude of Bohr effect. Hb M Milwaukee-I showed a increased Bohr effect in half ferric state, but in totally reduced state both the Bohr effect and affinity were approximately the same as Hb. A. Hb M Iwate showed much higher affinity for EIC than Hb A in the totally reduced state, while affinity was lower in the half ferric state.

DISCUSSION

We have studied the properties of ligand binding on carefully prepared half ferric and totally reduced Hbs M using EIC, which needs not equilibration with gas phase and is a nonoxidizing ligand. Our results indicated that the cooperativity in ligand binding was lost in the Hbs M, in which proximal histidine is replaced by tyrosine, while the Hbs M which have substitution at or near distal histidine show heme-heme interaction. The results are summarized in Table I.

Table I. Equilibrium of Hemoglobins M with Ethylisocyanide

Hemoglobin	Substitution	Half ferric			Totally reduced		
		n	Ligand affinity	Bohr effect	n	Ligand affinity	Bohr effect
Hb M Iwate	α Proximal his—>tyr	1.0-1.1	very low (1/5)	lost	1.0-1.1	high (3 fold)	normal
Hb M Hyde Park	β Proximal his—>tyr	1.0-1.1	high (2 fold)	normal	1.0-1.1	high (4 fold)	decreased
Hb M Saskatoon	β Distal his—>tyr	1.3	normal	normal	1.6	high (3 fold)	normal
Hb M Milwaukee-I	β (E11) val—>glu	1.3	low (1/2)	increased (1.5 fold)	2.0	normal	normal
Hb A					2.4		

Hb M Milwaukee-I and Hb M Saskatoon showed a definite but small heme-heme interaction in half ferric state and the value of 1.3 for n is approximately the same as that for valency hybrid hemoglobin (Banerjee and Cassoly 1969), and the cooperativity is enhanced when all the hemes are reduced and are capable of binding ligands. The Hill's n of 2.0 for Hb M Milwaukee-I is comparable to that of 2.4 for Hb A. Normal Bohr effect of Hb M Milwaukee-I, which shows a large Bohr effect in half ferric state, may be the result of a break of abnormal bonding between ferric heme and the side chain of glutamic acid (Perutz et al., 1972). From the properties of EIC binding, the structure of abnormal β chains in Hb M milwaukee-I in totally reduced state seems to be similar to that of Hb A. According to a model proposed by Perutz (1970), the loss of cooperativity in Hb M Iwate and Hb M Hyde Park are associated with their quaternary structure (Greer 1971). The former is considered to be frozen in the T state and the latter is shifted to the R state even after deoxygenation. When the hemes in abnormal chains of Hb M Iwate are reduced, quaternary structure seems to change to the R state. The reduction of heme iron might weaken the bond between the mutated tyrosine and iron, and the constraints in tertiary structure of abnormal chains might have been abolished. The only data which does not agree with our results are those reported by Gersonde et al. (1973). They reported a large Hill's n value of 1.8 in CO binding of half ferric Hb M Iwate. We could not repeat their diffusion method, but determined CO equilibria spectrophotometrically by the method of Hayashi et al. (1966). The maximum value we obtained for the Hill's n was 1.2 for Hb M Iwate both in the half ferric and totally reduced states.

It is interesting that the ESR spectra of β chains in Hb M Hyde Park changes with the alteration in ligand state of α chains, but no heme-heme interaction was observed in totally reduced state. The change in spin state derived from quaternary state of globin seems not to be associated with the ligand binding property. From our results it is suggested that proximal histidine is essential for high cooperativity in ligand binding.

REFERENCES

Anderson, N.M., Antonini, E., Brunori, M., and Wyman, J. (1970). Equilibrium of human hemoglobin with ethylisocyanide: further evidence for cooperativity in hemoglobin dimers. J. Mol. Biol. 47: 205.

Banerjee, R. and Cassoly, R. (1969). Oxygen equilibria of human hemoglobin valency hybrids. J. Mol. Biol. 42: 351.

Bemski, G. and Nagel, R.L. (1968). Electron spin resonance of four human hemoglobins. Biochim. Biophys. Acta 154: 592.

Gersonde, K., Overkamp, M., Sick, H., Trittelvitz, E., and Junge, W. (1973). β-Chain allostery in the frozen quaternary T-structure of Hemoglobin M Iwate. Eur. J. Biochem. 39: 403.

Greer, J. (1971). Three-dimentional structure of abnormal human Hemoglobin M Hyde Park and M Iwate. J. Mol. Biol. 59: 107.

Hayashi, A., Suzuki, T., Shimizu, A., Morimoto, H., and Watari, H. (1967). Changes in EPR spectra of M-type abnormal hemoglobins induced by deoxygenation and their implication for the heme-heme interaction. Biochim. Biophys. Acta 147: 407.

Hayashi, A., Suzuki, T., Imai, K., Morimoto, H., and Watari, H. (1969).Properties of Hemoglobin M Milwaukee-I variant and its unique characteristic. Biochim. Biophys. Acta 194: 6.

Hayashi, N., Motokawa, Y., and Kikuchi, G. (1966). Studies on relationships between structure and function of Hemoglobin M Iwate. J. Biol. Chem. 241: 79.

Perutz, M.F., Pulsinelli, P.D., and Ranney, H.M. (1972). Structure and subunit interaction of Hemoglobin M Milwaukee. Nature New Biol. 237: 259.

Perutz, M.F. (1970). Stereochemistry of cooperative effects in hemoglobin. Nature 228: 726.

Ranney, H.M., Nagel, R.L., Heller, P., and Udem, L. (1968). Oxygen equilibrium of Hemoglobin M Hyde Park. Biochim. Biophys. Acta 160: 112.

Suzuki, T., Hayashi, A., Shimizu, A., and Yamamura, Y. (1966). The oxygen equilibrium of Hemoglobin M Saskatoon. Biochim. Biophys. Acta. 127: 280.

van Slyke, D.D., and Plazin, J. (1961). Micromanometric analyses. The Williams and Wilkins co.

DISCUSSION

Dr. Perutz: Have you tested any of the other hemoglobin M's for the heme-heme interaction of the kind that is produced on the ferric hemes by ligation of the ferrous hemes with ligand? You showed the effect on Hb Hyde Park which had been demonstrated before. Did you try with Saskatoon to see whether it would show a similar effect, for instance?

Dr. Sugita: I showed ligand binding of totally reduced Saskatoon.

Dr. Perutz: I'm talking about the ESR... You repeated it on Hyde Park; I wondered if you tried it on any of the other hemoglobin M's?

Dr. Sugita: I didn't measure the EPR spectrum of Saskatoon but Dr. Morimoto did under some conditions at high pH, the EPR spectrum seems to change with the ligation state of the normal chain. But the change is much smaller than that for Hyde Park.

Dr. Perutz: Yes. Did you try it on Milwaukee?

Dr. Sugita: No. I did not try it.

Dr. Perutz: In Milwaukee, Dr. Ho found changes in the NMR spectrum and I found interesting changes in optical spectra, so I wondered whether you tried the ESR?

Dr. Sugita: I didn't try it but all the results by Dr. Morimoto showed no change in ESR spectra.

Dr. Perutz: In Milwaukee?

Dr. Sugita: Yes.

Dr. Perutz: How strange. So Saskatoon shows something but Milwaukee does not?

Dr. Sugita: Yes.

Dr. Ho: By using the technique of electron nuclear double resonance (ENDOR), Dr. George Feher and coworkers reported that upon oxygenation of the α chains of Hb M Milwaukee one of the histidine-^{14}N endor lines of the abnormal ferric β hemes is shifted to higher frequencies by 100 kHz [Ann. N. Y. Acad. Sci. 222, 86 (1973)]. This EPR spectral shift indicates that a primary event at the α chain produces a structural change in the β chain. This finding supports our earlier NMR results on Hb Milwaukee, namely there is a spectral change in the hyperfine shifted proton resonances of the ferric β hemes upon addition of CO to the α chains of this mutant hemoglobin [Lindstrom, Ho, and Pisciotta, Nature New Biol. 237, 263 (1972)]. More recently, Dr. Leslie Fung and I have carried out additional proton NMR experiments on Hb M Milwaukee. We have observed the co-existence of oxy and deoxy quaternary structures of Hb M Milwaukee at 80% oxygen saturation (of the α chains) in 0.1M Bis-Tris at pH 7 and 30°C. Our NMR results are consistent with Dr. Sugita's findings that there are interactions between the two α chains in this naturally occurring valency hybrid (i.e. n = 1.3).

Dr. Salhany: We've looked at the EPR spectrum as I mentioned yesterday on nitroso-hemoglobins and there is an interesting observation with stripped Kansas. It is in the T state as NO hemoglobin independent of pH. Neither the 14 ppm line nor the EPR spectrum showed any significant change when we raised the pH, yet there was an optical spectral change. So there seems to be some unusual disjunction between the EPR changes and some optical spectral changes.

Dr. Perutz: Did you find that you had loss of heme in hemoglobins Hyde Park or Saskatoon?

Dr. Sugita: The ratio of the absorption peak at the 280 and 430 nm, I think, showed no heme loss.

Dr. Perutz: We had a meeting in Naples last April where someone reported heme lost in both of these proteins. It may have been the German group. Did you have trouble with that?

Dr. Sugita: No.

Dr. Kilmartin: I would like to make a few comments on this nice presentation. If the Bohr effect of a half oxidized hemoglobin is normal, that is a value of 2.0 protons per tetramer at pH 7.4, then the Bohr factor Δ log p50/Δ pH will be twice as large as normal because this factor measures the protons released per ligand bound and only two ligands bind per tetramer in these M hemoglobins. Thus the increase in the Bohr factor for Hb Milwaukee over normal hemoglobin means that this mutant has a normal Bohr effect.

I would also like to say that our results on Hb Iwate-Kankakee obtained from Heller are completely in agreement with Dr Sugita's and show the absence of heme-heme interaction and Bohr effect in the oxygen equilibrium curve.

USE OF GLOBIN COMPLEMENTARY DNA IN STUDIES OF GLOBIN GENES AND mRNA.

Arthur I. Skoultchi

Department of Cell Biology
Albert Einstein College of Medicine
Bronx, New York 10461

INTRODUCTION

It is generally acknowledged that a prerequisite for our understanding of the mechanisms of cellular differentiation and development in higher organisms is a detailed knowledge of the way in which gene expression is controlled. Among the several approaches which must be brought to bear on these problems are studies of the control of specific messenger RNA synthesis. Such studies are greatly facilitated if a specific reagent can be used to identify and quantitate the amount of a particular mRNA sequence present in a RNA preparation. In bacteria a suitable reagent was obtained by constructing an episome bearing a single bacterial gene (Attardi et. al., 1963). DNA-RNA hybridization was then used to measure the amount of specific mRNA transcribed. With the recent demonstration (Ross et. al., 1972a; Verma et, al., 1972; Kacian et. al., 1972) that RNA dependent DNA polymerase ("reverse transcriptase") can be used to synthesize a complementary DNA copy (cDNA) of globin mRNA such studies became feasible in eukaryotes.

Because of the large DNA content of the eukaryotic genome (Mirsky and Ris, 1951), and the existence of reiterated DNA sequences (Britten and Kohne, 1968; Wetmur and Davidson, 1968) considerable interest has also been generated in determining the number of copies of specific structural genes in animal cell DNA. While in certain instances such measurements can be made by DNA-RNA hybridization with a purified, radioactively labeled mRNA (Kedes and Birnsteil, 1971; Bishop et. al., 1972), a simpler, more general approach involves the use of a cDNA copy of the mRNA.

The purpose of this review is to summarize the properties of globin mRNA and the cDNA copy prepared from it, and to indicate how the cDNA can be used to study globin genes and mRNA.

ISOLATION AND PROPERTIES OF GLOBIN MESSENGER RNA

RNA isolated from the polyribosomes of avian and mammalian reticulocytes contains a component sedimenting at about 9S with many of the properties expected of the messenger RNA for globin. The early work of Chantrenne and collaborators provided circumstantial evidence for its identification as mRNA (Chantrenne et. al., 1967). Lingrel and collaborators were the first to provide comprehensive evidence that reticulocyte 9S RNA encodes the synthesis of globin. By using cell-free protein synthesizing systems prepared from rabbit, guinea pig and duck reticulocytes these workers demonstrated that 9S RNA isolated from mouse reticulocytes directs the synthesis of mouse alpha and beta globin chains (Lingrel et. al., 1971). Subsequently it was shown in a number of laboratories that 9S RNA from rabbit reticulocytes causes a specific synthesis of globin when added to various heterologous protein synthesizing systems, including those from mouse ascites cells (Housman et. al., 1971), wheat germ (Roberts and Patterson, 1973), and frog oocytes (Lane et. al., 1971). These systems, in contrast to the reticulocyte lysates used in the earlier work, do not contain endogenous globin synthesizing capacity.

Two general methods are available for purification of globin mRNA. In both cases polyribosomes are prepared from a reticulocyte lysate by sedimentation through sucrose gradients. Treatment of the polyribosomes with sodium dodecyl sulfate followed by sucrose gradient centrifugation leads to the resolution of a minor peak at 9S (Chantrenne et. al., 1967), which can be further purified by a second zone sedimentation. Alternatively, treatment of the polyribosomes with EDTA releases globin mRNA in a ribonucleoprotein particle which sediments at 15S-20S in sucrose gradients. (Chantrenne et. al., 1967; Labrie, 1969; Pemberton et. al., 1972). The 9S RNA obtained from this particle by sodium dodecyl sulfate treatment followed by sucrose gradient centrifugation has been reported to be free of the contaminants present in preparations made directly from polyribosomes (Lanyon et. al., 1972). In either case the 9S RNA can be further purified by chromatography on oligo (dT)-cellulose (Aviv and Leder, 1972) or poly U-Sepharose (Lanyon et. al., 1972). These latter procedures are used to separate molecules which contain polyadenylate segments (e.g., globin mRNA, see below) from others which lack these sequences (e.g., ribosomal RNA).

Globin mRNA isolated by these methods is a mixture of the mRNAs for the alpha and beta chains of hemoglobin. Separation of the two species of mRNA has been achieved by treatment of rabbit reticulocytes with the isoleucine analogue O-methylthreonine which blocks aminoacylation of isoleucine tRNA. In certain species of rabbits the distribution of isoleucine residues in the alpha and beta chains is such that this treatment causes beta chain mRNA to accumulate preferentially in heavier polyribosomes whereas alpha chain mRNA accumulates in lighter polysomes. Isolation of the mRNAs from the separated polysome fractions yields β mRNA about 10-20% contaminated with α mRNA, and α mRNA contaminated with 20-30% β mRNA (Temple and Housman, 1972). A more highly purified preparation of α mRNA (about 90% free of β mRNA) can be isolated from a ribonucleoprotein particle present in the post ribosomal fraction of rabbit reticulocyte lysates (Jacobs-Lorena and Baglioni, 1972).

The best preparations of globin mRNA migrate as a single diffuse band in polyacrylamide gels (Lanyon et. al., 1972; Morrison et. al., 1974). Electrophoresis in formamide containing polyacrylamide gels resolves two bands in the 9S RNA region (Gould and Hamlyn, 1973; Morrison et. al., 1974; Kazazian et. al., 1974). Evidence has been presented that the slower moving component contains primarily the beta globin mRNA, whereas the faster moving component is enriched for alpha globin mRNA (Morrison et. al., 1974; Kazazian et. al., 1974).

Estimates of the molecular weight of 9S RNA by polyacrylamide gel electrophoresis fall in the range of 200,000 - 230,000 daltons (Gaskill and Kabat, 1971; Pemberton et. al., 1972; Gould and Hamlyn, 1973;), although a value of about 170,000 daltons has been obtained for mouse 9S RNA by analytical ultracentrifugation (Williamson et. al., 1971). A molecular weight of 200,000 - 230,000 daltons corresponds to a RNA chain length of 590-675 nucleotides. The number of nucleotides required to code for rabbit alpha and beta globin chains (141 and 146 amino acid residues respectively, Eck and Dayhoff, 1967) is 423 and 438 nucleotides respectively, suggesting that globin mRNA may contain about 200 nucleotides in excess of those required for coding. Globin mRNAs contain an adenylic acid-rich sequence (poly A) of about 60 residues, presumably at or near the 3' end of the molecule. (Lim and Canellakis, 1970; Gorski et. al., 1974) Poly (A) segments of about 150 nucleotides have been isolated from newly synthesized globin mRNAs of duck erythroblasts (Pemberton and Baglioni, 1972). Evidence for another normally untranslated region of at least 100 nucleotides in alpha globin mRNA has been obtained by analysis of three human hemoglobin variants with elongated alpha chains. The amino acid sequence data are consistent with the elongated alpha chains having arisen by mutations in or near the normal alpha chain termination codon, allowing read-through into a normally untranslated polynucleotide sequences between the chain termination codon and the 3' terminal poly A tract (Clegg et. al., 1971; Clegg et. al., 1974). Recent nucleotide sequence data of human globin mRNA confirm this hypothesis (Marotta et. al., 1974).

SYNTHESIS AND PROPERTIES OF GLOBIN cDNA

RNA tumor viruses contain a DNA polymerase ("reverse transcriptase") which can be purified from the virions and is capable of utilizing a variety of non-viral RNA molecules as templates (Verma et. al., 1971; Kacian et. al., 1971). Initiation of DNA synthesis requires the presence of a primer which binds to the template by hydrogen bonds (Baltimore and Smoler, 1971). The primer is covalently attached to the newly synthesized DNA (Smoler et. al., 1971). The property which globin mRNA shares with most messengers, of having a poly(A) segment at its 3' end, makes it a particularly suitable template for "reverse transcriptase". Synthesis of a complementary DNA copy (cDNA) of the globin messenger was achieved with purified DNA polymerase from avian myeloblastosis virus (Verma et. al., 1972; Kacian et. al., 1972; Ross et. al., 1972a). DNA synthesis was almost completely dependent upon the presence of a short homopolymer of thymidilate, oligo(dT)$_{10-20}$, which primes initiation of transcription by pairing with the poly(A). In most studies double stranded DNA synthesis is prevented by including actinomycin D in the reaction mixture. The DNA product in this case consists mostly of DNA strands complementary to the globin mRNA template. The cDNA can be recovered free of the mRNA template by treatment of the reaction mixture with 0.3N NaOH (100°C; 5 min.) and chromatography on Sephadex G-150.

The mean molecular weight of globin cDNA is about 120,000 - 145,000 daltons (Bishop and Freeman, 1974; Harrison et. al., 1974), corresponding to a chain length of 360-440 nucleotides. The cDNA contains a poly(T) sequence of about 40 nucleotides, presumably at the 5' end of the molecule (Bishop and Freeman, 1974). Comparison of the chains lengths of globin cDNA and globin mRNA (600-650 nucleotides) indicates that 55-70% of the mRNA sequence is represented in the DNA copy. A direct measurement was made by hybridization of radioactively labeled duck globin mRNA with increasing amounts of cDNA. In the presence of excess cDNA about 75% of the labeled globin mRNA was rendered ribonuclease resistant, indicating that some molecules of cDNA are transcribed from three-fourths of the mRNA sequence (D. Housman and A. Skoultchi, unpublished results). The sequences in the mRNA which are not transcribed probably lie at the 5' end of the messenger molecule. Other results indicate that globin cDNA contains transcripts of the alpha and beta chain mRNAs in approximately equal amounts. No additional sequences are present in the cDNA in amounts greater than 10% (Housman et. al., 1974). Chain specific globin cDNAs have been prepared by using the separated mRNAs for alpha and beta globin as templates in the reverse transcription reaction (Housman et. al., 1973; Kacian et. al., 1973). The chain specific cDNAs can be used to quantitate the amounts of mRNA for the individual globin chains in cellular RNA (see below).

MEASUREMENT OF GLOBIN GENE FREQUENCY

The somatic cells of higher organisms often devote a large proportion of their protein synthetic activity towards the production of a single protein species (e.g., hemoglobin in erythroid cells). In principle, this might be accomplished by specific replication (amplification) of the required gene(s) in the differentiating cell types. Alternatively, the required gene(s) might be present in multiple copies in the DNA of all cells (reiteration). The ribosomal RNA genes provide an example of DNA sequences which are both reiterated in all cells and amplified in a specific cell type, the oocyte (reviewed by Birnsteil et. al., 1971). Evidence for other reiterated sequences in animal cell DNA has come from studies of DNA reassociation reactions. When denatured DNA is placed in solution under conditions which promote reannealing, the rate of reassociation of a specific sequence is dependent upon the concentration of the specific complementary strands. Kinetic analysis of the reassociation of mammalian DNAs shows three transitions corresponding to the three major frequency classes of DNA sequences: the highly repetitive sequences with a reiteration frequency of about 10^6, the intermediate repetitive sequences each present in about 10^3 copies, and the bulk of the DNA which consists of single copy DNA sequences (Britten and Kohne, 1968). By including in the reassociation mixture a small amount of radioactively labeled mRNA or cDNA copy of the mRNA, it is possible to follow the reassociation kinetics of a specific gene sequence. The analysis can be used to calculate the number of copies of the specific gene in genomic DNA. An important parameter in such a study is the amount of mRNA or cDNA added. A sufficiently small quantity of mRNA or cDNA must be used so that the concentration of the specific sequence in the mixture is not appreciably increased.

The first measurements of globin gene frequency were made by DNA-RNA hybridization in RNA excess, using radioactively labeled globin mRNA as a probe for the globin gene sequences. The results of these studies led to estimates of about 50,000 copies of globin genes in mouse and chicken DNA (Williamson et. al., 1970; Sanchez de Jimenez et. al., 1971). In retrospect these estimates are clearly four orders of magnitude too high and demonstrate the inherent difficulties of RNA excess hybridization with eukaryotic DNA. The results are best explained by hybridization of a minor component of the RNA preparation with a family of repetitive DNA sequences. Subsequently, the technique of DNA-RNA hybridization in DNA excess was used. The kinetics of hybridization of duck globin mRNA to DNA from duck red blood cells indicated an upper limit of five globin genes in this DNA (Bishop et. al., 1972).

The availability of a cDNA copy of globin mRNA provided a new method for following the reassociation of globin gene sequences, which has certain advantages over the use of labeled mRNA. Since the cDNA is synthesized in vitro from radioactively labeled nucleotides higher specific activities can be attained. True conditions of vast DNA excess are therefore more easily achieved. The DNA-RNA hybridization reactions must be corrected for differences in the rate constants of hybridization and DNA renaturation (Bishop, 1972). Such corrections should not be necessary when a cDNA probe is used. Finally, the cDNA is more stable than RNA at the high temperatures required for annealing. The amount of radioactive cDNA annealed to complementary sequences in nuclear DNA is most often determined by treatment of the reassociation mixture with nuclease S_1. This enzyme digests single-stranded DNA sequences much more rapidly than DNA-DNA duplexes and DNA-RNA hybrids (Sutton, 1971).

The results of experiments in which globin cDNA was annealed with an excess of various animal cell DNAs in general confirm the conclusion that there are at most only a few copies of the globin genes in the animal cell genome. Annealing of duck globin cDNA with duck DNA gave values of less than 5 copies (Packman et. al., 1972) and 2-3 copies (Bishop and Rosbash, 1973). In the mouse a value of less than 2 copies was obtained (Harrison et. al., 1974). In two of these studies annealing of globin cDNAto DNA from both erythroid and non-erythroid cells was compared. The measured number of globin gene copies in all cases was approximately the same (Packman et. al., 1972; Harrison et. al., 1974). These results clearly indicate that the globin genes are neither substantially reiterated in all cells nor specifically amplified in differentiating erythroid cells.

ASSAY OF GLOBIN mRNA CONTENT

The simplest method for determining mRNA content is to hybridize increasing amounts of RNA with a constant amount of radioactively labeled cDNA and estimate the smallest amount of RNA which produces maximum hybridization of the cDNA. The amount of globin mRNA in the RNA sample can be calculated from this estimate since the mRNA input should be equal to the cDNA input at the point of saturation. It is important that each reaction be incubated for a length of time sufficient for hybridization to proceed to completion. In this case the extent of hybridization, not its rate, will be measured. The proportion of the input cDNA which hybridizes is determined by treatment of the hybridization mixture with the S_1 nuclease.

Figure 1A shows the results of a typical titration experiment using purified mouse globin mRNA and ^{3}H-mouse globin cDNA. Complete hybridization of the cDNA is obtained with about 0.5 ng of the purified mRNA preparation. Total

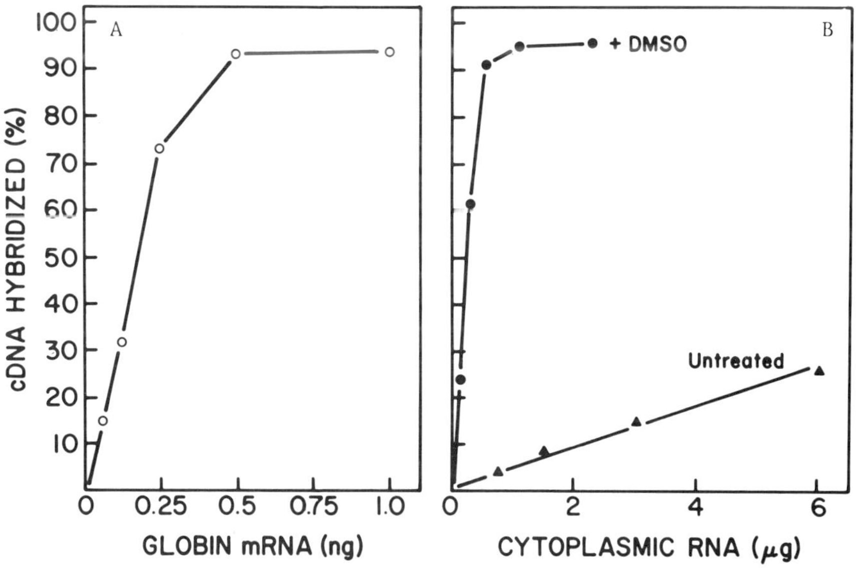

Figure 1. Hybridization between mouse RNA and mouse globin [^{3}H]cDNA. Each reaction mixture contained 245 cpm [^{3}H]cDNA and the amounts of RNA indicated in the figure, in a final volume of 5 μl. Further details of the hybridization procedure and S_1 nuclease digestion were as previously described (Housman et. al., 1973). Acid precipitable radioactivity in a blank reaction mixture containing no RNA was 20 cpm after treatment with S_1 nuclease. Total cytoplasmic RNA was prepared by phenol-chloroform extraction (Perry et. al., 1972) of the post-nuclear supernatant fraction from detergent-lysed cells. (A) Purified mouse globin mRNA; (B) Total cytoplasmic RNA from untreated (x—x) Friend erythroleukemic cells (clone 745A) and from Friend cells grown in the presence of 2% (v/v) dimethylsulfoxide for 90 hours (•—•).

cytoplasmic RNA extracted from murine erythroleukemic cells was assayed for globin mRNA content (Fig. 1B). The erythroleukemic cells, originally isolated by Friend and co-workers from a mouse infected with Friend leukemia virus, have been shown to undergo erythroid differentiation in cell culture. The synthesis of normal adult mouse hemoglobin is markedly enhanced when the cells are grown in the presence of dimethylsulfoxide (DMSO) (Friend et. al., 1971; Boyer et. al., 1972). About 0.5μg of cytoplasmic RNA from DMSO-treated cells is required for complete hybridization of the mouse globin cDNA (Fig. 1B). Saturation of the cDNA with RNA from untreated cells can be obtained, but about fifty times more RNA is required.

Comparing the amount of RNA from treated cells required for maximal hybridization (0.5 μg) with that for the purified mRNA (0.5 ng), indicates that about 0.1% of the total cytoplasmic RNA from treated cells is globin mRNA. In mouse reticulocytes 1-2% of total RNA is globin mRNA (Williamson et. al., 1971; Young et. al., 1974). By performing similar titration experiments with RNA from cells treated with DMSO for various lengths of time, Ross et. al., (1972b) demonstrated that globin mRNA gradually accumulates in the cells during the course of several days growth in the presence of DMSO. Further experiments are necessary to determine the mechanisms which govern the accumulation of globin mRNA in these cells.

Globin mRNA in Thalassemia

The thalassemia syndromes are inherited disorders of man in which there is absent or decreased synthesis of one of the two globin chains of adult hemoglobin. When globin mRNA isolated from α thalassemic reticulocytes (Hb H disease) is used to program a heterologous cell-free protein synthesizing system, much less α chain is synthesized than β chain (Benz et. al., 1972; Grossbard et. al., 1973). An opposite result was observed with RNA from β thalassemic reticulocytes (Nienhuis and Anderson, 1971; Benz and Forget, 1971; Dow et. al., 1972). Since these studies utilized an assay procedure which depends upon the functional activity of the mRNA, they cannot rule out the possibility that the thalassemic reticulocytes contain normal amounts of functionally deficient mRNA for the affected chain. DNA-RNA hybridization experiments provide a direct measurement of globin mRNA content which does not depend upon the ability of the RNA to function as a messenger.

It is possible to isolate rabbit globin α mRNA and β mRNA which is 80-90% pure with respect to contamination by the mRNA for the opposite chain (see above). Chain specific cDNAs have been prepared by using the purified rabbit mRNAs as templates in the reverse transcription reaction. Because there is sufficient cross-hybridization between human globin mRNA and rabbit globin cDNA, these chain specific probes can be used to quantitate the ratio of α mRNA to β mRNA in human reticulocyte RNA (Housman et. al., 1973; Kacian et. al., 1973). Control experiments were performed with rabbit mRNAs and rabbit cDNAs to show that there is no cross-hybridization between α mRNA and β-chain cDNA and between β mRNA and α-chain cDNA (Housman et. al., 1974).

In order to determine the ratio of α mRNA to β mRNA in a human RNA sample, increasing amounts of the RNA are hybridized separately with α-chain cDNA and with β-chain cDNA. The minimum amount of RNA required for maximum hybridization of each probe is determined. The ratio of the two values gives a direct measurement of the ratio of α mRNA to β mRNA in the sample. An analysis of this type was performed with reticulocyte RNA from patients with homozygous α thalassemia (Hb H disease) and homozygous β thalassemia, and from a nonthalassemic patient with hemolytic anemia (Housman et. al., 1973). The same amount of RNA from the nonthalassemic reticulocytes was required for maximum hybridization of α-chain cDNA as for β-chain cDNA, indicating that the relative amounts of α and β mRNA in this sample are about equal. Approximately six times as much RNA from α-thalassemic reticulocytes was required for saturation of α-chain cDNA as for β-chain cDNA, indicating a marked deficiency of α mRNA relative to β mRNA in this patient's reticulocytes.

The initial hybridization experiments with RNA from β-thalassemic reticulocytes indicated only a minor deficiency of β mRNA relative to α mRNA. It was noted, however, that in a cell-free protein synthesizing system this RNA preparation promotes the synthesis of substantial amounts of γ chains. Because there is a good deal of homology between human γ and β globin chains, the possibility was raised that γ mRNA in this sample was hybridizing with the rabbit β-chain cDNA, giving falsely high results for β mRNA content. In order to eliminate these difficulties two changes were made in the determination of β mRNA. A cDNA copy of human β mRNA was synthesized, using as template the mRNA from α-thalassemic reticulocytes which contains primarily β mRNA contaminated with less than 15% α mRNA. Secondly, the stringency of the hybridization conditions was increased by raising the hybridization temperature to 78°C. The effect of this increase in temperature is to eliminate imperfectly formed hybrids, such as those which might otherwise occur between γ mRNA and β-chain cDNA. Using these more rigorous hybridization conditions it was possible to demonstrate a 10-fold deficiency of β mRNA relative to α mRNA in the β-thalassemic reticulocytes (Housman et. al., 1973). Similar experiments were performed with RNA samples from reticulocytes of two unrelated patients with homozygous β° thalassemia (A_2 variety) and also with pooled reticulocyte RNA from three siblings with homozygous δ-β thalassemia. In both syndromes Hb A synthesis is not detected. The hybridization results indicated a virtual absence of β mRNA in these patients' reticulocytes (Forget et. al., 1974).

In conclusion, in the two studies outlined here, as well as in a third study in which similar DNA-RNA hybridization techniques were used (Kacian et. al., 1973), the thalassemic reticulocytes of all patients studied to date exhibit either a marked quantitative deficiency or complete absence of the mRNA for the affected globin chain. Other types of experiments have been performed which suggest the presence of significant amounts of β mRNA in β°-thalassemic reticulocytes of patients from the Ferrara region. Cell-free synthesis of normal β globin chains was reported when ribosomes from reticulocytes of these individuals are incubated with a supernatant fraction from nonthalassemic reticulocytes (Conconi et. al., 1972; Rowley and Kosciolek, 1972). It will be of interest to examine reticulocyte RNA from such patients by the hybridization methods described here.

DISCUSSION

Two basic types of measurements utilizing globin cDNA have been outlined in the preceding sections: (1) DNA-DNA annealing for the detection of globin gene sequences in animal cell DNA, and (2) DNA-RNA hybridization for quantitative estimation of globin mRNA content. Both methods can be used to answer numerous other questions of importance to the biology of animal cells. In the following report in this volume, for example, the chain specific globin cDNAs have been used to demonstrate a deletion of the DNA sequences coding for α-chain mRNA in homozygous α thalassemia, hydrops fetalis. Similar experiments need to be performed to determine whether a corresponding deletion of the β globin gene occurs in β°-thalassemia. DNA-RNA hybridization of globin cDNA has been used to localize globin mRNA in cells by *in situ* hybridization (Harrison et. al., 1973). DNA-DNA *in situ* renaturation with globin cDNA is potentially useful for localizing the sites of globin genes on the chromosomes. By comparing the hybridization of globin cDNAs and globin mRNAs from several species, it is possible to study the evolutionary relationships of globin genes in mammals (Gummerson and Williamson, 1974). Finally, the globin cDNA has been used recently to identify a likely nuclear intermediate in the synthesis of globin mRNA (Macnaughton et. al., 1974). No doubt then this reagent will continue to be of central importance in future studies of globin genes and mRNA.

SUMMARY

The existence of a poly(A) segment at or near the 3' end of globin mRNA makes it a particularly suitable template for the DNA polymerase ("reverse transcriptase") of RNA tumor viruses. As much as 75% of the globin mRNA sequence is transcribed into a complementary DNA copy (cDNA). The use of globin cDNA as a probe for measuring globin gene frequency in animal cell DNA has been reviewed. All indications are that globin genes are present in only a few copies in the genome of both erythroid and non-erythroid cells. Globin cDNA also can be used to measure the globin mRNA content of cellular RNA preparations. The chain specific cDNAs which can be synthesized from purified α-globin mRNA and β-globin mRNA have been used to quantitate the relative amounts of the two mRNAs in reticulocytes from thalassemic individuals. The results reviewed here indicate that there is either a marked quantitative deficiency or virtual absence of the mRNA for the affected globin chain in thalassemic reticulocytes.

ACKNOWLEDGEMENTS

I thank Drs. B. G. Forget and D. Housman for preparations of mouse globin mRNA and cDNA and for many stimulating hours of discussion and experimentation. The author is a recipient of an American Cancer Society Research Faculty Award, FRA-124.

REFERENCES

Attardi, G., Naono, S., Rouviere, J., Jacob, F., and Gros, F., (1963). Cold Spring Harbor Symp. Quant. Biol. 28:363.

Aviv, H. and Leder, P. (1972). Proc. Natl. Acad. Sci. USA 69:1408.

Baltimore, D., and Smoler, D. (1971). Proc. Natl. Acad. Sci. USA 68:1507.

Benz, E.J. and Forget, B.G., (1971). J. Clin. Invest. 50: 2755.

Benz, E.J., Swerdlow, P.S. and Forget, B.G., (1972). Blood 40:430 abstr.

Birnsteil, M.L., Chipchase, M., and Speirs, J., (1971). Progr. Nucleic Acid Res. Mol. Biol. 11:351.

Bishop, J.O., (1972). Biochem. J. 126:171.

Bishop, J.O., Pemberton, R. and Baglioni, C. (1972). Nature 235:231.

Bishop, J.O. and Freeman, K.B., (1973). Cold Spring Harbor Symp. Quant. Biol. 38:707.

Bishop, J.O. and Roshbash, M., (1973). Nature New Biol. 241:204.

Boyer, S.H., Wuu, K.D., Noyes, A.N., Young, R., Scher, W., Friend, C., Preisler, H.D., and Bank, A. (1972). Blood 6:823.

Britten, R.J. and Kohne, D.E. (1968). Science 161:529.

Chantrenne, H., Burny, S., and Marbaix, G. (1967). Progr. Nucl. Acid Res. Mol. Biol. 7:173.

Clegg, J.B., Weatherall, D.J. and Milner, P.F. (1971). Nature 234:337.

Clegg, J.B., Weatherall, D.J., Contopolon-Griva, I., Caroutsos, K., Poungouras, P., and Tsevrenis, H., (1974). Nature 251:245.

Conconi, F., Rowley, P.T. Del Senno, L., Pontremoli, S., and Volpato, S., (1972). Nature New Biol. 238:83.

Dow, L.W., Kacian, D., Terada, M., Metafora, S., Spiegelman, S., Marks, P.A. and Bank, A., (1972). J. Clin. Invest. 51:24a abstr.

Eck, R.V. and Dayhoff, M.O. (1967). Atlas of Protein Sequence and Structure.

Forget, B.G., Benz, E.J., Skoultchi, A., Baglioni, C., and Housman, D., (1974). Nature 247:379.

Gould, H.J. and Hamlyn, P.H., (1972). FEBS Letters 30:301.
Grossbard, E., Terada, M., Dow, L.W. and Bank, A., (1973). Nature New Biol. 241:209.
Gummerson, K.S. and Williamson, R., (1974). Nature 247:265.
Harrison, P.R., Conkie, D. and Paul, J., (1973). FEBS Letters 32:109.
Harrison, P.R., Birnie, G.D., Hell, A., Humphries, S., Young, B.D., and Paul, J., (1974). J. Mol. Biol. 84:539.
Housman, D., Pemberton, R. and Taber, R. (1971). Proc. Natl. Acad. Sci. USA 68:2716.
Housman, D., Forget, B.G., Skoultchi, A., and Benz, E.J., (1973). Proc. Natl. Acad. Sci. USA 70:1809.
Housman, D., Skoultchi, A., Forget, B.G., and Benz, E.J., (1974). Ann. N.Y. Acad. Sci., in press.
Jacobs-Lorena, M., and Baglioni, C. (1972). Proc. Nat. Acad. Sci. USA 69:1425.
Kacian, D.L., Watson, K.F., Burny, A., and Spiegelman, S., (1971). Biochim. Biophys. Acta. 246:365.
Kacian, D.L., Spiegelman, S., Bank, A., Terada, M., Metafora, S., Dow, L., and Marks, P.A. (1972). Nature New Biol. 235:167.
Kacian, D.L., Gambino, R., Dow, L.W., Grossbard, E., Natta, C., Ramirez, F., Spiegelman, S., Marks, P.A., and Bank, A., (1973). Proc. Natl. Acad. Sci. USA 70:1886.
Kazazian, H.H., Snyder, P.G. and Cheng, T., (1974). Biochim. Biophys. Res. Commun. 59:1053.
Kedes, L.H. and Birnsteil, M.L. (1971). Nature 230:165.
Labrie, F., (1969). Nature 221:1217.
Lane, C.D., Marbaix, G., and Gurdon, J.B. (1971). J. Mol. Biol. 61:73.
Lanyon, W.G., Paul, J., and Williamson, R. (1972). Eur. J. Biochem. 31:38.
Lingrel, J.B., Lockard, R.E., Jones, R.F., Burr, H.E., and Holder, J.W. (1971). Ser. Haematol. 4:37.
Macnaughton, M., Freeman, K.B. and Bishop, J.O., (1974). Cell 1:117.
Marotta, C.A., Forget, B.G., Weissman, S.M., Verma, I.M., Mc Caffrey, R.P., and Baltimore, D. (1974). Proc. Natl. Acad. Sci. USA 71:2300.
Mirsky, A.E. and Ris, H. (1951). J. Gen. Physiol. 34:451.

Morrison, M., Brinkley, S., Gorski, J., and Lingrel, J.B. (1974). J. Biol. Chem. 249:5290.
Nienhuis, A.W. and Anderson, W.F., (1971). J. Clin. Invest. 50:2458.
Packman, S., Aviv, H., Ross, J., and Leder, P., (1972). Biochem. Biophys. Res. Commun. 49:813.
Pemberton, R.E., Housman, D., Lodish, H.F. and Baglioni, C. (1972). Nature New Biol. 235:99.
Perry, R.P., LaTorre, J., Kelley, D.E. and Greenberg, J.R., (1972). Biochim. Biophys. Acta 262:220.
Roberts, B.E. and Patterson, B.M. (1973). Proc. Natl. Acad. Sci. USA 70:2330.
Ross, J., Aviv, H., Scolnick, E., and Leder, P. (1972a). Proc. Natl. Acad. Sci. USA 69:264.
Ross, J., Ikawa, Y., and Leder P., (1972b). Proc. Natl. Acad. Sci. USA 69:3620.
Rowley, P.T., and Kosciolek, B., (1972). Nature New Biol. 239:234.
Sanchez de Jimenez, E., Dominguez, J.L., Webb, F.H., and Bock, R.M., (1971). J. Mol. Biol. 61:59.
Smoler, D., Molineaux, I., and Baltimore, D., (1971). J. Biol. Chem. 246:7697.
Sutton, W.D., (1971). Biochim. Biophys. Acta 240:522.
Temple, G.F., and Housman, D.E. (1972). Proc. Natl. Acad. Sci. USA 69:1574.
Verma, I.M., Meuth, N.L., Bromfield, E., Manly, K.F., and Baltimore, D. (1971). Nature New Biol. 233:131.
Verma, I., Temple, G.F., Fan, H. and Baltimore, D. (1972). Nature New Biol. 235:163.
Wetmur, J.G. and Davidson, N. (1968). J. Mol. Biol. 31:349.
Williamson, R., Morrison, M., and Paul, J., (1970). Biochem. Biophys. Res. Commun. 40:740.
Williamson, R., Morrison, M., Lanyon, G., Eason, R. and Paul, J. (1971). Biochem. 10:3014.
Young, B.D., Harrison, P. R., Gilmour, R.S., Birnie, G.D., Hell, A., Humphries, S. and Paul, J., (1974). J. Mol. Biol. 84:555.

DISCUSSION

Dr. Winter: It is known that the alpha to beta synthesis ratio in thalassemia apparently changes in marrow cells versus circulating cells. Do you have any evidence now that would show whether this messenger RNA deficiency is progressing during the lifetime of the differentiating cells?

Dr. Skoultchi: Really not. All these experiments were done with reticulocytes and you need a fair quantity of material to do these experiments. It's not clear that they could be done very easily with bone marrow preparation, but I suppose that's being thought about.

HOMOZYGOUS α THALASSEMIA (HYDROPS FETALIS): EVIDENCE FOR DELETION OF THE α STRUCTURAL GENE

Y.W. Kan*, J.M. Taylor*, A.M. Dozy*, H.E. Varmus*, L.E. Lie-Injo*, J. Ganesan**, and D. Todd†

*University of California, San Francisco
**Institute for Medical Research, Kuala Lumpur
†University of Hong Kong, Hong Kong

In thalassemia, the defect in synthesis of the α and β globin chain has been demonstrated to be the result of deficiencies of the α and the β globin chain mRNA respectively (1-9). The mechanism of the deficiency has not previously been defined. It could be due to defective production of the affected mRNA or to the production of an abnormal RNA which is rapidly destroyed. In addition the types of thalassemia in which the affected globin chain is absent in the homozygous state, (viz. homozygous β^0 thalassemia and homozygous α thalassemia associated with hydrops fetalis) could also be the result of deletion of the structural gene of that globin chain.

The presence of globin structural genes may be detected by DNA-DNA hybridization with radioactive copies of DNAs (cDNA) complementary to the globin mRNA. Since the differences in amino acid sequence between the beta, gamma, and delta chains are relatively small, their respective mRNAs may also be fairly similar in structure. On the other hand, the amino acid sequence of the α chain (and hence the nucleotide sequence of its mRNA) is quite dissimilar to those of the non-α chains. Detection of the α globin structural gene by cDNA complementary to α globin mRNA is less likely to be affected by the structure genes for the non-α globin chains. We have performed this type of experiment and found that in homozygous α thalassemia there is a loss of the DNA in the region of the α globin structural gene.

MATERIALS AND METHODS

Two Chinese infants from Hong Kong and Malaysia with homozygous α thalassemia were studied. They had the classical features of hydrops fetalis and hemoglobin Barts ($\gamma 4$) was the major component on electrophoresis (10). In addition, a stillborn baby without thalassemia served as control. DNA was prepared from the livers of these infants by SDS, pronase digestion and phenol extraction and reduced in size to about 2×10^6 daltons by limited depurination (11).

Messenger RNA was prepared from reticulocyte rich blood from patients with hemoglobin H disease and from non-thalassemic patients with autoimmune hemolytic anemia. These RNAs were transcribed into cDNA with RNA-directed DNA polymerase from Rous sarcoma virus, as follows: 0.1 M Tris-HCl pH 8.1, 0.008 M $MgCl_2$, 0.02 M β. mercaptoethanol, 80 μM dATP, 80 μM TTP, 80 μM dGTP, 0.8 μM dCTP (^{32}-P) (115 Ci/mmole), 0.1 unit/ml of polymerase, 0.4 μg/ml RNA, in a total volume 3 ml, incubated at 37°C for 120 minutes. The nucleic acids were extracted with SDS, pronase and phenol, and the RNA hydrolysed with alkali. The cDNAs were annealed to their respective template RNA. The cDNA which annealed to the RNA was isolated by batchwise elution from hydroxylapatite. The cDNA transcribed from the mRNA of an individual with hemoglobin H disease was used after this step for probing β globin sequences. The probe for β globin sequences was prepared by annealing the cDNA from the patients with autoimmune hemolytic anemia to hemoglobin H mRNA under such conditions that 70% of the cDNA was annealed. The unannealed fraction was isolated by hydroxylapatite and Sephadex G-50 chromatography, and subjected to the adsorption procedure three more times.

The cDNAs were annealed to normal or hemoglobin H mRNA under the following condition: 0.3 M NaCl, 0.001 M EDTA, 0.02 M Tris-HCl, pH 7.4 at 68°. They were annealed to the liver DNA under the following conditions: 5 mg/ml cell DNA, 240 cpm ^{32}P globin cDNA, 0.5 M NaCl, 0.002 M EDTA, 0.04 M Tris-HCl, pH 7.4 at 68°. Incubations were performed in 80 μl volumes mixtures under mineral oil from 20 minutes to 120 hours. Annealing was also assayed with hydroxylapatite. The details of these methods have been given elsewhere (12).

RESULTS

In Figure 1 the specificities of the α and β probes were tested by measurement of their rates of annealing to mRNAs from a nonthalassemic patient and a patient with hemoglobin H disease. Both cDNAs annealed at equal rates to the former RNA which contains α and β globin sequences in equal amount. In contrast, the β cDNA annealed at a rate 10 times more rapidly to the hemoglobin H mRNA than the α cDNA. This was consistent with the result of translation obtained when this preparation of hemoglobin H mRNA was assayed in a cell-free system from Krebs ascites tumor. It directed the synthesis of 9 times more β globin chain than α chain.

The annealing of these cDNAs to cellular DNA prepared from the livers of the hydropic and the stillborn infants is shown in Figure 2. The β cDNA annealed at the same rate and to the same extent to the DNA from the hydropic and the nonthalassemic infants. In contrast, the α cDNA annealed to a much less extent to the DNA of both hydrops in comparison to the nonthalassemic control.

DISCUSSION

Homozygous α thalassemia associated with hemoglobin Barts is a condition which is not compatible with life. The affected infants are severely anemic, grossly edematous,

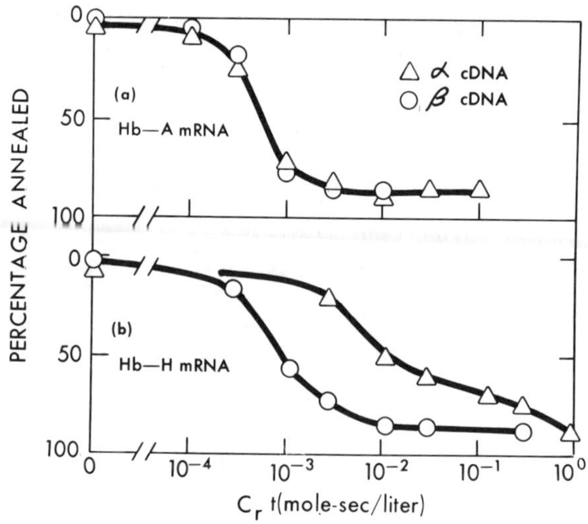

Fig. 1. Annealing of α and β globin cDNA to mRNA.

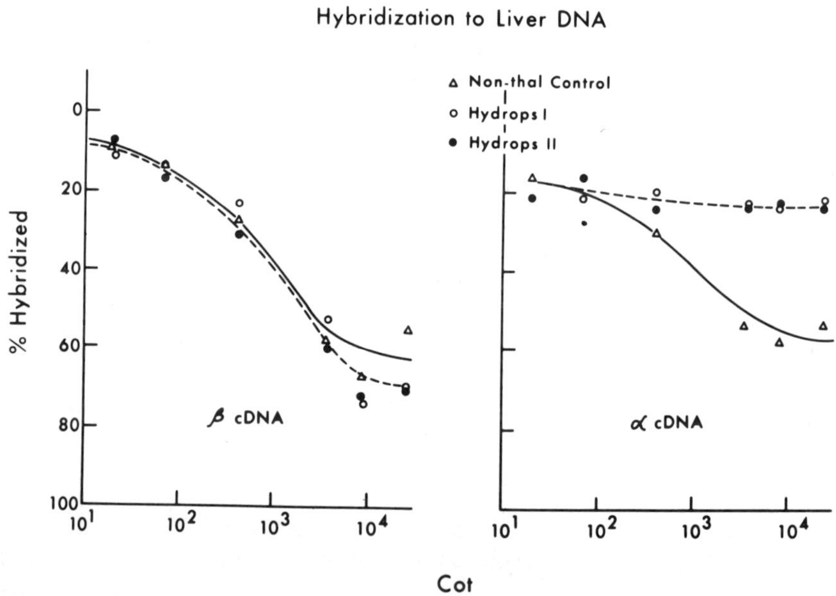

Fig. 2. Annealing of α and β globin cDNA to liver DNA from two hydrops and a nonthalassemic control.

and have massive enlargement of the liver and the placenta. The major hemoglobin component is hemoglobin Barts ($\gamma 4$). No α chain is detectible.

It has been shown that the mRNA isolated from the reticulocytes of these infants are deficient in α globin mRNA activity when assayed in the cell-free system and by hybridization with α and β globin mRNA specific cDNAs (19). The results of the experiments reported here show that the absence of α mRNA is the result of the lack of DNA sequences normally found in α globin mRNA. The extent of involvement of the α structural gene cannot be deduced accurately with these experiments, since the average size of the cDNA used was about 380 nucleotides in length. The α mRNA is about 650 nucleotide long (13), 60 to 100 of which are contained in the 3' poly-A segment (14), which is preceded by at least 93 nucleotides encoding for the normally untranslated Constant Spring region (15). Since cDNAs are copied from the 3' end, the probes used in these experiments must have extended only partially into the translated region of the mRNA. Thus we can conclude from these studies that the α structural gene homologous to the 3' portion of the α globin mRNA is deleted.

There is evidence that the α structural gene may be duplicated (16). The extent of reduction of annealing by the α cDNA is consistent with the conclusion that if there are two loci for α chain synthesis, the loss in α globin sequences must have affected both loci.

The small amount of annealing of the α cDNA that occurred may be due to some β cDNA present in the α probe. Alternatively, it may also be due to cross hybridization of the α cDNA with the gene for the zeta globin chain, the amino acid composition of which is somewhat similar to the α chain (17).

Alpha thalassemia is not uncommon in the Mediterranean area, in Africa and Asia (18). However, the severe form of homozygous α thalassemia associated with hydrops occurs almost exclusively in the Far East. Typically, this is the offspring of a mating between two individuals with α thalassemia trait or α thalassemia-1 (18) which is characterized by microcytosis of the red blood cells. Outside of the Far East, this type of matings have been found not infrequently to produce offsprings with hemoglobin H disease (19). Thus the deletion of α globin structural gene reported here and in Singapore and Thailand (20) may only be applicable to the severe type of homozygous α thalassemia found in the Orientals. Alpha thalassemia may well be caused by mechanisms other than deletion which allow for some α globin chain synthesis. These two types may be analogous to β^0 and β^+ forms of homozygous β thalassemia and referred to as α^0 and α^+ respectively. Perhaps in the Orient, α^0 is the commoner type and results in hydrops in the homozygous state. Elsewhere, the α^+ type predominates, and hence results in hemoglobin H rather than hydrops.

ACKNOWLEDGMENT

Supported by grants from the National Institute of Health, John A. Hartford Foundation Inc., a Senior Dernham Fellowship from the American Cancer Society (J.M.T.) and USPHS Research Career Development Awards (Y.W.K. and H.E.W.)

REFERENCES

1. Nienhuis, A.W. and Anderson, W.F. J. Clin. Invest. 50:2458, 1971.

2. Benz, E.J., Jr. and Forget, B.G. J. Clin. Invest. 50: 2755, 1971.

3. Dow, L.W., Terada, M., Natta, C., Metafora, S., Grossbard, E., Marks, P.A. and Bank, A. Nature New Biology 243:114, 1973.

4. Benz, E.J., Jr., Swerdlow, P.S. and Forget, B.G. Blood 42:825, 1973.

5. Grossbard, E., Terada, M., Dow, L.W., and Bank, A. Nature New Biology 241:209, 1973.

6. Housman, D., Forget, B.G., Skoultchi, A. and Benz, E.J. Jr. Proc. Nat. Acad. Sci. (USA) 70:1809, 1973.

7. Kacian, D.L., Gambino, R., Dow, L.W., Grossbard, E., Natta, C., Ramirez, F., Spiegelman, S., Marks, P.A. and Bank, A. Proc. Nat. Acad. Sci. (USA) 70:1886, 1973.

8. Kan, Y.W., Dozy, A.M., Holland, J.H. Blood 42:99, 1973.

9. Kan, Y.W., Todd, D., Holland, J.H., and Dozy, A.M. J. Clin. Invest. 53:37a, 1974.

10. Lie-Injo, L.E. Blood 20:581, 1962.

11. Tibbets, C., Johansson, K., and Philipson, L. J. Virol. 12:218, 1973.

12. Taylor, J.H., Dozy, A.M., Kan, Y.W., Varmus, H.E., Lie-Injo, L.E., Ganesan, J. and Todd, D. Nature 251:392, 1974.

13. Williamson, R., Crossley, J., and Humphries, S. Biochemistry 13:703, 1974.

14. Lim, L. and Canellakis, E.S. Nature 227:710, 1970.

15. Clegg, J.B., Weatherall, D.J. and Milner, P.F. Nature 234:337, 1971.

16. Lehmann, H. Lancet ii:635, 1970.

17. Huehns, E.R. Personal communication.

18. Wasi, P., Na-Nakorn, S., and Pootrakul, S. Clinics in Haematology 3:383, 1974.

19. McNiel, J.R. J. Med. Assoc. of Thailand 53:153, 1971.

20. Ottolenghi, S., Lanyon, W.G., Paul, J., Williamson, R., Weatherall, D.J., Clegg, J.B., Pritchard, J., Pootrakul, S. and Wong, H.B. Nature 251:389, 1974.

DISCUSSION

Dr. Charache: I was wondering using the copy DNA technique, have you or do know of anyone who has tried to unravel the difference between β-thalassemia minor, intermedia, and major?

Dr. Kan: Beta thalassemia is a more difficult problem because delta chain and beta chain are so similar that some cross hybridization is to be expected. Furthermore, since we believe that there is only one locus for beta chain synthesis, I don't think this sort of study will be useful to differentiate the severity of the disease.

Dr. Perutz: Would you like to comment on the relationship between your results and Weatherall's?

Dr. Kan: Dr. Weatherall together with Dr. Williamson's group in Glasgow studied hydrops from Singapore and Thailand and they obtained the same result.

Dr. Perutz: It is very interesting how the research proceeded backwards in thalassemia research. First, everybody looked for amino acid changes and found none, and then for messenger, and finally for the gene.

Dr. Kan: I think it has to do with the techniques available. We knew how to measure protein synthesis for a long time. When the cDNA came along, mRNA was first studied because it is relatively easily available in the reticulocytes. Because we are searching for a sequence which is represented once or twice in the DNA, these studies are again a little more difficult.

RED BLOOD CELL METABOLISM

Chairman: K. R. Tanaka

EFFECT OF INTRACELLULAR pH(pHi) CHANGE ON RED CELL GLYCOLYSIS

Shigeki Minakami[1], Akio Tomoda[1] and Sachiko Tsuda[2]

[1]Department of Biochemistry, Kyushu University School of Medicine, Fukuoka 812, [2] Higashi-Tsukushi Junior College, Kitakyushu 805, Japan.

INTRODUCTION

Remarkable effect of hydrogen ion concentration on red cell glycolytic rate has been noticed as early as in 1914 by Rona and Wilenko. The effect was studied by many investigators, notably by Murphy(1960) who rightly suggested that "the enzymic reaction involving the conversion of fructose-6-PO_4 to fructose-1,6-PO_4 is a likely site of the pH-effect", which was later confirmed by us with direct determination of the intermediates (Minakami and Yoshikawa,1966). Another marked effect of pH-change on red cell was the change in 2,3-diphosphoglycerate (DPG) concentration, which was shown by Rapoport and Guest (1939) and confirmed and extended by us(Asakura et al.,1966a). These observations remind us strict control of pH as essential in red cell study.

Relatively little attention has been paid to intracellular pH(pHi), though metabolism and function of red cells may depend mainly on cell pH rather than on extracellular pH(pHe) and the difference of pH across the membrane may change. During study on lactate formation at various conditions of red cells, we noticed that glycolytic rate as well as concentration of DPG increased in anaerobic condition(Asakura et al.,1966b). From the observations that treatment of deoxygenated cells with carbon monoxide depressed glycolytic rate to the same extent as that with oxygen, and the pH-glycolytic activity curve shifted to alkaline side by oxygenation of the cells, we explained the phenomenon to be due to pHi-change by oxygenation of hemoglobin. The pHi-change was later directly demonstrated by Duhm and Gerlach(1971). Duhm(1971) has also demonstrated effect of DPG concentration on pHi of red cells, which fits beautifully to that calculated from the classical theory of the Donnan-equilibrium. Another implication of intracellular pH on red cell glycolysis has been shown by Tsuboi and Fukunaga(1970) that glycolytic rate increased when suspending saline solution is replaced by non-electrolyte solution such as iso-osmotic cellobiose medium.

In the present communication, pHi of red blood cells as measured by 5,5' -dimethyloxazolidine-2,4-dione(DMO) method of Waddel and Butler(1959) were studied at various conditions of red cells in connection with glycolytic process. Cells used were 1) preserved blood, 2) cells suspended in citrate containing medium and 3) those suspended in iso-osmotic sucrose solution. From these observations, we would like to stress the necessity of considering pHi, not only in study of red cell metabolism but also in practical fields such as blood preservation.

METHODS

Determination of Intracellular pH

ACD blood was kept in a refrigerator after addition of 4 uCi of ^{14}C-5,5'-dimethyloxazolidine-2,4-dione(DMO) per 100 ml of the blood. Samples were taken out at intervals by sterile syringes and pHi was calculated essentially according to Calvey(1970) from pHe, extra- and intracellular water content(Ve,Vi), radioactivities in plasma and whole blood (Cp,Cb) and pKa of DMO at 4°C(6.52 as determined by titration).

$$pHi = pKa + \log[\{Cb/Cp \cdot Vi - Ve/Vi\} \times \{1 + 10^{(pHe - pKa)}\} - 1]$$

The pHe(pH of the suspension) was measured by a Hitachi-Horiba Expanded Scale pH-Meter F-5 at 4°C with a combination electrode. It was standardized with primary standards(NBS Phosphate D and Phthalate) at 4°C. Plasma was separated by a refrigerated centrifuge and DMO extracted either from whole blood or plasma was measured for radioactivity with a liquid scintillation counter. The extracellular water content was calculated from hematocrit value with correction of intercellularly trapped water which amounted 2 % of packed cells. The intracellular water was the difference between the total water and the extracellular water.

The pHi at 37°C was similarly obtained by using ^{14}C-DMO which was added at least 10 min before separation of plasma, except that pHe determination and centrifugation were carried out at 37°C. The pH-meter was standardized at the temperature. The pKa value of DMO at 37°C was 6.13(Waddel and Butler,1959).

Study of Glycolysis

One day old ACD blood obtained from Fukuoka Red Cross Blood Bank was used. Red cells were washed with saline and incubated at 37°C under a pH-stat. Glycolytic intermediates and nucleotides were determined as described in previous publication(Minakami et al.,1965) except DPG which was assayed essentially according to Rose and Liebowitz(1970).

Table I. Effect of Temperature on pH of ACD Blood and Plasma

		Mean ± S.E.M.(n=9)
ACD Blood	pH at 4°C	7.43 ± 0.043
	pH at 37°C	6.93 ± 0.028
	ΔpH*	0.50 ± 0.022
ACD Plasma	pH at 4°C	7.40 ± 0.047
	pH at 37°C	7.10 ± 0.038
	ΔpH*	0.30 ± 0.015

*The difference of pH measured at 4°C and 37°C of each sample.

RESULTS AND DISCUSSION

pH of Blood Preserved in ACD Medium

We first studied pH of ACD blood, since its importance in blood preservation has been well-known. The first problem we encountered was temperature for the pH-measurement and we decided to carry out the measurement at 4°C, since it is the temperature at which the blood is preserved. Looking at literatures, we noticed that an adequate considerations has not been bestowed in the field of blood preservation for the effect of temperature on pH. Most investigators carry out the measurement at 37°C and some at room temperature. These pH values give us relatively little information, since the red cells will be in plasma of physiological pH as soon as the blood is transfused to body and since we are interested in stability of red cells during storage in a refrigerator. This is clearly shown by Beutler and Duron(1965) that there is little difference in the pH optimum for preservation of red cell ATP at 37°C and at 4°C when the actual hydrogen concentration at the temperature of storage is taken into consideration.

Fig.1 shows change of pHe and pHi of ACD blood during storage, which was measured at 4°C. The blood pH was about 0.5 unit higher than those reported by previous investigators who measured at 37°C, in good agreement with that reported by Beutler and Duron(1965). Unexpected observation is that the intracellular pH was higher than the blood pH, in apparent contradiction to the usual concept that the pHi of red cells is lower than the pHe(Tsuda et al.,1972). These observations can be explained by the temperature at which the pHi was measured and presence of citrate anion in ACD medium as shown below.

Remarkable effect of temperature on pH of whole blood and plasma has been noticed since introduction of blood pH-measurement(Yoshimura and Fujimoto,1937; Rosenthal,1948). The pH of ACD blood and ACD plasma at 4°C and 37° were shown in Table I. This change of pH is due to large negative temperature coefficient of pKa of proteins. The observation that

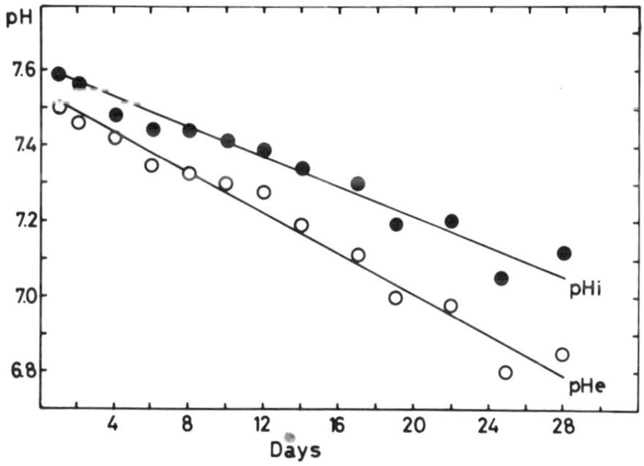

Figure 1. The extracellular pH(pHe) and the intracellular pH (pHi) at 4°C of ACD blood stored in a refrigerator.

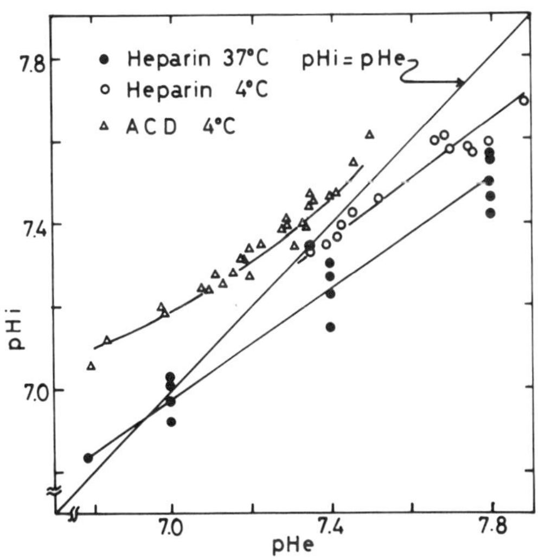

Figure 2. The pHe-pHi curves of heparinized blood(37°C and 4°C) and ACD blood(4°C). The pHe of heparinized blood was adjusted by NaOH or lactic acid solution. Left half of the curve for ACD blood at 4°C was that of stored ACD blood.

temperature effect for whole blood is larger than that for plasma, indicates that increase of proton inside the cells is greater than that in plasma, suggesting more pronounced change of cell pH by temperature change than that of blood.

Effects of temperature and citrate on red cell pH are shown in Fig. 2. When intracellular pH of heparinized blood was measured at 37°C, the result was essentially in agreement with those reported by previous investigators(Waddel and Bates 1968, as review). When both extracellular and intracellular pH were measured at 4°C, a line was obtained which is approximately parallel to that at 37°C but with upward shift. This shows that cell pH shifts to alkaline side when cooled, and extent of the shift is more than that of blood pH. The line for ACD blood shifts further upward compared with the line for heparinized blood at the temperature. These observations can be explained by the Donnan equilibrium.

If decrease in the dissociation of protein anions inside the cells is greater than that outside of the cells, which happens when blood is refrigerated, the Donnan ratio:

$$r = [Cl^-]_i/[Cl^-]_o = [H^+]_o/[H^+]_i$$

increased, so that the intracellular pH at given blood pH shifts to alkaline side. Similar consideration can be applied to the effect of citrate. When citrate, impermeable anion (Garby,1965), is added to blood, the Donnan ratio increases, so that cell pH shifts further to alkaline side. Effect of citrate on cell pH has been observed by Funder and Wieth (1966).

Preliminary experiments to measure ATP and DPG in blood preserved at various conditions showed that maintenance of these two important components depended on the pH inside the cells. Cell pH of about 7.4 at 4°C seemed to be an appropriate condition for maintenance of both ATP and DPG in heparinized blood, though further study is necessary, with due consideration of plasma pH and other factors. It should be stressed that the cell pH of ACD blood during storage is not acidic as sometimes misunderstood from the blood pH at 37°C.

The present result also tells us about considerations of temperature at which heparinized blood is to be handled. Biochemists have a habit to keep and handle biological samples at low temperature. The intracellular pH of heparinized blood increased to as high as pH 7.8 when it was cooled to 4°C, which caused decrease in ATP and increase in DPG.

Effect of Citrate on Glycolysis

If addition of citrate to blood cause increase of cell pH as indicated above, glycolytic rate is supposed to change by the addition. When citrate was added to red cell suspension incubated at 37°C under a pH-stat at pH 7.4 to a final concentration of 33 mM, the lactate formation increased about 20 % (Tomoda et al.,1973). This citrate effect on glycolytic rate depended on pH of the suspension and it was almost negligible at pH 8.0. The possibility that this citrate-effect is due to change of intracellular pH was shown by the pHe-glycolytic rate curve(Fig.3). With addition of citrate, the curve shifed 0.2 unit to acidic side, which can be explained by the shift of cell pH to alkaline side. This was confirmed by the direct measurement with DMO method.

Another confirmation for the shift of cell pH was given by measurement of glycolytic intermediates shown in Fig. 4. When citrate was added to red cell suspension, glucose 6-phosphate decreased and fructose diphosphate increased. This pattern is similar to that observed when pH of the suspension shifts to alkaline side(Minakami and Yoshikawa,1966). Occurrence of cross-over at phosphofructokinase is the most sensitive indication to suggest the possible change of pH.

Tsuboi and Fukunaga(1970) observed acceleration of glycolysis by replacing saline suspending medium with iso-osmotic citrate solution. They explained this phenomenon by acceleration of ATP break-down, since they observed accompanied ATP decrease. In the present experiment, decrease of ATP was not observed by addition of citrate. Change of glycolytic rate as well as that of glycolytic intermediate pattern could be explained by change of intracellular pH.

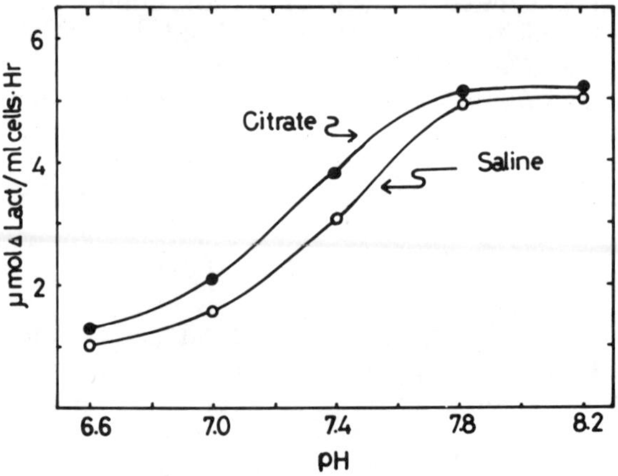

Figure 3. The pHe-glycolytic activity curves of red cells with or without citrate. The cells were incubated in 120 mM NaCl, 5 mM KCl, 1 mM $MgCl_2$, 2 mM sodium phosphate and 10 mM glucose under a pH-stat. Sodium citrate-citric acid solution (1 M) was added to a final concentration of 33 mM. Hematocri value was 20-30 %. Lactate formation before and after the addition of citrate was measured.

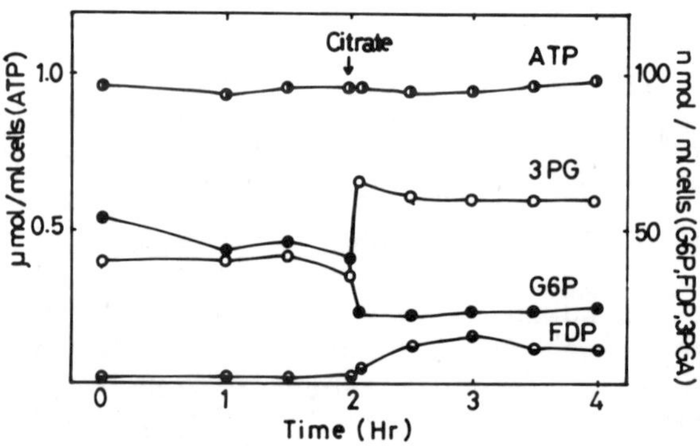

Figure 4. Changes of glycolytic intermediates and ATP by the addition of citrate at pH 7.4. Experimental conditions were as in Fig. 3.

Glycolysis of Red Cells in Sucrose Solution

Another condition which causes change of red cell pH is the replacement of saline with iso-osmotic non-electrolyte solution. This is due to the exchange of cellular Cl^- with OH^- of the medium. When red blood cells were added to isotonic sucrose solution, almost instantaneous decrease of medium pH was observed, which was then followed by the slow increase (Jacob and Parpart,1933;Wilbrandt,1940;LaCelle and Rothstein, 1966). This is the reflection of pH change inside the cells: rapid initial increase of cellular pH and the subsequent slow decrease. Fig. 5 shows the relation of pHe and pHi, which is measured by DMO-method, 30 min after the addition of cells into isotonic sucrose solution. Slight decrease of cell pH was observed with time.

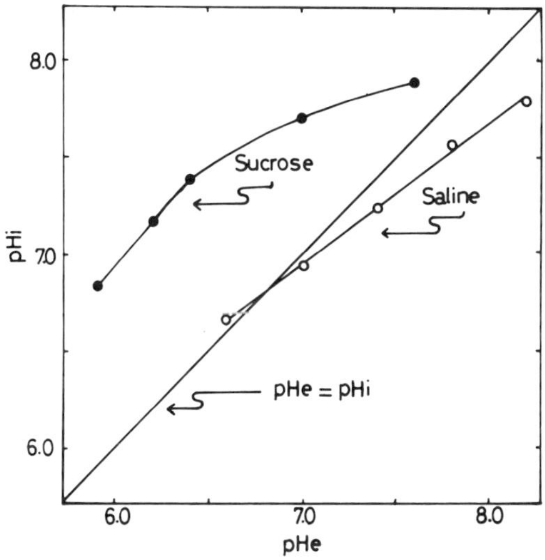

Figure 5. The pHe-pHi curves of red cells suspended in saline and in isotonic sucrose solution. Composition of saline was as in Fig. 3. Packed red cells were preincubated for 15 min at 37°C, suspended in a solution(250 mM sucrose, 5 mM KCl, 1 mM $MgCl_2$, 2 mM sodium phosphate and 10 mM glucose) to 5-7 % hematocrit and incubated with ^{14}C-DMO under a pH-stat. Plasma was separated 30 min after suspension.

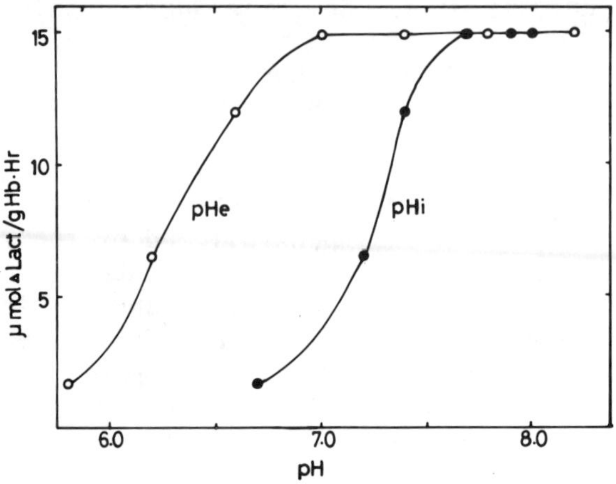

Figure 6. The pH-glycolytic activity curve of red cells in sucrose medium. The cells were incubated as in Fig. 5 and the pHe curve was obtained. The pHi curve was calculated from the pHe curve and the pHe-pHi curve in Fig. 5.

The increase of glycolytic rate by addition of sucrose was observed by de Verdier and Garby(1968) and by us(Minakami, 1968), but it was at first considered to be due to osmotic swelling and shrinking of the cells. Tsuboi and Fukunaga(1970) has shown activation of glycolysis in isotonic medium containing apparent inert solutes of limited cell permeability such as sucrose and cellobiose. Tsuboi(1974) explained this phenomenon by both intracellular change of pH and activation of membrane ATPase in non-electrolyte media.

Fig. 6 shows the pH-glycolytic rate curve of red cells suspended in the sucrose solution. The rate was half-maximal at about pH 6.4, in contrast to that of the saline suspension which is about pH 7.4. This anomalous pH curve can be explained by shift of cell pH shown in Fig. 5. Normal pH curve was obtained when it was plotted against intracellular pH.

Another indication of cell pH change was obtained from

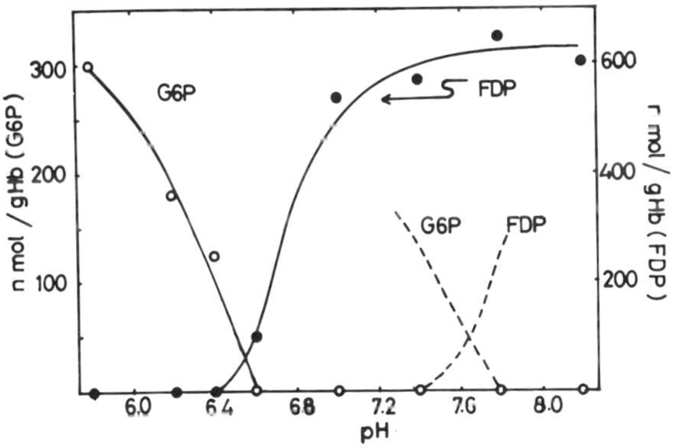

Figure 7. Dependence of glucose 6-phosphate(G6P) and fructose diphosphate(FDP) on pHe of red cells suspended in isotonic sucrose solution. Conditions of incubation were as in Fig. 5. Concentrations of G6P and FDP were those 15 min after suspending in sucrose solution. Dotted lines indicate those of the cells incubated in saline medium.

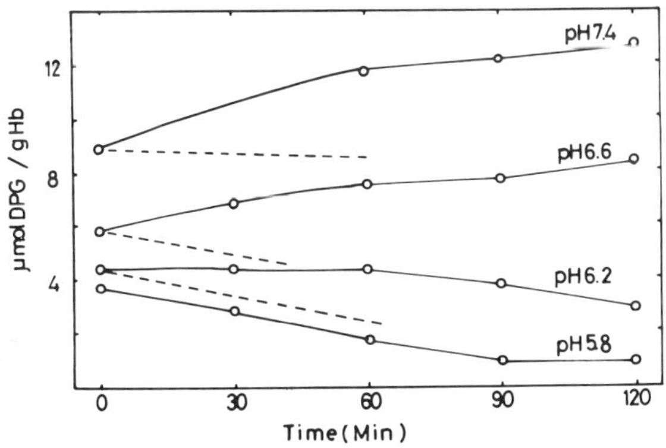

Figure 8. Change of 2,3-diphosphoglycerate in red cells suspended in sucrose medium of various pHe. Dotted lines indicate those of the cells incubated in saline solution.

changes of glycolytic intermediates. As shown in Fig. 7, glucose 6-phosphate increased when the suspension was acidified to lower than pH 6.6 and fructose diphosphate increased when pH was elevated to above pH 6.4. This is in contrast to the suspension in saline medium, which was shown by dotted lines. Apparent shift of the pH was about 1 unit, which is in good agreement with the shift of cell pH shown in Fig.5 and 6. Similar conclusion may be obtained from the measurement of DPG. Even at pH 6.6, DPG tended to increase, in contrast to the saline suspension which is shown by dotted lines(Fig. 8).

Although above mentioned results indicate that the acceleration of glycolytic rate is mainly due to shift of intracellular pH, the contribution of ATP break-down could not be neglected. When ATP determination were made, its level rapidly decreased in less than 5 min after the addition of red cell into the sucrose solution. Since this rapid decrease did not correspond to the amount of fructose diphosphate and triose phosphates increased, it may be due to the activation of ATPase by the organic cell impermeates as described by Tsuboi(1974).

SUMMARY

The intracellular pH(pHi) of red blood cells was measured by 5,5'-dimethyloxazolidine-2,4-dione(DMO) method and discussed in connection with glycolytic activity, in order to provoke attention to the necessity of considering pHi in study of metabolism and blood preservation. The initial pHi of ACD blood at 4°C was about pH 7.5 and higher than the blood pH(pHe). The high pHi is due to low temperature and presence of citrate in medium. Stimulation of glycolysis was observed when citrate was added to red blood cell suspension at constant pHe(7.4 at 37°C). This can be explained by the shift of pHi. Similarly, effect of sucrose to accelerate glycolysis can be explained mainly by the shift of pHi.

ACKNOWLEDGEMENT

Competent technical assistance of Miss Miltes Oba is

acknowledged. Her present address is Instituto Paranaense de Patologia Clinica,Londrina,Parana, Brasil. Authors express their thanks to Dr.M.Yoshinari of Fukuoka Red Cross Blood Bank for his generous supply of ACD blood. Part of this study was aided by Scientific Research Fund of Ministry of Education.

REFERENCES

Asakura,T.,Sato,Y.,Minakami,S.,and Yoshikawa,H.(1966a). pH-Dependency of 2,3-diphosphoglycerate content in red blood cells. Clin.Chim.Acta 14:840

Asakura,T.,Sato,Y.,Minakami,S.,and Yoshikawa,H.(1966b). Effect of deoxygenation of intracellular hemoglobin on red cell glycolysis. J.Biochem. 59:524

Beutler,E.,and Duron,O.,(1965). Effect of pH on preservation of red cell ATP. Transfusion 5:17

Calvey,T.N.(1970). Intracellular pH in mature and immature rabbit red cells. Quart.J.Exp.Physiol.55:238

de Verdier,C.-H.,and Garby,L.(1968). Glycolysis in shrunken and swollen erythrocytes. Folia Haemat. 89:418

Duhm,J.(1971). Effects of 2,3-diphosphoglycerate and other organic phosphate compounds on oxygen affinity and intracellular pH of human erythrocytes. Pflügers Arch.326:341

Duhm,J.,and Gerlach,E.(1971). On the mechanisms of the hypoxia-induced increase of 2,3-diphosphoglycerate in erythrocytes. Studies on rat erythrocytes in vivo and on human erythrocytes in vitro. Pflügers Arch. 326:254

Funder,J.,and Wieth,J.O.(1966). Chloride and hydrogen ion distribution between human red cells and plasma. Acta Physiol.Scand. 68:234

Garby,L.(1961/62). Citrationenpermeabilität der roten Blutkörperchen. Folia Haemat. 78:295

Jacobs,M.H.,and Parpart,A.K.(1933). Osmotic properties of the erythrocytes VI. The influence of the escape of salts on hemolysis by hypotonic solutions. Biol.Bull. 65:512

LaCelle,P.,and Rothstein,A.(1966). The passive permeability of the red blood cell to cations. J.Gen.Physiol. 50:171

Minakami,S.(1968). Regulation of glycolysis in human red cells. Application of "crossover" theorem. In Deutsch,E., Gerlach,E.,and Moser,K.,eds. "Metabolism and membrane permeability of erythrocytes and thrombocytes". Georg Thieme Verlag, Stuttgart. p. 10.

Minakami,S.,Suzuki,C.,Saito,T.,and Yoshikawa,H.(1965). Determination of glycolytic intermediates in human erythrocytes. J.Biochem. 58:543

Minakami,S.,and Yoshikawa,H.(1966). The effect of active cation transport, pH and inorganic phosphate concentration on erythrocyte glycolysis. J.Biochem. 59:145

Murphy,J.R.(1960). Erythrocyte metabolism. II. Glucose metabolism and pathways. J.Lab.Clin.Med. 55:286

Rapoport,S.,and Guest,G.M.(1939). The decomposition of diphosphoglycerate in acidified blood:its relation to reactions of glycolytic cycle. J.Biol.Chem. 129:781

Rona,P.,and Wilenko,G.G.(1914). Beiträge zur Frage der Glykolyse. IV. Biochem.Z. 60:1

Rose,Z.W.,and Liebowitz,J.(1970). Direct determination of 2,3-diphosphoglycerate. Anal.Biochem. 35:177

Rosenthal,T.B.(1948). The effect of temperature on the pH of blood and plasma in vitro. J.Biol.Chem. 173:25

Tomoda,A.,Tsuda,S.,and Minakami,S.(1973). Acceleration of red cell glycolysis by citrate due to intracellular pH enhancement. Experientia 29:539

Tsuboi,K.K.(1974). Regulation of erythrocyte glycolysis. Membrane mediated activation induced in low electrolyte medium. Biochim.Biophys.Acta 352:307

Tsuboi,K.K.,and Fukunaga,K.(1970). Relationship of solute permeability to erythrocyte glycolysis. Biochi.Biophys. Acta 196:215

Tsuda,S.,Kakinuma,K.,and Minakami,S.(1972). Intracellular pH of red cells stored in acid citrate dextrose medium. Experientia 28:1481

Waddell,W.J.,and Bates,R.G.(1969). Intracellular pH. Physiol.Rev. 49:285

Waddell,W.J.,and Butler,T.C.(1959). Calculation of intracellular pH from the distribution of 5,5'-dimethyl-2,4-oxazolidinedione(DMO). Application to skeletal muscle of the dog. J.Clin.Invest. 38:720

Wilbrandt,W.(1940). Ionenpermeabilität der Erythrocyten in Nicht-leiterlösungen. Pflügers Arch. 243:537

Yoshimura,H.,and Fujimoto,T.(1937). Studies on the blood pH estimated by the glass electrode method VI. J.Biochem. 25:493

DISCUSSION

Dr. Diederich: How does the red cell pH measured by the DMO method compare with that measured by the freeze-thaw lysis?

Dr. Minikami: By DMO method we get the values about 0.1 units higher than that by the hemolysis method. There are discussions about which is the true intracellular pH.

Dr. Brain: This is a very fascinating paper because it has profound bearing on many of the studies being carried out on red cell metabolism. I think if my memory is right, Dr. Baglinni and coworkers showed that red cells in isotonic bis Tris buffer showed a very comparable shift and rise in pH. It has been of some concern to me--though I don't know whether Dr. Zelda Rose will comment about this--whether in fact phosphate which is being used in 10mM or even higher amounts as a so-called ideal buffer might not also be accompanied by a rise in pH. If anyone is interested in the possible interaction with various compounds affecting red cell metabolism, it's obviously of great importance to distinguish between the possible pH effects and the specific effects of compounds like phosphate.

Dr. Minakami: We are interested in the phosphate effects as to whether part of it can be explained by pH change or not, but so far we have not observed changes with high concentration of phosphate.

Dr. Duhm: May I comment on the question whether inorganic phosphate can influence the red cell pH? In extensive studies of Deuticke and Gerlach and of other authors it has been shown that inorganic phosphate penetrates relatively rapidly through the human red cell membrane although much slower than chloride, for instance. Upon addition of inorganic phosphate to the suspension one has to expect, therefore, only a transient rise of the red cell pH lasting for about 30-60 minutes or even for shorter times. However, one has to take into account that considerable species differences exist.

Dr. Minakami: I expected the change on the ground you mentioned, but I could not obtain convincing results.

Dr. Diederich: At the risk of asking a ridiculous question, is there a compositional difference in the red cell 4° versus 37° that explains the reversal of pH? We normally think of the lower pH inside the red cell. You are saying that this is completely reversed. Is that all a temperature phenomenon or did I misunderstand what you said? For instance having a red cell pH at 7.5 with a whole blood pH of 7.4, now is that a function of temperature?

Dr. Minakami: Yes, I think so. I would like to give an example of the temperature effect. Dr. Rapoport's group showed the changes of glycolytic intermediates by the change of temperature from 4°C to 37°C. Their crossover plot can be explained almost completely by the change in pH: they observed an increase in glucose-6-phosphate and a decrease in fructose diphosphate by warming up cooled red blood cells to 37°.

Dr. Duhm: If I understood you right, the fact that the red cell pH was higher than the extracellular pH in ACD blood temperature has to be interpreted to be due mainly to the presence of citrate in the ACD blood?

Dr. Minakami: Yes. However, if we compare the heparinized blood at 37° and the ACD blood at 4°C., the difference of pH_i can be explained by two factors: 1) the effect of temperature and 2) the effect of citrate. The effect of temperature is bigger than that of citrate.

Dr. Tanaka: Dr. Diederich, was that your question as to which component is really the primary one?

Dr. Diederich: I have difficulty thinking about the pH inside the red cell being higher than outside the red cell. It is difficult to conceptualize a higher red cell pH than whole blood, that's my only point. Can this be explained by temperature only? The red cell functions at 37° so that doesn't cause me great difficulty, but it is very hard for me to understand how the Donnan equilibrium can explain the red cell you reported at 4°.

Dr. Salhany: It is probably explicable because the pK's of the proteins are temperature dependent, so you change the temperature and change the pK's and what might be happening is that relative to the inside the outside pK's are different. I looked at Bis-Tris in the past and what happens if I recall is that Bis-Tris raises the pH_i because it is a nondiffusable buffer and the Donnan equilibrium shifts such that the pH_i rises.

Dr. Brewer: The ACD solution for blood storage has been arrived at empirically as a good preservative. I always assumed that it was because it slowed down glycolysis, partly because of the decrease in pH_i. Now you say the pH_i is really about 7.8. Should I assume that as we search for other blood preservatives we should try to obtain a similar pH, based upon the success of ACD?

Dr. Minakami: That's a point I want to make; but not 7.8; around 7.5 or 7.6.

Dr. Brain: I think the temperature effect is an interesting one because we certainly observed that if you spin cells at 4°C, wash them, and resuspend them in an appropriate buffer, there are perturbations in the levels of glycolytic intermediates which after an hour or so return to normal values. Perhaps the lesson is that we should be cautious about the buffers we use; they shouldn't be impermeable, but we also shouldn't really lower the temperature of cells. We should wash them, if not at 37°, certainly at room temperature as we are having effects which are very significant for the metabolism of the cells.

Dr. Minakami: We are also working on the platelets and leukocytes and we prefer to treat them at room temperature. We do not want to cool them down, due to the change in pH_i.

Dr. Tanaka: Yes, I think that is a very practical point. As long as one is able to do the experiments in a relatively short period of time.

Dr. Meyers: I have noted effects of temperature on red cells, but I have not given them the importance which you have. If we store red cells at 4° overnight and take certain measurements 12 hours later, would you advise that we adjust the pH when they return to ambient temperature? Are these pH-temperature changes you speak of reversible?

Dr. Minakami: The pH of blood shifts to about 8.0 when cooled down to 4°C. In this condition, the level of ATP is reduced to half after 10 hours. We can keep ATP, if we adjust the pH at 4°C. The change of pH by temperature is essentially reversible but that of ATP is not due to deamination. The simplest way is to use acidic solution such as ACD, even for several hours' storage.

Dr. Tanaka: Are there any other comments or questions? Thank you very much, Dr. Minakami.

STUDIES ON 2,3-DIPHOSPHOGLYCERATE: EFFECTS ON HEMOGLOBIN, GLYCOLYSIS, AND ON BUFFERING PROPERTIES OF HUMAN ERYTHROCYTES

Jochen Duhm

Physiologisches Institut

Universität München, München, Germany

The most prominent function of 2,3-diphosphoglycerate (DPG) in erythrocytes of man and many other mammalian species consists in decreasing the oxygen affinity of hemoglobin. However, DPG alters not only the oxyhemoglobin dissociation curve but also influences the binding of CO_2 and hydrogen ions to hemoglobin (cf. recent reviews 4,8,26,35).

Another effect of DPG not directly related to hemoglobin function concerns its inhibitory effect on a number of glycolytic enzymes (11,12,40,48). Enzymes of pentose and nucleotide metabolism are also inhibited by DPG (5,20,30,45). These inhibitory effects are caused either by interactions of DPG with the enzyme proteins or by the Mg^{++}-chelating property of DPG, or by both. Furthermore, DPG affects red cell metabolism due to its influence on the Gibbs-Donnan equilibrium of penetrating ions and on the red cell pH, respectively (19,21,44). Finally, DPG might alter the buffering power of erythrocytes since the pK_2 values of the two phosphate groups are within the physiological pH range (9,13).

This report deals with three of the properties of DPG mentioned above. First, an attempt is made to gain insight into the mutual interactions of DPG, CO_2, hydrogen ions, KCl and oxygen with the hemoglobin molecule at high hemoglobin concentrations in terms of measurements of P_{50} values; particular emphasis will be directed to the question whether fully oxygenated hemoglobin binds DPG. Secondly, the mechanism of the inhibition by DPG of red cell glycolysis is studied in order to differentiate inhibitory effects mediated by changes of the intracellular pH (19) from those caused by direct enzyme inhibition (32-34,40). Finally, it will be shown that high red cell DPG concentrations can affect the buffering properties of blood in a way opposite to that to be expected.

EFFECTS OF DPG, CO_2 AND KCl ON THE OXYGEN AFFINITY AND THE BOHR EFFECT OF HUMAN HEMOGLOBIN

The purpose of these studies was to quantify the effects of DPG and CO_2 on the oxygen affinity and the Bohr effect of human hemoglobin at hemoglobin concentrations and pH values close to those prevailing in the intact erythrocyte. In addition, the effects of increased KCl concentrations on the interactions of DPG, CO_2, H^+ and oxygen with the hemoglobin molecule were studied. Some of the results were already presented elsewhere (23-25).

The data summarized in Figure 1 demonstrate the effects of changes of DPG concentration and of pH on the P_{50} of solutions containing about 70% of the hemoglobin concentration in intact erythrocytes. The P_{50} value - given as log P_{50} - increased both with rising DPG concentration and with lowering of the pH. Elevation of DPG concentration from <0.1 to 8 mM resulted in an increase in the negative slope of the lines relating log P_{50} and pH, indicating changes in the Bohr coefficient $\Delta \log P_{50}/\Delta pH$. With

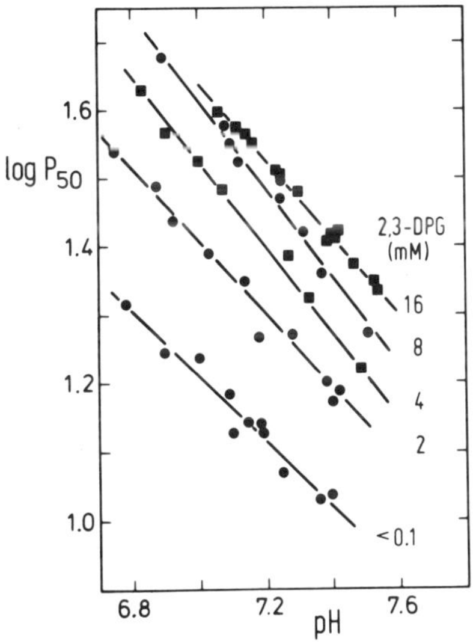

Figure 1

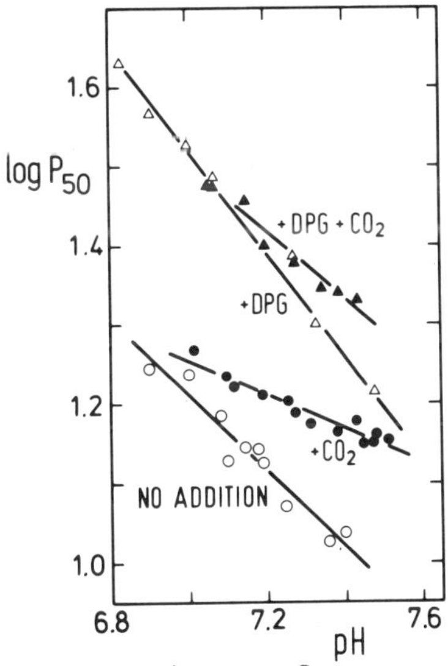

Figure 2

Figure 1: Effects of DPG on the P_{50} and the Bohr effect of human hemoglobin (37°C, P_{CO_2} <1 mmHg, 170 mmoles Cl^-/l water, 3.5±0.1 mmoles Hb_4/l solution).-Washed human erythrocytes were hemolyzed by freezing in liquid nitrogen and thawing. Membranes were removed using toluene. The hemolysates were dialyzed (4°C, 2-3 days) against solutions containing 130 mM KCl and 18 mM $NaHCO_3$ until the molar ratio of total phosphate to hemoglobin was less than 0.1. Aliquots of 0.1 ml of the hemoglobin solutions were equilibrated with water-saturated gas mixtures of known composition for 15 min. O_2 saturations were determined spectrophotometrically (21). The P_{50} valus (O_2 pressures in mmHg at 50% O_2 saturation of hemoglobin) were calculated from Hill plots computed from 3-5 measurements of O_2 saturation in the range of 20-80% HbO_2 (21). The pH was varied by addition of 0.3 M $NaHCO_3$ or 0.3n HCl.

Figure 2: Effects of 4 mM DPG and 40 mmHg CO_2 on the P_{50} and the Bohr effect of human hemoglobin (37°C, 3.5 mM Hb_4). For experimental details see legend of Figure 1.

further elevation of DPG concentration the slope decreased again. These findings demonstrate that the effects of DPG on the O_2 affinity and the Bohr effect of hemoglobin in concentrated solutions correspond to those observed in more diluted systems (9,50).

In Figure 2 the effects of physiological concentrations of DPG and CO_2 alone and of simultaneous addition of both effectors on the relation between the P_{50} and pH are compared. Both DPG and CO_2 decreased the oxygen affinity, whereas the Bohr effect was affected by the two agents in the opposite direction, namely increased by DPG and decreased by CO_2. The efficiency of one agent became considerably reduced in the presence of the second one, indicating that DPG and CO_2 mutually influence their action on the hemoglobin molecule. These resuls agree closely with observations on solutions containing 2 mM hemoglobin (35).

In the following only P_{50} values and Bohr coefficients computed from regression lines like those shown in Figures 1 and 2 shall be considered. Figure 3 demonstrates the effects of DPG, CO_2 and elevated KCl concentrations on the P_{50} at pH 7.2. Apparently, increasing DPG concentrations reduced the oxygen affinity in a curvilinear manner in the absence and the presence of the other effectors. CO_2 increased the P_{50}, the effect being more pronounced at the lower Cl^- concentration than at the higher one. The effect of Cl^- on the P_{50} tended to vanish at high DPG concentrations. The effect of DPG did not disappear at 670 mM Cl^-. This latter observation is in contrast to results obtained on more diluted hemoglobin solutions (9). At the moment it cannot be decided whether this discrepancy is due to a hemoglobin concentration effect (29) or to other differences in experimental conditions.

Calculation of DPG-Binding Constants of Hemoglobin from P_{50} Values

Although calculations using all the determinations of O_2 saturation underlying the data given in Figures 1 to 3 might provide more information concerning the functional properties of hemoglobin (31), an attempt was made to calculate binding constants from P_{50} values. Before going into details it should be pointed out that the binding constants to be calculated in the following have to be regarded with certain reservations: First, the ionic strength was not kept constant in the experiments since the addition of DPG was not counterbalanced by removal of KCl. Secondly, the experimental error, amounting to about ± 1.5% saturation and ± 1 mmHg for the determinations of O_2 saturation and P_{50} values, must be considered. Thirdly, the changes of O_2 solubility in water resulting from alterations of the ionic strength have not been taken into account. Finally a number of assumptions had to be made which might cause some unexpected error.

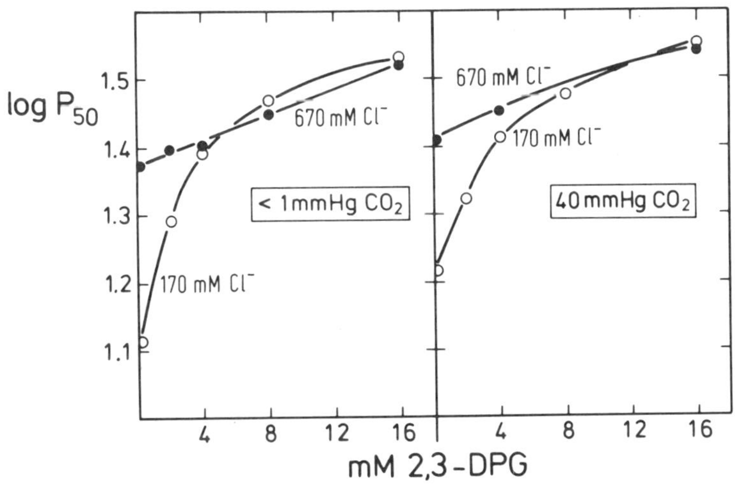

Figure 3: P_{50} of human hemoglobin as affected by DPG, CO_2 and KCl (37°C, 3.5 mM Hb_4, pH 7.2).

It was assumed that all 4 O_2 molecules bind at once to the hemoglobin tetramer, i.e. that no intermediates exist other than Hb and $Hb(O_2)_4$. This assumption of an infinite strength of tertiary-quaternary interaction certainly does not meet the properties of the hemoglobin molecule. The error introduced appears to be small, however, since the sum of the concentrations of the two hemoglobin species mentioned seems to exceed by far the concentrations of the other possible intermediates with 1-3 O_2 molecules bound (49). Furthermore, the latter three intermediates might exhibit one of the two quaternary conformations characteristic for Hb and $Hb(O_2)_4$. Secondly it was assumed that the DPG effect is due to a preferential binding of the anion to one of the two quaternary conformations which each has one binding site. Thus, binding of DPG to both Hb and $Hb(O_2)_4$ is permitted.

Under these assumptions the binding of O_2 to hemoglobin in the absence and presence of DPG can be described by equations (1) and (2), and the binding of DPG to deoxy- and oxyhemoglobin by equations (3) and (4):

$$Hb + 4O_2 \rightleftharpoons Hb(O_2)_4 \quad (1)$$

$$Hb + HbDPG + DPG + 4O_2 \rightleftharpoons Hb(O_2)_4 + Hb(O_2)_4DPG + DPG \quad (2)$$

$$Hb + DPG \rightleftharpoons HbDPG; \qquad K_3 = \frac{[HbDPG]}{[Hb]\,[DPG]} \quad (3)$$

$$Hb(O_2)_4DPG + DPG \rightleftharpoons Hb(O_2)_4DPG; K_4 = \frac{[Hb(O_2)_4DPG]}{[Hb(O_2)_4]\,[DPG]}. \quad (4)$$

At the P_{50}

$$K_1 = \frac{1}{(P_{50})^4}, \quad \text{and } K_2 = \frac{[Hb(O_2)_4]\,[Hb(O_2)_4DPG]}{[Hb]\,[HbDPG]\,(P_{50}^{+})^4}$$

when O_2 concentrations are substituted by O_2 pressure (P_{50} and P_{50}^{+} are the P_{50} values determined in the absence and presence of DPG). By dividing K_1 by K_2 one obtains:

$$\frac{(P_{50}^{+})^4}{(P_{50})^4} = \frac{[Hb(O_2)_4]}{[Hb]}$$

The two unknown quantities $[Hb(O_2)_4]$ and [Hb] in this equation can be substituted by using equations (3) and (4) when taking into account that the P_{50}

$$[Hb_t]/2 = [Hb(O_2)_4] + [Hb(O_2)_4DPG] = [Hb] + [HbDPG],$$

where Hb_t indicates the total concentration of hemoglobin. After appropriate rearrangements and taking logs one obtains

$$\log P_{50}^{+} - \log P_{50} = 0.25 \log \frac{1 + [DPG]\,K_3}{1 + [DPG]\,K_4} \quad (5)$$

For the left side of this equation measured values are available (see **Figure** 3). On the right side we find the binding constants of deoxy- and oxyhemoglobin for DPG (K_3 and K_4), and the concentration of free DPG. The latter can be calculated from the known total DPG concentration by the equation

$$[DPG_t] = [HbDPG] + [Hb(O_2)_4DPG] + [DPG]$$

when inserting the values for [HbDPG] and $[Hb(O_2)_4DPG]$. These two quantities are equal to

$$\frac{[Hb_t]/2 \cdot [DPG] \cdot K}{1 + [DPG] \cdot K}$$

where K is K_3 and K_4 in the case of [HbDPG] and $[Hb(O_2)_4DPG]$. Thus, only K_3 and K_4 are unknown which can be varied independently of each other to obtain the best fit of equation (5).It may be mentioned that other authors (18,49) obtained an equation similar to equation (5). In the equation of Szabo and Karplus which was derived in an entirely different way (49) the constant factor is given as 0.27. On the basis of the concept outlined this value would indicate that less than 4 O_2 molecules are bound to fully oxygenated hemoglobin.

The binding constants approximated by this procedure are summarized in Table 1. Before discussing the values given in this Table the attention may be directed to Figure 4. In this graph the best fits of equation (5) obtained for P_{50} values determined under two different experimental conditions are shown as examples. The closed symbols refer to values obtained assuming that both deoxy- and oxyhemoglobin can bind DPG. The values indicated by the open symbols are obtained assuming that only deoxyhemoglobin binds DPG. It appears that the closed symbols fit very well with the theoretical relation (solid lines), whereas the open symbols (connected by broken lines) show a systematic devia-

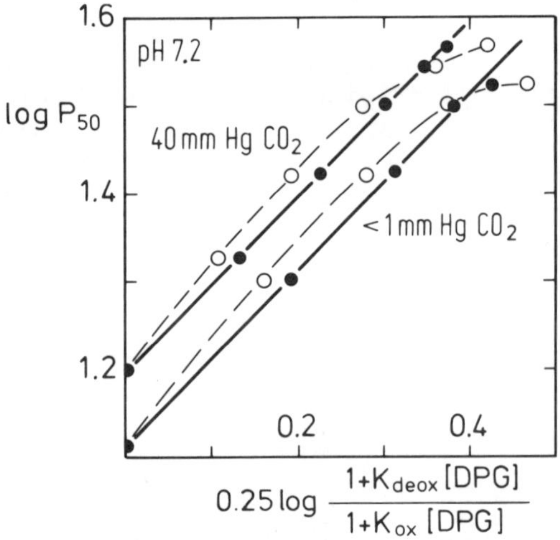

Figure 4: Dependency of log P_{50} on the concentration of free DPG.- The experimental values were determined at pH 7.2 (37°C, 170 mM Cl^-, 3.5 mM Hb_4). K_{deox} and K_{ox} and the concentrations of free DPG were calculated as described in the text (cf. data given in Table 1). For further details see text.

tion and a greater scattering. Thus, the results strongly suggest that oxyhemoglobin exhibits a definite affinity for DPG.

In Table 1 the binding constants calculated under the two assumptions are compared. It may be noted that the DPG and hemoglobin concentrations given in the Figures as μmoles/ml solution were converted to μmoles/ml water for the calculations which were performed using a Wang computer 600-6. A mean water content of the solutions of 73% was determined experimentally. First the results shall be considered, which were obtained when binding of DPG to both hemoglobin conformations was assumed. It turned out that oxyhemoglobin exhibits a definite affinity for DPG at the lower KCl concentration but not at the higher one. The results meet the postulate that the ratio of the DPG binding constants of deoxy- and oxyhemoglobin should exceed a value of 20 (10): The binding constants of deoxyhemoglobin were found to be 60 to 80 times greater than those of oxyhemoglobin in the absence of CO_2, whereas in the presence of CO_2 this factor ranged between 36 and 53, indicating that CO_2 affects DPG binding to oxyhemoglobin to a lesser extent than to deoxyhemoglobin (29). CO_2 exhibited a profound effect on the binding constants, especially at the higher pH values. This result is in accordance with direct measurements of binding of DPG or CO_2 to hemoglobin (6,7,16,28,29, 39). The binding constants of the two hemoglobin conformations decreased with rising pH to a similar extent, indicating that the binding sites in oxy- and deoxyhemoglobin exhibit similar pK values.

When binding of DPG to oxyhemoglobin was not allowed much smaller binding constants were obtained (Table 1). Thus, the great influence of even a weak binding of DPG to oxyhemoglobin on the magnitude of the effect of DPG on the oxygen affinity of hemoglobin becomes apparent. The standard deviations of the

Table 1: Association constants of Hb and $Hb(O_2)_4$ For DPG (K_{deox} and K_{ox}, liters/mole) calculated from P_{50} values determined at 37°C (3.5 mM Hb_4). For details see text.

	P_{CO_2} <1 mmHg		P_{CO_2} = 40 mmHg	
Cl^- concentration (mM)	170	670	170	670
pH 6.9				
K_{deox}	15 500	130	4 700	./.
K_{ox}	218	0	88	
S_D	0.02	0.01	0.002	
K_{deox} when $K_{ox} \stackrel{!}{=} 0$	4 920		2 320	
S_D	0.05		.03	
pH 7.2				
K_{deox}	9 800	125	2 850	100
K_{ox}	164	0	66	4
S_D	0.006	0.01	0.003	0.003
K_{deox} when $K_{ox} \stackrel{!}{=} 0$	3 640		1 320	85
S_D	0.04		0.04	0.002
pH 7.5				
K_{deox}	7 000	95	800	./.
K_{ox}	84	0	22	
S_D	0.03	0.03	0.01	
K_{deox} when $K_{ox} \stackrel{!}{=} 0$	3 620		540	
S_D	0.04		0.02	

S_D is the standard deviation of the differences between the experimental values (left side of the equation) and the values calculated from the right side of the equation

$$\log P_{50,DPG_t=x} - \log P_{50,DPG_t=0} = 0.25 \log \frac{1 + K_{deox}\,[DPG]_{free}}{1 + K_{ox}\,[DPG]_{free}}$$

differences between the experimental values (left side of equation (5)) and the calculated values (right side of equation (5)) (S_D in Table 1) were smaller by a factor of 2 to 10 when binding also to oxyhemoglobin was permitted. Accordingly, the results strongly suggest that DPG is bound also to oxyhemoglobin. The affinity of oxyhemoglobin for DPG, however, appears to be much smaller than previously reported (17,28). The conclusion that oxyhemoglobin exhibits a definite affinity for DPG derived here from measurements of P_{50} values is in accordance with recent conclusions derived from studies on the oxygen-linked binding of H^+ to hemoglobin as affected by DPG (14,37).

Influence of DPG, CO_2 and KCl on the Bohr Effect of Human Hemoglobin

The effects of DPG, CO_2 and elevated KCl concentrations on the Bohr coefficient are summarized in Figure 5. In the absence of CO_2 and at the lower KCl concentration the Bohr coefficient first increased with rising DPG concentration and then decreased with further elevation of DPG levels (cf. Figure 1); the maximum of the effect was observed at molar ratios of DPG to hemoglobin of 2 to 3 (9, 50). Elevation of KCl concentration decreased the Bohr coefficient in the absence of CO_2 at all DPG levels and the maximum observed at the lower KCl concentration disappeared. Interestingly, all the four curves shown in Figure 5 tend to level off at a Bohr coefficient of about -0.5.

In the presence of CO_2 the Bohr coefficient was lowered and no maximum was observed. The KCl effect on the Bohr coefficient of stripped hemoglobin was reversed in the presence of CO_2, i.e. increasing salt concentration increased the Bohr coefficient (right panel of Figure 5). In the presence of DPG the "normal" KCl effect was observed, i.e. a decrease of the Bohr coefficient. This decrease was much smaller in the presence than in the absence of CO_2.

When taking into account that the change of the P_{50} resulting from a change of H^+ activity can be regarded as the reciprocal phenomenon of the oxylabile binding of hydrogen ions (51), the observed alterations of the Bohr effect can be explained on the basis of the present knowledge as follows (cf. reviews 4,8,35): The Bohr effect (only the alkaline Bohr effect is discussed here) is enhanced by DPG due to the preferential binding of DPG to deoxyhemoglobin and the consecutive increase of the pK values of the cationic groups of hemoglobin involved in DPG binding. On the other hand, the influence of DPG on the Bohr effect might simply be interpreted as a consequence of the higher affinity of hemoglobin for DPG at lower pH values. The decrease of the Bohr effect occurring with elevation of the molar ratio of DPG to hemoglobin above a value of 3 could be due to the increased binding of DPG to oxyhemoglobin at high DPG concentrations. Such a binding would counterbalance the effect of DPG on deoxyhemoglobin (41).

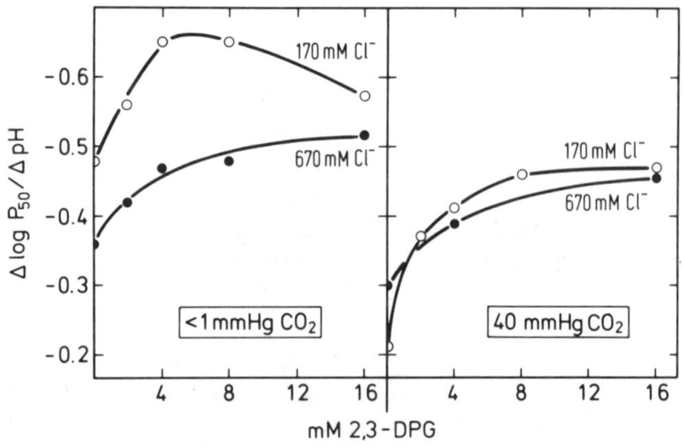

Figure 5: Effects of DPG, CO_2 and KCl on the Bohr coefficient of human hemoglobin. Experimental conditions as described in the legend of Figure 1.

The decrease of the Bohr coefficient caused by CO_2 has been interpreted as being due to the oxygen-linked carbamate formation (43). The influence of DPG on the CO_2-induced alterations of the Bohr effect should then be a result of a reduction of the amount of oxylabile carbamate in the presence of DPG (6, 7,39).

The influence of increased KCl concentrations on the Bohr effect in the absence of other effectors can be explained analogously as the DPG effect when assuming that Cl^- is bound preferentially to the deoxyconformation (2,3,4,15,35) and that oxyhemoglobin exhibits a lower affinity for the anion. Then one must accept that the measurements have been performed in a concentration range where the binding of Cl^- to oxyhemoglobin becomes increasingly significant (15). The effects of elevated KCl concentrations on the interactions of DPG and CO_2 with hemoglobin can be explained by KCl-induced inhibition of DPG binding (9) (see Table 1) and by a reduction of oxylabile CO_2 binding to hemoglobin in the presence of high KCl concentrations (24).

EFFECT OF DPG ON GLYCOLYSIS IN HUMAN ERYTHROCYTES

As already mentioned in the introduction, the rate of glycolysis is decreased in human erythrocytes containing high concentrations of DPG (19, 32-34, 40). The present studies were performed to analyse quantitatively the contribution of the two possible inhibitory effects to the total inhibition of red cell glycolysis by DPG (i.e. of inhibitory effects mediated by pH changes and by direct inhibition of rate limiting enzymes). The experimental approach consisted in measurements of glycolytic rates and of concentrations of glycolytic intermediates in human erythrocytes with normal or elevated concentrations of DPG, the intracellular pH of which had been varied between pH 6.8 and 7.3.

The effect of very high DPG levels on the rates of glucose consumption and of lactate production are shown in Figure 6 in dependence of the extracellular pH and of the intracellular pH, respectively. In this Figure the glycolytic flux rates have been related to hemoglobin on a molar basis in order to eliminate apparent changes in the rate of glycolysis resulting from changes in the red cell water content consecutive to changes of the extracellular pH and of the red cell DPG content (19,22). First the results obtained at different extracellular pH values will be considered. As shown in Figure 6 A, DPG inhibited markedly both glucose consumption and lactate production at all extracellular pH values. The magnitude of this effect increased with rising pH. Thus, the normal dependency of red cell glycolysis on the extracellular pH is almost completely lost in the "high-DPG" cells.

A completely different picture was obtained when the rates of glucose consumption and of lactate production were related to the intracellular pH (Figure 6 B): The characteristic pH dependency of the normal red cell glycolysis reappeared in the "high-DPG" cells. Obviously, the inhibition of glycolysis in "high-DPG" cells is far less pronounced at a given intracellular pH than at a given extracellular pH. At the normal values for the extracellular and intracellular pH of 7.4 and 7.2, for instance the rates of glucose consumption and of lactate production (the latter values are given in parantheses) were reduced in the "high-DPG" cells by about 70% (40%) and 40% (10%), respectively. Thus, one must conclude that the DPG-induced fall of the red cell pH contributes markedly to the reduction of the glycolytic rate in "high-DPG" cells. It is apparent, however, that another inhibitory effect must be involved.

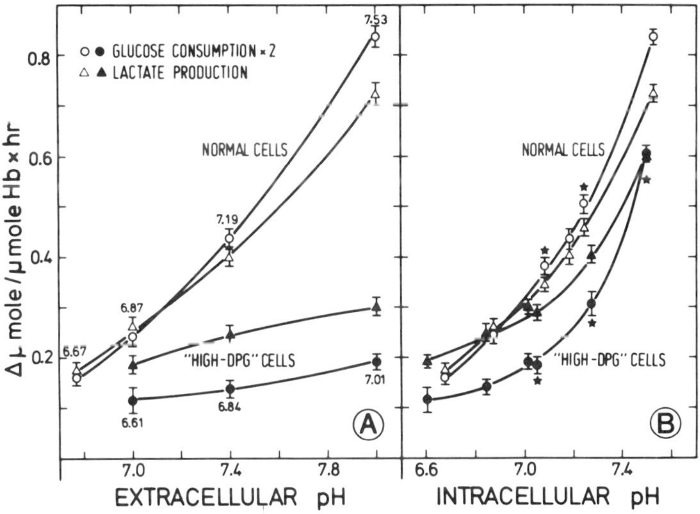

Figure 6: Effects of the extracellular and intracellular pH on glucose consumption x 2 (circles) and lactate production (triangles) in normal and "high-DPG" erythrocytes (37°C, mean values ± 1 SEM from 5-7 experiments).- DPG levels were elevated above the normal value of 4-5 μmoles/g cells to 20-25 μmoles/g cells ("high-DPG" cells) by preincubation in a medium containing (mM) inosine, 10, pyruvate, 10, inorganic phosphate, 75, and NaCl, 35 (37°C, hct 10-15%, incubation time 100 min) (19). The cells were then washed three times and incubated at 37°C in Locke solution for 60 min. After three further washings the cells were finally incubated in Locke solution for 5 hours (37°C, hct 30-35%). The intracellular pH was determined as described (21).
Ⓐ: Values determined at different extracellular pH values. The numbers below and above the two pairs of curves indicate the intracellular pH of the two types of erythrocytes.
Ⓑ: Values determined at different intracellular pH values. The asterisks indicate experiments in which 100 mM of NaCl of the suspension medium were replaced by 68 mM tri-sodium citrate in order to elevate the red cell pH (cf. 27).

To characterize the possible inhibitory effects of DPG on rate limiting glycolytic enzymes in intact erythrocytes the concentrations of selected glycolytic intermediates were determined in normal and "high-DPG" cells. As shown in Figure 1, the shapes of the dependencies on the intracellular pH of the concentrations of G-6-P, F-1,6-P, DAP+GA-3-P, and 3-PG were similar in normal and "high-DPG" cells, indicating that the regulatory properties of the enzyme phosphofructokinase are not altered in the presence of high DPG concentrations. The concentrations of G-6-P tended to be lower in "high-DPG" cells. This finding suggests that the enzyme hexokinase might be inhibited in the "high-DPG" cells.

The concentrations of F-1,6-P, and of DAP+GA-3-P were found to be almost identical in the two types of cells (Figure 7). The concentrations of 3-PG, however, were higher in "high-DPG"cells then

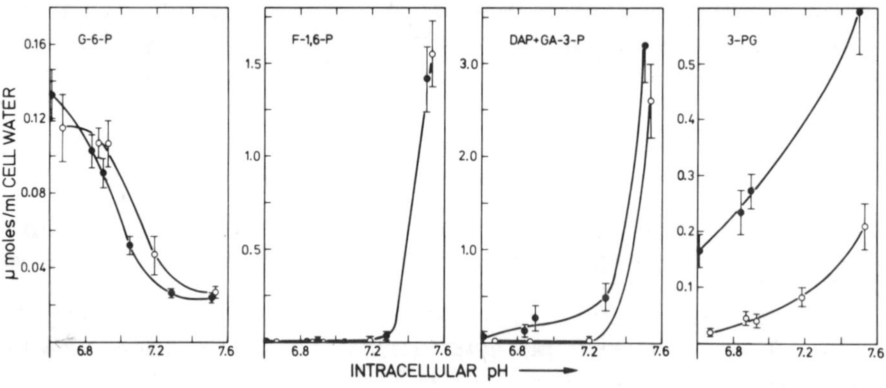

Figure 7: Effect of the red cell pH on glycolytic intermediates in normal erythrocytes (open circles) and "high-DPG" cells (closed circles). The values (means $\pm$ 1 SEM, 4-7 experiments) were determined after 5 hours of incubation. For experimental details see legend of Figure 6.

in normal erythrocytes. It is reasonable to assume that the concentrations of PEP were elevated to a similar extent since the reactions catalyzed by the enzymes enolase and phosphoglycerate mutase are close to the thermodynamic equilibrium in human erythrocytes (38); furthermore, the two reactions are not inhibited by DPG (48). Thus it is concluded that the enzyme pyruvate kinase is inhibited in "high-DPG" cells. It seems unlikely, however, that an inhibition of pyruvate kinase - an enzyme which controls the lower part of the glycolytic chain - can be made responsible for the reduction of glucose consumption in "high-DPG" erythrocytes (cf. 42).

In order to assess more in detail the possible inhibitory effect of elevated DPG concentrations on the hexokinase reaction, red cell glycolysis was studied under conditions where the hexokinase becomes the rate limiting enzyme for glucose degradation. This is true for cells with very low G-6-P levels due to the presence of methylene blue (1). The data shown in Figure 8 demonstrate that glucose consumption was inhibited in the "high-DPG" cells by 30-40% even in the presence of methylene blue. The

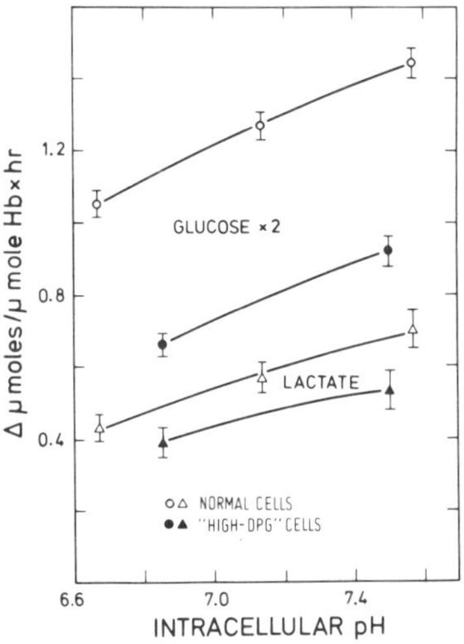

Figure 8: Glucose consumption x 2 and lactate production in normal erythrocytes (open symbols) and "high-DPG" cells (closed symbols) in the presence of 1 mM methylene blue. For experimental details see legend of Figure 6. Mean values (± 1 SEM) from 4 experiments.

absolute rates were considerably higher in the presence of methylene blue than in the absence of the redox dye, most probably due to the low G-6-P concentrations which were found to range between 0.015 and 0.025 µmoles/ml cell water (not shown) at all pH values, no significant differences being observable in the two types of erythrocytes. These results strongly indicate that the enzyme hexokinase is inhibited by elevation of DPG concentration in intact erythrocytes.

From all these findings it is concluded that about 50% of the inhibition of glycolysis in the "high-DPG" cells can be accounted for by the DPG-induced decrease of the red cell pH. This fall of the red cell pH leads to a reduction of the glycolytic rate due to the properties of the enzyme phosphofructo kinase. The remaining part of the inhibitory effect must be attributed to an inhibition by DPG of the enzyme hexokinase. The concentrations of ATP and inorganic phosphate were found to be slightly higher in "high-DPG" cells (27); thus, concentration changes of these meabolites cannot be made responsible for the reduction of the glycolytic flux in "high-DPG" cells. Also the enzyme pyruvate kinase appears to be inhibited in "high-DPG" cells. Other glycolytic enzymes like phosphofructo kinase, aldolase, GAPDH and phosphoglycerate kinase which are susceptible to an inhibition by DPG (11, 40,48) seem not to be inhibited significantly upon elevation of red cell DPG concentration above the normal value.

EFFECT OF DPG ON THE BUFFERING PROPERTIES OF HUMAN ERYTHROCYTES

In the studies described in the preceding section it was observed that the pH change in the red cell suspensions observed after addition of small amounts of NaOH for neutralization of the lactic acid formed was greater in the suspension of "high-DPG" cells than in those of normal erythrocytes, especially at high pH values. This phenomenon is in contrast to that what one might expect, namely a greater buffering capacity of red cell suspensions containing high concentrations of the buffer DPG (pK_2 of the two phosphate groups 6.95-7.1 (9,13)). Therefore, titration studies were performed in which normal and "high-DPG" cells suspended in Locke solution were titrated with 0.3n HCl. Aliquots of 50 to 100 µl of titrant were added stepwise to 5 ml samples of red cell suspensions, and the resulting pH changes were continuously measured using a digital pH meter (PHM 64, Radiometer, Copenhagen). The pH reached a new stable value after each addition of titrant within 1 to 2 min (pH change about 0.1 units per titration step).

The buffer values (added acid per hemoglobin tetramer per pH change) determined in these studies are summarized in Figure 9A. At pH values above 7,

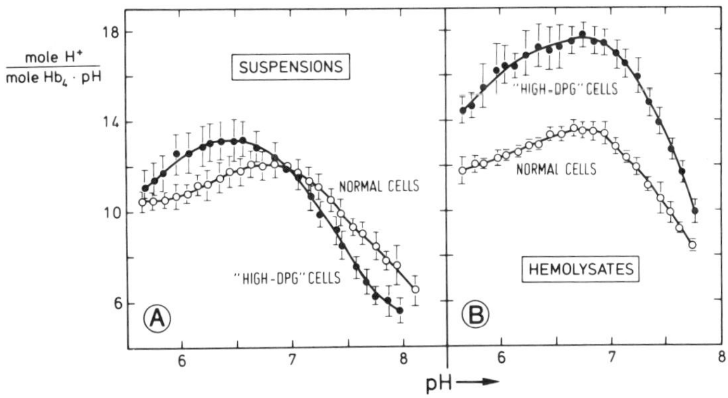

Figure 9: pH dependency of the buffer value of intact and hemolyzed suspensions of normal or "high-DPG" erythrocytes (37°C, solutions in contact with room air). The cells were suspended in Locke solution (1 mM PO_4) and the hemoglobin concentration was adjusted to 2.2 mM Hb_4. Mean values ± 1 SD from 6-10 experiments on blood of 5 different donors.

the buffering capacity of "high-DPG" cell suspension was lower than that of normal cells. Below this pH value the situation was reversed. When the cell suspensions were first hemolyzed by freezing and thawing and then titrated, an entirely different picture was observed (Figure 9B): The hemolysates of the "high-DPG" cell suspensions exhibited a greater buffering capacity than those of normal cells at all pH values. This is what one would anticipate from the presence of about three extra DPG molecules per hemoglobin tetramer (46).

By comparing the curves given in Figure 9 it becomes evident that the apparent pK values of the hemolysates of the two types of cells are identical. This holds not true for suspensions of intact cells where the apparent pK of "high-DPG" cells is decreased from 6.8 to 6.5. Furthermore it appears that the maximal buffer value of the red cell contents of normal and "high-DPG" cells is reduced by 10% and 25% when determined in suspension of intact erythrocytes. These effects must be caused by the presence of the intact red cell membrane in the erythrocyte suspensions.

In interpreting the phenomena observed one has to consider that the red cell DPG content alters the Donnan distribution of penetrating ions across the red cell membrane (21,44). Due to this effect the change of the red cell pH resulting from a given change of the extracellular pH (Δ pHi/Δ pHe) is lowered in "high-DPG" cells as shown in Figure 10. At an extracellular pH of 7.4, for instance Δ pHi/Δ pHe amounts to about 0.8 in suspensions of normal cells, and only to 0.5 in "high-DPG" cell suspensions (see Figure 10); this difference increases with rising extracellular pH values.

Thus, the elevated buffering capacity of the red cell contents is not fully reflected by the buffer value due to the "stability" of the red cell pH in "high-DPG" erythrocytes. The efficiency of this effect may be estimated as follows: At an extracellular pH of 8.0, for instance, the red cell pH is 7.5 in normal cells and 7.0 in "high-DPG" erythrocytes (see Figure 6). At these pH values the buffer values of the hemolysates of the suspensions are about 10 and 17 (see Figure 9 B). Thus, one would expect the buffering capacity of the "high-DPG" cell suspensions to be 70% higher than that of suspensions of normal erythrocytes. However, the red cell pH follows the changes of the extracellular pH with 70% in normal cells and only with 30% in "high-DPG" cells at an extracellular pH of 8.0 (see Figure 10). Accordingly, a theorectical buffering capacity of 7 and 5.1 can be calculated for suspensions of normal and "high-DPG" erythrocytes (0.7x10 and 0.3x17). These values correspond to a decrease of the buffer value of "high-DPG" cell suspension by about 25%, and not to the expected increase of 70%. The calculated values agree well with the values actually determined (see Figure 9A). Similar agreement was obtained when such calculations were performed for other extracellular pH values. Thus it is concluded that the paradox of a

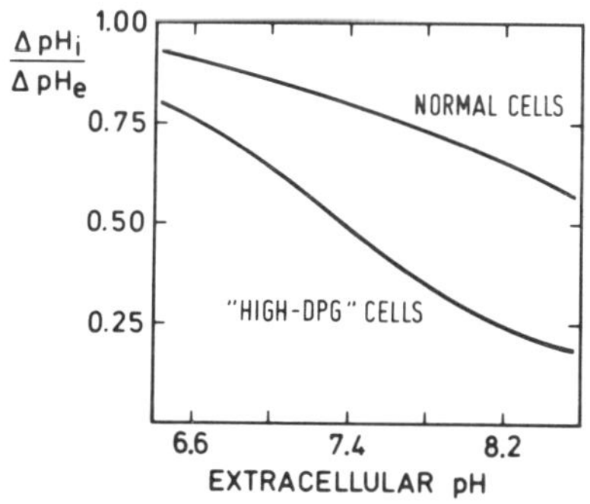

Figure 10: Relation between the change of the red cell pH resulting from a change of the extracellular pH and the extracellular pH in normal and "high-DPG" erythrocytes. The curves were calculated from data already published (21).

decreased buffer power of "high-DPG" cell suspensions at pH values above 7 can be fully explained by the Donnan effect of DPG.

In the system studied bicarbonate and plasma proteins were not present. Since these two buffers contribute with more than 50% to the total buffering capacity of human blood, only a minimal decrease of the buffer power against metabolically induced acid base disturbances of human blood containing "high-DPG" erythrocytes is to be expected. The same holds true for respiratory changes of acid base status as shown in Figure 11: No significant change of the slope of CO_2 titration curves resulting from an increase of the red cell DPG content could be detected. Thus it appears that no harm for acid base metabolism is to be anticipated from an infusion of "high-DPG" cells into man for therapeutical or experimental purposes.

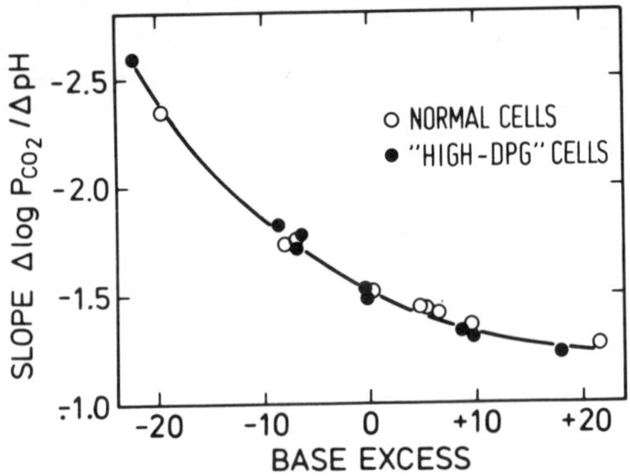

Figure 11: Dependency of the slope of CO_2-titration curves on base excess of whole human blood containing normal or "high-DPG" erythrocytes (37°C, 2.2 mM Hb_4). The titration curves were obtained by using an acid base analyzer (BMSMk2, Radiometer, Copenhagen) and gas mixtures containing 2, 4, 5.6, 8 or 10% CO_2 in O_2 prepared by gas mixing pumps (Wösthoff, Bochum).

Table 2: Effects of DPG on human erythrocytes

A) On Hemoglobin

Primary effect:	Preferential binding to deoxyhemoglobin
Secondary and tertiary effects:	Changes in the allosteric equilibrium and in the quaternary and tertiary structure of hemoglobin
	Decrease of O_2 affinity
	Changes in tissue oxygenation (?) and cardiac output (?)
	Changes of pK values of hemoglobin and DPG
	Change of the Bohr effect
	Decrease of CO_2 binding to hemoglobin
	Decrease of oxylabile carbamate
	Release of ATP from hemoglobin
	Change in the activity of DPG mutase (?)

B) On Red Cell Enzymes

Primary effect:	Interaction with the proteins or chelation of Mg^{++}
Secondary effects:	Inhibition of glycolysis
	Inhibition of DPG synthesis
	Activation of phosphoglycerate mutase
	Alteration of other metabolic pathways (?)

C) On the Red Cell Membrane

Primary effect:	Chelation of Ca^{++}
Secondary effect:	Change in red cell flexibility (?)

D) On the Donnan Distribution of Penetrating Ions

Primary effect:	Alteration of the Donnan ratio due to the charge and the osmotic activity of DPG
Secondary and tertiary effects:	Decrease of the red cell pH
	Decrease of red cell Cl^- and HCO_3^- concentrations
	Change in the oxygen affinity of hemoglobin
	Change in the activity of pH-dependent metabolic pathways
	Decrease of the red cell water content
	Increase of red cell hemoglobin concentration
	Decrease of hematocrit
	Increase of osmotic resistance
	Decrease of $\Delta pH_i / \Delta pH_e$
	Change in the buffering power of red cells

In concluding it may be stated that DPG exerts a great number of effects on human erythrocytes. These effects can be separated in primary and secondary ones as shown in Table 2. However, it appear that we are far apart from a complete understanding of the complex actions of the phosphate anion on the human red blood cell. This holds true for many physico-chemical phenomena as well as for the most important physiological question whether displacements of the oxygen dissociation curve of blood induce the physiological changes which can be anticipated theoretically.

REFERENCES

1) Albrecht,V., Roigas,H., Schultze,M., Jacobasch, G., and Rapoport,S. (1971) Eur.J.Biochem. 44-50
2) Antonini,E., and Brunori,M. (1970) Ann.Rev. Biochem. 39:977-1042
3) Arnone,A. (1972) Nature 237:146-149
4) Arnone,A. (1974) Ann.Rev.Med. 25:123-130
5) Askari,H., and Rao,S.N. (1968) Biochim.Biophys. Acta 151:198-203
6) Bauer,Ch. (1969) Life Sciences 8:1041-1046
7) Bauer,Ch. (197o) Resp.Physiol. 10:10-19
8) Bauer,C. (1974) Rev.Physiol.Biochem.Pharmacol. 70:1-31
9) Benesch,R.E., Benesch,R., and Yu,C.I. (1969) Biochemistry 8:2567-2571
10) Benesch,R.E., Benesch,R., Renthal,R., and Gratzer,W.B. (1971) Nature (New Biology) 234:174-17
11) Beutler,E., Matsumoto,F., and Guinto,E. (1974) Experientia 30:190-192
12) Brewer,G.H. (1969) Biochim.Biophys.Acta 192: 157-161
13) De Bruin,S.H., and Janssen,L.H.M. (1973) J.Biol.Chem. 248:2774-2777

14) De Bruin,S.H., Rollema,H.S., Janssen,L.H.M. and Van Os,A.J. (1974) Biochem.Biophys.Res.Commun. 58:204-209
15) De Bruin,S.H., Rollema,H.S., Janssen,L.H.M.and Van Os,A.J. (1974) Biochem.Biophys.Res.Commun. 58:210-215
16) Caldwell,P.R.B., Nagel,R.L., and Jaffe,E.R.(1971) Biochem.Biophys.Res.Commun. 44:1504-1509
17) Chanutin,A. and Hermann,E. (1969) Arch.Biochem. Biophys. 131:180-184
18) Damaschun,G., Damaschun,H., Müller,J.J., Pommerening,K., and Ruckpaul,K. (1973) VIIth International Berlin Symposium on Structure and Function of Erythrocytes, Abstract Volume pp. 104-108
19) Deuticke,B., Duhm,J., and Dierkesmann,R. (1971) Pflügers Arch. 326:15-34
20) Dische,Z., and Igals,D. (1963) Arch.Biochem. Biophys. 101:489-493
21) Duhm,J. (1971) Pflügers Arch. 326:341-356
22) Duhm,J. (1972) in: Oxygen Affinity of Hemoglobin and Red Cell Acid Base Status (M.Rørth, P.Astrup, eds) Munksgaard: Copenhagen and Academic Press: New York, pp. 583-594
23) Duhm,J. (1973) in: Oxygen Transport to Tissue, Adv.Exp.Med.Biol. 37A (H.I.Bicher,D.F.Bruley,eds.) Plenum Press: New York-London, pp. 179-186
24) Duhm,J. (1973) Pflügers Arch. 343:R3 (abstract)
25) Duhm,J. (1973) in: Erythrocytes, Thrombocytes, Leucocytes; Recent Advances in Membrane and Metabolic Research, (E.Gerlach, K.Moser,E.Deutsch, W.Wilmans, eds.) G.Thieme: Stuttgart, pp.149-157
26) Duhm,J. and Gerlach,E. (1974) in: The Human Red Cell in Vitro (T.Greenwalt, G.A.Jamieson, eds), Grune and Stratton:New York-London,pp. 111-148
27) Duhm,J.,Biochim.Biophys.Acta, in press
28) Garby,L., Gerber,G., and DeVerdier,C.-H. (1969) Europ.J.Biochem. 10:110-115
29) Garby,L. and DeVerdier,C.-H. (1972) in: Oxygen Affinity of Hemoglobin and Red Cell Acid Base Status (M.Rørth,P.Astrup,eds) Munksgaard:Copenhagen and Academic Press:New York, pp. 236-242

30) Hershko,A., Razin,A., and Mager,J. (1969) Biochim.Biophys.Acta 184:64-76
31) Herzfeld,J. and Stanley,H.E. (1974) J.Mol.Biol. 82:231-265
32) Keitt,A.S. (1971) Clin.Res. 19:4o (abstract)
33) Keitt,A.S. (1971) Final Report. Office of Naval Research Contract N00014-68-A-0173-0004. Springfield,Va.: National Technical Information Service, June 30, 1971 (AD-725 858).
34) Keitt,A.S. (1972) in: Proceedings of a Conference of the Committee on Red Blood Cell Preservation, National Research Council, June 5-6
35) Kilmartin,J.V. and Rossi-Bernardi,L. (1973) Phys. Rev. 53:836-89o
36) Kilmartin,J.V., Breen,J.J., Roberts,G., and Ho,C. (1973) Proc.Nat.Acad.Sci.USA 70:1246-1249
37) Kilmartin,J.V. (1974) FEBS letters 38:147-148
38) Minakami,S. and Yoshikawa,H. (1966) J.Biochem. (Tokyo) 59:139-150
39) Pace,M., Rossi-Bernardi,L. (1970)Biochem.J.119:67
40) Ponce,J., Roth,S., and Harkness,D.R. (1971) Biochim.Biophys.Acta 250:63-74
41) Riggs,A.(1971)Proc.Nat.Acad.Sci.USA 68:2062-2065
42) Rose,M.A., Warms,J.V.B.(1966)J.Biol.Chem.241: 4848-4854
43) Rossi-Bernardi,L. and Roughton,F.J.W. (1967) J.Physiol. 189:1-29
44) Salhany,J.M., Keitt,A.S.,and Eliot,R.S. (1971) FEBS letters 16:257-261
45) Sammons,D.W., Henry,H., and Chilson,O.P. (1970) J.Biol.Chem. 245:2109-2113
46) Siggaard-Andersen,O. (1971) Scand.J.Clin.Lab. Invest. 27:351-360
47) Siggaard-Andersen,O., Salling,N., Nörgaard-Pedersen,B.,and Røhrt,M. (1972) Scand.J.Clin.Lab.Invest. 29:185-320
48) Srivasta,S. and Beutler,E. (1972) Arch.Biochem. Biophys. 148:249-255
49) Szabo,A.,Karplus,M.(1972)J.Mol.Biol. 72:163-197
50) Tomita,S.,Riggs,A.(1971)J.Biol.Chem.246:547-554
51) Wyman,J.(1964)Advan.Protein.Chem. 19:223-286

DISCUSSION

Dr. Salhany: I wish to make a point about this business about binding to oxyhemoglobin. It may be possible that binding to oxyhemoglobin occurs because of some finite population of fully liganded T state. You could get binding of DPG if this species forms. However, the question is a quantitative one.

Dr. Duhm: I do not know whether Dr. Perutz would agree that 1/60th to 1/40th of 100% oxygenated hemoglobin exists in the deoxy conformation.

Dr. Perutz: That seems unlikely. According to some data recently published by Imai and Yonetani, the effect of DPG on the fourth Adair constant must be very small. The situation is rather similar to the pH effect shown by John Kilmartin this morning. You have a large difference in K_1 but hardly any difference in K_4.

Dr. Kilmartin: The protein concentration of these conditions is very low and the pH is quite high so I don't think we would expect any binding to the oxy form. On the other hand in the red cell, where the protein concentration is very high DPG probably binds to the oxy form.

Dr. Perutz: For reasons of mass equilibrium.

Dr. Kilmartin: Yes.

Dr. Perutz: Because the protein concentration is so much higher than in these experiments.

Dr. Kilmartin: Yes, if you have a binding constant of, say, 100 then DPG would bind significantly to the oxy form on the red cell, but you wouldn't see any binding under these conditions of low protein concentration.

Dr. Ho: Last year, Dr. Lindstrom and I reported that DPG can affect the conformation of E11 valines in HbCO A [Biochemistry 12, 134 (1974)] suggesting that DPG can bind to HbCO A. Where does DPG bind to HbCO A?

Dr. Duhm: What I hoped to achieve by the calculations of binding constants from P_{50} values was to contribute to the resolution of the discrepancy in the binding data published in the literature. The results obtained indicate--at least to me--that binding constants of oxyhemoglobin for DPG are much smaller--even in concentrated hemoglobin solutions--than those directly determined by Dr. Garby and by some other authors. However, one should be careful, as I already pointed out, in drawing definite conclusions from the data since the concept underlying the calculations does not meet completely the properties of the hemoglobin tetramer.

Dr. Kilmartin: Could I just make another point? Surely from the measurements of log P_{50}, all you can really measure is the difference in the binding constants between the oxy and deoxy forms of hemoglobin rather than the absolute binding constants to these two forms.

Dr. Duhm: Then, I could be able to calculate the ratio of the two binding constants.

Dr. Kilmartin: Yes, that's what I mean, it seems to me you can't really tell what the absolute number will be, just the ratio.

Dr. Duhm: You're right. I think it would be better to analyze all the data in terms of a more general concept considering all the 3-5 single determinations of O_2 saturation in the range of 70-80% Hb O_2 underlying the P_{50} values given in the Figures.

Dr. Brewer: I would like to point out that there are differences in the situation of high DPG cells obtained by incubation, as opposed to those obtained when, say, an individual is exposed to hypoxia. We find for instance, that during altitude exposure or in anemia the pH_i does not go down as a result of DPG buildup. It is high, if anything. The G6P levels also tend to be high, so there are some differences.

Dr. Duhm: I think this is a very good point you made because--and this must be noted--I dealt with red cells the DPG content of which had been acutely elevated. When we incubate the cells for longer times, say for more than 24 hours, then they begin to gain a part of the water they lost, most probably due to increased potassium leakage resulting from the elevated concentration of potassium in the cell water, or from other reasons. The result would then be that the concentrations in the cell water of hemoglobin and DPG will decrease again. Accordingly, the red cell pH will rise a little bit and the relation between the extracellular pH and the red cell pH determined in the acute experiment will no longer be true for chronic (high DPG" cells. However, the red cell pH remains lower in chronic "high DPG" cells than in normal cells. This fall of the red cell pH should be accompanied by an increase of the G-6-P concentration (when determined on a water basis) similar to that shown in Figure 7.

Dr. Ho: Dr. Perutz, could you repeat the X-ray diffraction study by putting molecules into single crystals of carbon monoxy hemoglobin?

Dr. Perutz: I can't do it with the crystallization methods we have at the moment but I think that this is what I ought to try to do; develop methods of crystallization of hemoglobin at low ionic strength where one can do just that.

Dr. Minakami: Your metabolic study is very interesting for me. I have one question. What is the ATP and ADP concentrations of the DPG-rich cells--elevated or decreased?

Dr. Duhm: The results obtained referring to this question are shown in the Figure below. After the DPG accumulation period very high ATP concentrations were observed as to be expected from the cell shrinkage. After an additional five hours of incubation in Locke solution with substrates other than glucose (37°C.) the ATP concentrations in the "high DPG" cells had approximated the values found in normal cells. In both types of cells the same typical dependency of ATP levels on the red cell pH were observed. At the moment we do not know whether an as yet unknown regulatory process determining the level of ATP is the reason for this phenomenon, or whether we are dealing with an accidental finding which would not be observed after longer times of incubation. It may be noted that ATP levels did not further decrease in "high-DPG" cells incubated at an extracellular pH of 7.4 in the time interval between the 5th and 24th hour of incubation. I doubt, however, that we have observed a new regulatory mechanism. The reason why is that experiments designed to clarify this question showed that the ATP concentration--when determined on a water basis--experimentally increased by cell shrinkage resulting from addition of NaCl to the suspension medium remained elevated during a four-hour incubation period, i.e. ATP levels did not decrease in cells shrunken due to addition of NaCl to the suspension medium as in cells shrunken due to elevation of DPG concentration. Now, this discrepancy might be due to the differences in the glycolytic rates

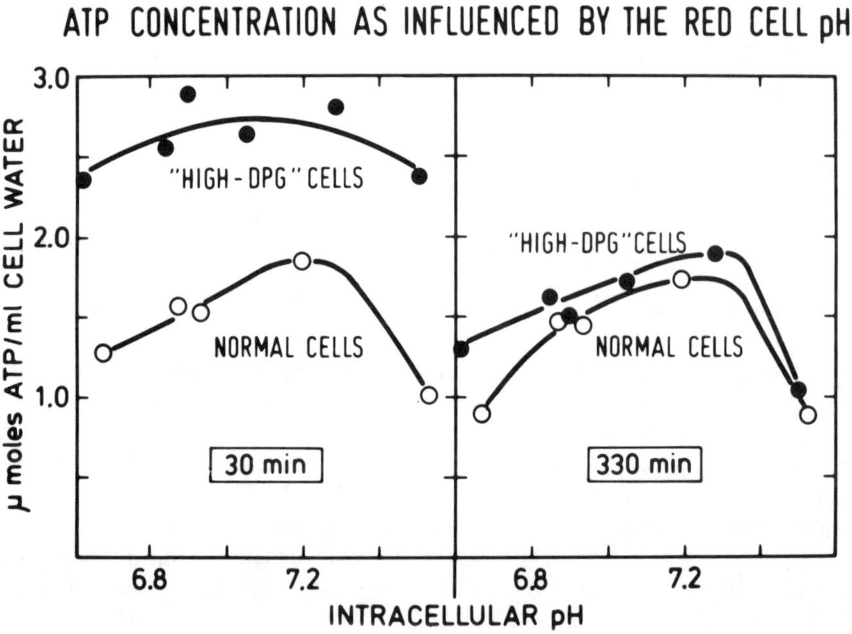

in the two types of shrunken cells: the glycolytic flux is increased in the NaCl-shrunken cells and decreased in the "high DPG" cells. The pH dependency of ADP and AMP levels I cannot remember at the moment; however, the concentrations of both nucleotides remained below 0.4 μ moles/ml cell water under all experimental conditions.

Dr. Grindlay-Moore: What was your comment on the explanation for the 3-PG increase under increased pH?

Dr. Duhm: As far as the well known dependency of DPG concentration on the red cell pH is concerned, the general accepted explanation seems to be that the 3-PG levels increase with rising pH due to the properties of the enzyme pyruvate kinase. This enzyme is not saturated with respect to PEP under normal conditions. Thus, an increased flux at an elevated pH through the reaction catalyzed by the pyruvate kinase can only be achieved by a rise of PEP concentration. As a result of this, 3-PG levels must increase since the reactions catalyzed by the enolase and by the phosphoglycerate mutase are close to the thermodynamic equilibrium, as has been clearly demonstrated by Minakami and Yoshikawa. The increase of ADP concentration occurring upon elevation of the red cell pH above a value of 7.2 apparently is not of a sufficient magnitude to allow a sufficient increase of the flux through the reaction catalyzed by the PK. The elevation of 3-PG concentration in "high DPG" cells led us to conclude that the PK is inhibited in these cells, since the reactions catalyzed by the enolase and PGK are at the equilibrium and since both enzymes are not inhigited by DPG. A further argument favouring this conclusion is that the same metabolic patterns can be observed in pyruvate kinase deficient erythrocytes, which have both elevated 3-PG and elevated DPG concentration, at least the classic type of PK deficient cells.

ROLE OF IN VIVO PYRUVATE KINASE ACTIVITY: A. INHERITANCE OF ELEVATED RED CELL ATP LEVELS B. RED CELL MALARIAL PARASITE INTERACTIONS

Fred J. Oelshlegel, Jr., Barry J. Sander, and George J. Brewer

Department of Human Genetics, University of Michigan Medical School, Ann Arbor, Michigan

INTRODUCTION

Red cell glycolytic control has been the subject of some rather intensive study during the last several years. In brief, it is known that the route of perhaps 90% of the glucose consumed by the erythrocyte is that of the Embden-Meyerhof Pathway. In the process of Embden-Meyerhof glycolysis there is a net production of 2 ATP[1] molecules for each molecule of glucose consumed. ATP, of course, has an important role in maintaining red cell shape, deformability, cation transport, resynthesis of purine nucleotides, and

---

[1]Abbreviations: ATP, adenosine triphosphate; GLU, glucose; G6P, glucose-6-phosphate; F6P, fructose-6-phosphate; FDP, fructose-1,6-diphosphate; DHAP, dihydroxyacetone phosphate; GAP, glyceraldehyde-3-phosphate; 1,3 DPG, 1,3-diphosphoglycerate; 2,3 DPG, 2,3-diphosphoglycerate; 3PG, 3-phosphoglycerate; 2PG, 2-phosphoglycerate; PEP, phospho-enolpyruvate; PYR, pyruvate; LACT, lactate; ADP, adenosine diphosphate; AMP, adenosine monophosphate; Pi, inorganic phosphate; NAD and NADH, nicotinamide adenine dinucleotide, oxidized and reduced forms; NADP and NADPH, nicotinamide adenine dinucleotide phosphate, oxidized and reduced forms.

synthesis of glutathione. As has been emphasized in the last several years, there is a two-enzyme shunt unique to red cell glycolysis that produces the intermediate, 2,3 DPG. Red cell oxygen affinity is in large part determined by 2,3 DPG. Thus red cell metabolism and function are tightly interrelated through ATP and 2,3 DPG.

There are several different research approaches one might take in attempting to understand red cell metabolism. One such approach is to break open the red cell and study its parts in detail. This approach as represented by the vast literature on red cell enzymes has done much to increase our knowledge of red cell glycolytic control. A second approach to the study of red cell metabolism involves perturbing intact red cells *in vitro*, observing the effects of such perturbations on the levels of red cell metabolites, and then making conclusions about red cell metabolic control from such observations. Again this approach, as pioneered by Minakami's group (Yoshikawa and Minakami, 1968), has greatly expanded our understanding of red cell glycolytic control. There's a third approach to understanding red cell glycolysis which is a bit different from the above two approaches. This third approach stems from the philosophy that we're all ultimately interested in the true *in vivo* control of red cell metabolism and function. That is, within the whole organism, what red cell enzymes have a major influence on the cell's ATP and 2,3 DPG levels? For this it seems that one could gain a good idea of such *in vivo* control by seeking red cell biochemical perturbations that are those of mother nature herself. We have had the opportunity to study two such perturbations and will review our studies to date in this paper. One of the perturbations studied is a genetic one. That is, we have carried out some studies on a unique family in which some individuals have an inherited alteration in red cell metabolism. The second perturbation we'll discuss is that caused by the malaria parasite.

MATERIALS AND METHODS

For the studies involving human subjects, blood was drawn from an antecubital vein into "Vacutainer" tubes

(Becton-Dickinson, Rutherford, New Jersey). For studies involving monkeys, blood was drawn via a heparinized syringe from the femoral vein. The monkeys were anesthetized with ketamine hydrochloride (Parke Davis, Co., Detroit, Michigan). For studies involving glycolytic intermediates, the heparinized blood was precipitated immediately with perchloric acid (Oelshlegel et al., 1972). For studies involving enzyme assays the blood was drawn into acid-citrate-dextrose tubes and stored at 4° C until used.

The method of preparation and assay of extracts for the glycolytic intermediate studies is a modification (Oelshlegel et al., 1972) of that described by Minakami et al. (1965). Assays of 2,3 DPG and ATP were carried out on trichloroacetic acid extracts of the blood (Brewer and Powell, 1966; Keitt, 1971).

Enzyme assays (Vmax) were carried out by standard methods (Beutler, 1971; Brewer et al., 1964). The pyruvate kinase assay was performed as described by Beutler (1971) with the exception that the hemolysate was prepared and dialyzed according to the method of Brewer et al. (1964). Michaelis constants (K_m) for PEP were determined by the traditional Lineweaver-Burk method on the same hemolysate. For the K_m determinations, FDP was present at 100 μM concentration in the assay cuvette. All assays were performed on a Gilford Model 2400-S Linear Recording Spectrophotometer.

Gel electrophoretic studies of pyruvate kinase were performed as described by Brewer (1970).

Both mice and monkey malaria red cell infections were initiated by inoculation of parasitized blood. The *Plasmodium berghei* strain (a rodent malaria) used was originally obtained from Dr. P.E. Thompson of the University of Georgia, Athens. The *P. knowlesi* strain (a simian malaria) was obtained from Dr. G.J. McCormick of the Walter Reed Army Medical Center, Washington, D.C.

RESULTS AND DISCUSSION

A. Inheritance of Elevated Red Cell ATP Levels

This family has been discussed previously (Brewer, 1965). It had been shown that certain members of this family possess an autosomally inherited allele that somehow leads to elevated red cell ATP. Since the mechanism for the increased red cell ATP was never elucidated, we decided to restudy this family in hopes of finding clues for this mechanism. A partial pedigree of this family is depicted in figure 1. All members of the family appeared normal clinically. Subjects II-2 (normal red cell ATP) and III-3 (elevated red cell ATP) were studied most intensively. We studied this pair in particular because aside from the ATP differences they were quite similar in that they lived together, were of the same sex (males), were similar in genotype, were close in age, and were cooperative.

Our initial approach in attempting to elucidate the reason for elevated ATP in those individuals so affected was to compare the levels of red cell glycolytic intermedi-

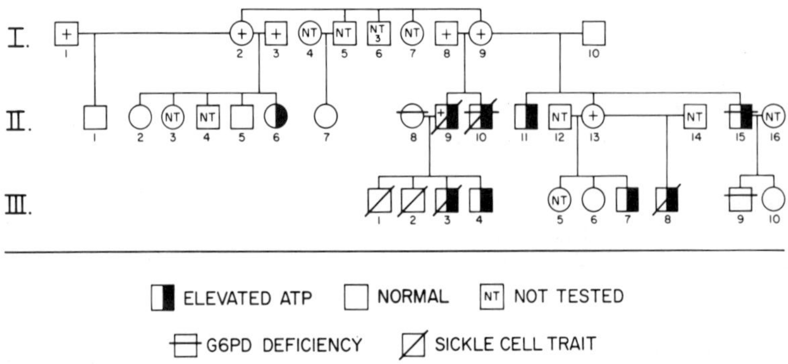

Figure 1. Partial pedigree of family with the allele determining elevated red cell ATP levels. Female II-8 of the pedigree is only partially deficient in G6PD activity.

ates found in the elevated ATP family members to those found in the normal ATP family members. Using this approach we found that an abnormal glycolytic intermediate pattern existed in the elevated ATP individuals. This is represented in figure 2. Considering the data in figure 2 plus studies of additional family members (a total of five elevated ATP individuals and three normal ATP individuals with several duplicates done on blood drawn on different days) statistically significant differences between the two groups of subjects in 2,3 DPG, 2PG, PEP, and of course, ATP were observed. The groups did not significantly differ in G6P, F6P, FDP, DHAP, AMP, and ADP. There was also much overlap between blood PYR and LACT levels between the two groups of subjects. (These latter intermediates vary considerably according to the subject's resting state. The data in figure 2 represent values obtained on six family members in one session with all family members under a similar activity state.) The plot of figure 2 can be interpreted in a fairly straightforward way, that is, in terms of the elevated ATP individuals having a higher _in vivo_ activity of pyruvate kinase. This arises from the principle that if the _in vivo_ activity of an enzyme is increased (in this case, pyruvate kinase)-- the steady state level of its substrate (PEP) should be decreased as well as the steady state level of its product (PYR) should be increased. Glycolytic regulation is, of course, complex and extrapolation to _in vivo_ conditions based on the measurements of glycolytic intermediates should be cautious. However, our interpretation of this as indicative of elevated _in vivo_ pyruvate kinase activity would be consistent with the hypothesis of Zürcher et al. (1965) that increased pyruvate kinase activity should lead to decreased PEP, 2PG and 3PG. The decreased 3PG should, in turn, lead to decreased 2,3 DPG since 3PG is a product inhibitor of the 2,3 DPG → 3PG step and an activator of the 1,3 DPG → 2,3 DPG step. Decreased 3PG should also shift the phosphoglycerate kinase steady state equilibrium in the direction of increased ATP. In addition, it seems that more ATP would be obtainable from the increased pyruvate kinase activity itself (refer to pathway at top of figure 2).

There is evidence that increased pyruvate kinase activity, does, indeed, lead to increased red cell ATP (Zürcher et

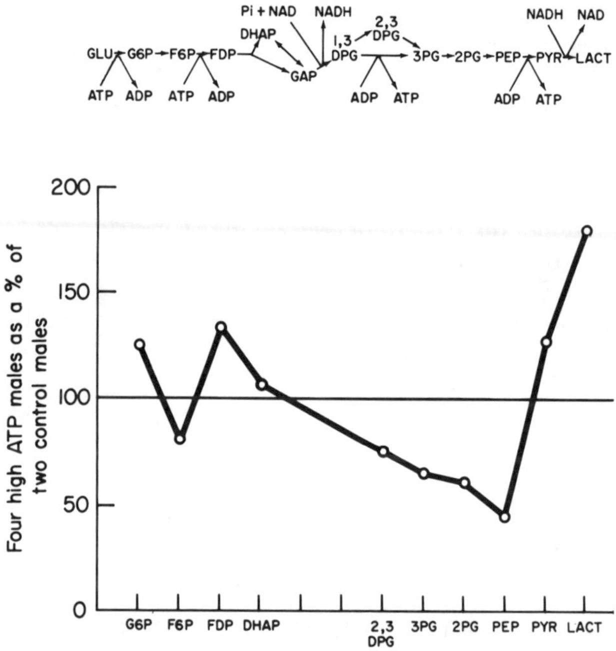

Figure 2. Red cell glycolytic plot comparing four elevated ATP males (II-10, II-11, III-3, and III-4 of figure 1) to two normal ATP males (III-1 and III-2 of figure 1). The glycolytic intermediates are listed on the horizontal axis in their order of appearance in the glycolytic pathway. On the vertical axis, the average of each intermediate for the elevated ATP individuals is expressed as a percentage of the corresponding average for the normal ATP individuals. In all, intermediate determinations were performed on eight family members (see text).

al., 1965). Zürcher's group have identified a family with increased pyruvate kinase activity associated with increased red cell ATP. They did not measure all the above intermediates on their family. They did, however, measure red cell glucose consumption and found no major glucose consumption differences in their normal ATP and elevated ATP individuals

viduals. Glucose consumption is very useful in interpreting plots such as that of figure 2. Thus far we have measured red cell glucose consumption on one normal ATP individual and one elevated ATP individual of our family and find them both to be within our normal range.

We performed the more traditional red cell enzyme assays on members of our family, fully expecting an increased pyruvate kinase Vmax activity as found in the family of Zürcher et al., but were a bit surprised by the results. These assay results are diagramed in figure 3. As can be seen in the figure, we found no Vmax differences for several key red cell enzymes between the elevated and the normal ATP family members. There were, however, marked differences in the pyruvate kinase values, the elevated ATP individuals having lower pyruvate kinase activities. This seemed to contrast somewhat with the predicted higher _in vivo_ activity obtained from the glycolytic intermediate data.

It seemed that one interpretation consistent with these two observations would be that the elevated ATP individuals have an altered pyruvate kinase which is more active _in vivo_ in spite of a lower than usual Vmax. This would require the altered pyruvate kinase to be kinetically more efficient than usual. For example, it might have a lower K_m for at least one of its substrates. An alternate interpretation would be that the association between the glycolytic pattern and pyruvate kinase Vmax activity is not directly a causal one but is due to an unrecognized third primary factor. Preliminary kinetic studies on the red cell pyruvate kinase of some of our family's individuals make us feel the first interpretation mentioned is most likely since it allows us to explain all our data in the simplest manner. Table I summarizes the K_m data obtained for PEP on the pyruvate kinase activity of red cell hemolysates of selected family members. Thus, the one pyruvate kinase kinetic property studied (K_m for PEP) does suggest that the high ATP subjects have an altered pyruvate kinase which could be more efficient _in vivo_ than its normal counterpart. Calculations based on an estimated _in vivo_ PEP level of 20 μM indicated that the K_m differences reported in the results section are enough to yield a calculated _in vivo_ velocity in the altered enzyme

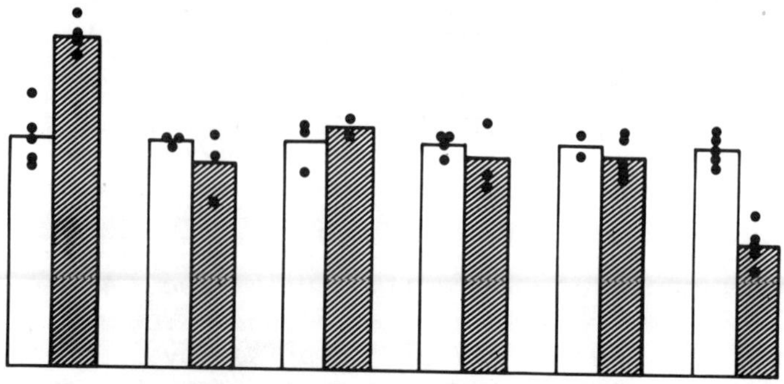

Figure 3. Relative red cell enzyme activities of elevated ATP subjects (shaded) compared to normal ATP subjects (unshaded). With the exception of the pair of bars on the left, the bars represent relative average enzyme Vmax's--obtained by standard methods. The bars on the left illustrate the ATP levels found in some family members. The black dots represent individual values. Abbreviations: HK, hexokinase; G6PD, glucose-6-phosphate dehydrogenase; 6PGD, 6-phosphogluconate dehydrogenase; PFK, phosphofructokinase; PK, pyruvate kinase.

Table I--Pyruvate Kinase Michaelis Constants

Subject		K_m (PEP) μM	
III-3	(Elevated ATP)	60 ± 12.5	(4 determinations)
II-2	(Elevated ATP)	71	(1 determination)
III-2	(Normal ATP)	122 ± 10	(4 determinations)
III-1	(Normal ATP)	122 ± 26	(2 determinations)

Subjects are those illustrated in figure 1. Michaelis constants are expressed as mean ± standard deviation.

that is nearly equal to--but not greater than--that of the normal enzyme. More kinetic studies are, of course, needed to be done on the altered enzyme before an _in vivo_ velocity can be estimated with any reasonable degree of certainty. The _in vivo_ activity of the altered (and normal) enzyme should most properly be assessed under simulated physiologic conditions in the presence of various metabolites, phosphate compounds, and substrates and products (of physiologic concentration). However, until this can be done, we would speculate that the altered pyruvate kinase is more active than the normal enzyme under _in vivo_ conditions.

B. Red Cell-Malarial Parasite Interactions

There has been much interest in the role of red cell ATP in malaria infections. (It should be remembered that during part of its life cycle, the malaria organism is a single cell parasite growing within the red cell.) There are indications from previous studies that malaria organisms favor red cells with high ATP. That is, in humans the rate of malarial parasitemia is proportional to the initial ATP of the host cell (Brewer and Powell, 1965). In monkeys, maximum parasitemia is proportional to host red cell ATP levels (Eaton and Brewer, 1969). _In vitro_, ATP has a favorable effect on the culturing and growth of the parasite (Trager, 1950). Also, on the average, blacks have lower red cell ATP than whites (Brewer, 1967). This latter finding has been speculated to be due to the strong malaria selection pressure the black genotype has been subjected to, resulting in a red cell that is a bit less desirable to the parasite, that is, a red cell with decreased ATP levels (Brewer, 1967).

We used the glycolytic intermediate approach to see if malaria-infected red cells have a perturbed glycolytic pattern. Figure 4 demonstrates what we have found in monkeys. It can be seen that the heavily infected monkey red cells have increased ATP and decreased DPG, PEP and so forth. This is reminiscent of the pyruvate kinase activation pattern seen in the ATP family study. Control monkeys bled and treated in a manner similar to the malaria-infected monkeys did not show this pattern. Further, this degree of parasitemia is reached in too short a time for a reticulocyte response. Thus these patterns are most likely caused by the presence within the red cell of the parasite itself and not caused by some more indirect hematological response. A plot consistent with elevated pyruvate kinase activity was also seen with mouse malaria (figure 5). Glucose consumption was greatly increased in both the monkey and the mouse malaria systems.

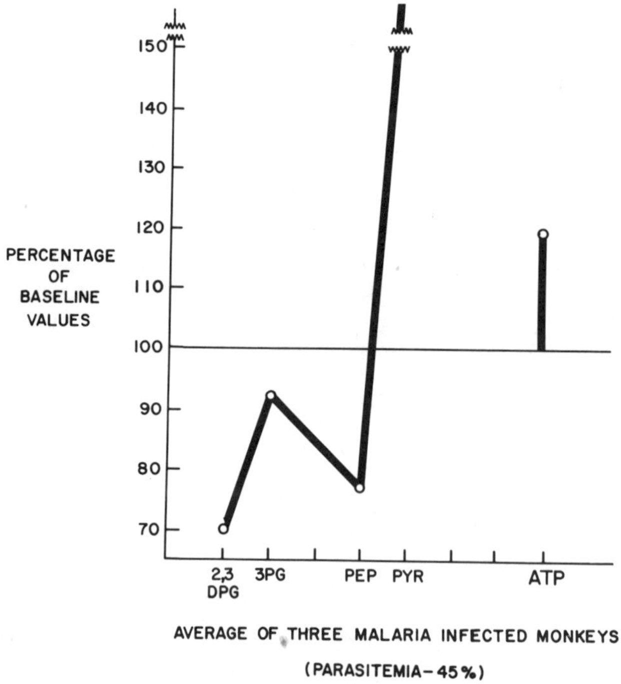

Figure 4. Glycolytic plot comparing three P. knowlesi-infected rhesus monkeys to their uninfected baseline values. For each monkey the level of each red cell intermediate is expressed as a percentage of the monkey's preinfected value. The average percentage for all three monkeys are then plotted to give the points on the figure.

Unlike the ATP family study, when we assayed for pyruvate kinase activity we found no surprises. As figure 6 summarizes, there were clear increases in pyruvate kinase Vmax activity in both the monkey and the mouse malaria systems.

These studies did tell us that there is increased pyruvate kinase activity in malaria-infected red cells, but they did not tell us the source of the activity. Was it more host related or more parasite related? Since the red cell can't

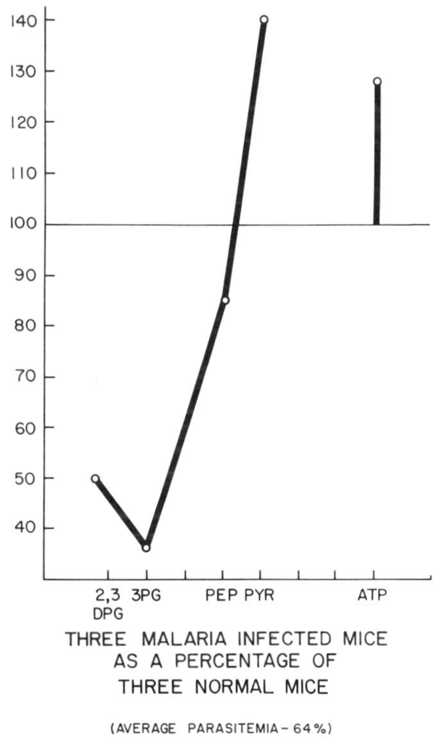

Figure 5. Glycolytic plot comparing intermediate levels found in the pooled blood of three P. berghei infected mice (Small blood volumes did not allow us to use the same animal as his own control as was done with the monkeys.)

synthesize new enzyme it seemed more likely that the increased enzyme activity came from the parasite. However, there did exist the possibility that the parasite had somehow activated the normal red cell enzyme. Some gel electrophoretic studies provide evidence that the parasite perturbs red cell metabolism by introducing a pyruvate kinase isozyme of its own. Figure 7 is a schematic of what was found for malaria-infected and non-infected red cell hemolysates subjected to starch gel electrophoresis and stained for pyruvate kinase activity. It can be seen that in both the monkey and the mouse systems a new pyruvate kinase isozyme is present

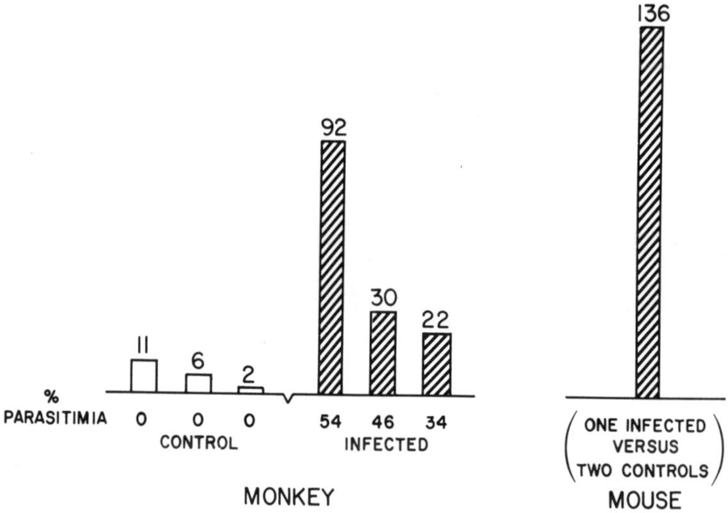

Figure 6. Pyruvate kinase Vmax activity in malaria infected red cells of monkeys and of mice. The monkey activities are expressed as a percent increase (numbers above the bars) over preinfection values. It can be seen that control monkeys (treated much like the infected animals in terms of blood drawing and such) showed only very small increases in activity compared to the large increases seen in infected monkeys. The infected mouse pyruvate kinase activity is expressed on the basis of uninfected mice. (Small blood volumes did not allow us to use the same mouse as his own control as was done in the monkeys.)

in infected red cells which was not present in uninfected red cells. Presumably these new isozymes are of parasitic origin.

In summarizing our malaria studies we can say that it looks like the malarial parasite introduces a new pyruvate kinase isozyme into the red cell. This isozyme then perturbs red cell metabolism in such a way that ATP is increased at the expense of a decrease in DPG. For the parasite this seems ideal since it can utilize ATP but presumably has no use for DPG.

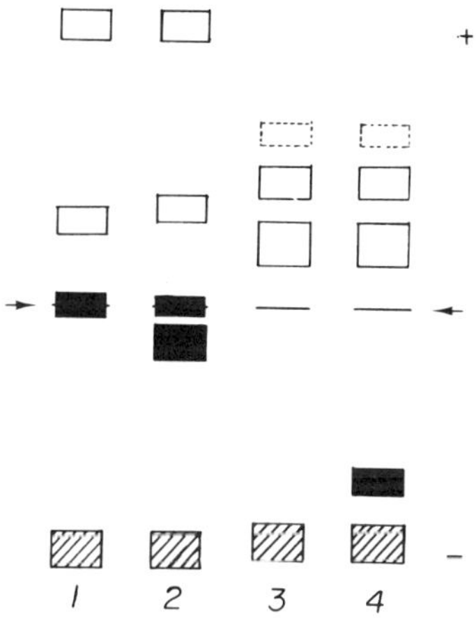

Figure 7. Schematic of pyruvate isozymes found in various samples. The solid bands represent pyruvate kinase activity; the unfilled bands represent adenylate kinase activity; and the hatched bands represent hemoglobin bands. Slot 1 = hemolysate of healthy mouse; Slot 2 = hemolysate of P. berghei-infected mouse; Slot 3 = hemolysate of healthy monkey; and Slot 4 = hemolysate of P. knowlesi-infected monkey. (The adenylate kinase bands were discerned by staining the opposite face of the gel. This is necessary because the pyruvate kinase stain also stains for adenylate kinase. Presumably the healthy monkey's pyruvate kinase band is buried under the adenylate kinase band much as in the human situation (Brewer, 1970).)

CONCLUSIONS

We have studied two conditions in which *in vivo* red cell glycolysis has been perturbed. In both cases it appears that the *in vivo* activity of pyruvate kinase has been increased, and both studies demonstrate the general importance of pyruvate kinase as a regulator of certain features of red cell metabolism. These studies have shown that an *in vivo* increase in pyruvate kinase activity can lead to marked changes in the steady state levels of red cell glycolytic intermediates most notably an increase in ATP and a decrease in DPG. This suggests that DPG and ATP are at least partially determined in a reciprocal manner according to the *in vivo* pyruvate kinase activity. This is important, because these two intermediates have quite different functions as already discussed. The ATP family study has not only lead to the elucidation of a possible mechanism by which red cell ATP is elevated in this genetic condition but has also demonstrated the lesson that *in vivo* and *in vitro* (Vmax) enzyme activities do not necessarily have to be directly related. The malaria studies have provided information as to one way this intracellular parasite perturbs and presumably controls red cell metabolism in a direction favorable to its own growth and development.

SUMMARY

We have carried out two separate projects which demonstrate the effect of pyruvate kinase perturbations on red cell metabolism. These studies emphasize the important regulatory role of pyruvate kinase in glycolysis.

A.--Certain members of a family with inherited elevated red cell ATP levels were found to have a red cell glycolytic intermediate pattern consistent with increased activity of pyruvate kinase. However, associated with the elevated ATP individuals were lower than normal *in vitro* red cell pyruvate kinase activities (Vmax) rather than higher than normal, as might be expected. A preliminary study suggests that the elevated ATP individuals have a red cell pyruvate kinase with altered kinetic properties. We speculate that this altered pyruvate kinase is more active than the normal enzyme under in vivo conditions.

B. In monkeys heavily infected with Plasmodium knowlesi and mice heavily infected with P. berghei we have found an increase in red cell ATP. We have evidence that these malaria parasites introduce a pyruvate kinase isozyme into their host red blood cells in amounts sufficient to alter red cell glycolysis. We suggest that this alteration in red cell glycolysis is in a direction favorable to the parasite because it will increase red cell ATP at the expense of red cell 2,3 DPG. The data we have gathered which are consistent with these suggestions are: 1) glycolytic intermediate data implying an increase in in vivo pyruvate kinase activity in infected red cells; 2) an increase in in vitro pyruvate kinase activity (Vmax) in hemolysates of infected cells; and 3) gel electrophoretic patterns showing a new pyruvate kinase isozyme in infected cells.

REFERENCES

Beutler, E. (1971). Red Cell Metabolism. A Manual of Biochemical Methods. Grune and Stratton, New York.

Brewer, G.J. (1965). A new inherited abnormality of human erythrocytes-elevated erythrocytes adenosine triphosphate. Biochem. Biophys. Res. Commun. 18:430.

Brewer, G.J. (1967). Genetic and population studies of quantitative levels of adenosine triphosphate in human erythrocytes. Biochem. Genet. 1:25.

Brewer, G.J. (1970). An Introduction to Isozyme Techniques. Academic Press, New York.

Brewer, G.J., and Powell, R.D. (1965). A study of the relationship between the content of ATP in human red cells and the course of falciparum malaria. A new system that may confer protection against malaria. Proc. Nat. Acad. Sci. 54:741.

Brewer, G.J., and Powell, R.D. (1966). The adenosine triphosphate content of glucose-6-phosphate dehydrogenase-deficient and normal erythrocytes, including studies of a glucose-6-phosphate dehydrogenase-deficient man with "elevated erythrocytic ATP". J. Lab. Clin. Med. 67:726.

Brewer, G.J., Powell, R.D., Swanson, S.H., and Alving, A.F. (1964). Hemolytic effect of primaquine. XVII. Hexokinase activity of glucose-6-phosphate dehydrogenase-deficient and normal erythrocytes. J. Lab. Clin. Med. 64:601.

Eaton, J.W., and Brewer, G.J. (1969). Red cell ATP and malaria infection. Nature 222:389.

Keitt, A.S. (1971). Reduced nicotinamide adenine dinucleotide-linked analysis of 2,3 diphosphoglyceric acid: Spectrophotometric and fluorometric procedures. J. Lab. Clin. Med. 77:470.

Minakami, S., Suzuki, C., Saito, T., and Yoshikawa, H. (1965). Studies on erythrocyte glycolysis. I. Determination of the glycolytic intermediates in human erythrocytes. J. Biochem. 58:543.

Oelshlegel, F.J., Jr., Brewer, G.J., Penner, J.A., and Schoomaker, E.B. (1972). Enzymatic mechanisms of red blood cell adaptation to anemia. In Hemoglobin and Red Cell Structure and Function (G.J. Brewer, ed.). Adv. Exp. Med. Biol. 28:377.

Trager, W. (1950). Studies on the extracellular cultivation of an intracellular parasite (avian malaria). I. Development of the organisms in erythrocyte extracts and the favoring effects of adenosine triphosphate. J. Exp. Med. 92:349.

Yoshikawa, H., and Minakami, S. (1968). Regulation of glycolysis in human red cells. Folia. Haematol. 89:357.

Zürcher, C., Loos, J.A., and Prins, H.K. (1965). Hereditary high ATP content of human erythrocytes. Bibl. Haematol. 23:549.

DISCUSSION

Dr. Duhm: You have observed an increase of the total concentration of adenine nucleotides in the first part of the study, and I think that an activation of the enzyme pyruvate kinase cannot fully explain this phenomenon, because the enzymes involved in degradation and synthesis of adenine nucleotides must contribute in determining the total level of adenine nucleotides.

Dr. Oelshlegel: We found no differences in the ADP and AMP levels between the high and the normal ATP individuals in our family. Total adenine would, of course, be increased in the high ATP individuals due to their ATP levels. Since pyruvate kinase is an ATP producing enzyme, it seems reasonable to assume that it may have an important role in determining total adenine levels. Our data would support this. The genetic evidence would also support this. That is, those individuals with high ATP also have an altered pyruvate kinase (as judged by Vmax data). In light of this genetic evidence, attempts to involve other adenine nucleotide related enzymes would require hypotheses more circumvented than our hypothesis that the altered pyruvate kinase is responsible for the increased ATP.

Dr. Duhm: The second question is whether the change in the activity of pyruvate kinase in the red cells of your patient can be in some way related to the two types of pyruvate kinase deficiency recently separated by Schröter.

Dr. Oelshlegel: These people are not PK deficient. There is no hemolysis, and it looks like the *in vivo* PK is increased. So, don't confuse this with a clinically deficient PK person.

Dr. Eaton: Fred, I'm a little curious about something. That is, if one extrapolates from the 92% increase in PK activity you saw in the monkey with mild *P. knowlesi* infection to what it might be in 100% infected red cells (and, therefore, in a parasite), the activity of the enzyme would be tremendous. Yet in your starch gel electrophoresis patterns, one doesn't see the heavy staining that one might expect in the PK band. Do you have an explanation for this?

Dr. Oelshlegel: I do. Most of what you saw on the gels with the monkey samples was adenylate kinase. If you compare the control monkey PK band it is usually somewhat weaker than the infected monkey pyruvate kinase. And the infected mouse pyruvate kinase band was pretty obviously increased.

Dr. Minakami: Probably you observed the increase of lactate formation in vitro in malaria infected red cells. If so, it might be better to add the rate of lactate formation in your crossover plot. The reason is, you may have a similar pattern by the decrease of phosphofructokinase activity. The levels of DPG and ATP depend mainly on the ratio of phosphofructokinase and pyruvate kinase activities, so without discussing the overall glycolytic rate, it's difficult to say whether pyruvate kinase is activated or not.

Dr. Oelshlegel: Flux is increased. The glucose consumption as well as lactate production in malaria infected cells is greatly increased. Further, in the malarial studies (as well as in the ATP family studies) we found no changes in phosphofructokinase Vmax activities.

Dr. Rasmussen: I wasn't clear, was the glucose consumption in your high ATP cells increased, decreased, or unchanged?

Dr. Oelshlegel: I didn't say. This family does not live near Ann Arbor, and by the time we get the blood here, glucose consumption may not be too reliable. (We precipitate samples for DPG and other intermediates on the spot.) The little bit of glucose consumption work I did do on some people did not reveal much difference in glucose consumption between high and low ATP people. But don't hold me on that. Zürcher also found normal glucose consumption in his high ATP individuals.

Dr. Rasmussen: You didn't measure that or lactate production, either one? If not, then the crossover data can't be interpreted.

Dr. Oelshlegel: No. We tried to measure glucose consumption. We didn't see much difference between the two. But we believe we can tentatively interpret the patterns. After all, we have found a structurally different PK, and the intermediate patterns are consistent with increase in our PK activity.

Dr. Tanaka: Are you explaining the elevated ATP on the basis of a lower Km for PEP, is that correct?

Dr. Oelshlegel: I'm speculating that the enzyme is kinetically altered.

Dr. Tanaka: There are some PK variants with a lower Km for PEP which have a decreased ATP, and there is clinical hemolytic disease. How would you reconcile your results with these patients? And don't you think the high ATP ordinarily should have an inhibiting effect? Did you determine the Ki for ATP?

Dr. Oelshlegel: No, we didn't measure the Ki for ATP.

Dr. Brewer: I believe the pyruvate kinase variants producing hemolysis that have a lower Km for PEP must have some other abnormality, such as an abnormal Km_{ADP}, reduced Vmax. I think Dr. Oelshlegel measured the Km for ADP, and found it to be normal.

Dr. Oelshlegel: We did Km's for ADP. They were similar between high and normal ATP individuals.

Unidentified Speaker: Did you look at the sodium-potassium transport across these cells?

Dr. Oelshlegel: We measured content. Again, we haven't studied this exhaustively, but we didn't see much difference in red cell sodium or potassium content.

Dr. Miller-New York: More important perhaps than the Km for ATP is the inhibitory effect of ATP on your enzyme? What was the Ki ATP? We know with the G6PD model, for instance, that NADP and NADPH may critically control the activity of this enzyme. I'd be very interested to know whether this enzyme was more inhibited by ATP and perhaps some other system was involved to explain your results. The other question I had has to do with the fact that some of your patients had G6PD deficiency, or sickle cell trait as well as the high ATP. How do these other abnormalities fit in?

Dr. Oelshlegel: That's why we picked these particular two subjects, because they both had similar genotypes except for the ATP differences. Dr. Brewer has already studied the interaction of high ATP and G6PD deficiency. As I said, we haven't measured Ki for ATP. That's obviously something we should look at. There are many more kinetic studies to do.

Dr. Brewer: I would like to comment that this is a family revisited. We studied them back in the early 1960's. One of the G6PD deficient people underwent typical hemolysis in response to primaquine in spite of twice normal levels of ATP. There was no interaction as far as we could tell. I would like to comment on the Ki for ATP business within this family. I think one would be searching for a lessened Ki_{ATP} rather than a greater one, as an explanation for this variant, because you have to explain why the situation is apparently one of a greater PK activity *in vivo.*

MALARIA-INDUCED ERYTHROCYTE OXIDANT SENSITIVITY

Nina L. Etkin and John W. Eaton

Department of Medicine
University of Minnesota
Minneapolis, Minnesota

INTRODUCTION

Numerous human populations have had extended exposure to endemic malaria. Many of these same populations display a high frequency of variants of the X-linked enzyme, glucose-6-phosphate dehydrogenase (G-6-PD). These frequent variants are generally characterized by diminished G-6-PD activity, and erythrocytes from hemizygous males or homozygous females show a marked sensitivity to additional oxidant stress (reviewed in Eaton and Brewer, 1974).

The geographic coincidence of endemic malaria and high frequencies of G-6-PD deficiencies suggests that the deficiencies somehow protect against fulminant malaria infection (for reviews, see Livingstone, 1967; 1971). More direct evidence supporting this conjecture comes from the investigations of Luzzatto et al. (1969) who noted that, in red cells from females heterozygous (and, therefore, mosaic) for the African (A-) form of G-6-PD deficiency, G-6-PD normal erythrocytes were 2-80 times more likely to contain malaria parasites than were G-6-PD deficient cells. Furthermore, Allison and Clyde (1961) and Gilles et al. (1967) found lower parasite counts among G-6-PD deficient children under the age of 5 years than among G-6-PD normal controls of the same age. Lastly, Gilles and Taylor (1961) have reported a lack of G-6-PD deficient children among 30 cases of severe P. falciparum infection.

The accumulated evidence, then, suggests that the G-6-PD deficient erythrocyte is either less likely to be infected by the malaria merozoite or that, once infected, the deficient red cell is less capable of supporting the growth and maturation of the parasite. Because no differences have been reported between erythrocyte membranes from G-6-PD deficient and normal subjects, we considered it likely that the G-6-PD deficient red cell was, in some way, a suboptimal environment for the developing parasite.

The cardinal characteristic of G-6-PD deficient red cells is a marked sensitivity to oxidant stress; we therefore hypothesized that the malaria parasite itself might generate oxidants within the infected red cell. Such oxidants would have predictably deleterious effects upon these oxidant-sensitive erythrocytes. Using an analogue of human malaria - P. berghei in mice - we have investigated the effects of parasitization upon oxidation and reduction processes within infected erythrocytes. The results which we report here partially confirm the initial hypothesis and, further, suggest that the parasite may disrupt other portions of the metabolism of infected red cells.

METHODS

Swiss White mice were inoculated with P. berghei (NYU-2 strain) according to standard techniques (Ladda,1969). Infected erythrocytes were obtained by axillary incision and aspiration 8-12 days following inoculation, at which time 20-70% of the erythrocytes were infected. No attempt was made to quantify the proportions of various stages of parasite maturation within these samples, but little variation was noted microscopically.

Prior to all experimental procedures (except methemoglobin determinations on non-incubated blood), as many white cells as possible were removed by filtration of the samples through glass wool, washing of erythrocytes in Hanks balanced salt solution, and aspiration of the residual buffy coat. The separation of malaria parasites from host erythrocytes was accomplished by ammonium chloride lysis (Martin et al., 1971) and subsequent washing of the free parasites in 0.154M KCl with 0.32mM $KHCO_3$ (alkaline potassium chloride).

Methemoglobin was measured by a previously reported modification of the Evelyn Malloy procedure (Eaton et al., 1973). The sensitivity of malaria infected erythrocytes to additional oxidant stress was determined by the incubation of infected and control erythrocytes with sodium ascorbate (Jacob and Jandl, 1966). In the present studies, erythrocytes were washed four times in Hanks balanced salt solution and resuspended to an hematocrit of about 1% (v/v) in Hanks balanced salt solution with 5mM tris(hydroxymethyl)aminomethane (Tris) and 25mM sodium ascorbate, pH 7.40. Dilute cell suspensions and the presence of Tris buffer were necessary for the maintenance of pH at 7.4 during prolonged incubation. Following incubation at 37°C, the erythrocytes were thrice washed in 100 volumes of cold saline (to remove ascorbic acid which will interfere with methemoglobin determinations).

The generation of H_2O_2 within infected red cells was detected through the interaction of 3-amino-1,2,4-triazole (hereafter, aminotriazole) with erythrocyte catalase. Aminotriazole combines irreversibly with catalase:H_2O_2 complex I and permanently inactivates the enzyme (Margoliash et al., 1960) (Figure 1). The extent of formation of the catalase: aminotriazole complex is, thus, a reflection of the presence of intracellular H_2O_2 (Cohen and Hochstein, 1964). To measure the formation of this complex, we employed both the binding of ^{14}C-aminotriazole to elements of the cytoplasm of the infected erythrocyte and determinations of the progressive inactivation of erythrocyte catalase in the presence of 50mM (non-isotopic) aminotriazole. Catalase activity was determined as previously described (Eaton et al., 1972).

NAD(P)H oxidation was measured by a modification of the technique of Baehner et al. (1970). Incubations were

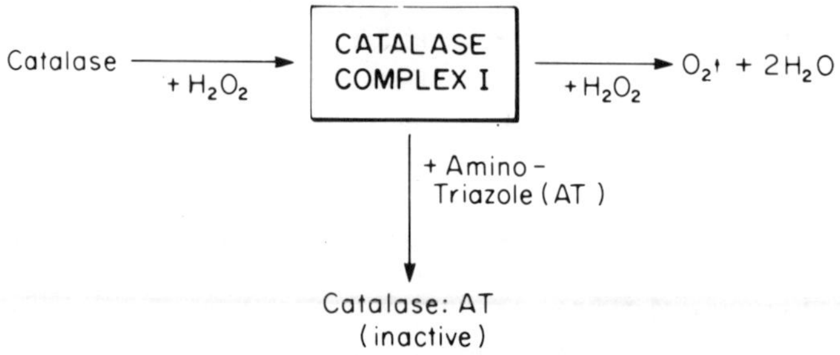

Figure 1. The reaction of catalase with H_2O_2 and aminotriazole.

performed using whole parasite suspensions (dialyzed 18 hours against large volumes of alkaline KCl) and with parasite homogenates made from the latter preparations. Whole parasites or homogenates were incubated at 37°C in a final concentration of 3mg parasite protein per ml in a reaction buffer containing 1mM NADH, 1mM KCN, 0.130M KCl, 0.25mM $KHCO_3$, 0.017M KH_2PO_4, pH 7.0. The amount of NADH oxidized was determined through the periodic removal of an aliquot of the reaction solution, dilution of this aliquot 1:14 with 0.1M potassium phosphate buffer, pH 7.0, and measurement of absorbance at 340nm.

RESULTS

Red cells from malaria infected mice were found to have up to 5 times the normal concentration of methemoglobin (Figure 2) and the level of methemoglobin *in vivo* was directly related to the percentage of infected erythrocytes ($r = 0.879$, $p<0.001$; $n = 13$) (Figure 3).

Upon incubation of infected and control mouse red cells for 2 hours with sodium ascorbate, the former evidenced marked accumulations of methemoglobin (Figure 4). Erythrocytes from those animals with the highest parasite rates tended to form the most methemoglobin during these *in vitro* incubations.

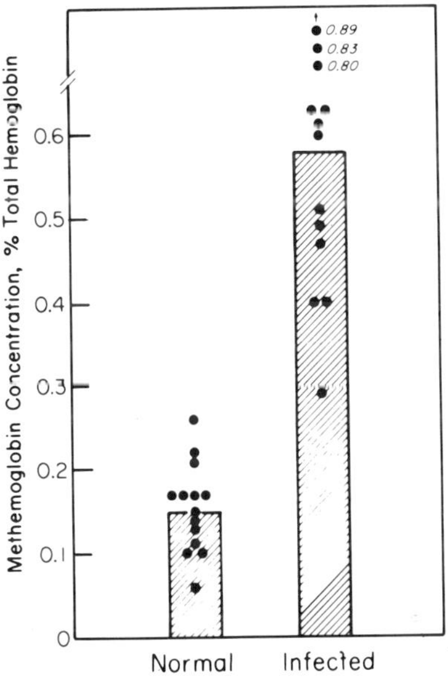

Figure 2. In vivo methemoglobin concentrations in normal and P. berghei infected mice. Each point represents the value from one animal.

The intimate relationship between the accumulation of methemoglobin in vivo and the severity of the malaria infection suggested that the oxidation of hemoglobin was occurring primarily or solely within infected red cells. This raised the intriguing possibility that the parasite itself might be generating oxidants within infected erythrocytes. As an initial test of this, we incubated infected and control erythrocytes with ^{14}C-aminotriazole. Red cells were incubated 2 hours in Hanks balanced salt solution with 5mM Tris, pH 7.4 at 37°C with 2 x 10^{-6}M ^{14}C-aminotriazole (New England Nuclear) and subsequently washed 6 times in saline. Analysis of lysates made from these erythrocytes revealed that malaria infected red cells incorporate approximately four times as much aminotriazole as do uninfected control cells (Figure 5).

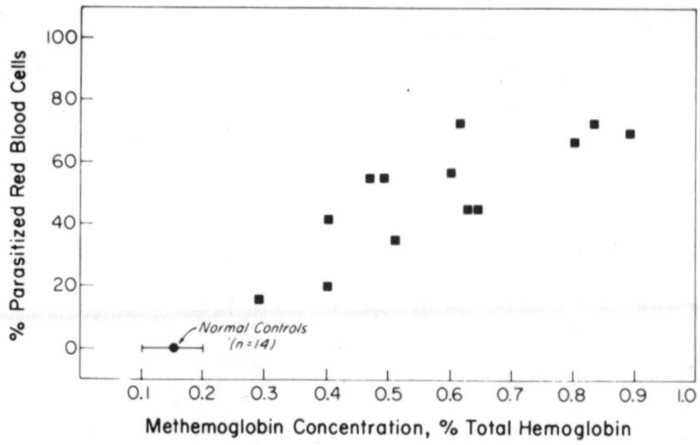

Figure 3. The relationship between percent parasitized red cells and methemoglobin concentration in normal and P. berghei infected mice. The horizontal bar through the normal mean indicates 1 standard deviation.

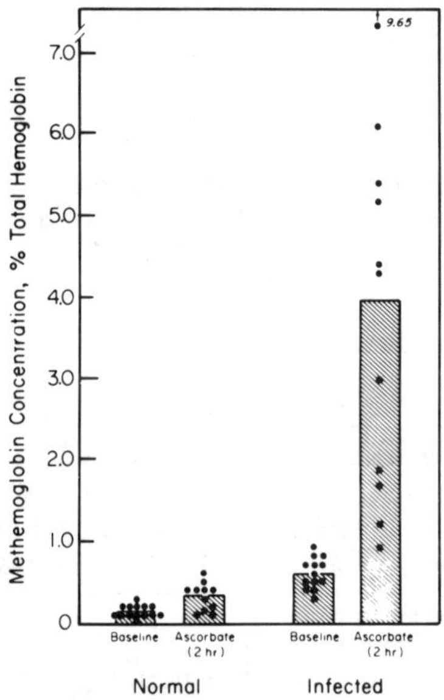

Figure 4. Methemoglobin concentrations in normal and P. berghei infected mouse red cells before and after 2 hours of incubation with sodium ascorbate. See text for experimental details.

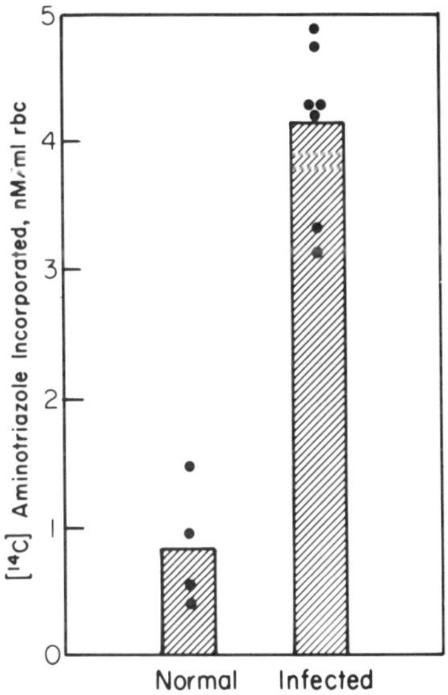

Figure 5. The incorporation of ^{14}C-aminotriazole by normal and P. berghei infected mouse red cells.

Furthermore, preferential ammonium chloride lysis of infected cells (but not parasites) showed that more than 95% of the ^{14}C-aminotriazole taken up by infected erythrocytes is localized in the host cell cytoplasm. However, the amount of aminotriazole incorporated greatly exceeded the molar amount of intracellular catalase (assuming that catalase accounts for about 0.1% of total intracellular protein). Therefore, lysates prepared from similarly incubated erythrocytes were chromatographed on Sephadex G-200 to define the way in which intracellular aminotriazole was partitioned. It was found that the majority of the globin-bound (i.e., acid acetone precipitable) counts were associated with the catalase peak. However, some of the radioactivity was also bound to a protein of molecular weight approximately 60,000 daltons (possibly hemoglobin), and a great deal was present as free, apparently unbound, aminotriazole.

We therefore turned to the progressive inactivation of catalase by non-isotopic aminotriazole as a more direct measure of the generation of intracellular oxidants. During these incubations, malaria infected erythrocytes showed a progressive decrease in intracellular catalase activity, while control red cells showed no change over a period of 90 minutes (Figure 6). Similar incubations were performed with parasite-rich and parasite-poor red cells centrifugally separated from the same initial sample. In these samples, as in samples from animals with varying levels of infection, the extent of aminotriazole-induced catalase inactivation closely paralleled the degree of parasitemia, demonstrating that the inactivation was probably restricted to infected erythrocytes. Aminotriazole-induced catalase inactivation did not occur when samples were incubated under nitrogen or

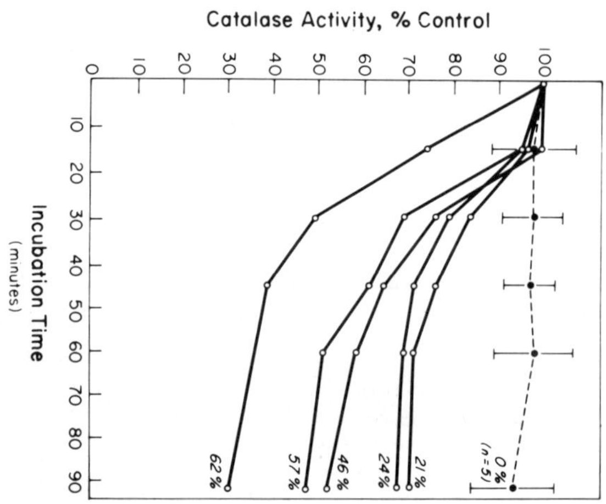

Figure 6. Changes in catalase activity induced by incubation of normal and P. berghei infected mouse red cells with 50mM aminotriazole. Numbers at the right hand ordinate indicate the percent infected erythrocytes in each sample.

when ethanol (0.45M) was present. The inactivation is, therefore, dependent upon molecular oxygen and, further, is blocked by the presence of a peroxidatic donor which limits the availability of catalase:H_2O_2 complex I.

The inactivation of catalase by aminotriazole in infected erythrocytes indicated that oxidants were being generated within the infected cell, presumably by the malaria parasite itself. In addition, the accumulation of methemoglobin within infected cells implied that NADH and/or NADPH levels might be diminished. One enzyme in particular - NAD(P)H oxidase - will both oxidize NAD(P)H and produce H_2O_2 (Baehner et al., 1970). This enzyme is normally present within neutrophils and is of importance in the generation of the H_2O_2 required for the phagocytic killing of ingested bacteria. The malaria parasite is analogous to the human white cell, in that it phagocytically consumes elements of the cytoplasm of the host erythrocyte. We therefore measured the oxidation of NAD(P)H by isolated P. berghei.

Preliminary analyses of isolated parasites and parasite homogenates indicate that P. berghei has significant levels of one or more enzymes which will oxidize NADH (Table 1). This NADH oxidation is cyanide-insensitive, independent of substrates other than NADH and O_2, and is blocked by brief boiling of whole parasite preparations. The oxidation of NADH by these parasites is, in all respects, similar to that found in guinea pig and human neutrophils (Baehner et al., 1970). Furthermore, very preliminary studies in our laboratories suggest that the parasite will oxidize NADPH at a comparable rate. We cannot, however, definitely ascribe this NAD(P)H oxidation to "NAD(P)H oxidase" because our system will not allow the detection of the small amounts of H_2O_2 which might be generated under these experimental conditions.

DISCUSSION

The malaria parasite undoubtedly inflicts several kinds of metabolic stress upon the host red cell. Among these stresses may be consumption of host red cell ATP (Brewer and

Table 1. NADH oxidation by isolated preparations of P. berghei.

Sample	NADH oxidized (uM/gm protein/hour)* Mean	Range
Whole parasites (n = 5)	55	44-71
Parasite homogenates (n = 3)	39	30-46
Whole parasites, heated to 100°C for 5 minutes (n = 3)	4	2-7
Membranes from uninfected red cells (n = 3)	4	2-6

*Uncorrected for red cell membrane contamination.

Powell, 1965; Eaton and Brewer, 1969), as well as phagocytosis of elements of the erythrocyte cytoplasm (reviewed in Peters, 1969). Our results suggest several additional ways in which the parasite may damage the host red cell.

We find that the parasite itself generates oxidants within infected erythrocytes and also diminishes the ability of the infected cell to prevent or repair oxidant damage. In mouse erythrocytes infected with P. berghei, these phenomena may be partially explicable on the basis of parasite-mediated oxidation of red cell NADH and, probably, NADPH. Such oxidation would be expected to have several effects: (1) The diminished availability of NADH will decrease the ability of the infected cell to reduce methemoglobin through NADH-methemoglobin reductase (diaphorase I). (2) The increased concentrations of NAD may act to accelerate glycolysis in general and, perhaps, the regeneration of ATP in particular. In view of the dependence of the parasite upon host cell ATP, this process might be of adaptive value to the parasite during its growth and reproduction. (3) The parasite-mediated oxidation of NADPH will accelerate the pentose phosphate pathway (a phenomenon which we have previously observed in P. berghei infected erythrocytes) and hinder the regeneration of GSH from GSSG. (4) If, as we now suspect, H_2O_2 is a byproduct of the NADH and NADPH oxidation, this process will not only diminish the ability of the cell to repair oxidant damage but will, simultaneously, oxidize a portion of intracellular hemoglobin to methemoglobin.

Insofar as P. berghei in mice is similar to P. falciparum and P. vivax in humans, our results suggest a biochemical basis for the protection against fulminant malaria infection which is thought to be afforded by inherited deficiencies of erythrocyte G-6-PD. The G-6-PD deficient red cell would be relatively intolerant of the oxidation of NAD(P)H and the intracellular generation of oxidants. Cumulative oxidant damage to the infected, deficient erythrocyte would lead to the rapid destruction of both the host cell and the developing parasite.

Our results also suggest that certain antimalarial drugs may preferentially damage the infected red cell as well as the parasite itself. Most antimalarials which act upon the endoerythrocytic form of the parasite also exert an oxidant stress (Cohen and Hochstein, 1964; Fraser and Vesell, 1968). Therefore, the sum of parasite-induced and drug-induced erythrocyte oxidation might very well mimic G-6-PD deficiency and result in an analogous, premature destruction of both the cell and the developing parasite.

SUMMARY

P. berghei infected mouse red cells accumulate methemoglobin in vivo and are more sensitive to exogenous oxidants in vitro. In the absence of added oxidants, catalase within infected cells is readily inactivated by 3-amino-1,2,4-triazole, a reaction which requires the presence of H_2O_2. These phenomena are at least partially attributable to parasite-mediated NADH (and, probably, NADPH) oxidation, which diminishes the ability of the infected cell to prevent and repair oxidant damage. To the extent to which P. berghei is similar to human malarias, these data suggest a biochemical basis for the selective advantage of G-6-PD deficiency and, further, may help explain the mode of action of certain antimalarial drugs.

ACKNOWLEDGEMENTS

Supported by NIH grants HL-15169-9 and HL-16833, and by a grant-in-aid from the University of Minnesota Graduate School. Completely unsupported by the U.S. Army Medical Research and Development Command. We thank Elaine Berger for frequent advice and invaluable help with all aspects of this work. Finally, we wish to thank Dr. Coy Fitch, without whose parasite this work would have been impossible.

REFERENCES

Allison, A. C. and Clyde, D. F. (1961). Malaria in African children with deficient erythrocyte glucose-6-phosphate dehydrogenase. Brit. Med. J. 1:1346.

Baehner, R. L., Gilman, N. and Karnovsky, M. L. (1970). Respiration and glucose oxidation in human and guinea pig leukocytes: comparative studies. J. Clin. Invest. 49:692.

Brewer, G. J. and Powell, R. D. (1965). A study of the relationship between the content of adenosine triphosphate in human red cells and the course of falciparum malaria: a new system that may confer protection against malaria. Proc. Nat. Acad. Sci. 54:741.

Brewer, G. J. and Coan, C. C. (1969). Interaction of red cell ATP levels and malaria, and the treatment of malaria with hyperoxia. Mil. Med. 134:1056.

Cohen, G. and Hochstein, P. (1964). Generation of hydrogen peroxide in erythrocytes by hemolytic agents. Biochem. 3:895.

Eaton, J. W. and Brewer, G. J. (1969). Red cell ATP and malaria infection. Nature, 222:389.

Eaton, J. W., Boraas, M. and Etkin, N. L. (1972). Catalase activity and red cell metabolism. In G. J. Brewer (ed.) Hemoglobin and Red Cell Structure and Function, Plenum Press, New York, pp. 121-131.

Eaton, J. W., Kolpin, C. F., Swofford, H. S., Kjellstrand, C.-M. and Jacob, H. S. (1973). Chlorinated urban water: a cause of dialysis-induced hemolytic anemia. Science 181:463.

Eaton, J. W. and Brewer, G. J. (1974). Pentose phosphate metabolism. In D. Surgenor (ed.) The Red Blood Cell, Academic Press, New York, pp. 435-471.

Fraser, I. M. and Vesell, E. S. (1968). Effects of metabolites of primaquine and acetanilid on normal and glucose-6-phosphate dehydrogenase-deficient erythrocytes. J. Pharm. Exper. Therap. 162:155.

Gilles, H. M. and Taylor, B. G. (1961). The existence of glucose-6-phosphate dehydrogenase deficiency trait in Nigeria and its clinical implications. Ann. Trop. Med. Parasitol. 55:64.

Gilles, H. M., Fletcher, K. A., Hendrickse, R. G., Lindner, R., Reddy, S., and Allan, N. (1967). Glucose-6-phosphate dehydrogenase deficiency, sickling, and malaria in African children in southwestern Nigeria. Lancet 1:138.

Jacob, H. S. and Jandl, J. H. (1966). A simple visual screening test for glucose-6-phosphate dehydrogenase deficiency employing ascorbate and cyanide. New Eng. J. Med. 274:1162.

Ladda, R. L. (1969). New insights into the fine structure of rodent malarial parasites. Mil. Med. 134:825.

Livingstone, F. B. (1967). Abnormal Hemoglobins in Human Populations. Aldine, Chicago.

Livingstone, F. B. (1971). Malaria and human populations. Ann. Rev. Gen. 5:33.

Luzzatto, L., Usanga, E. A. and Reddy, S. (1969). Glucose-6-phosphate dehydrogenase deficient red cells: resistance to infection by malaria. Science 164:839.

Margoliash, E., Novogrodsky, A. and Schejter, A. (1960). Irreversible reaction of 3-amino-1,2,4-triazole and related inhibitors with the protein of catalase. Biochem. J. 74:339.

Martin, W. J., Finerty, J. and Rosenthal, A. (1971). Isolation of Plasmodium berghei (malaria) parasites by ammonium chloride lysis of infected erythrocytes. Nature New Biol. 233:280.

Peters, W. (1969). Recent advances in the physiology and biochemistry of plasmodia. Trop. Dis. Bull. 66:1.

Pollack, S. and George, C. J. N. (1966). Glucose-6-phosphate dehydrogenase deficiency and malaria: II. The mechanism of oxidative drug action in Plasmodium berghei infections. In A. Corradetti (ed.) Proceedings of the First International Congress of Parasitology. Pergamon Press, Milano, Vol. I, pp. 252-253.

Pollack, S., George, J. N. and Crosby, W. H. (1966). Effects of agents simulating the abnormalities of the glucose-6-PD-deficient red cell on Plasmodium berghei malaria. Nature 210:33.

DISCUSSION

Dr. Tanaka: Thank you for an interesting paper. Are there any comments or questions?

Dr. Brewer: I wondered if you have considered the possibility that the parasite might be generating superoxide which could then serve as a source of the peroxide and also other radicals? In such a case you might end up with a number of possibly damaging radicals. Also, you mentioned that the antimalarials affecting the erythrocytic stages produce oxidant stress, but one of the most effective is chloroquine, which really doesn't do much to the cell. It doesn't cause G6PD type hemolysis, for instance.

Dr. Eaton: It doesn't appear to, you're right. Concerning the nature of the oxidants produced by the parasite, we have no idea of the origins of the peroxide in this case. It may well come out first as superoxide, be converted by superoxide dismutase to peroxide and then we detect it. I don't know.

Dr. Babior: I have two questions related to permeability. One is whether the difference in amino triazole binding by infected and normal red cells relates to the ease with which it gets into the two cell populations, and the other is a question of whether the NADH is oxidized extracellularly by H_2O_2 or some other oxidizing agent excreted by the malaria parasite? Do you know which experiment I'm talking about?

Dr. Eaton: In response to the first question, we've incubated infected red cells with amino triazole, spun them down, and looked at the partition of the label after about 30 minutes of incubation. It appears to be fairly freely permeable to the red cell, so that I doubt whether a change of permeability explains this result. Secondly, I can't rule out the possibility that the parasite is oxidizing NADH outside of its membrane (although this would not alter our conclusions). However, the fact that this process is dependent solely upon the presence of NADH and oxygen, and is cyanide insensitive suggests that we are dealing with an enzyme very similar to NADH oxidase.

Dr. McCord: Have you assayed superoxide dismutase levels in infected cells relative to the level in normal cells? The reason I ask this is because the cytoplasmic mammalian superoxide dismutases are reasonably sensitive to inactivation by hydrogen peroxide, and if hydrogen peroxide accumulates and is produced at high levels in an infected cell, you might expect that there would be some decrease of this activity which normally is extremely stable and doesn't decrease.

Dr. Eaton: As I understand it, the inhibition of superoxide by H_2O_2 is a transient one; isn't that correct?

Dr. McCord: No. It's irreversibly deactivated.

Dr. Eaton: I was unaware of that and, no, we haven't assayed superoxide dismutase.

Dr. Tanaka: We will be hearing about selenium and glutathione peroxidase tomorrow from Dr. Hoekstra, but I was just wondering, if you made your mice selenium deficient, which would inhibit glutathione peroxidase, what might happen in your model.

Dr. Eaton: We might expect, unless the selenium deficiency adversely affected the parasite itself that the oxidant damage inflicted by the parasite would be intensified; however, that's just speculation.

Dr. Jacob: Dr. McCord's question stimulates a speculation on my part. That is, since peroxide inhibits superoxide dismutase, and catalase deficiency further potentiates this inhibition, I would expect that iron deficiency which diminishes red cell catalase would protect one from malaria. Has this epidemologic correlation, in fact, been made?

Dr. Eaton: I've heard about interactions between protein deficiency and malaria, but not iron deficiency that I can remember.

CYCLIC NUCLEOTIDE-MEMBRANE PROTEIN INTERACTION IN THE REGULATION OF ERYTHROCYTE SHAPE AND SURVIVAL: DEFECT IN HEREDITARY SPHEROCYTOSIS

Harry S. Jacob, Yoshihito Yawata, Noburo Matsumoto, Steven Abman, and James White

Minneapolis, Minnesota
University of Minnesota Medical School

INTRODUCTION

Ultrastructural studies with highly diverse cells have implicated fibrous proteins in the regulation of cell shape. These proteins, which may assume microtubular or microfilamentous conformations, are frequently located at, or near, the cell membrane. Perhaps the best studied association of such tubules and filaments with cell shape has been noted in the platelet (White, 1968), in which microtubular structures, just beneath the cell membrane, are obvious when the platelet manifests its normal discoid shape; when these microtubules are caused to disappear as with cooling or by treatment with various drugs which denature fibrous proteins, the platelet concomitantly becomes spheroidal. Analogous observations have been made in other cell types as diverse as amoeba and human fibroblasts in tissue culture. It seems reasonable to predict that similar membrane-associated, fibrous proteins might be critical to red cell shape, since these cells also undergo reversible disc-sphere transformations (Nakao et al., 1961). If so, it would seem equally logical to seek a defect in this system in hereditary spherocytosis, in which red cells are abnormally shaped and rigid, leading to their specific sequestration in the filter meshwork of the spleen.

That the red cell membrane contains a protein which can assume a filamentous conformation has been demonstrated by Marchesi and Steers (1968). Thus, about 20% of membrane protein, after solubilization at low ionic strength, aggregates into long microfilaments when ionic strength is increased. This protein, named "spectrin," appears as a filamentous fuzz at the inner aspect of the intact red cell membrane. The present studies indicate that spectrin is crucial to red cell shape, and that its integrity requires phosphorylation by ATP in a reaction catalyzed by cyclic nucleotides. Furthermore, we have found this phosphorylation to be defective in hereditary spherocytosis.

We previously demonstrated (Jacob et al., 1972) that vinblastine, colchicine or strychnine, known denaturants of fibrous proteins, reproduce all the typical characteristics of hereditary spherocytes when added to normal red cells. Thus, these cells manifest the characteristically abnormal morphology, sodium permeability and osmotic fragility of hereditary spherocytes, and if reinjected with a chromium-51 label, they behave in vivo like hereditary spherocytes, as well.

These previous studies strengthened our hypothesis that mutations in vinblastine -- reactive, fibrous proteins underlie the hereditary spherocytosis syndrome. We have gathered further support in the present studies by expanding to red cells the recent studies by others (Sheppard, 1971; Hsie and Puck, 1971; Johnson et al., 1971 Roisen et al., 1972; Kram and Tomkins, 1973) that fibrous proteins are regulated by the cyclic nucleotides, 3'5' AMP and 3'5' GMP; this regulation has been found to modulate the shape and permeability of cells in tissue culture. Thus, the microtubule denaturants, vinblastine or colchicine, alter the shape and membrane transport of tissue-cultured cells in a manner which is specifically and competitively inhibited by the cyclic nucleotides. The present studies demonstrate that an analogous competitive interaction affects red cell shape as well, and that such interaction is defective in hereditary spherocytosis.

METHODS

Fresh heparinized blood from normal human or rat donors was centrifuged and buffy coats removed. The erythrocytes were washed 3 times in phosphate-buffered isotonic saline (pH 7.4; [PO_4]=12mM; [glucose]=14mM) and resuspended in buffer to hematocrit of 30. Various saline-dissolved nucleotides were added to the washed cell suspensions 5-60 minutes before vinblastine or colchicine, which were added, in turn, as described previously (Jacob et al., 1972). Radiolabelled ^{22}Na uptake was measured by adding 0.05 uc of ^{22}Na (Amersham Searle) to 2.0 ml of the cell suspensions which were then incubated for 2 hours at 37°C; the erythrocytes were thrice washed rapidly in 0.1 M $MgCl_2$ and analyzed by flame photometry for total erythrocyte Na content and by gamma-spectrometry for radioactivity. Erythrocyte morphology was examined by scanning electron microscopy with a Cambridge stereoscan electron microscope. Erythrocyte survival and organ sequestration were studied by reinjection of Na_2 $^{51}CrO_4$-labelled rat erythrocytes into Sprague-Dawley, Bartonella-free animals. Erythrocyte membranes were prepared, exposed to ATP- $\gamma^{32}P$, solubilized in SDS, and electrophoresed on polyacrylamide gels by methods slightly modified from those used by Guthrow et al. (1972).

RESULTS AND DISCUSSION

That cyclic nucleotides interact with vinblastine-reactive proteins to modulate red cell shape is shown in Fig. 1. After exposure to vinblastine, sphering and cupping of red cells occur (left, Fig. 1). This conformational change is completely inhibited if vinblastine-treated cells are simultaneously incubated with either cyclic 3'5' AMP (cAMP) or 3'5' GMP (cGMP) (right, Fig. 1). In contrast, the physiologically-inactive cyclic 2'3' nucleotides do not prevent sphering and cupping (not shown).

This protective role of cyclic nucleotides in intact cells is further documented in Fig. 2. The usual increase in osmotic fragility induced by vinblastine is prevented by cyclic 3'5' GMP (right, Fig. 2). Non-cyclic 5' GMP has

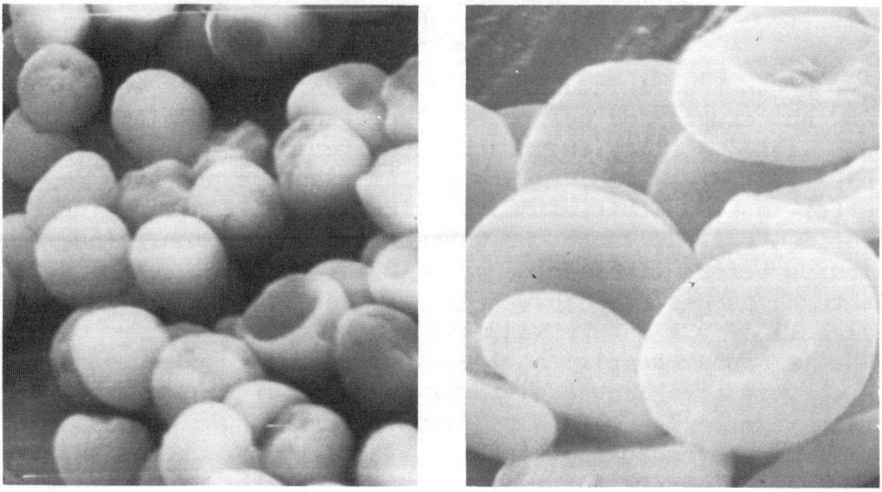

Figure 1. Inhibition of vinblastine-induced erythrocyte sphering and cupping by cGMP. LEFT: Erythrocytic cups and spheres form after 2-hour incubation with vinblastine (0.28 mM) at 37°C. RIGHT: normal morphology persists if cyclic 3'5' GMP (10mM) is added 15 minutes before vinblastine. Cyclic 3'5' AMP is as effective as cyclic 3'5' GMP in preventing shape changes, whereas cyclic 2'3' GMP and cyclic 2'3' AMP are completely ineffective. Completely analogous results were obtained if colchicine (1 mM) was used to induce erythrocyte sphering.

slight, if any, protective effect. Analogous results are obtained utilizing sodium permeability as a measure of red cell membrane alteration (left Fig. 2). Vinblastine or colchicine treatment increased by up to 5 times the uptake of radiolabeled ^{22}Na from the medium into erythrocytes (Jacob et al., 1972); cGMP and cAMP (not shown) prevent this increment, and double reciprocal plots (left, Fig. 2) indicate the antagonism follows competitive kinetics; cGMP inhibits with a Ki=4.9mM more efficiently than cAMP (K_i=5.9 mM). Again, the non-physiologic 2-3 cyclic nucleotide congeners were inactive.

As might be predicted from these studies on shape, permeability, and fragility, cyclic nucleotides also inhibit

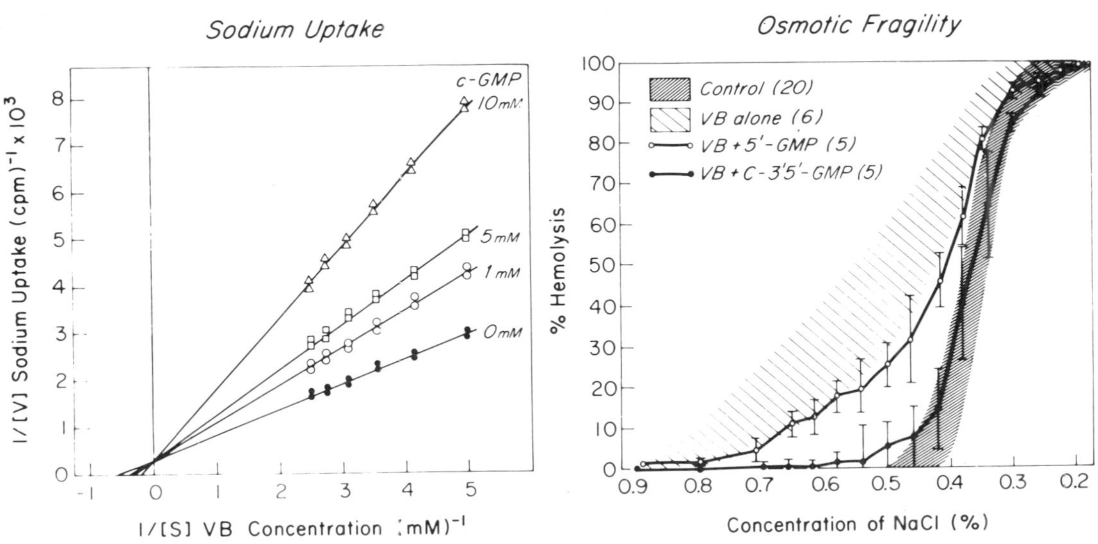

Figure 2. Cyclic 3'5' GMP competitively inhibits ^{22}Na uptake and prevents increased osmotic fragility of vinblastine (VB)-treated erythrocytes. LEFT: ^{22}Na uptake during incubation of erythrocytes for 2 hours at 37° C with various concentrations of vinblastine; cyclic 3'5'GMP inhibits the induced leakiness with competitive kinetics. RIGHT: Addition of 10 mM cyclic 3'5' GMP (closed circles) prevents increases in the osmotic fragility of erythrocytes incubated with 0.28 mM vinblastine for 2 hours at 37° C; non cyclic 5' GMP (open circles) has slight, if any, inhibitory effect. Brackets are ± S.D. Analogous results were obtained if colchicine replaced vinblastine in these experiments.

the splenic entrapment and destruction of vinblastine-treated red cells (Fig. 3). Vinblastine-treated rat red cells, when reinfused after chromium-51 labeling, rapidly disappear from the circulation; however, if cGMP is simultaneously present with the vinblastine, red cell survival remains normal (left, Fig. 3). Concomitant with the loss of circulating radioactivity, labeled red cells accumulate solely in the rat spleens, unless cGMP is simultaneously present in which case abnormal swquestration is prevented (middle and right, Fig. 3).

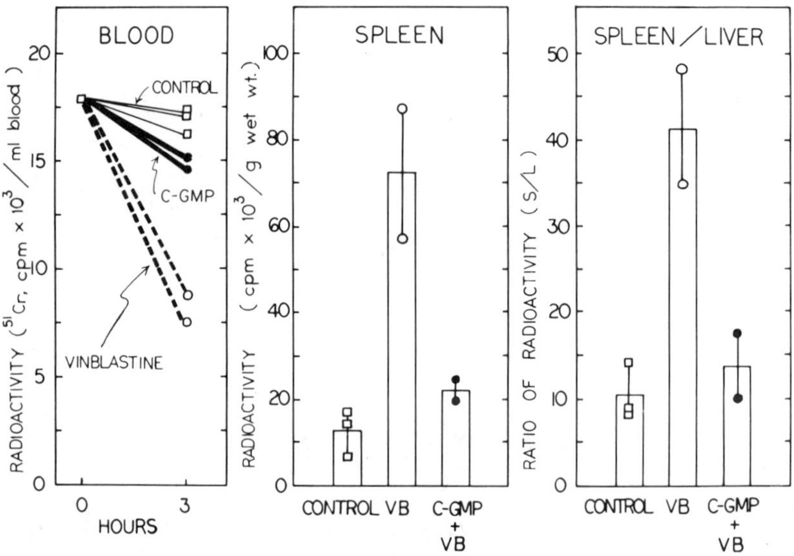

Figure 3. Cyclic 3'5' GMP inhibits vinblastine-induced destruction (left) and splenic sequestration (middle and right) of ^{51}Cr-labeled red cells. Radiolabeled rat red cells incubated for 2 hours with 1 mM vinblastine disappear rapidly from the circulation and are sequestered in the spleen after reinjection into autologous animals (open circles). Cyclic 3'5' GMP (10 mM) added simultaneously with vinblastine prevents these deleterious effects (closed circles).

All of these effects on intact erythrocytes can at the subcellular level be demonstrated to specifically involve spectrin. When red cell membrane proteins are analyzed by SDS polyacrylamide gel electrophoresis after vinblastine treatment, only spectrin is denatured (Fig. 4). Spectrin is easily identified, as it typically migrates most slowly as 2 narrowly separated bands of molecular weight approximately 200,000. Its location is well shown in gels of untreated red cell membrane proteins (top, Fig. 4). After vinblastine exposure, spectrin solely is noted to be lost (middle, Fig. 4). Moreover, the ability of cyclic nucleotides to inhibit vinblastine's deleterious effects on red cells is completely reflected at the subcellular level in that cyclic GMP prevents the denaturation and loss of spectrin from solubilized red cell membranes (lower, Fig. 4). Cyclic AMP protects equally well (not shown).

In other tissues cyclic nucleotides function by catalyzing a protein kinase reaction, which utilizes ATP to

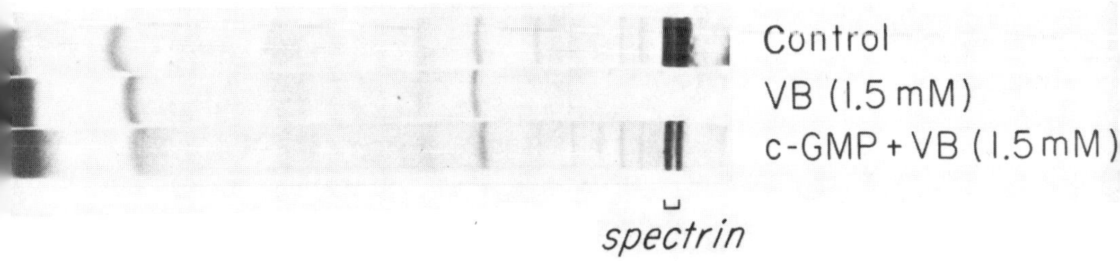

Figure 4. Cyclic nucleotides inhibit the specific denaturation of spectrin by vinblastine. Spectrin, the double-banded protein is easily identified in SDS gels of untreated red cell membrane proteins (top). Vinblastine incubation removes spectrin solely (middle) - an effect prevented by the simultaneous presence of cyclic 3'5' GMP. Cyclic 3'5' AMP is equally effective (not shown).

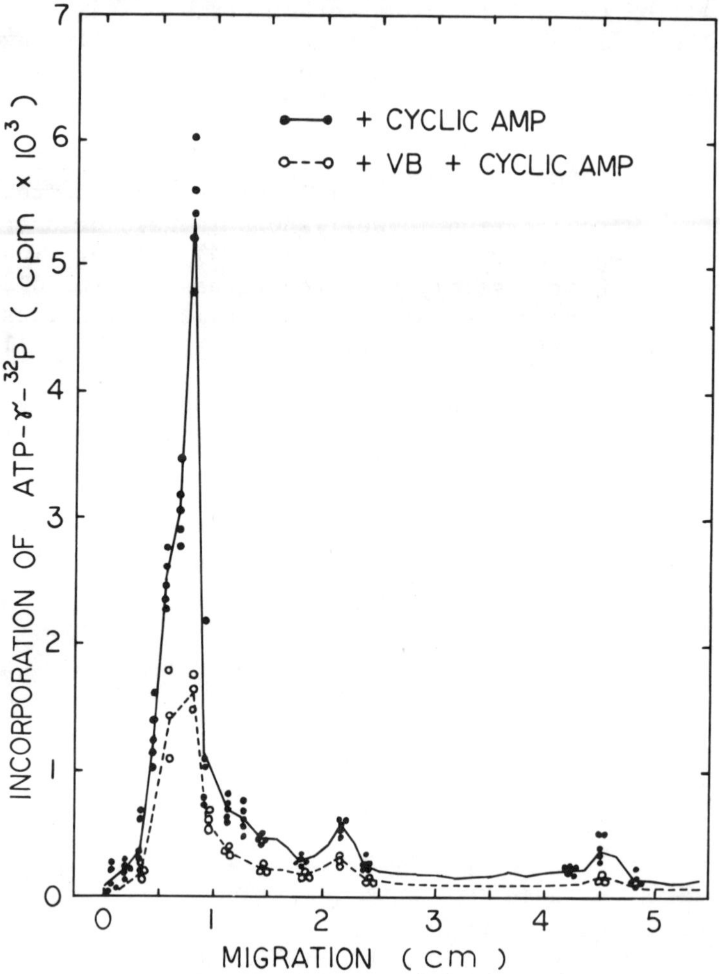

Figure 5. Vinblastine inhibition of cyclic AMP-dependent spectrin phosphorylation. SDS polyacrylamide gels of membrane proteins extracted from ghosts incubated with ATP-γ32p and cyclic AMP were cut into short segments and analyzed for radioactivity. Most activity is associated with spectrin, the slowest-migrating, shouldered peak (black circles). Exposure of ghosts to vinblastine inhibits spectrin labeling (open circles).

phosphorylate various protein substrates. Others have demonstrated this reaction to be intact in red cells (Guthrow et al. 1972; Rubin and Rosen, 1973). In our hands when red cell membranes are phosphorylated by radioactive ATP in the presence of cyclic nucleotides, and the constituent proteins of the membranes analyzed by SDS gels, nearly all of the radioactivity is associated with spectrin (Fig. 5). Consistent with its ability to specifically denature spectrin, vinblastine markedly inhibits this phosphorylation, (dashed line, Fig. 5). From these studies we can define spectrin as a vinblastine-denaturable, fibrous protein whose function is probably importantly regulated by its phosphorylation through a cyclic nucleotide-catalyzed protein kinase.

Further evidence that normal red cell shape and plasticity depend upon spectrin and its phosphorylation was gathered by studies with heated red cells. It is well known that red cells when briefly heated at 50°C become typical microspherocytes, similar to those seen in hereditary spherocytosis (Harris et al. 1957). Just as in the hereditary syndrome, heated cells are specifically sequestered in the spleen; in fact such cells have been utilized for clinical splenic scanning (Wagner et al. 1962). As is the case with vinblastine, red cell membrane proteins, extracted after brief incubation of red cells at 50°C, are specifically depleted of spectrin (insert, Fig. 6). As might be predicted, progressive diminution in phosphorylation of membrane protein (mainly spectrin) occurs with such heating (Fig. 6). Phosphorylation both in the unstimulated state and with added cyclic nucleotides, is diminished during heat-induced spectrin depletion.

Since ultracentrifugation studies by us (Jacob et al., 1971), and electrophoretic analyses by others (Limber et al., 1970); Hayashi et al., 1974), have suggested that mutant membrane proteins may be present in hereditary spherocytes, we were particularly interested in whether ATP-dependent membrane phosphorylation might be defective in this disease. Such phosphorylation is indeed deficient as measured in membranes from 6 consecutive patients with hereditary

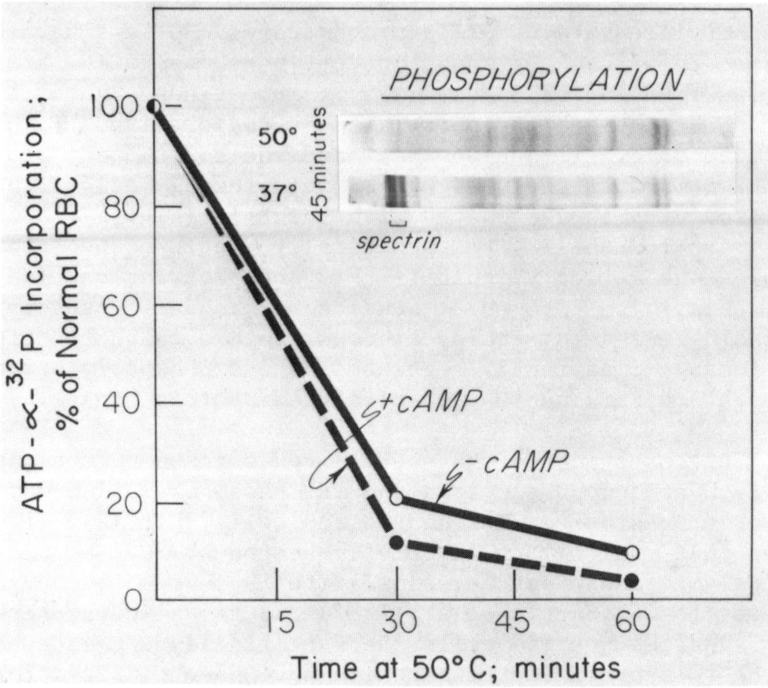

Figure 6. Concomitant loss of spectrin and membrane phosphorylation by ATP-32p in heat-induced microspherocytes. The SDS gel of membrane proteins from red cells heated 30 minutes at 50° C (top, insert) but not at 30° C (bottom, insert) demonstrates solitary loss of spectrin. A progressive decrease in ^{32}P-phosphorylation of ghosts prepared from red cells preheated for increasing periods is noted both with (closed circles) and without (open circles) added cyclic AMP.

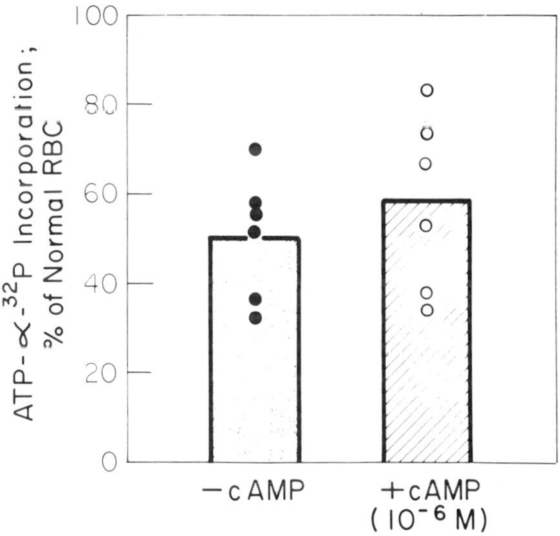

Figure 7. Decreased ATP- γ^{32}P phosphorylation of hereditary spherocytosis red cell membranes. A roughly 50% decrement in radiophosphorylation is noted in membranes from 6 consecutive spherocytosis patients either with (right) or without (left) added cyclic AMP.

spherocytosis. A roughly 50% decrement in labelling, as compared to normal cells, is found (left, Fig. 7) and stimulation of phosphorylation with cyclic nucleotides does not correct the deficiency (right, Fig. 7). These results are similar to those preliminarily reported by Greenquist and Shohet (1973) in 3 other patients. Since the most defective cells in this disease might be expected at any time to be entrapped in the spleen, it is of interest that the most severe abnormality of phosphorylation we have yet observed -- that being only 30% of normal -- occurred in hereditary spherocytes drained from the splenic pulp at the time of splenectomy of one of the portrayed patients.

SUMMARY

Spectrin, a filamentous protein located at the interior of red cell membranes, is specifically denatured by vinblastine or by brief heating at 50° C. With spectrin loss, sphering, rigidity, cation leakiness, and specific splenic sequestration of red cells result. By catalyzing spectrin's phosphorylation with radioactive ATP, cyclic AMP or cyclic GMP stabilizes the protein against denaturation. This phosphorylation reaction is inherently diminished in red cell membranes from patients with hereditary spherocytosis. From these studies we would conclude that spectrin underlies, and is critical to, normal red cell shape. For proper function, its phosphorylation by ATP is required in a reaction catalyzed by cyclic nucleotides. This process is genetically defective in hereditary spherocytosis resulting in the shortened red cell survival of this disease.

REFERENCES

Greenquist, A. and Shohet, S.B. (1973). ATP dependent phosphorylation of a membrane protein in normal and hereditary spherocytosis red cells. Blood 42:997.

Guthrow, C.D. Jr., Allen, J.E., and Rasmussen, H. (1972). Phosphorylation of an endogenous membrane protein by an endogenous, membrane-associated cyclic adenosine 3', 5'-monophosphate-dependent protein kinase in human erythrocyte ghosts. J. Biol. Chem. 247:8145.

Harris, I.M., McAlister, J.M., and Prankerd, T. A. J. (1957). The relationship of abnormal red cells to the normal spleen. Clin. Sci. 16:223.

Hayashi, S., Koomoto, R., Yano, A., Ishigami, S., Tsiyino, G., Salki, S., and Tanaka, T. (1974). Abnormality in a specific protein of the erythrocyte membrane in hereditary spherocytosis. Biochem. Biophys. Res. Comm. 57:1038.

Hsie, A.W., and Puck, T.T. (1971). Morphological transformation of Chinese hamster cells by dibutyryl adenosine cyclic 3' :5'-monophosphate and testosterone. Proc. natl. Acad. Sci. U.S.A. 68:358.

Jacob, H., Amsden, T., and White, J. (1972). Membrane microfilaments of erythrocytes: alteration of intact cells reproduces the hereditary spherocytosis syndrome. Proc. Natl. Acad. Sci. U.S.A. 69:471.

Johnson, G.S., Friedman, R.M., and Pastan, I. (1971). Restoration of several morphological characters of normal fibroblasts in sarcoma cells treated with adenosine-3':5'-cyclic monophosphate and its derivatives. Proc. Natl. Acad. Sci. U.S.A.68:425.

Kram, R., Tomkins, G.M. (1973). Pleiotypic control by cyclic AMP: Interaction with cyclic GMP and possible role of microtubules. Proc Natl. Acad. Sci. U.S.A.70:1659.

Limber, G.K., Davis, R.F., and Baberman,S. (1970). Acrylamide gel electrophoreses studies of human erythrocyte membrane. Blood. 36:111.

Marchesi, V.T., and Steers, E. Jr. (1968). Selective solubilization of a protein component of the red cell membrane. Science 159:203.

Nakao, M., Nakao, T., Yamazoe, S. et al. (1961). Adenosine triphosphate and shape of erythrocytes. J. Biochem. 49:487.

Roisen, F.J., Murphy, R.A., and Broden, W.G. (1972). Dibutyrl cyclic adenosine monophosphate stimulation of colcemid-inhibited axonal elongation. Science 177:809.

Wagner, H.N. Jr., McAfee, J.G., and Winkelman, J.W. (1962). Splenic disease diagnosis by radioisotope scanning. Arch. Int. Med. 109:673.

White, J.G. (1968). Fine structural alterations induced in platelets by adenosine diphosphate. Blood 31:604.

DISCUSSION

Dr. Rasmussen: That's a beautiful theory, Dr. Jacob. The only problem is that there is no cyclic AMP in the normal red cell. And there is no evidence that we have been able to find of any factor, hormonal or otherwise that will alter the concentration of cyclic AMP in the human red cell. By the most sensitive test which we can make, the concentration is clearly less than 10^{-9} molar and the concentration of cyclic AMP which you employ are anywhere from 10^{-6} to 10^{-2} molar. So, I believe that spectrin is involved in the way you suggest, but I doubt that the cyclic nucleotides are the factors that are regulating it in the normal human red cell.

Dr. Jacob: We are aware of the controversy in various laboratories as to how much cyclic nucleotide can be found in human red cells and how much adenyl cyclase is demonstrable in ghosts; perhaps this controversy is irrelevant, however. We are particularly interested in the possibility that cyclic nucleotides are provided to the red cell from its immediate environment. I would remind you that the spleen is an organ in which red cells spend a good deal of time. We have preliminary evidence that the cyclic nucleotide levels in blood drained from the splenic pulp is very high. This coupled with the well-known abnormalities in red cell shape which occur after splenectomy suggest to us that the spleen (and probably other areas of the microvasculative as well) may well "nurse" red cells, providing them with their needed cyclic nucleotides.

Dr. Rasmussen: Well, I don't think there is any real controversy about the fact that in adult human red cells there is no cyclic. There are a few statements in the literature to the contrary, but if you track those down and confront the investigators, they do admit that that is not correct. There is some in human reticulocytes. So if you get a blood that has a very high reticulocyte level, you may see cyclic AMP but in adult cells there is none. Now the other problem is that Rosen and co-workers have shown that apparently exogenous cyclic AMP in intact erthyrocytes will not catalyse the protein kinase. They take cells from the same individual, prepare ghosts, and activate the protein kinase with a Km for activation around 10^{-6}M cyclic. If they take intact cells and repeat the experiment, they can not show a change in membrane phosphorylation.

Dr. Jacob: I hesitate to join you in doubting other investigator's published results but am interested in your evidently private information. On another tack can you tell me what the permeability of cyclic nucleotides in the intact red cell is? We and others obtain active phosphorylation of membranes utilizing ghosts with 10^{-6} - 10^{-8} molar cyclic nucleotides. On the otherhand we need 10^{-3} to 10^{-2} molar to get effects on shape, sodium permeability, etc., in intact cells.

Dr. Rasmussen: We have tried to do that using theophylline-treated cells and labeled cyclic AMP. The rate of penetration is extremely slow. Even after something upwards of thirty minutes incubation, if we start with 10^{-3}M cyclic outside and then wash the cells with a phosphodiesterase to remove all the external cyclic, we have less than 10^{-6}M and probably closer to 10^{-7}M cyclic inside. So it doesn't go in very readily at all. That is the argument that Rosen et al are making: That if you add it outside, you don't catalyse the phosphorylation inside. Now, Friday, in fact, we'll show that with very low doses of cyclic, you do get an effect on the red cell, but I don't think it is because it is acting on the inside of the membrane.

Dr. Jacob: In addition to the possibility that an external supply of cyclic nucleotide may be important we believe that tiny amounts of cyclic nucleotides in a strategic local (at the interior of the membrane where large amounts of ATPase are produced) may be important in red cell shape. An inability to measure relatively large amounts of intracellular nucleotides would not in that case be very telling.

Dr. Rasmussen: I wouldn't accept that view, unless. . .

Dr. Jacob: You don't believe that rapid turnover of strategically located cyclic nucleotides is even a possibility?

Dr. Rasmussen: I think you have to have a certain concentration that will activate the protein kinase and the Km for activation of that enzyme is in the range of 10^{-6}M. Clearly this is a concentration that is very easy to measure by the Gilman assay or by using labeled adenine and so on. The best estimate that we can get is 10^{-8}M or less in human cells exposed to theophylline. That is two orders of magnititude too low. It wouldn't matter how rapidly the pool is turning over, unless for some reason in the intact membrane, the Km for activation is two orders of magnititude lower than that of the isolated ghosts. That is the only way that I can see that it would work.

Dr. Jacob: Then you are faced with the problem of why there is an active protein kinase capable of phosphorylating endogenous membrane proteins in the red cell membrane.

Dr. Rasmussen: Yes, it's a problem.

Dr. Jacob: I prefer to believe its presence signifies an important function.

Dr. Rasmussen: Well, that's an act of religious faith and what one has to look for is factual evidence in science.

Dr. Jacob: It is an act stimulated by a sense of biology. I believe the burden of proof is on one who claims an active system is vestigial or extraneous.

Dr. Rasmussen: One ought to be able to measure the activator.

Dr. Jacob: Unless it is turning over rapidly or is supplied from exogenous sites, such as the spleen.

Dr. Rasmussen: It has got to be there in a concentration sufficient to activate the system regardless of the rate of turnover.

Dr. Salhany: I have a non-controversial question. Is it true that spectrin is a polymer? If so, I was wondering what you meant by denaturation.

Dr. Jacob: The evidence is that spectrin actually precipitates; it polymerizes into a denatured macromolecular structure. Solubilized red cell membrane protein is visually precipitated by vinblastine or high concentrations of calcium, which may be the relevant situation *in vivo*.

Dr. Salhany: By precipitation, you mean it is polymerizing into an insoluble complex?

Dr. Jacob: Yes

Dr. Salhany: You don't mean unfolding the protein?

Dr. Jacob: No, with vinblastine it actually precipitates into macromolecular structures.

Dr. Greenquist: I had a question regarding vinblastine precipitation also. I was wondering why cyclic GMP actually prevents the precipitation of spectrin by the vinblastine. Why should that be so? Is it just a physical precipitation reversed by cyclic GMP or cyclic AMP?

Dr. Jacob: I assume that phosphorylation of this protein is inhibiting its denaturation.

Dr. Salhany: Is there a time-dependent process involved in preventing the precipitation?

Dr. Jacob: I have not studied this.

Dr. Salhany: So it appears to be just a physical process.

Dr. Jacob: It might be.

Dr. Perutz: I wonder how much is known about the parameters of spectrin as a fiber? Can you see a repeating structure in the electronmicroscope? What is its subunit molecular weight? Has it been characterized in any way?

Dr. Jacob: I don't think repeating units have been observed. The subunit molecule appears in SDS gels with an apparent M. weight of about 220,000.

Dr. Perutz: Can you see any repeat in the EM?

Dr. Greenquist: There is sort of a problem here. Fuller has recently reported six N-terminals for material in the spectrin area. Fairbanks has used all kinds of denaturants and hasn't been able to break it down into any smaller components than you will see in an SDS gel. So, it does seem to be around 200,000 molecular weight or greater. It doesn't go down to smaller molecular weights in guanidine and other denaturants.

Dr. Jacob: I believe there is recent evidence taht there is a smaller molecular weight protein which is thought to be a portion of spectrin.

Dr. Rasmussen: There are supposed to be three proteins in this complex now. One is the spectrin, the area #2 of Fairbanks. Another has all the properities of actin and is there in about 10% of the amount of spectrin, and that appears in Fairbank's gel, either in region 4 or 5, I don't remember. And another protein that's either 4 or 5 and the nature of that isn't known. In answer to your question, Dr. Perutz, you don't see any crystalline kind of structure of this complex in the intact cell. And no one has gotten a complex of these three proteins to crystallize in vitro. They form a fiber; a fibrous matrix in vitro, but if you look at it in the electron microscope, its just a complex and rather disarrayed fibrous matrix.

Dr. Perutz: No repeat along the fiber axis?

Dr. Rasmussen: Not that one can tell.

Dr. Perutz: Yes. Is anything known about the amino acid composition. In view of the molecular weight of 200,000, I wonder if it bears any resemblance to myosin?

Dr. Rasmussen: It doesn't have much resemblance to myosin. It was first thought that it had a resemblance to actin, but it is quite clear that it does not. It's fairly hydrophobic.

Dr. Perutz: Thank you very much. So it's a mystery how it works?

Dr. Tanaka: How about in hereditary elliptocytosis? Have you had a chance to look at that?

Dr. Jacob: No. Have you Dr. Greenquist?

Dr. Greenquist: We have looked at two hereditary elliptocytos patients and we haven't found any abnormality in the phosphorylation in those patients.

Dr. Jacob: Were these hemolyzing patients or just patients with morphologically abnormal red cells?

Dr. Greenquist: They were both hemolyzing.

Dr. Jacob: That's peculiar. I think many of us feel that patients with hereditary elliptocytosis that actually hemolyze really have forme fruste hereditary spherocytosis with similar protein abnormalities. For instance, there are many families in which one member would be diagnosed as having hereditary spherocytosis and another as elliptocytosis. There may be different elliptocytotic syndromes; I think at least one has the same defect in membrane structrual protein found in spherocytosis, but simply is not as severe.

Dr. Tanaka: Thank you Dr. Jacob and the discussants for a lively opening this morning.

A MEMBRANE PERMEABILITY ALTERATION RESULTING IN DESICCYTOSIS AND HEMOLYTIC ANEMIA

Bertil E. Glader, Normand Fortier, and Maurice Albala
Dept. of Pediatrics, Harvard Medical School, Boston, Mass., Dept. of Hematology, St. Vincent's Hospital, Worcester, Mass., Dept. of Hematology, Rhode Island Hospital, Providence, R.I.

Hemolytic anemia due to abnormalities in cation permeability have been described by several investigators (1,2, 3). In each of these previous reports the membrane lesion has been characterized by a marked increase in cation permeability which was greater for Na than K. As a consequence of this defect, these cells gained Na in excess of K lost, total cation content increased, cell water increased, and osmotically fragile "hydrocytes" were formed. We recently have observed another patient with hemolytic anemia and increased permeability to cations. In this case the membrane was more leaky to K than Na. Consequently these cells lost total cation, cell water decreased, and osmotically resistant "desiccytes" were produced.

The patient we have studied is a 21 year old white female with a life-long history of anemia and jaundice. Prior to her splenectomy at 6 years of age, she received several blood transfusions. Subsequently, she has not been transfused and her anemia has remained stable (hemoglobin 10.0 gm%, hematocrit 27.5, red blood cell count 2.7 x 10^6 cells/ µl, MCV 106 μ^3, MCH 37.4 pg, MCHC 36.4 g/100 ml). At 13 years of age she had a cholecystectomy, and at 16 she became pregnant and delivered a term male infant. Overall her clinical course has been uneventful. Her son (now 3 years old) also has anemia, hepatosplenomegaly, and jaundice. Although he has not been studied in detail, his hemolytic anemia appears to be identical to that of his mother. No other family members have been available for study.

The patient's peripheral blood contained abnormal cells consistent with her post-splenectomy status. In addition many RBC's appeared dehydrated and contained areas at the cell periphery where hemoglobin seemed to be puddled. Unlike some other permeability abnormalities, stomatocytosis was not a characteristic of these erythrocytes. The usual laboratory evaluation of this hemolytic anemia failed to identify any known hemoglobin or metabolic abnormality. The 2,3-DPG level (4.0 μMole/ml RBC) was within normal limits, but was less than expected for the degree of anemia. The osmotic fragility curve was shifted to the right, indicating the presence of a resistant population of cells.

The Na and K content of the RBC's from our patient and her son are seen in Table 1. In contrast to normal cells, these RBC's contained more Na and less K. The total cation content also was less than normal. The cell water content was measured with tritiated water and corrected for trapped plasma with ^{14}C-sucrose. In contrast to the normal water content (69-72% cell water) the RBC's of the propositus were dehydrated (58% cell water).

Table 1

Red Blood Cell Cation and Water Content

	Na	K	Na + K	Cell H_2O
	----(meq/1 RBC)--------			--(%)---
Patient (R.D.)	18.6	58.1	77.7	58.7
Son (A.D.)	16.0	59.1	81.2	-
Control	7.0	92.0	99.0	69.1
Normal	(5-12)	(90-103)		(69-72)

Table 2

Net Na and K Fluxes With and Without Ouabain

(meq/1 RBC/hr)	Control			Patient		
	Na	K	Na + K	Na	K	Na + K
No ouabain	+0.8	-0.7	+0.1	+1.1	-2.4	-1.3
+ ouabain	+2.7	-1.8	+0.9	+4.9	-4.9	0
"Pump"	1.9	1.1		3.8	2.5	
Na:K pump	1.9/1.1 = 1.73			3.8/2.5 = 1.52		

In order to gain insight into the pathophysiology of this cation abnormality, net Na and K flux measurements were made (Table 2). Control cells incubated in a glycylglycine-buffered salt solution manifested a slight Na increase (0.8 meq/1 RBC/hr) and a similar K loss (0.7 meq/1 RBC/hr). The net effect of these fluxes was a slight cation gain equivalent to 0.1 meq/1 RBC/hr. When ouabain (10^{-4}M) was added to inhibit the Na-K pump, control cells gained Na (2.7 meq/1 RBC/hr), lost K (1.8 meq/1 RBC/hr), and there was a net gain of 0.9 meq of cation/ml RBC/hr. "Pump" activity was calculated as the ouabain-induced difference in net flux. Control RBC's pumped Na at a rate of 1.9 meq/1 RBC/hr, and K was transported at a rate of 1.1 meq/1 RBC/hr. The cation pump was normally coupled in a Na:K ratio of 1.73. In contrast, RBC's from the propositus, incubated under conditions which were approximately steady-state for control cells, lost K (2.4 meq/1 RBC/hr) in excess of Na gained (1.1 meq/1 RBC/hr). Consequently, these cells lost approximately 1.3 meq of total cation per hour. When ouabain was added, Na influx increased further but there was an equivalent K efflux. The net effect of the cardiac glycoside was such that there was no change in total cation content. Calculated Na

Table 3

Na and K Permeability in Ouabain Treated RBC's

	Control	Patient
Potassium		
Passive efflux (^{39}K)	1.6	3.4
Mean ^{39}K gradient	130.0	94.1
"P" constant	.0123	.0362
Relative "P"	1.0	3.0
Sodium		
Passive influx (^{23}Na)	2.9	4.3
Mean ^{23}Na gradient	142.3	128.3
"P" constant	.0204	.0335
Relative "P"	1.0	1.6

and K active transport were increased in the patient's RBC's and this increased pump activity was appropriate for the elevated internal Na concentration (4). Furthermore, the patient's cation pump was normally coupled with a Na:K ratio of 1.52.

When ouabain is added to inhibit the active transport of Na and K, these cations passively traverse the membrane. The rate at which they cross the membrane is related to the concentration gradient between the cell and extracellular medium, and "p", the intrinsic permeability properties of the membrane (including membrane potential):

$$\text{Passive membrane transport} = \text{"p"} \times \text{mean cation gradient}$$

$$\frac{\text{Passive membrane transport}}{\text{Mean cation gradient}} = \text{"p"}$$

This value "p" was calculated for both Na and K in ouabain-treated cells in which the passive flux and mean cation gradient were known (Table 3). The relative "p" for a given cation is a comparison of the patient's "p" value compared to that of the control. The patient's RBC's were 3 times more permeable to K than the control, and 1.6-fold more permeable to Na. The ratio of Na:K permeability was 1.66 in control cells, and 0.93 in RBC's of the propositus. Thus, K permeability of this patient's red cells was greater than that of the control, as well as being greater than the Na permeability of her own cells.

Other K-losing syndromes have been described for erythrocytes. In red cell pyruvate kinase deficiency (5), metabolically depleted cells (6), irreversibly sickled cells (7) and in the presence of propanolol (8), there is a marked K loss in excess of Na gain, and a resultant decrease in total cation content and cell water. In each of these cases, calcium is required for the induction of K and water loss. In contrast, RBC's of the propositus manifested no significant difference in the rate of K loss, with or without added calcium (1.5 mM). In common with other K-losing entities, however, our patient's red cells maintained K and water content when they were incubated in a 140 mM K-buffer. In fact, cell K, total cation content, and cell water were increased under these conditions, thus suggesting that membrane permeability to K influx also was enhanced.

In order to determine the relevance of these _in vitro_ cation changes to events _in vivo_, young and old RBC's were separated by centrifugation for 1 hour (Table 4). Control cells manifested little difference in the Na content of young (top) and old (bottom) RBC's; but the K content was decreased approximately 10 meq in the older cells. The patient's red cells manifested more marked changes in cation content. The bottom layer of RBC's contained approximately 8 meq less of Na, and 20 meq less K. Thus the patient's older cells had significantly less total cation and water. This cellular dehydration also was manifested by the increased MCHC (40.2) in the dense cells on the bottom. It was of interest that many of the patient's dense cells were

Table 4

Na and K Concentration in Separated Young and Old RBC's

	Retic	MCHC	Na	K	Na + K
			----(meq/1 RBC)----		
Control					
Top	4.0	33.8	8.5	98.7	107.2
Bottom	0	36.7	6.6	91.4	98.0
Patient					
Top	43	33.0	32.3	73.2	105.5
Bottom	25	40.2	24.0	53.0	77.0

reticulocytes, suggesting that the membrane defect also affected many young cells. The cation composition of the least dense cells on top had a decreased K concentration, but Na content was increased and the total cation and water content were normal.

In summary, we have presented a patient with a hemolytic anemia associated with altered permeability to cations. The pathophysiology of this disorder is best understood in juxtaposition to "hydrocytosis", another major permeability disorder. Hydrocytes manifest a markedly increased cation permeability which is greater for Na than K. The Na-K pump is stimulated to maintain the normal cation distribution, but it is unable to keep up with the accelerated leak. Consequently these cells gain more Na than they lose K, the total cation content increases, cell water increases, and these RBC's become osmotically fragile. In all cases of hydrocytosis associated with hemolysis, the response to splenectomy has been excellent. Presumably this reflects the effects of the adverse splenic environment on these metabolically active RBC's.

Table 5

	Hydrocytosis	Desiccytosis
Permeability	Na greater than K	K greater than Na
Cell Na + K	Increased	Decreased
Cell water	Increased	Decreased
Osmotic fragility	Increased	Decreased
Response to splenectomy	Good	?

The lesion in desiccytosis, in contrast, is characterized by an increase in permeability which is greater for K than for Na. The Na:K pump is appropriately stimulated for the internal Na concentration, but is unable to compensate for the excess K loss. Consequently, these cells lose total cation, cell water decreases, and osmotically resistant desiccytes are formed. The clinical response to splenectomy is not very impressive. Although our patient has not required blood transfusions subsequent to her splenectomy, the indications for her early blood transfusions are not known. In addition, her son (who has not been splenectomized) manifests the same degree of anemia.

The studies described in this report demonstrate the physiology of a membrane lesion which results in altered cation transport and hemolytic anemia. Further definition of the specific chemical lesion is currently under investigation.

References

1. Zarkowsky, H.S., Oski, F.A., Sha'afi, R., Shohet, S.B., and Nathan, D.G.: Congenital hemolytic anemia with high sodium, low potassium red cells. I. Studies of membrane permeability. New Engl. J. Med. (1968) 278:573-581

2. Oski, F.A., Naiman, J.L., Blum, S.F., Zarkowsky, H.S., Whaun, J., Shohet, S.B., Green, A., and Nathan, D.G.: Congenital hemolytic anemia with high sodium, low potassium red cells. Studies of three generations of a family with a new variant. New Engl. J. Med. (1969) 280:909-916

3. Dutcher, P.O., Segel, G.B., Feig, S.A., Miller, D.R., and Lichtman, M.: Stomatocytic RBC - A model of altered transport control. Blood (in press)

4. Segel, G.B., Feig, S.A., Glader, B.E., Müller, A., and Dutcher, P.: An essential role for phosphoglycerate kinase dependent red cell cation transport. American Society of Hematology, December, 1973, Program #16

5. Mentzer, W.C., Baehner, R.L., Schmidt-Schonbein, H., Robinson, S.H., and Nathan, D.G.: Selective reticulocyte destruction in erythrocyte pyruvate kinase deficiency. J. Clin. Invest. (1971) 50:688-699

6. Gardos, G., and Straub, F.B.: Uber die rolle der adenosintriphosphorsäure (ATP) in der K-permeabilität der menschlichen roten blutkörperchen. Acta Physiol. Acad. Sci. Hung. (1957) 12:1-8

7. Glader, B.E., and Nathan, D.G.: Comparison of membrane permeability abnormalities in reversibly and irreversibly sickled erythrocytes. Progress Report of the 1st National Symposium on Sickle Cell Disease, 1974, (in press)

8. Manninen, V.: Movement of sodium and potassium ions and their tracers in propanolol-treated red cells and diaphragm muscle. Acta Physiol. Scand. (1970) 355:1-76

DISCUSSION

Dr. Brain: This is a very fascinating patient. We described, admittedly rather briefly, a rather similar patient a number of years ago. We found a somewhat similar disturbance in red cell cation composition. However, in contrast to your patient, profound lowering of intracellular potassium and intracellular water was not associated with a rise in intracellular sodium. We found it difficult to account for the ability of the red cells to sustain their potassium level without a rise in intracellular sodium to activate the $Na^{+}K^{+}$ pump. We found comparable changes in cation and water content in young and old cells. The other feature which distinguished our patient from yours was that despite a splenectomy the red cells showed a striking increase in osmotic fragility.

Dr. Glader: It sounds like these cells are much more dehydrated than those we have described. I wonder if one doesn't reach a point where cell dehydration produces membrane injury and the cells actually become more osmotically sensitive. We see this with propanolol-induced cell dehydration, where there is initially a marked loss of potassium and water, but there is little or no hemolysis. After a period of time, some sodium enters these cells, and then they lyse. These are dehydrated cells which have apparently lost their ability to increase their volume appropriately. So, presumably, there is some membrane injury which occurs secondary to severe dehydration. Sounds like that is what you're seeing with your patient.

Dr. Miller: Dr. Glader and I have discussed this many times before, but perhaps it would be wise to discuss it in front of the open audience. Not all stomatocytes are hydrocytes.

Dr. Perutz: What is a stomatocyte?

Dr. Miller: A stomatocyte is a happy or sad looking cell with a slit rather than a central area of pallor, which is most beautifully seen in scanning electron microscopy. The cells are uni-concave rather than bi-concave. In the syndromes of stomatocytosis described by Oski and Zarkowsky, the cells certainly were hydrocytes. We studied a very large family with cation content very similar to Dr. Glader's patient's cells in which there was an increased loss of potassium over sodium gain as well. In fresh cells, the sodium was elevated and the potassium content was decreased, the cell water was slightly decreased; the osmotic fragility was decreased and further decreased with incubation. The response to splenectomy was poor. Thus there is a very great heterogeneity in the stomatocytosis syndromes.

Unidentified Speaker: I wondered if you had had a chance to look at sodium-potassium changes with prolonged incubation and metabolic deprivation in your cells?

Dr. Miller: No.

Dr. Brain: We carried out studies of erythrocyte metabolism in our patient and looked at factors influencing levels of glycolytic intermediates. This led us to the observation that our patient's red cells were remarkably unresponsive to the metabolic effects of raised concentrations of inorganic phosphate. In the light of Dr. Minakami's paper yesterday, I think one needs to be concerned about the intracellular pH when you get disturbances of cation concentration and water concentration. Unfortunately, we did not measure intracellular pH.

Dr. Glader: We measured the pH in this patient. I take that back, we didn't directly measure pH. Instead we determined the radioisotope chloride distribution ratio and, assuming a Donnan equilibrium, calculated the intracellular pH to be about 7.25, a little bit higher than our control of 7.20.

Dr. Orringer: I was a little concerned about your permeability calculations. You mentioned that in the steady state your control cells were losing about 0.7 mEq of potassium and gaining about 0.8 mEq of sodium per liter of cells per hour. Have you done any isotopic fluxes in your cells to determine permeability?

Dr. Glader: Yes, we have done isotopic fluxes, but I think they tend to confuse more than help us understand the pathophysiology. We're finding more and more that this is the case when we use isotopes. This particular patient has a high sodium-sodium exchange which is not ouabin-sensitive.

Dr. Orringer: When you wash your cells to measure cell content of sodium and potassium, do you wash them in magnesium chloride?

Dr. Glader: Yes.

Dr. Orringer: If these cells were more permeable to magnesium than normal cells, this certainly could give you altered cation and water content.

Dr. Glader: We haven't looked at magnesium permeability. I have no way of knowing that.

Dr. Orringer: Have you done osmotic fragility curves in the child who hasn't had a splenectomy? Clearly, post splenectomy states can give you a decreased fragility.

Dr. Glader: Yes. The child's hematologic status, both in terms of the abnormal cells in his peripheral smear and in a shift to the right in the osmotic fragility is somewhere intermediate between his mother and the control.

Dr. Jacob: In answer to the last questioner, I don't think there is any question that these cells are dehydrated, both morphologically and by osmotic fragility studies, so that magnesium might cause a slight artifact, but it is probably not very important, if it occurs at all. I have a question about filterability. If you dehydrate red cells as by suspension in hypertonic salt, do you in fact get decreased cell filterability in your system? One might expect up to a point that the smaller cells would go through a filter more readily until polymerization of hemoglobin occurred. If that is the case, do not your results imply that there is something inherently wrong with the rigidity of the membranes--not just a dehydrated cell?

Dr. Glader: This is an interesting concept. My prejudice is that cellular dehydration produces a viscous intracellular milieu, and this may have the same effect as a "rigid membrane." We're actually in the process of evaluating this possibility. I don't doubt that she has a rigid membrane and that may explain what we're seeing. Nevertheless, it seems plausible that cellular dehydration *per se* without altered-membrane rigidity, might give you decreased deformability.

Dr. Jacob: The MCHC is not very elevated--37 or so. Do you think hemoglobin would polymerize at such a concentration?

Dr. Orringer: I can answer Dr. Jacob. Teitel in 1969, using the old filterability technique showed that following dehydration cells filtered less well than euhydrated cells.

Dr. Tanaka: Your findings would suggest, along with other findings, that the red cell really doesn't have an osmoreceptor for water. Do you feel that water just always follows the cations?

Dr. Glader: Yes. I think that is what happens. Dog red cells probably have an osmosensitive mechanism.

Dr. Perutz: I just wondered whether it is technically feasible to probe deeper and see whether the sodium pump is defective in such abnormalities in membrane proteins?

Dr. Glader: That is exactly what we are doing. I think we have defined a physiological defect, we're looking for the chemical lesion right now. I don't think it is going to be in the cation pump. It appears from a variety of cells that Na, K ATPase is much more sensitive to the internal sodium than the external potassium. So I think the pump is working fine in this particular cell. I think the major question is why are particular cells permeable to potassium?

Dr. Perutz: Then may I ask a naive question, but one which may puzzle other non-clinicians in the audience here. What is the advantage of splenectomy?

Dr. Glader: In some hemolytic anemias, such as hereditary spherocytosis which Dr. Jacob talked about earlier, you have an ongoing hemolytic state and cells are frequently destroyed in the environment of the spleen. The spleen is a graveyard for red cells and if you can remove where the cells are destroyed you can increase the life span of these cells. Although abnormal cells may continue to circulate, they can live a pretty normal life in the absence of the spleen. For some hemolytic anemias due to metabolic abnormalities, or membrane abnormalities, splenectomy has been very beneficial. In this particular case, as well as in many cases where you have severe cellular dehydration, other reticuloendothelial tissue in the liver and elsewhere can remove the cells as well as the spleen. So there is really no big benefit from taking the spleen out.

STUDIES ON RED CELL ACETYLCHOLINESTERASE WITH SPECIAL REFERENCE TO AUTOIMMUNE HEMOLYTIC ANEMIA

Kouichi R. Tanaka, M.D.
Department of Medicine
Harbor General Hospital, Torrance,
and UCLA School of Medicine, Los Angeles, CA

Red cell acetylcholinesterase (E.C. 3.1.1.7.) (ACE) is of particular interest since this is the only enzyme located in the cell membrane that has reflected changes in activity with several clinical disorders. ACE activity is decreased in paroxysmal nocturnal hemoglobinuria (PNH) (DeSandre et al., 1956; Auditore and Hartmann, 1959), in ABO hemolytic disease of the newborn (Kaplan et al., 1964), in familial reduction in ACE activity (Johns, 1962), and in severe poisoning with specific anticholinesterase agents (Goldin et al., 1964). We have previously described subnormal levels of red cell ACE activity in autoimmune hemolytic anemia (AHA) (Tanaka et al., 1964) but there have been conflicting reports (Brabec et al., 1967; Sirchia et al., 1970; Herz et al., 1972). This report presents studies on red cell ACE and additional data to indicate that red cell ACE activity is usually decreased in AHA of the warm antibody type when ACE activity is related to red cell age. The significance of the depressed ACE activity in several hematologic disorders is discussed.

METHODS

Fresh venous blood was processed and assays for glucose-6-phosphate dehydrogenase were performed as previously described (Tanaka et al., 1962). Initially ACE activity was determined in duplicate by the method of Michel (1949) utilizing acetylcholine chloride as substrate in a barbital buffer at pH 8.0 at 25°C with a Radiometer pH meter. Subsequently, ACE activity was assayed colorimetrically with acetylthiocholine iodide as substrate in the presence of 5,5'-dithiobis (2-nitrobenzoic acid) in phosphate buffer at pH 8 (Ellman et al., 1961), utilizing a Gilford spectrophotometer unit at 412 nm at 37°C. Hexokinase was assayed as described by Valentine et al. (1967). The direct anti-globulin (Coombs) test was performed with rabbit anti-human globulin serum. Crystalline trypsin and γ-chymotrypsin, and crude bromelin, ficin, and papain were obtained from Calbiochem.

RESULTS

In Table I are presented our normal values for ACE activity by the method of Michel, and illustrative examples of increased and decreased activity as in sickle cell anemia and PNH, respectively. Two representative cases of hereditary spherocytosis show that ACE activity in hereditary spherocytosis is frequently elevated even after splenectomy when reticulocytosis is no longer present.

Table I. RED CELL ACETYLCHOLINESTERASE

	ACE Activity†	
	Δ pH/hour	% of Normal
Normals (29) (Range=.64-.93)	0.79 ± .08	100
Sickle cell anemia	0.98	124
PNH* (Case 1)	0.51	65
(Case 2)	0.16	20
HS**, presplenectomy (Case 1)	1.00	127
HS**, postsplenectomy (Case 2)	0.98	124

†Method of Michel
*PNH, paroxysmal nocturnal hemoglobinuria
**HS, hereditary spherocytosis

Table II. AUTOIMMUNE HEMOLYTIC ANEMIA (COOMBS POSITIVE)

Pt	Age	Sex	Retic(%)	G6PD	ACE Activity† Δ pH/hr	ACE Activity† % Normal	Diagnosis
				3.88*	.79	100	
P.G.	34	F	35.9	----	.47	59	2° to SLE
D.A.	45	M	14.1	6.19	.56	71	Idiopathic
A.M.	49	F	16.4	5.64	.32	41	Idiopathic
B.L.	21	F	15.5	6.79	.40	51	2° to SLE
E.G.	67	M	7.6	4.79	.50	63	2° to CLL
W.H.	59	M	5.3	4.49	.46	58	Idiopathic
C.H.	71	M	9.9	----	1.14	144	Idiopathic
S.F.	45	F	3.9	4.49	.64	81	2° to SLE
H.C.	48	F	20.3	7.02	.60	76	Idiopathic
J.H.	24	F	13.3	4.79	.78	99	Idiopathic
V.P.	56	M	3.6	6.16	.47	59	Idiopathic

*Upper limit of our normal range, expressed as μmoles of NADP reduced/10^{10} red cells/minute at 37°C.

†Method of Michel.

In Table II are summarized the initial 11 patients with Coombs positive autoimmune hemolytic anemia of the warm antibody type. It is to be noted that ACE activity as expressed in Δ pH/hour or in % of normal was decreased in comparison to the degree of reticulocytosis and elevated G6PD activities. Patient C.H. was a notable exception. His value was elevated on several assays. Patient V.P. had a normal ACE value upon recovery as did two other patients studied during remission. Patient A.M. had values in this range for 2 years. Study of her family demonstrated normal ACE values, thus excluding a familial low ACE.

As shown in Table III, a number of experiments were performed with the red cells of patient A.M. In order to exclude the possibility of unknown exposure to organophosphorous anticholinesterase compounds, the red cells were incubated with the oxime, pyridine 2-aldoxime methiodide. No increase in activity resulted. Simple experiments as shown failed to demonstrate the presence of an inhibitor or absence of an activator. Some attempts with elution

Table III. EXPERIMENTS ON RBC OF PT. A.M.

RBC + 2 - PAM 10^{-3} M
RBC Freeze thaw 25 X
RBC + high activity hemolysate
RBC + 56°C normal hemolysate
RBC + 1.2% NaCl 37°C 1 hr
RBC + large volume 0.9% NaCl 4°C 24-40 hrs
RBC + 0.9% NaCl pH 3.0 37°C 45 minutes
RBC + Normal serum 37°C 2 hrs
Pt. serum + Normal RBC 37°C 2 hrs

were unsuccessful in increasing the red cell ACE activity of this patient. Similar experiments with the erythrocytes of patient V.P. also gave negative results.

In further studies of over 500 subjects, ACE activity was determined by the method of Ellman et al. (1961). In Table IV are shown the normal value, mean value in a healthy adult of Japanese ancestry with hereditary deficiency of ACE which will be reported in detail elsewhere, and an unexplained persistently elevated ACE value in an adult without evidence of hematologic disease.

In Table V are shown the main groups constituting the 50 normal subjects as well as cord blood results. Red

Table IV. RED CELL ACETYLCHOLINESTERASE

	ACE Activity Mean ± SD
Normals (50)	14.0 ± 1.56
Hereditary deficiency of acetylcholinesterase (8 determinations over 6 year period)	8.4 ± 0.57
Subject S.T. (Mean of 3 determinations)	25.7

† Expressed as μmoles substrate utilized/10^{10} red cells/min at 37°C.

Table V. RED CELL ACETYLCHOLINESTERASE

Number	Subjects	ACE Activity†
50	Normals	14.0 ± 1.6
24	Normal males	13.6 ± 1.2
26	Normal females	14.4 ± 1.8
13	Normal Japanese	13.8 ± 1.7
15	Normal Caucasians	14.4 ± 1.6
10	Normal Filipinos	14.0 ± 1.9
5	Normal Chinese	13.5 ± 1.3
12	Cord blood	10.3 ± 1.8

†Mean ± S.D. Activity expressed as μmoles substrate utilized/10^{10} red cells/min at 37°C.

cells from an additional 19 Japanese subjects assayed by the method of Michel had ACE activity comparable to that of Caucasians.

Red cell ACE activities in elderly patients with non-hematologic disorders were comparable to that of younger subjects (Table VI).

Red cell ACE and hexokinase activities were determined in a variety of hereditary hemolytic anemias. Representative results are shown in Table VII. It is to be noted that as expected both ACE and HK activities are generally increased. The hexokinase deficiency patients of course have a relatively decreased hexokinase activity for the degree of reticulocytosis. The ACE/HK ratio was markedly

Table VI. RED CELL ACETYLCHOLINESTERASE

Number	Subject	ACE Activity†	Mean Age
38	Normals	100.0 ± 10.8	33.8
34	Patients* (Age 70-79)	97.8 ± 13.4	74.8
30	Patients* (Age 80-97)	110.4 ± 15.5	84.9

†Expressed as per cent of normal ± SD using method of Michel.

*Patients with non-hematologic disorders and with packed red cell volumes of 36% or over.

Table VII. RED CELL ACETYLCHOLINESTERASE IN HEREDITARY HEMOLYTIC ANEMIAS

Subject	Diagnosis	PCV	Retic(%)	ACE Activity†	HK†	ACE/HK
	Normal			14.0*	.26*	54
T.D.	G6PD Torrance	32	8.8	19.0	.32	59
D.L.	G6PD def	39	6.8	23.7	.69	34
R.N.	HK def	37	8.2	19.9	.22	90
P.M.	HK def	46	4.1	19.2	.15	128
C.C.	PFK def	42	5.5	20.6	.24	86
D.W.	PFK def	52	2.0	21.8	.23	95
K.R.	PK def	41	8.6	15.3	.31	49
L.M.	PK def	37	4.3	14.1	.28	50
G.M.	PK def**	29	56.7	34.5	.92	38
J.R.	PK def**	17	76.0	30.9	3.00	10
A.H.	Unstable hgb.	32	9.0	27.2	.77	35
R.P.	Hgb. CC_{Harlem}	30	5.3	14.3		

†Activity expressed as μmoles substrate utilized/10^{10} red cells/min at 37°C.

*S.D. for normal ACE is ± 1.6; for HK ± .07.

**Postsplenectomy

decreased only in the pyruvate kinase deficiency patient with an unusually elevated hexokinase value.

Studies on 11 patients with autoimmune hemolytic anemia are summarized in Table VIII. It is to be seen that the ACE/HK ratio is decreased in 9 of the 10 subjects. It is of interest that patient V.M. with cold agglutinin hemolytic disease has a normal ratio. Of the current total of 33 patients studied with autoimmune hemolytic anemia, 6 have had cold agglutinins. This group does not appear to have depression of ACE activity as consistently as the warm antibody type.

Serial studies on patient N.R. with idiopathic autoimmune hemolytic anemia are summarized in Table IX. The simultaneous determination of ACE and hexokinase activities

Table VIII. AUTOIMMUNE HEMOLYTIC ANEMIA (COOMBS POSITIVE)

Patient	Diagnosis	PCV	Retic(%)	ACE†	HK†	ACE/HK
	Normals (50)			14.0	.26	54
N.R.	Idiopathic 1969	18	22.7	14.2	1.64	8.7
N.R.	" 1974	28	20.0	10.7	.82	13.0
L.N.	Idiopathic	12	0.5	9.4	---	----
R.P.	Idiopathic	27	26.9	22.4	1.69	13.3
V.B.	Idiopathic	25	16.2	14.9	1.53	9.7
F.B.	Idiopathic	28	7.4	12.1	.88	13.8
C.H.	2° to L-dopa	29	8.4	10.1	.52	19.4
S.R.	2° to CLL	19	21.6	14.2	1.72	8.3
R.W.	2° to CLL	39	2.8	14.5	.53	27.6
B.G.	2° to lymphoma	25	4.1	14.8	.74	20.0
R.B.	Cold agglutinins	21	7.4	9.3	.96	9.7
V.M.	Cold agglutinins	31	6.2	27.5	.52	52.9

†Mean values for normals. Activity expressed as μmoles substrate utilized/10^{10} red cells/min at 37°C.

Table IX. Pt. N.R. AUTOIMMUNE HEMOLYTIC ANEMIA

Date	PCV	Retic(%)	Coombs	ACE	HK	ACE/HK
5-23-69	18	22.7	4+	14.2	1.64	8.7
6-13-74	28	20	4+	10.7	0.82	13.0
6-20-74	31	19	4+	10.8	1.13	9.6
6-27-74	38	7.6	4+	11.4	0.82	13.9
7-05-74	40	3.8	3+	13.5	0.63	21.4
7-12-74	42	2.6	1+	14.6	0.48	30.4
7-25-74	39	2.1	1+	12.5	0.43	29.1
8-15-74	39	1.7	2+	12.3	0.44	28.0
9-12-74	39	0.4	1+	11.6	0.34	34.1

and their ratios provide a more comprehensive view of her clinical disease.

Crystalline trypsin and γ-chymotrypsin and crude bromelin, ficin, and papain were used in a concentration of 1.5 mg/ml of washed normal red cell suspension and incubated at 37°C. ACE was determined on an aliquot at the time

Figure 1 RBC INCUBATION WITH PROTEOLYTIC ENZYMES (1.5 mq/ml)

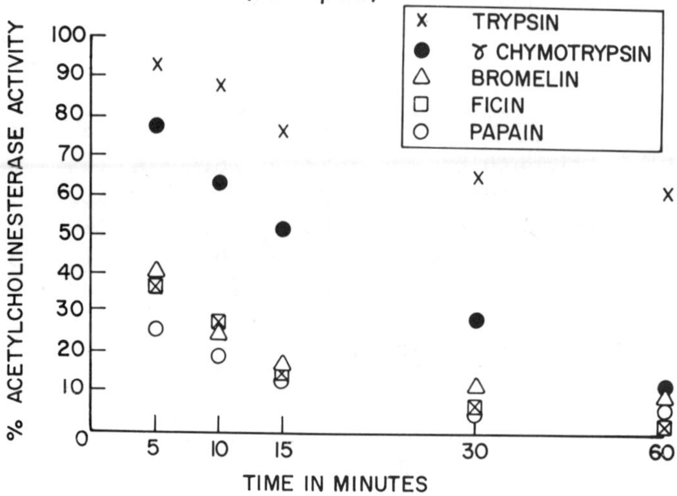

intervals indicated (Fig. 1) and expressed in terms of % ACE activity of the unincubated sample. The variable rate of decrease of ACE activity is similar to that previously described by others (Firkin et al., 1963; Herz et al., 1963; Perona et al., 1965). Crystalline carboxypeptidase also decreased ACE activity. In another experiment with ficin, which causes a very rapid loss of ACE activity, a small but measurable amount of ACE activity was found in the supernatant after one minute of incubation and a lesser amount after 5 minutes.

Incubation of normal red cells and PNH red cells with 0.085 molar penicillin or sodium cephalothin* in phosphate buffer pH 7.0 (Herz, 1967) for up to 24 hours resulted in a similar loss of ACE activity, more with cephalothin than with penicillin. Cephaloridine+ also decreased ACE activity in normal red cells to the same degree as penicillin.

As shown in Table X the acid serum test was positive with all proteolytic enzymes except for γ-chymotrypsin as previously demonstrated (Firkin et al., 1963).

---

*+Kindly supplied as Keflin and as Loridine, respectively, by The Lilly Research Laboratories.

Table X.

RBC Experiment				ACE Activity(%)	Acid Serum Test
Saline control not incubated				100.0	---------
Saline control, incubated 37°C 4 hrs				87.0	negative
Trypsin	1.5 mg/ml	"	"	46.1	positive
γ chymotrypsin	1.5 " "	"	"	12.4	negative
"	5.0 " "	"	"	9.5	negative
Ficin	1.5 " "	"	"	9.1	sl. pos.
"	5.0 " "	"	"	8.0	positive
Papain	1.5 " "	"	"	10.2	positive
Bromelin	1.5 " "	"	"	8.4	positive

In Table XI are listed patients with disorders that may be associated with decreased red cell ACE activity. The low values in PNH are well established, though variable among patients; ACE values in myelofibrosis with myeloid metaplasia are frequently low but not to the usually marked degree as in PNH. Centrifugation studies have shown the top young cells to have greater activity than the bottom older cells in myelofibrosis.

Table XI. DISORDERS ASSOCIATED WITH DECREASED RED CELL ACETYLCHOLINESTERASE ACTIVITY

Subject	Diagnosis	ACE Activity*
	Normals (38)	100
F.B.	Paroxysmal nocturnal hemoglobinuria	22
R.H.	Myelofibrosis with myeloid metaplasia	58
H.G.	DiGuglielmo's syndrome	70
A.S.	Refractory anemia, idiopathic	76
E.R.	Acute myelomonocytic leukemia	68
V.F.	Chronic uremia	73
R.K.	Cirrhosis with spur cell anemia	65
S.F.	Microangiopathic hemolytic anemia	70

*Activity expressed as % of normal utilizing method of Michel.

DISCUSSION

These studies confirm and extend our initial report that patients with warm antibody-sensitized red cells usually have decreased levels of red cell ACE when interpreted in comparison with known age related parameters such as glucose-6-phosphate dehydrogenase and hexokinase (Valentine et al., 1967). Unless examined in this manner, the significance of the ACE assay value may not otherwise be appreciated since ACE itself is a function of red cell age (Pritchard, 1949; Sabine, 1951). Other parameters such as creatine content may be useful as an indication of cell age (Griffiths and Fitzpatrick, 1967). Scott and Rasbridge (1971) related the ACE values of patients with a positive anti-globulin test to their creatine content and thereby were able to demonstrate that many ACE values were lower than would be expected for the age of the red cell population. The use of age related parameters is also helpful in evaluating the ACE values during the clinical course of the patient with AHA.

The type of antibody in AHA appears to be important in determining the ACE level. Red cells coated with IgG warm antibodies, with or without complement, are more likely to have reduced ACE activity than red cells sensitized by complement-binding cold antibodies (Sirchia et al., 1970; Scott and Rasbridge, 1971). Although in our patients the type of antibody was not examined systematically, a few observations have been made and appear to be consistent with these reports, which may account partly for the differences in ACE results described in the literature for AHA. Variability in enzyme determinations may also play a role; however, in our patients similar results were obtained with the electrometric method of Michel (1949) or the colorimetric technique of Ellman et al. (1961).

ACE is known to be decreased in cord blood (Burman, 1961). In the red cells of elderly subjects ACE was found to be normally active. Since a subject of Japanese ancestry was found to have hereditary deficiency of ACE, several different ethnic groups were examined. No apparent differences were noted. Details of studies on the family with hereditary deficiency will be described elsewhere, since it appears that no cases have been published since the case report of Johns in 1962.

The mechanism for the subnormal ACE activity in AHA remains unclear. No evidence for an inhibitor or absence of an activator could be shown. Since incubation of normal red cells with a number of proteolytic enzymes results in decreased ACE activity (Herz et al., 1963; Herz and Kaplan, 1974), it has been inferred that ACE is located at or near the outer surface of the cell membrane where the primary interaction between antibodies and erythrocytes occurs. This coupled with the finding of an abnormally rapid decline of ACE activity with cell aging (Scott and Rasbridge, 1971; Herz et al., 1972) suggests loss as a likely mechanism as previously proposed (Tanaka et al., 1964). This view is also consistent with the decreased red cell content of cholesterol and phospholipids during the active phase, but with normal values during remission of AHA as described by Brabec et al. (1969).

It may be suggested that in PNH, a population of red cells with severely defective membranes is produced to account for the usually very low ACE activity, whereas in AHA there is abnormally rapid loss due to the damaging effect of antibodies, particularly of the IgG type. Clinical states in which disordered erythropoiesis occurs, such as myelofibrosis with myeloid metaplasia, erythroleukemia, and refractory anemia, may be associated with some decrease in ACE activity due to mild abnormalities in membrane formation. ACE activity may be occasionally somewhat depressed in another group of disorders, such as in chronic uremia and microangiopathic hemolytic anemias; here one or more plasma factors or mechanical factors may play a role. Thus, the evaluation of red cell ACE activity in conjunction with proper age related parameters may be useful clinically and should improve our understanding of these disorders.

SUMMARY

These studies confirm and extend our initial report that patients with warm antibody-sensitized red cells usually have decreased levels of red cell acetylcholinesterase when interpreted in comparison with known red cell age related parameters. Accumulating evidence suggests that the low activity results from loss secondary to membrane damage by antibodies. ACE determination may be useful clinically and in the understanding of several hematologic disorders.

ACKNOWLEDGEMENTS

The author is grateful to the many physicians who have referred patients for study. This investigation was supported by grant AM 14898 from the National Institutes of Health. The competent technical assistance of Pansy Chao, Annie Gammon, Hugo Galmarini, and Mirta Galmarini is acknowledged.

REFERENCES

Auditore, J.V., and Hartmann, R.C. (1959). Paroxysmal nocturnal hemoglobinuria. II. Erythrocyte acetylcholinesterase defect. Amer. J. Med. 27:401.

Brabec, V., Michalec, C., Palek, J., and Kout, M. (1969). Red cell lipids in autoimmune hemolytic anemia. Blood 34:414.

Brabec, V., Palek, J., Mircevova, L., Friedmann, B., Vopatova, M., Kout, M., Michalec, C., and Volek, V. (1967). Red cell metabolism in autoimmune hemolytic anemia. Proc. 10th Congr. europ. Soc. Haemat., Strasbourg 1965; part II, p. 346.

Burman, D. (1961). Red cell cholinesterase in infancy and childhood. Arch. Dis. Childhood 36:362.

De Sandre, G., Ghiotto, G., and Mastella, G. (1956). l'acetilcolinesterasi eritrocitaria. II. Rapporti con le malattia emolitica. Acta Med. Patavina. 16:310.
Ellman, G.L., Courtney, K.D., Andres, V., Jr., and Featherstone, R.M. (1961). A new and rapid colorimetric determination of acetylcholinesterase activity. Biochem. Pharmacol. 7:88.
Firkin, B.G., Beal, R.W., and Mitchell, G. (1963). The effects of trypsin and chymotrypsin on the acetylcholinesterase content of human erythrocytes. Australasian Ann. of Med. 12:26.
Goldin, A.R., Rubenstein, A.H., Bradlow, B.A., and Elliot, G.A. (1964). Malathion poisoning with special reference to the effect of cholinesterase inhibition on erythrocyte survival. New Engl. J. Med. 271:1289.
Griffiths, W.J., and Fitzpatrick, M. (1967). The effect of age on the creatine in red cells. Brit. J. Haemat. 13:175.
Herz, F. (1967). Inactivation of erythrocyte acetylcholinesterase by penicillin. Nature 214:497.
Herz, F., and Kaplan, E. (1974). In vitro modifications of red cell acetylcholinesterase activity. Brit. J. Haematol. 26:165.
Herz, F., Kaplan, E., and Scheye, E.S. (1972). Red cell acetylcholinesterase deficiency in autoimmune hemolytic anemia and in paroxysmal nocturnal hemoglobinuria. Clin. Chim. Acta 38:301.
Herz, F., Kaplan, E., and Stevenson, J.H., Jr. (1963). Acetylcholinesterase inactivation of enzyme-treated erythrocytes. Nature 200:901.
Johns, R.J. (1962). Familial reduction in red-cell cholinesterase. New Engl. J. Med. 267:1344.
Kaplan, E., Herz, F., and Hsu, K.S. (1964). Erythrocyte acetylcholinesterase activity in ABO hemolytic disease of the newborn. Pediatrics 33:205.
Michel, H.O. (1949). An electrometric method for the determination of red blood cell and plasma cholinesterase activity. J. Lab. & Clin. Med. 34:1564.
Perona, G., Cortesi, S., Ghiotto, G., and De Sandre, G. (1965). Acetylcholinesterase in human erythrocytes

treated with trypsin, papain, or bromelin: its relationship with susceptibility to acid lysis *in vitro*. Brit. J. Haemat. 11:171.

Pritchard, J.A. (1949). Erythrocyte age and cholinesterase activity. Amer. J. Physiol. 158:72.

Sabine, J.C. (1951). The cholinesterase of erythrocytes in anemias. Blood 6:151.

Scott, G.L., and Rasbridge, M.R. (1971). Red cell acetylcholinesterase and adenosinetriphosphatase activity in patients with a positive antiglobulin test. Scand. J. Haemat. 8:53.

Sirchia, G., Ferrone, S., Mercuriali, F., and Zanella, A. (1970). Red cell acetylcholinesterase activity in autoimmune haemolytic anaemias. Brit. J. Haematol. 19:411.

Tanaka, K.R. Valentine, W.N., and Miwa, S. (1962). Pyruvate kinase (PD) deficiency hereditary nonspherocytic hemolytic anemia. Blood 19:267.

Tanaka, K.R., Valentine W.N. and Schneider, A.S. (1964). Red cell cholinesterase in Coombs positive autoimmune hemolytic anemia (AHA). Clin. Res. 12:110.

Valentine, W.N., Oski, F.A., Paglia, D.E., Baughan, M.A., Schneider, A.S., and Naiman, J.L. (1967). Hereditary hemolytic anemia with hexokinase deficiency. Role of hexokinase in erythrocyte aging. New Engl. J. Med. 276:1.

DISCUSSION

Dr. Bunn: Your observations may relate to the mechanism for membrane loss in autoimmune hemolysis, studied by Lo Buglio, Abramson, and Jandl. They demonstrated rosettes with monocytes that were specific for red cells coated with gamma globulin having class 1 and 3 heavy chain subtypes. It might be interesting to look at the eluates from your patients with Coomb's positive hemolytic anemia to see whether there was a correlation between decrease in red cell cholinesterase and particular subtypes of gamma G that are prone to form rosettes.

Dr. Tanaka: Thank you for your comment. We have just looked at Ig G, not the subtypes. We have looked at some to show that, as reported by others, the Ig G type does seem to be the type most frequently associated with a decrease in acetylcholinesterase. It certainly will be interesting to look at the subtypes.

Unidentified speaker: Would you tell me what the normal function of acetylcholinesterase is in the red blood cell?

Dr. Tanaka: I wish I could tell you that. I certainly don't know, and as far as I'm aware, in the literature no one has been able to explain the function of this enzyme.

Dr. Brain: I wondered in view of the possibility that you suggest that it's related to membrane loss, whether you've tried to correlate the activity with increase in osmotic fragility which, I think, would probably occur in some of these other spur cell hemolytic anemias in which you also say there's a loss. Sphering is a variable feature of acquired hemolytic anemia, and I wondered if there's a correlation.

Dr. Tanaka: Yes, we've done some studies, and the greater the degree of spherocytosis, the more likely it is that the activity is depressed. There is a correlation with spherocytosis based more on the work of others. For instance, the interesting situation that Herz and Kaplan initially described of ABO hemolytic disease being associated with decreased acetylcholinesterase where spherocytosis occurs, whereas usually in Rh hemolytic disease where spherocytosis does not occur, acetylcholinesterase is not decreased. So there seems to be a correlation with spherocytosis.

Dr. Greenquist: Is acetylcholinesterase activity reduced if you incubate red cell membranes with some appropriate antibody, such as anti-A or anti-B? In other words, does an antigen-antibody reaction reduce the enzymatic activity?

Dr. Tanaka: No. That's been done by others, and it does not decrease in these short-term *in vitro* experiments. Others have explained that in terms of trying to account for the depression by implicating the RE system. Something else is probably necessary which is not present in *in vitro* experiments, and some investigators have implicated the RE system as being probably necessary for loss of the membrane or actual damage sufficient to lose the acetylcholinesterase.

Dr. Brewer: Do you think it's possible that the red cell carries around certain enzymes to help in detoxifying substances? Is it a possible function for this enzyme to metabolize acetyl choline that escapes from the nervous system or other choline esters?

Dr. Tanaka: Well, that's certainly possible, but probably not the case. Other workers have considered it. I have not done any studies to try to prove or disprove that, but others have wondered about it and have not come up with an explanation so far.

Dr. Fuller: I wondered if you'd studied any patients who had an oxidant susceptible red cell before and after the oxidant stress--to see if they have Heinz body formation, and lose red cell membrane, and have a decrease in acetylcholinesterase?

Dr. Tanaka: I'm sorry. I have not done that.

Dr. Jacob: As I have already stated to Dr. Rasmussen, one should be cautious before assuming an active enzymatic system is simply vestigial. I am very intrigued, therefore, that acetylcholinesterase is elevated in hereditary spherocytosis, even after splenectomy. Do you have speculation as to why this should be within the framework that acetylcholinesterase is a potent cyclic nucleotide stimulator in other cells and the hereditary spherocyte manifests abnormalities in cyclic nucleotide metabolism.?

Dr. Tanaka: I can only speculate. My feeling would be that in hereditary spherocytosis, there is an abnormal membrane which has more acetylcholinesterase to begin with. I think it is a possibility that because the most likely defect in HS is in the membrane, that it is just carying more to start with, that is, it is formed with more acetylcholinesterase. In contrast, in PNH where the membrane is probably the primary defect, there is something wrong structurally initially, and perhaps that accounts for the decreased acetylcholinesterase.

Dr. Brewer: Have you by any chance taken a look at whether cyclic nucleotides affect the activity of acetylcholinesterase?

Dr. Tanaka: No, I have not. I'd like to make just one other comment about myeloid metaplasia. Others have described positive sugar water tests with cells of myeloid metaplasia, that is, myelofibrosis with myeloid metaplasia. Other workers have shown that the depression of acetylcholinesterase is more severe, the more severe the anemia is in myelofibrosis, indicating probably that there is a greater population of abnormal cells, and this would suggest that there is perhaps a relationship between diseases like myelofibrosis with decreased acetylcholinesterase and PNH, the latter having perhaps even more severely defective cells to begin with.

METHEMOGLOBIN REDUCTION IN NORMAL AND CONGENITAL METHEMOGLOBINEMIC ERYTHROCYTES

Yoshiki Sugita, Yoshimasa Yoneyama,
Takeshi Kitao, and Kenichi Hattori

Department of Biochemistry and Department of Medicine, Kanazawa University School of Medicine
Kanazawa, Japan

INTRODUCTION

Methemoglobin in human erythrocyte is reduced by several systems, and a NADH dehydrogenase that is lacking in congenital methemoglobinemia is considered to play a major role in the reduction (Scott, 1960; Scott *et al*. 1969). However, methemoglobin was one of the least active substrates for the enzyme. We have purified the NADH-dehydrogenase and found that cytochrome b_5 was the most effective electron acceptor and that the rate of methemoglobin reduction by the enzyme in the presence of cytochrome b_5 was rapid and approximately equal to the rate of cytochrome b_5 reduction (Sugita *et al*., 1971). Hultquist and Passon (1971) also reported the rapid reduction of methemoglobin by erythrocyte cytochrome b_5 and cytochrome b_5 reductase. However, the identity of the cytochrome b_5 reductase with the NADH dehydrogenase reported by Scott was not clear. In this paper we report the deficiency of cytochrome b_5 reductase activity in congenital methemoglobinemic erythrocytes, and some properties of the NADH dehydrogenase from normal and methemoglobinamic red cells.

METHODS

For the preparation of purified normal NADH dehydrogenase,

hemolysate was first treated by the method of Passon *et al.* (1972a) to remove hemoglobin. Washed cells were lysed by the addition of 3 volumes of water, adjusted to pH 6.0 with HCl, and the stroma was removed by centrifugation. From the supernatant fraction, most of the hemoglobin was removed by Amberlite CG-50. The solution was diluted with 8 volumes of water, adjusted to pH 7.0 with NaOH, and applied on a DEAE-cellulose column. After washing the column with 0.01 M phosphate buffer, pH 7.0, the enzyme was eluted by 0.2 M phosphate buffer, pH 7.0. The enzyme was purified further by ammonium sulfate fractionation (precipitate between 40 and 70% saturation), gel filtration on a Bio Gel P-100 column, DE-32 column (linear gradient from 0.01 to 0.2 M phosphate buffer, pH 7.7), hydroxylapatite column (linear gradient from 0.01 to 0.2 M phosphate buffer, pH 6.8), and Ampholine electrofocusing (pH 5-8).

For the separation of cytochrome b_5 reductase from the other diaphorase in red cell, a simple method of Kuma *et al.* (1972) was adopted. Red cells were treated with sodium nitrite and the enzymes were purified from the major methemoglobin fraction on a CM-cellulose column. The cytochrome b_5 reductase and the diaphorase were separated from each other on a DEAE-cellulose (DE-32) column. Enzyme activities were measured as described previously (Sugita *et al.*, 1971).

RESULTS

The substrate specificity of the major NADH dehydrogenase in red cell for electron acceptors are shown in Table I. Cytochrome b_5 was the most effective electron acceptor and the Vmax was about 700 times as great as that for methemoglobin and the Km value was less than one-fortieth of that for methemoglobin. As the redox potential of cytochrome b_5 is low compared with that of hemoglobin, it is considered that reduced cytochrome b_5 reduces methemoglobin nonenzymically in red cells. The effects of small amounts of cytochrome b_5 on methemoglobin reduction *in vitro* are given in Table II. Under the standard assay conditions for methemoglobin reduction, stimulation of the reaction was observed at the concentrations of cytochrome

Table I

Kinetic constants for electron acceptors

Electron acceptor	Km	Vmax
	M	μmole·min^{-1} per mg protein
Methemoglobin[a]	3.1×10^{-4}	0.231
Metmyoglobin	8.7×10^{-5}	0.151
Oxidized cytochrome c	3.7×10^{-5}	0.655
Oxidized cytochrome b_5	7.1×10^{-6}	162
2,6-Dichlorophenolindophenol	5.0×10^{-5}	79

[a]Values are given on a molar heme basis.

Table II

Rate of increase in oxygenated hemoglobin was measured at 576 nm. The change in absorbance at 576 nm caused by the reduction of cytochrome b_5 at the concentrations given in the table was negligible. The reduction of cytochrome b_5 in the assay system was calculated from Km, Vmax, and concentrations of cytochrome b_5, neglecting the association of methemoglobin to the enzyme.

Concentration of cyt. b_5	Rate of metHb reduction	Calculated rate of cyt. b_5 reduction
M	μmole·min^{-1}	μmoles·min^{-1}/mg
No addition	0.09	
2.7×10^{-7}	5.02	5.96
1.35×10^{-7}	2.97	3.03
0.27×10^{-7}	0.21	0.61

b_5 lower than that of 10^{-6}M in red cells reported by Passon et al. (1972a). The reduction rate of cytochrome b_5 at these small concentrations cannot be determined directly by the photometric assay. As shown in Table II, the rate of methemoglobin reduction is approximately equal to the calculated rate of cytochrome b_5 reduction.

The purified enzyme showed only an absorption maximum at 277 nm in the ultraviolet and visible regions. No peak characteristic of flavoprotein or suggesting the presence of heme could be observed. Other results suggesting that no flavin is present in the enzyme as a prosthetic group are; 1) less than 0.02 mole of flavin was detected per mole of enzyme by treatment with trichloroacetic acid, 2) neither FAD nor FMN stimulated the enzyme activity, and 3) atebrin, an inhibitor of flavin enzymes, did not affect either diaphorase activity or cytochrome b_5 reductase activity.

The molecular weight was estimated to be 28,000 by gel filtration method. Sodium dodecyl sulfate acrylamide gel electrophoresis demonstrated that the enzyme consists of subunits of the molecular weight of about 8,000.

To prove the deficiency of cytochrome b_5 reductase in congenital methemoglobinemic erythrocytes, cytochrome b_5 reductase activity as well as diaphorase activity were measured on both normal and methemoglobinemic red cells. The diaphorase activity in red cells of the propositus, a Japanese woman aged 36, was about 17% of that in normal red cells. Hemolysates were fractionated according to the method of Kuma et al. (1972). Elution patterns from DE-32 column are shown in Fig.1. Two peaks of NADH diaphorase activity were separated and called here diaphorase I and II. For methemoglobinemic red cells, activities of diaphorase I and II were 80% and less than 5% of those for the normal red cells, respectively. Fractions of methemoglobinemic diaphorase II were combined and concentrated. Both the diaphorase II preparations, normal and methemoglobinemic, showed cytochrome b_5 reductase activity with NADH as an electron donor. However, both the normal and methemoglobinemic diaphorase I showed no cytochrome b_5 reductase activity. The ratio of diaphorase activity to cytochrome b_5

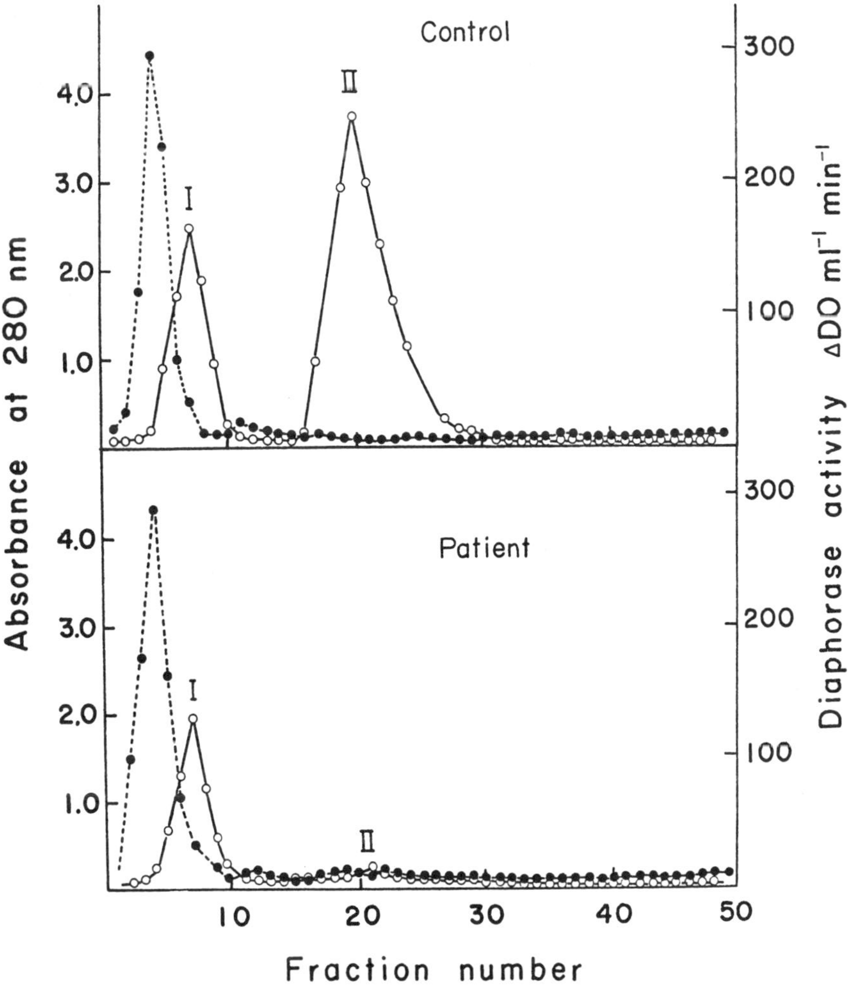

Figure 1. Fractionation of NADH diaphorases with DE-32 column chromatography. Enzyme solution from 60 ml of red cells were applied on a column (1.2 x 20 cm) and eluted with a linear gradient from 0.01 to 0.1 M of sodium phosphate buffer, pH 6.8, with 250 ml of each buffer. o—o, diaphorase activity; ●--●, absorbance at 280 nm.

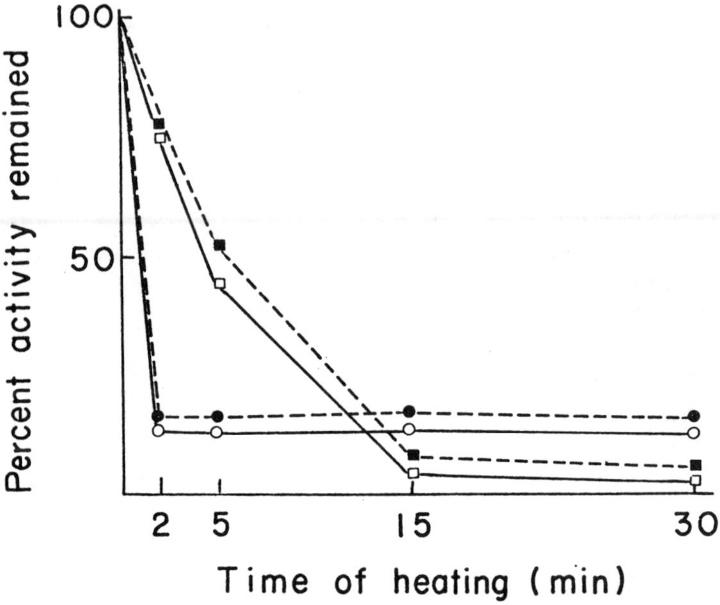

Figure 2. Heat stability of diaphorases. Enzymes were heated at 50° in a water bath at pH 7.5 for the time indicated, and remaining activity was measured. ○—○, normal diaphorase I; □—□, normal diaphorase II; ●--●, methemoglobinemic diaphorase I; ■--■, methemoglobinemic diaphorase II.

reductase activity was the same for both the diaphorases II.

The values of Km for 2,6-dichlorophenolindophenol and NADH with diaphorase I were 1.66 X 10^{-5}M and 9.1 X 10^{-5}M, respectively, for both of the normal and methemoglobinemic enzymes. The Km for the dye and NADH with diaphorase II were 6.7 X 10^{-5}M and 3.3 X 10^{-6}M, respectively, for both of these preparations. The heat stability, shown in Fig.2, and the effect of pH on enzyme activities of the diaphorase I and II were quite identical for the normal and methemoglobinemic preparations. No difference in acrylamide disc gel electrophoretic patterns was found between the normal and the methemoglobinemic diaphorases II.

DISCUSSION

The rate of methemoglobin reduction _in vitro_, in the presence of NADH, cytochrome b_5 reductase and cytochrome b_5 in the concentrations about the same as that in red cells, was equal to the rate of cytochrome b_5 reduction. This result suggests that the reduction of methemoglobin is accomplished through nonenzymatic reduction by cytochrome b_5, which is reduced enzymatically by NADH. In addition, the results that only diaphorase II which has cytochrome b_5 reductase activity is deficient in methemoglobinemic red cells, strongly support the hypothesis that cytochrome b_5 reductase plays a major role in physiological methemoglobin reduction in human erythrocytes. The plausible electron transfer reactions are summerized as follows.

NADH → Cyt b_5 reductase → Cyt b_5 → Methemoglobin

Cytochrome b_5 reductase from erythrocyte is distinct from that obtained from mammalian liver (Strittmatter and Velick, 1957) in that the former is a soluble enzyme and does not contain flavin as a coenzyme, whereas the latter is a particulate flavoprotein enzyme. A few papers report that diaphorases or methemoglobin reductase in red cells contained no flavin (Kajita _et al_., 1969: Adachi and Okuyama, 1972), but there are several reports describing the methemoglobin reductase as a flavoprotein enzyme. One mole of flavin was reported to be contained in 1.95 X 10^5, 7.2 X 10^5, and 2.8 X 10^5 g of enzyme protein by Scott _et al_. (1962), Hegesch and Avron (1967), and Passon and Hultquist (1972b), respectively. These flavin contents are too low for a flavoprotein as judged from the molecular weight of about 30,000 reported by most of the papers, and these amounts of flavin might be regarded as contamination.

Various abnormal electrophoretic mobilities have been reported for residual diaphorase activity in congenital methemoglobinemic red cells (West _et al_., 1967; Brewer _et al_., 1967; Kaplan and Beutler, 1967; Hsieh and Jaffe, 1971; Schwartz et al, 1972). The methemoglobinemic enzyme we have studied, however, was similar to the normal one in all the properties so far tested. Catalytic properties, namely the Km for the dye and NADH, effect of pH, and the ratio of diaphorase activity to cytochrome b_5 reductase activity, are all exactly the same for both the diaphorase II. Heat stability and electrophoretic mobility did not indicate any difference between the two enzymes. Although the possibility of substitution of an amino acid residue cannot be excluded, these results suggest that the low enzyme activity may be due to the decreasein the amount of enzyme protein rather than to the production of mutant enzyme protein.

Scott (1960) first reported the lack of diaphorase activity in homozygous methemoglobinemia. Scott *et al.* later showed four kinds of diaphorases in human red cells, but the effects of genetic defect on each of these enzymes were not clear. Kuma *et al.* (1972) found in methemoglobinemic erythrocytes only a major diaphorase was deficient and the other diaphorase activity was normal. We have shown that the major diaphorase (cytochrome b_5 reductase) consists of subunits. If there are two kinds of subunits and one is common to all the diaphorases, a mutation in the common subunit may cause the total loss of diaphorase activity in the affected erythrocytes.

REFERENCES

Adachi,K., and Okuyama,T. (1972). Studies on the reduced pyridine nucleotide dehydrogenase of bovine erythrocytes. Biochim. Biophys. Acta 268: 629.

Brewer,G.J., Eaton,J.W., Knutsen,C.S., and Beck,C.C. (1967). A starch-gel electrophoretic method for the study of diaphorase isozymes and preliminary results with sheep and human erythrocytes. Biochem. Biophys. Res. Commun. 29: 198.

Hegesch,E., and Avron,M. (1967). The enzymatic reduction of ferrihemoglobin. Biochim. Biophys. Acta 146: 397.

Hsieh,H.S., and Jaffe,E.R. (1971). Electrophoretic and functional variants of methemoglobin reductase in hereditary methemoglobinemia. J. Clin. Invest. 50: 196.

Hultquist,D.E., and Passon,P.G. (1971). Catalysis of methemoglobin reduction by erythrocyte cytochrome b_5 and cyto-

chrome b_5 reductase. Nature, New Biol. 229: 252.
Kajita,K., Kerwar,G.K., and Huennekens,F.M. (1969). Multiple forms of methemoglobin reductase. Arch. Biochem. Biophys. 130: 662.
Kaplan,J.C., and Beutler,E. (1967). Electrophoresis of red cell NADH- and NADPH-diaphorases in normal subjects and patients with congenital methemoglobinemia. Biochem. Biophys. Res. Commun. 29: 605.
Kuma,F., Ishizawa,S., Hirayama,K., and Nakajima,H. (1972). Studies on methemoglobin reductase. J. Biol. Chem. 247: 550.
Passon,P.G., Reed,D.W., and Hultquist,D.E. (1972a). Soluble cytochrome b_5 from human erythrocytes. Biochim. Biophys. Acta 275: 51.
Passon,P.G., and Hultquist,D.E. (1972b). Soluble cytochrome b_5 reductase from human erythrocytes. Biochim. Biophys. Acta 275: 62.
Schwartz,J.M., Paress,P.S., Ross,J.M., Di-Pillo,F., and Rizek,F. (1972). Unstable variant of NADH methemoglobin reductase in Puerto Ricans with hereditary methemoglobinemia. J. Clin. Invest. 51: 1594.
Scott,E.M. (1960). The relation of diaphorase of human erythrocytes to inheritance of methemoglobinemia. J. Clin. Invest. 39: 1176.
Scott,E.M., and McGraw,J.C. (1962). Purification and properties of diphosphopyridine nucleotide diaphorase of human erythrocytes. J. Biol. Chem. 237: 249.
Scott,E.M., Duncan,I.W., and Ekstrand,V. (1965). The reduced pyridine nucleotide dehydrogenases of human erythrocytes. J. Biol. Chem. 240: 581.
Sugita,Y., Nomura,S., and Yoneyama,Y. (1971). Purification of reduced pyridine nucleotide dehydrogenase from human erythrocytes and methemoglobin reduction by the enzyme. J. Biol. Chem. 246: 6072.
Strittmatter,P., and Velick,S.I. (1957). The purification and properties of microsomal cytochrome reductase. J. Biol. Chem. 228: 785.
West,C.A., Gomperts,B.D., Huehns,E.R., Kessel,I., and Asbby,J.R. (1967). Demonstration of an enzyme variant in a case of congenital methemoglobinemia. Br. Med. J. 4: 212.

FORMAL DISCUSSION

THE METHEMOGLOBIN REDUCTION SYSTEM OF ERYTHROCYTES

Donald E. Hultquist, Richard H. Douglas, and Richard T. Dean

Department of Biological Chemistry
The University of Michigan
Ann Arbor, Michigan 48104

The very slow catalysis of methemoglobin reduction by isolated methemoglobin reductase and the lack of correlation between rate of methemoglobin reduction in intact cells and the amount of reductase in these cells (1) suggest that the catalysis by reductase is not rate-limiting and that the process of methemoglobin reduction is more complicated than had been imagined.

Several years ago we demonstrated that NADH-methemoglobin reductase has properties similar to those of liver microsomal cytochrome b_5 reductase and we proposed that the enzyme be named "erythrocyte cytochrome b_5 reductase" (2). Like the liver reductase, our preparation of erythrocyte reductase contained FAD as prosthetic group (a finding in disagreement with the results just reported by Dr. Sugita). The liver and erythrocyte reductases show very similar substrate specificity, both with respect to electron donors and electron acceptors. Whereas the catalysis of methemoglobin is very slow, reduction of cytochrome b_5 proceeds rapidly. Dr. Dan Reed in my lab detected and isolated a soluble cytochrome b_5 from human erythrocytes and this protein serves as an excellent substrate for erythrocyte cytochrome b_5 reductase (Table I).

The question then arose, "In the intact cell do electrons flow from reductase through cytochrome b_5 to methemo-

Table I. Substrate specificity of erythrocyte cytochrome b_5 reductase. Rates in 0.05 M Tris-HCl buffer, pH 8.1, containing 0.5 mM EDTA, are compared on a per electron basis.

Electron acceptor	Relative rate with NADH
Ferricyanide	8.1
Dichlorophenolindophenol	2.45
Human erythrocyte cytochrome b_5	1.00
Bovine erythrocyte cytochrome b_5	0.35
Cytochrome *c*	0.012
O_2	0.0041
Glutathione	0.0025
Methemoglobin	0.0005

globin rather than directly from reductase to methemoglobin?" In a reconstitution experiment, Dr. Passon and I showed that the rate of methemoglobin reduction by NADH and reductase was stimulated dramatically by the addition of physiological amounts of erythrocyte cytochrome b_5 (3). The rate of reduction was first order with respect to the cytochrome b_5 concentration. We believe that in the intact cell, as well as in the reconstituted system, methemoglobin reduction proceeds by the pathway:

NADH → Reductase(FAD) → Cytochrome b_5 → Methemoglobin,

and that the reduction of methemoglobin by ferrocytochrome b_5 is the rate-limiting step. The overall rate is independent of O_2, $O_2^{\bullet -}$, and H_2O_2.

We have isolated in homogeneous form cytochrome b_5 from human and bovine erythrocytes and initiated a study of the chemical structures of these proteins. The water-soluble erythrocyte cytochrome b_5 is a smaller molecule than the water-insoluble cytochrome b_5 of liver microsomes. Tryptic degradation of bovine erythrocyte cytochrome b_5 yields a hemepeptide which co-migrates on disc gel electrophoresis with the hemepeptide obtained by tryptic degradation of bovine liver microsomal cytochrome b_5 (residues 9 through 90 of Fig. 1). The amino acid composition of the erythrocyte and liver tryptic hemepeptides are identical within experimental error (Table II).

10
NH_2-(Asx,Glx,Glx,Glx,Ala,Ser)-Ser-Lys-Ala-Val-Lys-Tyr-Tyr-Thr-
20
Leu-Gln-Gln-Glu-Ile-Lys-His-Asn-Asn-Ser-Lys-Ser-Thr-Trp-Leu-
30 40
Ile-Leu-His-Tyr-Lys-Val-Tyr-Asp-Leu-Thr-Lys-Phe-Leu-Glu-Glu-
50
His-Pro-Gly-Gly-Glu-Glu-Val-Leu-Arg-Glu-Gln-Ala-Gly-Gly-Asp-
60 70
Ala-Thr-Glu-Asp-Phe-Glu-Asp-Val-Gly-His-Ser-Thr-Asp-Ala-Arg-
80
Glu-Leu-Ser-Lys-Thr-Phe-Ile-Ile-Gly-Glu-Leu-His-Pro-Asp-Asp-
90 99
Arg-Ser-Lys-Ile-Thr-Lys-Pro-Ser-Glu-Ser-[Hydrophobic]-COOH

Fig. 1. The structure of bovine liver microsomal cytochrome b_5. From the data of Ozols and Strittmatter (4,5).

Table II. Comparison of amino acid compositions of tryptic hemepeptides derived from erythrocyte and liver cytochrome b_5.

Amino acid	Liver[a]	Erythrocyte
Ala	4	4.3
Arg	3	2.7
Asp	9	8.9
Glu	13	12.9
Gly	6	6.4
His	5	4.6
Ile	4	3.7
Leu	8	7.8
Lys	6	5.3
Met	0	0.2
Phe	3	3.0
Pro	2	2.2
Ser	4	4.2
Thr	6	5.9
Tyr	4	3.4
Val	4	4.0

[a]From the studies of Ozols and Strittmatter (4,6).

The amino acid composition of the intact bovine erythrocyte cytochrome b_5 is in good agreement with the composition of the 99-residue segment of bovine liver microsomal cytochrome b_5 which begins at the N-terminus (Fig. 1). The results suggest that soluble cytochrome b_5 of erythrocytes differs from microsomal cytochrome b_5 only in that the hydrophobic tail which extends from residue 100 to the C-terminus is absent. We propose that soluble cytochrome b_5 as well as soluble cytochrome b_5 reductase are derived from the microsomal proteins by proteolysis which occurs as the endoplasmic reticulum of immature erythroid cells is solubilized during erythropoiesis.

This work was supported by U.S. Public Health Service Grant AM-09250.

REFERENCES

1. Kanazawa, Y., Hattori, M., Kosaka, K. and Nakao, K. (1968). The relationship of NADH-dependent diaphorase activity and methemoglobin reduction in human erythrocytes. Clin. Chim. Acta *19*:524.

2. Passon, P. G. and Hultquist, D. E. (1972). Soluble cytochrome b_5 reductase from human erythrocytes. Biochim. Biophys. Acta *275*:62.

3. Hultquist, D. E. and Passon, P. G. (1971). Catalysis of methemoglobin reduction by erythrocyte cytochrome b_5 and cytochrome b_5 reductase. Nature New Biol. *229*:252.

4. Ozols, J. and Strittmatter, P. (1969). Correction of the amino acid sequence of calf liver microsomal cytochrome b_5. J. Biol. Chem. *244*:6617.

5. Ozols, J. (1974). Cytochrome b_5 from microsomal membranes of equine, bovine, and porcine livers. Isolation and properties of preparations containing the membranous segment. Biochemistry *13*:426.

6. Strittmatter, P. and Ozols, J. (1966). The restricted tryptic cleavage of cytochrome b_5. J. Biol. Chem. *241*:4787.

DISCUSSION

Dr. Duhm: I would like to ask you both, Dr. Sugita and Dr. Hultquist, whether there is any evidence that the reductase or the flavins or the cytochrome b_5 are bound or built in to the red cell membrane? I am asking because there are several unexplained findings in the literature, for instance, those of Passow and Mishra and those of Arese indicating that there exists a system in the red cell membrane which can transfer electrons over the membrane.

Dr. Sugita: I think both the cytochrome b_5 reductase and cytochrome b_5 in the erythrocyte exist in soluble fraction.

Dr. Perutz: I wonder if Dr. Hultquist can tell us if there's any relationship between the sequence of the erythrocyte cytochrome b_5 and that of the cytochrome whose crystal structure was solved by Scott Mathews?

Dr. Hultquist: Everything we know about the chemistry of the red cell cytochrome b_5 I have told you. Dr. Mathews, when he gets back from sabbatical and when we send him 2 mg of the red cell cytochrome b_5, will attempt to get the three dimensional structure. All we know is the amino acid composition. We are in the process of doing tryptic digestions of the apoprotein to get some evidence as to the sequence.

Could I just make one comment on the question on the membrane reductase (the NADH cytochrome _c_ reductase of red cell stroma)? We have tried to show that it's related to the methemoglobin reductase. We can find no evidence for any relationship between either the particulate or soluble form of the stromal cytochrome _c_ reductase and cytochrome b_5 reductase.

SICKLE CELL HEMOGLOBIN AND SICKLE CELL ANEMIA

Chairman: C. L. Conley

Sickle Cell Hemoglobin and Sickle Cell Anemia

C. Lockard Conley

The Johns Hopkins University School of Medicine

Baltimore, Maryland

All of the pleiotropic effects of the sickling mutation are attributable to the amino acid substitution in the beta chain of hemoglobin. Polymerization of the abnormal molecules may well be responsible for every one of the untoward manifestations. Other abnormal properties of hemoglobin S have been noted (1), but their pathophysiologic significance, if any, has not been established. Geneticists tend to think of a heritable disease as caused by a mutant protein that is deficient in carrying out its usual biologic function. But hemoglobin S is functionally adequate in the transport of oxygen. It would be harmless except for the accident of its tendency to polymerize when deoxygenated. The pathologic reaction is intermolecular rather than intramolecular; if there were only one molecule of hemoglobin per red cell, the disease could not occur.

Sickle cell anemia is said to be inherited as an autosomal recessive trait, but that statement is true only in a statistical sense. The mutant gene may be either dominant or recessive depending upon environmental and genetic factors. A person heterozygous for the sickling gene may have severe sickle cell anemia if additionally he has generalized hypoxemia, as occurs in cyanotic congenital heart disease (2). That fact actually was predicted in 1927 by Hahn and Gillepsie (3), the first to recognize the relationship of the oxygenation of hemoglobin to the sickling phenomenon. The sickling gene also is dominant if the carrier is heterozygous for other genetically determined abnormalities such as beta thalassemia, hemoglobin C or hemoglobin D_{Punjab}. There is abundant evidence that the proximate determinant of illness in the carrier of hemoglobin S is the occurrence of sickling of the red cells within the circulation (4). High concentrations of sickle hemoglobin in erythrocytes are quite harmless if the hemoglobin molecules do not polymerize. We do not know how many red cells must sickle to produce symptoms, but there is no doubt that clinical disorders, when they do occur, are related to intravascular sickling.

It is the environment of the hemoglobin S molecules in each individual red cell that determines whether sickling of that cell occurs. And red cells are not all alike. Water content, pH, and 2,3 DPG concentration vary from cell to cell, as a function of cell age among other factors. There is a wide variation in concentration of fetal hemoglobin among the erythrocytes in a sample of blood, variably influencing propensity to sickling. While hemoglobin F tends to lessen the tendency of cells to sickle, hemoglobins C, D_{Punjab} and O_{Arab} interact with hemoglobin S to enhance polymerization. These are gene product interactions - not gene interactions per se.

As the red cells flow through the capillary circulation, they are variably deoxygenated, depending on rates of blood flow, tissue oxygen tensions, pH and other factors, many of which cannot be measured.

When red cells containing sickle hemoglobin become rigid and deformed (Messer and Harris (5) demonstrated that rigidity precedes deformation), they are destroyed more rapidly than normal red cells. It is not the hemolytic anemia that is the cause of the major hazard to life of patients with sickle cell anemia. The sickling red cells in some way occlude blood vessels producing ischemia and infarction. Some patients with sickle cell anemia go for long periods of time, sometimes years, without symptoms referable to vascular occlusions. What are the precipitating events that cause these occlusions to occur? In a given patient symptoms may occur simultaneously in widely separated areas, suggesting that there has been some predisposing systemic change. A possibility, often suggested, is that some change in the character of the blood itself facilitates the vascular blockade; but it is equally possible that vascular changes producing alterations in blood flow are responsible.

For years febrile illness has been recognized as one antecedent of sickle cell crisis. Sydenstricker and his associates in 1923 (6) demonstrated the temperature dependence of the sickling phenomenon. Yet we do not know today whether elevation of body temperature enhances the tendency of red cells to sickle in vivo, because of the complexity of the many concomitant reactions. In fever metabolism is increased and oxygen consumption accelerated, carbon dioxide production is enhanced and there are remarkable changes in the circulation of the blood. How individual red cells in various areas of the body are affected by all of this is not known. Certainly areas of the body in which blood flow is sluggish and oxygen tension low are predisposed to vascular occlusive lesions. The portal circulation of the kidney and the countercurrent mechanism in the renal medulla presumably lead to enhanced deoxygenation, increased cell concentration and increased osmolarity, factors that might be expected to cause trouble in the renal papilla, where indeed vascular occlusions commonly occur. The character of the circulation in the spleen and bone marrow - the oxygen tension, pH, cell concentration and perhaps other factors - must foster vascular occlusions by sickled erythrocytes. Much of the blood supply of the liver comes through the portal vein, in which the blood is not fully oxygenated. We know little about oxygen tension, rate of blood flow and other critical factors in the hepatic circulation in sickle cell anemia, but the liver is a common site of involvement in these patients.

We do not even know whether the vascular lesion in sickle cell anemia is originated by blockade of a few small blood vessels by very few sickled erythrocytes, or whether there is primarily a "log jam" effect of many sickled cells. In this regard it is noteworthy that sickle cell crises can be prevented if about half of the red cells in the circulation are replaced by normal cells (7).

Approaches to treatment of sickle cell anemia are rational when they are based on efforts to prevent the polymerization of hemoglobin molecules. But many therapeutic efforts have been devoted to alleviation of sickle cell crises. Here a wholly unjustified assumption seems to have been made. The assumption is that if sickle cells could be immediately unsickled in some way, the pain and other symptoms of a crisis would be dramatically relieved. There is, in fact, no objective support for this concept and it is only a speculation. Many of the lesions of the sickle cell crisis are infarcts; tissue is dead and must be removed and replaced. It seems unlikely that any specific or non-specific agent will rapidly correct these lesions. A lesson that must be repeatedly emphasized is that therapeutic efforts are extremely difficult to evaluate when they are directed at variable and self-limited conditions such as sickle cell crises. Medical journals abound with favorable reports of the therapeutic effects of many agents on the sickle cell crisis, but actually none has stood the test of an adequately performed controlled trial.

In the discussions that follow, we will hear about explorations of some of the questions that I have mentioned.

References

1. Asakura, T., Ohnishi, T., Friedman, S. and Schwartz, E.: Abnormal precipitation of oxyhemoglobin S by mechanical shaking. Proc. Nat. Acad. Sci. 71: 1594, 1974.
2. Smith, E.W. and Conley, C.L.: Clinical manifestations of sickle cell diseases. Conference on Hemoglobin. National Academy of Sciences - National Research Council Publication No. 557, pg. 276, 1958.
3. Hahn, E.V. and Gillespie, E.B.: Sickle cell anemia. Report of a case greatly improved by splenectomy. Experimental study of sickle cell formation. Arch. Intern. Med. 39: 233, 1927.
4. Charache, S. and Conley, C.L.: Rate of sickling of red cells during deoxygenation of blood from persons with various sickling disorders. Blood 24: 25, 1964.
5. Messer, M.J. and Harris, J.W.: Filtration characteristics of sickle cells: Rates of alteration of filterability after deoxygenation and reoxygenation, and correlations with sickling and unsickling. J. Lab. Clin. Med. 76: 537, 1970.
6. Sydenstricker, V.P., Mulherin, W.A. and Honseal, R.W.: Sickle cell anemia. Report of two cases in children, with necropsy in one case. Amer. J. Dis. Child. 26: 132, 1923.
7. Charache, S.: The treatment of sickle cell anemia. Arch. Intern. Med. 133: 698, 1974.

SURFACE ACTIVITY OF HEMOGLOBIN S

Danek Elbaum, John Harrington, Ronald L. Nagel

Department of Medicine, Division of Hematology
Albert Einstein College of Medicine
Bronx, New York 10461

Studies by Asakura et al. (1) and Roth et al. (2) have shown that oxyhemoglobin S and A exhibit very different rates of mechanical precipitation. Precipitation of proteins by shaking appears to be caused by a complex set of factors and surface denaturation has been suggested (2) to be involved in this process. In order to gain some insight into understanding of the mechanism of mechanical precipitation, we have studied the kinetics of hemoglobin (Hb) film formation in the hope that this technique will generate, in addition, some information about the conformation of different mutants and conformers of human hemoglobins.

The pioneer work of Gorter, Harkins and Langmuir, reviewed by James and Augenstein (3), demonstrated that proteins were able to adsorb to liquid-air interfaces. Although some of the factors participating in the formation of these protein films and some of their properties are known (4), the system is far from completely understood.

Hemoglobin surface properties have been studied only to a limited extent. Jonxis (5) (using a technique different from the one employed in this paper) studied the spreading of different animal hemoglobins. His main conclusion was that the time of unfolding for different animal hemoglobins is different (independent from the differences in isoelectric point) and that the ligand state of hemoglobin had a clear influence on the rate of spreading in a water-air interface.

The present paper will examine the kinetics of the change in surface tension induced by the hemoglobin film formation from a dilute subface solution. Hemoglobin S and other mutants, in different ligand states, have been examined.

METHODS

Protein films can be studied by spreading the protein in the water-air interface or by following their rate of formation after injecting the protein solution in the subface (6) by the changes in surface tension (π). We have selected, as the initial approach, the latter method and the corresponding π-t isotherms will be described.

Surface tension measurements were made by the Wilhelmy hang-plate technique as described by Colacicco and Rapport (7). Changes in surface pressure ($\Delta\pi = \gamma - \gamma_o$) were determined after measurement of surface tension in the presence of the protein film ($-\gamma$) and in its absence (γ_o). A Platinum plate suspended from a tension balance (RG Automatic electrobalance, CAHN Instrument Corp.) was used.

The kinetics of surface pressure alteration was measured at constant area of 22.42 cm^2 in circular glass dish. All measurements, except the ones mentioned in the text, were obtained at 22°C.

The platinum blade was flamed and surface cleaned with a capillary tube attached to a suction pump before every measurement. The alterations of surface pressure were monitored on a chart recorder as a function of time.

The ability of a protein to form a film by absorption from its solution was studied by injecting 10λ of 3.2g% of hemoglobin solution into the subface of 30cc of 0.15M phosphate buffer, pH 7.35, followed by gentle mechanical stirring. Deoxy experiments were conducted in a globe box in an atmosphere of N_2.

Isolation of Hb F was accomplished by column chromatography (8) and the preparation of isolated chains by the method of Geracci et al (9).

RESULTS

Oxyhemoglobin A is capable of adsorbing into the water-air interface forming a protein film, in about 5 minutes, as can be seen in the π-t isotherms of Fig. 1.

The single amino acid substitution of Hb S (β6Glu → Val) confers on the oxy form of this protein a new property: an accelerated adsorption to the interface as compared with oxy Hb A (Figure 1).

Not so surprisingly, Hb F (which differs from Hb A in 40 sequence sites) is also different from A, in regard to protein film formation, and exhibits slower $\Delta\pi$ kinetics.

A second question is how the quaternary conformation states (R and T or oxy and deoxy) influence film formation. In Figure 2, it can be observed that the rate of deoxy Hb S film formation is slower and reaches equilibrium at a lower surface tension (about 10 dynes/cm) as compared to oxy Hb S (about 18-20 dynes/cm). In addition, deoxy Hb S surface tension kinetics are quite similar to deoxy Hb A. In other words, the significant difference between Hb A and S with respect to surface activity is the behavior of the oxy conformers of both hemoglobin. Oxy A is slower than the deoxy form while oxy S is faster than the deoxy form. The behavior of Hb A is entirely consistent with the spreading results of Jonxis (5).

Changes within the R state of Hb S did not have any consequence for the kinetics of surface film formation. Met Hb S and CO Hb S are indistinguishable from oxy Hb S (Figure 3).

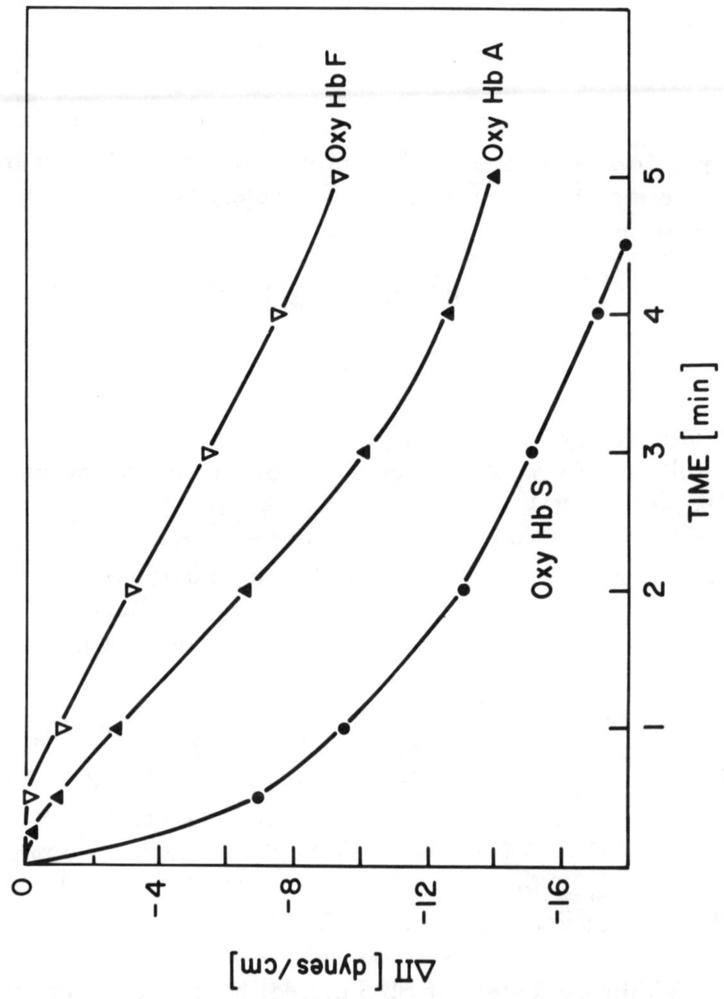

Figure 1. π -t isotherms of oxyhemoglobin A, F and S. Temperature 22°C.

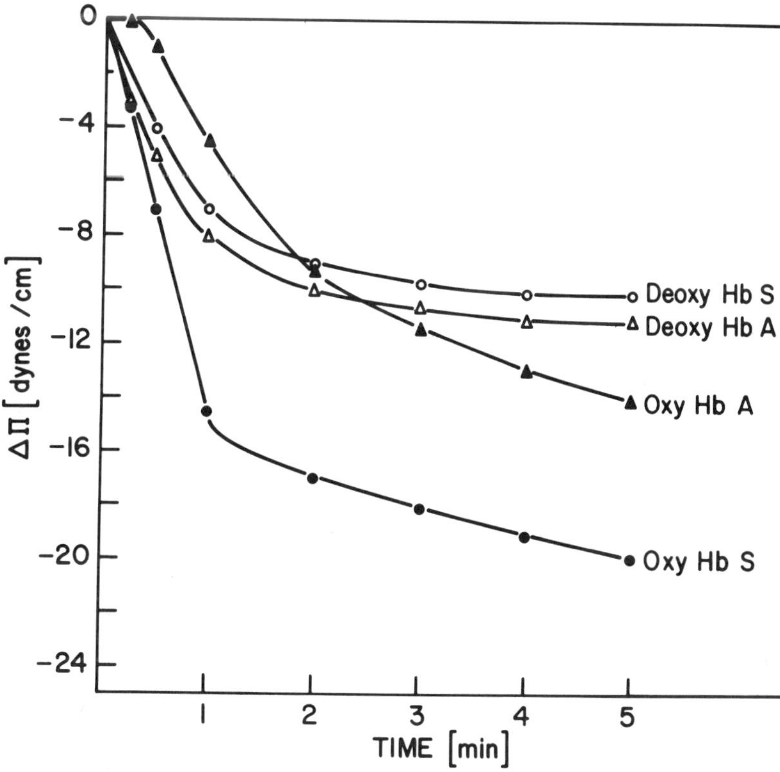

Figure 2. π -t isotherms for Hemoglobin A and S in oxy and deoxy state. Temperature 22°C.

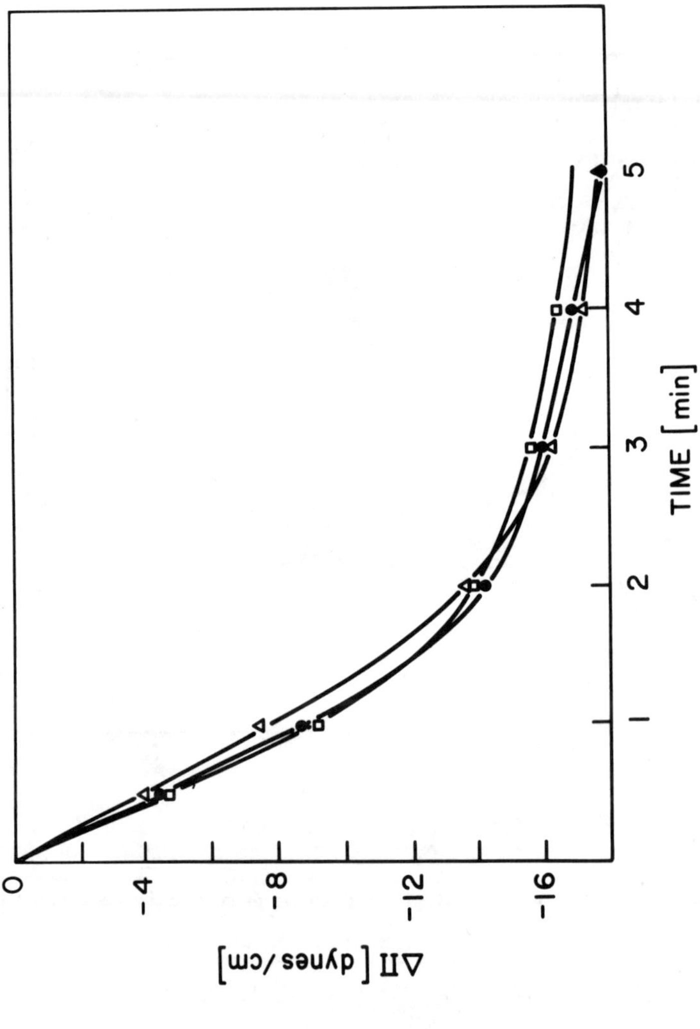

Figure 3. π –t isotherms for oxy Hb S (●), Met Hb S (△) and CO Hb S (□). Temperature 22°C.

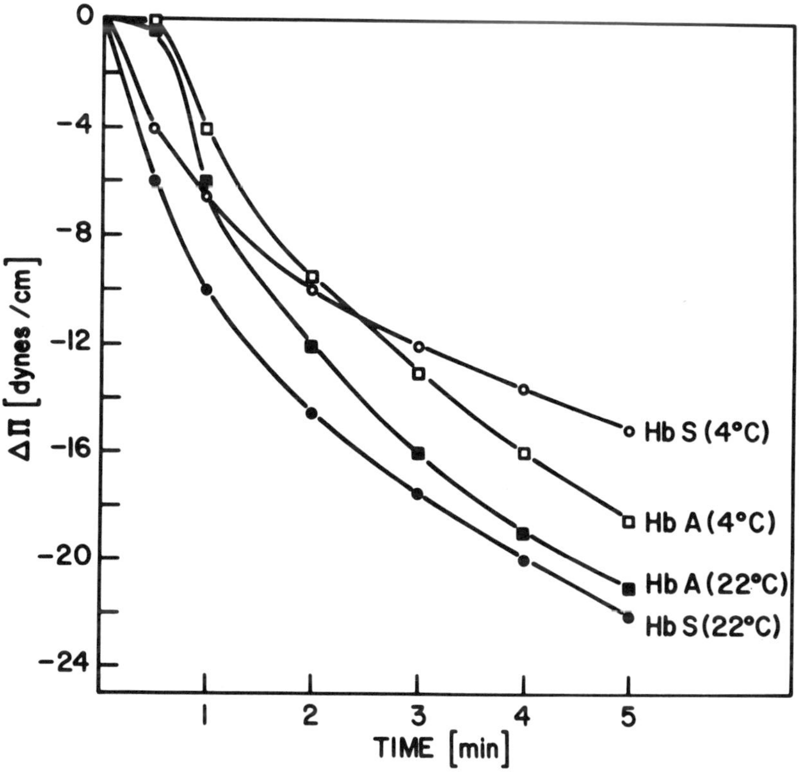

Figure 4. △ surface tension versus time at two temperatures (4° and 22°C) for Hb A and Hb S.

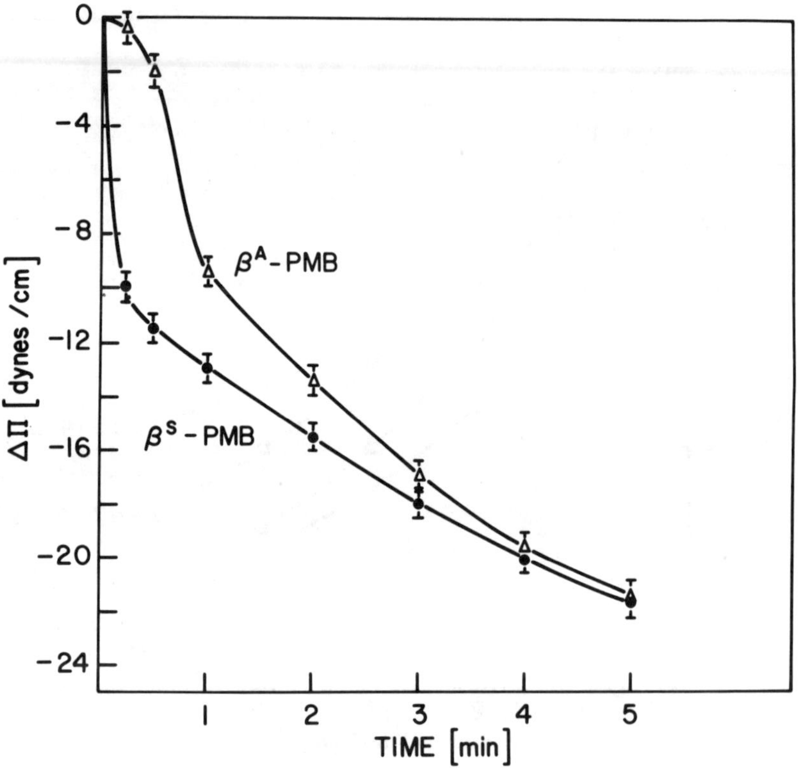

Figure 5. π-t isotherms of isolated PMB β^A and β^S chains. Temperature 22°C.

In Figure 4 are depicted the effect of temperature on the rate of film formation (on alteration of surface tension), comparing oxy Hb A and oxy Hb S at 4° and 22°C. The relatively small alteration in surface activity for oxy Hb A at 4° is in contrast to the significant decrease found for oxy Hb S at the lower temperature.

In order to clarify the role played by the substitution within the β chain of Hb S, the surface activity of monomeric oxy β^{S} PMB and oxy β^{A} PMB chains were studied (Figure 5). While both β chains have faster kinetics than their corresponding tetramer, oxy β^{S} PMB is considerably faster than oxy β^{A} PMB.

DISCUSSION

The data presented here should be interpreted in connection with two interrelated questions:

a) Can the surface activity of oxy Hb S explain the mechanical precipitability of this mutant?

b) What is the mechanism of the difference in surface activity between Hb A and Hb S?

In relation to the first question, one can see that a number of parameters influence surface tension in the same way that they influence mechanical precipitability: Oxy Hb S is more precipitable than oxy Hb A. Correspondingly, oxy Hb S forms protein films faster and reaches a larger $\Delta\pi$ at equilibrium.

No difference has been observed between the mechanical precipitability of deoxy Hb S and oxy Hb A. Correspondingly, their $\Delta\pi$ rates are similar.

There is no difference among oxy, CO and metHb S in their mechanical precipitability. No difference exists in their surface activity. Moreover, low temperature inhibits the precipitability of oxy Hb S. This low temperature has also a definitive effect on the surface activity of oxy Hb S.

Finally, the mechanical precipitability of oxy Hb S is shared by the β^S isolated chains. Correspondingly, a faster protein film formation rate is found also in β^S PMB chains as compared to β^A PMB chains.

All this suggests that surface activity may very well be one of the underlying bases for the increased mechanical precipitability of oxy Hb S. Nevertheless, one should avoid reducing the problem, at this time, exclusively to differences in surface activity.

It is likely that mechanical precipitability involves: a) formation of a protein film; b) surface unfolding of the protein with structural modification and possible aggregation; c) breaking of the film and precipitation of denatured protein aggregates. While the first two aspects are reflected in changes of surface activity, oxy Hb S could conceivably, in addition, form faster and larger aggregates of denatured material. This second aspect deserves further experimental inquiry.

The second question, the mechanism of the differences in surface activity between Hb A and Hb S, is more difficult to answer. Langmuir and Schaeffer (10) have described an equation which relates protein concentration at the film surface (n) with bulk concentration of the macromolecule (C_b), diffusion coefficient D at time t

$$n = 2C_b \sqrt{\frac{Dt}{\pi}}$$

At the first stage of formation of the film, assuming no barrier at the surface and when the local concentration of the protein below surface is low and the material absorbed do not leave the film, this equation may be used to generate some information about the kinetics of surface tension alteration. This relationship was successfully used by Evans et al. (4) to predict theoretical π -t isotherms derived from pressure-concentration data of modified β-casein, but in this system considerable differences in aggregation are observed. It has been experimentaly shown by Mac Ritchie and Alexander (11) that in the initial stages of film pressure alteration, in the absence of significant film pressure the bulk diffusion accounts very reasonably for the observed kinetics of adsorption of albumin at the interface, while in the later stages the observed rates are much slower than calculated, suggesting, according to the authors, the building up of a barrier associated with the film pressure.

In the case of hemoglobin, no experimental determination of D has been obtained for deoxy A and Hb S. Nevertheless, it is highly unlikely that diffusion constants will differ enough to explain the different rates observed between Hb A and Hb S.

Another parameter that can be eliminated is the influence of the isoelectric point differences between these hemoglobin mutants or their conformers. Although this parameter may modify to some extent the rate of film formation (faster rate as one approaches pI), the data can hardly be explained on the basis of this factor.

We turn, then, to the behavior of the hemoglobin molecules, once they have reached the interface, to find the basis of the differences observed.

The most important event is the unfolding of the protein to accommodate to the new requirements of the water-air interface. Different proteins have different rates of unfolding and they unfold to different extents (12).

Jonxis, studying the compressability of maximally spread animal hemoglobins, found that 1 mgm of protein covers an area of 9400 cm^2 (or about 10,000 A^2 per molecule). This implies quite a bit of uncoiling, but also suggests that the extent of uncoiling is the same for different hemoglobins. However, when he studied the time of maximum spreading many differences were apparent among different animal hemoglobins. This opens the possibility that the rate or type of uncoiling could be the basic difference between the surface activity of oxy Hb S and oxy Hb A. Further work in this area should involve obtaining π/area isotherms and time of spreading as a measure of unfolding time.

In any case the results described here suggest that the conformation of oxy Hb S is distinct and different from oxy Hb A. All extrapolation for polymer model building of the 2A structure of Hb A to Hb S seems unwarranted at this junction. In addition, the physiological relevance of Hb surface activity should be a reasonable area of future exploration. Particularly attractive seems to be the potential correlation between Hb S surface activity and its abnormal interaction with the irreversibly sickled cell membrane (12).

SUMMARY

The surface activity (measured as surface pressure (π) vs. time isotherms) of Hb A and Hb S were studied to understand the basis of different rates of mechanical precipitation exhibited by these two hemoglobins. The π-t isotherms indicate that oxy Hb S forms a protein film at a faster rate than oxy Hb A. Hb F in contrast, forms the film with a slower rate. In addition, ligand state has a definite effect on the phenonema: oxy Hb S is faster than oxy Hb A but deoxy Hb S is quite similar to deoxy Hb A. In addition, isolated oxy β^S chains are more surface active than deoxy β^S chains.

These and other findings suggest that surface tension kinetics and equilibrium differences between oxy Hb A and oxy Hb S may well be the basis for their differences in mechanical precipitability.

A possibility, based on previous work, suggest that time or type of uncoiling on the surface could be the basis for these differences.

The mechanism for the surface activity of oxy Hb S can not be understood without additional data (π/Area isotherms) describing time and type of uncoiling on the surface.

Acknowledgment

The assistance and advice of Dr. Giuseppe Colaccico are gratefully acknowledged. We are indebted to Dr. German Camejo, who helped in the initial stages of this work.

Supported by NHLI-2-2920-B, NIH AM 15053, HRC U-2339, and 5-PO 1-GM 19100. Dr. Elbaum is an NIH fellow.

REFERENCES

1. Asakura, T., Agarwal, P.L., Relman, D.A., McCray, J.A., Chance, B., Schwartz, E., Friedman, S. and Lubin, B.H. (1973): Mechanical instability of the oxyhemoglobin S. Nature 244:437.
2. Roth, E.F., Elbaum, D. and Nagel, R.L. (1974): Observations on the mechanical precipitation of oxy Hb S and other mutants. Blood. (in press).
3. James, L.K. and Augenstein, L.G. (1966): Adsorption of enzymes at interfaces: film formation and the effect of activity. Adv. Enzymes 28:1.
4. Evans, M.T.A., Mitchell, J., Mussellwhite, P.R., Irons, L. (1970): The effect of the modification of protein structure on the properties of proteins spread and adsorbed at the air-water interface. Adv. Exp. Med. and Biol. 7:1.
5. Jonxis, J.H.P. (1939) CCXVII: On the spreading of different hemoglobins, muscle hemoglobins and cytochrome C. Biochemistry 33:1743.
6. Colacicco, G. (1969): Applications of monolayer techniques to biological systems: symptoms of specific lipid-protein interactions. J. Colloid and Interface Sci. 29:345.
7. Colacicco, G. and Rapport, M.M. (1966): Lipid monolayers: action of phospholipase A from crotalus atrox and naga naga snake venoms on phosphatase choline and phosphatide choline. J. Lipid Res. 7:258.
8. Allen, D.W., Schroeder, W.A. and Balog, J. (1958): Observations on the chromatographic heterogeneity of normal fetal human hemoglobin. J. Am. Chem. Soc. 80:1628.
9. Geraci, G., Parkhurst, L.J. and Gibson, Q.H. (1969): Preparation and properties of α and β chains from human hemoglobin. J. Biol. Chem. 244:4664.
10. Langmuir, I. and Schaeffer, V.J. (1938): Activities of urease and

pepsin monolayers. J. Am. Chem. Soc. 60:1351.
11. McRitchie, F. and Alexander, A.E. (1963): Kinetics of adsorption of proteins at interfaces. J. Colloid Sci. 18:453.
12. Fischer, S., Nagel, R.L., Bookchin, R.M., Roth, E.F., and Tellez-Nagel, I. (1974): The binding of hemoglobin to membranes of normal and sickle erythrocytes. Biochim. Biophys. Acta. (in press).

DISCUSSION

Dr. Perutz: May I say a few words about the problem that Dr. Nagel has brought up and about Asakura's paper. May I begin recalling the experimental facts. Oxyhemoglobin A is isomorphous with Hb S in the crystalline state. Any gross differences in solution are therefore unlikely. When Asakura first suggested structural differences I proposed an alternative intrepretation derived from other work in Philadelphia by Englander and his colleagues. This group published a paper in the Journal of Biological Chemistry showing by detuerium exchange that the folded and unfolded forms of CO hemoglobin are in dynamic equilibrium in solution. The behavior of proteins and especially of abnormal hemoglobins indicates the influence of amino acid substitutions on this equilibrium. The introduction of uncompensated internal charges or of large nonpolar hydrophobic side chains on the surface biases the equilibrium toward the unfolded form. The latter also favour aggregation of the unfolded chains. The burying of hydrophobic groups in the interior is the main principle which underlies the folding of polypeptide chains. I therefore suggested that you do not need to postulate a different conformation for oxy Hb S in order to explain its denaturation by shaking. By the principle of Ockham's razor one should make do with the minimum number of assumptions. You do not need to assume a different conformation. All you need to assume is that the substitution of a glutamic acid residue at the surface by the nonpolar valine changes the equilibrium toward the unfolded form. Hence anything that will make the unfolded molecules stick together and precipitate, such as agitation or spreading a surface film, will shift the equilibrium to the unfolded form.

Dr. Nagel: I am certainly not at differences with you as to the importance of unfolding in the surface activity of proteins. As I stated in my presentation, we think that it is the main event. The differences between oxy Hb S and oxy Hb A probably involve differences in the type and/or rate of unfolding to the proper surface active conformation. But if oxy Hb S is capable of unfolding differently than oxy Hb A, it suggests to us a difference in the initial conformation of these two proteins. Not a big difference in conformation, as the one that can be detected by changes in crystal habit, but a subtle one, that can be detected by sensitive methods, as surface tension characteristics or NMR. Surface tension changes by protein film formation may prove to be a very sensitive method for studying conformation. We have seen changes in the surface activity of Hb stored 3 days in the refrigerator, when, at the same time, ORD was unable to distinguish the sample from a fresh solution.

Dr. Ho: I would like to show four slides of our recent proton NMR studies on the conformations of several surface amino acid residues on the sickle cell hemoglobin molecule. Before I show these slides, I would like to discuss with you some of our recent NMR investigations of the internal structure of the Hb S molecule. I do not have slides for this part of the discussion. Dr. Leslie Fung and Mrs. Allison Lin (who is a graduate student in my laboratory) have carried out extensive NMR studies comparing the structures of Hb S and Hb A. We have found no observable differences in the hyperfine shifted proton resonances between deoxy Hb A and Hb S in solution or in the ring-current shifted proton resonances between Hb A and Hb S in both CO and oxy forms. These NMR measurements are very sensitive to the heme environment in deoxy and CO (or oxy) forms. Due to the very long rotational correlation time of a gelled sample, the proton resonances of a gelled deoxy Hb S sample are too broad to provide information about the heme environment in the sample. We then examined the NMR spectra of the supernatant of the gelled deoxy Hb S samples and have found them to be indistinguishable from those of deoxy Hb A samples. Hence, we may conclude that there is probably no difference in the heme environments between Hb A and Hb S in the deoxy and oxy (or CO) forms.

As you know, there are 36 histidines per human hemoglobin molecule. With the exception of the proximal and distal histidines, the rest of the histidines are on the surface of the hemoglobin molecule. Hence, these histidines are good markers for monitoring the surface conformational differences between Hb A and Hb S. The first slide, which was obtained by Dr. Leslie Fung, shows the aromatic proton resonances of deoxy Hb A and Hb S in 0.1M Bis-Tris at pD 7.0 and at 30°C. The two hemoglobins are at the same concentration, pH, and ionic strength. There are differences in the histidine resonances between Hb A and Hb S. Slide 2 shows the aromatic proton resonances of Hb A and Hb S in CO form under the same experimental conditions. Again, there are significant differences in the histidine proton resonances between HbCO A and HbCO S suggesting that there are conformational differences among some of the histidine residues between these two proteins. These resonances are very sensitive to pH and ionic strength, so one has to be very careful in controlling the experimental conditions. Recently, Dr. Toshio Asakura reported that the oxy form of Hb S is readily precipitated out upon shaking and that the addition of inositol hexaphosphate (IHP) to HbO_2 S or HbCO S can stabilize the Hb S molecule against mechanical precipitation. The next slide provides a structural interpretation for Dr. Asakura's findings. This slide shows the effect of IHP on the aromatic proton resonances of HbCO S. In the absence of IHP, you can see that there are significant differences in the histidine proton resonances between HbCO A and HbCO S. When you add IHP to Hb A and Hb S in the CO form, the aromatic proton resonances of these two proteins become indistinguishable. This finding suggest that the binding of IHP to HbCO S can change the conformations of the surface residues and thus can alter the surface properties of the sickle cell hemoglobin molecule. This result may also be relevant to Dr. Perutz's finding. Dr. Perutz found that crystals of HbO_2 A and HbO_2 S are isomorphous. Dr. Perutz, you crystallize your protein at a very high salt concentration so you may have modified the surface conformation of HbO_2 S in such a way to make it indistinguishable from that of HbO_2 A. The next slide compares the aromatic proton resonances among Hb A, Hb S, and Hb Deer Lodge (NA2β2 His→Arg), and Hb Mälmo (FG4β97 His→Glu) in the CO form. Our results show that the single amino acid substitution at β6 in Hb S can alter several histidine resonances. By making further spectral assignments to specific histidine residues in the Hb S molecule, we hope to gain more insight into the conformations of the surface residues in the sickle cell hemoglobin and to relate these altered conformations to the functional properties of Hb S.

Dr. Charache: It's my recollection that Dr. Asakura found that the higher salt concentration, the greater was the precipitation. Do I have that part straight? Have you tried Dr. Muryama's idea; substituting propane for air at the top and saturating the fluid with propane to see what happens?

Dr. Nagel: No.

Dr. Charache: Have you tried putting the Hb S solution in a vial that has no air in it and shaking the insides of it with sonication or something like that. In other words, is it shaking the molecules or is it the air fluid interface that is doing it?

Dr. Nagel: We have done experiments in that direction, but I'm not prepared to discuss any of the results. Once we are satisfied with the technique, I'll be able to discuss it.

Dr. Charache: You must have tried the effect of alkylation?

Dr. Ho: In collaboration with Dr. Nagel and Dr. Roth, Dr. Fung and I have found that nitrogen mustard preferentially alkylates the β_2 histidine in the Hb S molecules.

Unidentified Speaker: The polymerization of Hb S is bad, causing the sickling. This property of oxy Hb S, that is of precipitability, is that thought to be bad too? I see for example that your Hb C-Harlem has the greatest amount of precipitability.

Dr. Nagel: I apologize if anybody understood from my presentation that we were suggesting that the surface activity of Hb S has a pathological effect by favoring the formation of Heinz bodies. Asakura has interpreted his mechanical precipitation experiments in that direction, but we do not believe that this is the case. My references to the potential functional significance of the surface activity of Hb S were exclusively limited to the interactions of Hb S with the red cell membrane. This aspect should be further looked at.

Dr. Perutz: Dr. John White of the Royal Postgraduate Medical School at Hammersmith Hospital, London, just published a paper showing that it is not bad. It's not responsible for Heinz body formation.

Dr. Nagel: I'm not surprised.

THE PREPARATION OF CYANATE DERIVATIVES OF SICKLE CELL HEMOGLOBIN

M. Perrella, D. Bresciani, G. Guglielmo, V. Russo, F. Rossi, L. Rossi-Bernardi, P. Righetti*, and J. V. Kilmartin**
Cattedra di Enzimologia, University of Milan
20133 Milan, Italy

Cyanate combines with the 4 amino groups of valine 1α of horse and human hemoglobin in a specific carbamylation reaction (1-3). A necessary step in analyzing the mechanism of action of cyanate in the treatment of sickle cell anemia is to prepare derivatives of HbS specifically reacted at the terminal α-amino groups of the α and β chains with cyanate, and to study their functional properties. This paper reports experimental details to prepare gram quantities of such derivatives.

MATERIALS AND METHODS

Hemoglobin was obtained from heparinized normal or sickle cell blood by the method of Adair and Adair (4). Resins for chromatographic separations were obtained from: DE-52 and CM-52, Whatman Biochemicals Ltd.; Sephadex G-25F, DEAE-Sephadex A50, and CM-Sephadex C50, Pharmacia; and Biorex 70 (200-400 mesh), Bio-Rad Laboratories. Cystamine hydrochloride and mercaptoethanol (ME) were obtained from Fluka AG. Dithioth-

* Cattedra di Biochimica Generale, University of Milan, 20133 Milan, Italy
** Medical Research Council Laboratory of Molecular Biology, Cambridge CB2, 2QH, England

reitol (DTT) and parahydroxymercuribenzoic acid, sodium salt (pMB) from Sigma. Analar grade reagents were used throughout. Potassium cyanate was recrystallized from 50% ethanol at 50°.

The compositions of the buffers used were as follows:
50 mM TRIS-HCl, pH 8.3, 250 ml 1 M TRIS and 90 ml 1.2 N HCl to 5 liters with H_2O;
50 mM TRIS-HCl, pH 7.9, 250 ml 1 M TRIS and 135 ml 1.2 N HCl to 5 liters with H_2O;
50 mM TRIS-HCl, pH 7.6, 250 ml 1 M TRIS and 147 ml 1.2 N HCl to 5 liters with H_2O;
33 mM TRIS-HCl, pH 8.5, 165 ml 1 M TRIS and 60 ml 1 N HCl to 5 liters with H_2O;
50 mM TRIS-HCl, pH 8.9, 250 ml 1 M TRIS and 1.9 ml 37% HCl to 5 liters with H_2O;
0.2 M Na phosphate (molarity referred to Na^+), pH 6.0, 21.2 g/liter $NaH_2PO_4 \cdot 2H_2O$ and 4.56 g/liter Na_2HPO_4;
25 mM Na phosphate, pH *ca* 8.5, 44.7 g $Na_2HPO_4 \cdot 12H_2O$ in 5 liters H_2O;
50 mM Na phosphate, pH 7.1. Dilute 1:10 350 g $Na_2HPO_4 \cdot 12H_2O$ and 75 g $NaH_2PO_4 \cdot H_2O$ in 5 liters;
50 mM Na phosphate, pH 6.8. Dilute 1:10 278 g $Na_2HPO_4 \cdot 12H_2O$ and 131 g $NaH_2PO_4 \cdot H_2O$ in 5 liters;
10 mM Na phosphate, pH 6.6, 0.36 g/liter Na_2HPO_4 and 0.77 g/liter $NaH_2PO_4 \cdot 2H_2O$;
10 mM K phosphate, pH 7.8, 0.68 g/liter KH_2PO_4 and 0.298 g/liter KOH.

Other buffers were made by suitable dilution and acid-base titrations of those listed above. The pH was measured at 20° with reference to NBS standards. Equilibration of hemoglobin samples with buffers was carried out by gel-filtration on properly sized columns of Sephadex G25 fine. All work was carried out on the carbonmonoxy form of hemoglobin. Great care was taken to store samples under CO by bubbling CO into the containers for 1 to 2 min. Foaming was prevented by the addition of a trace of octyl alcohol. During column chromatography the space between the resin top and the rubber bung was filled with CO at 12 hour intervals. All chromatographic purifications were done at 4°. Column elution profiles were recorded at 280 mm using an LKB automated collector. The ODs of the pooled fractions were usually measured at 540 mm using a Beckman Acta III spectrophotometer. Hemoglobin concentration (either in tetrameric or monomeric form) was determined using a coefficient $E^{1\%}_{1cm} = 9.03$ at 540 nm for COHb. Methemoglobin concentration was measured according to Kilmartin and Rossi-Bernardi (3). Concentration of hemoglobin samples was carried out using an Amicon ultrafiltration apparatus and PM 10 Diaflo membranes.

Purification of Hemoglobins A_o and S_o

Purification of HbA_o from HbA_2 (2 to 4%), HbA_3 and other minor components (*ca* 10%) was carried out according to Huisman and Dozy (5) using a Sephadex A50 column (10 x 45 cm) equilibrated with 50 mM TRIS-HCl buffer, pH 7.6. The hemoglobin sample (5 to 10 g) was loaded on the column at a concentration of *ca* 5% following gel-filtration. The flow rate was kept at 1 ml/hr per cm^2 until clear resolution of the fastest (HbA_2) and the slowest (HbA_3) bands was attained. The flow rate was then increased to 2 ml/hr per cm^2. HbS from homozygote sickle cell blood containing less than 10% contaminants was used without further purification. HbS from heterozygote sickle cell blood was freed of contaminants such as HbA_o, HbA_2, and HbF by a similar chromatography procedure on Sephadex A50. The hemoglobin sample in 50 mM TRIS-HCl buffer, pH 8.3, was loaded on the column (10 x 45 cm) equilibrated with the same buffer. At this pH HbA_2 moves slowly down the column. HbS was eluted by using a 3 liter/3 liter pH gradient from pH 8.3 to pH 7.9. The flow rate was the same as described above. At pH 7.9 HbA_o and HbF are firmly bound to the resin.

Preparation of the Cyanate Double-Blocked Derivative ($\alpha_2^c\beta_2^{Sc}$) of Hemoglobin S

The basic procedure used by Kilmartin and Rossi-Bernardi (3) for human hemoglobin was followed to prepare $\alpha_2^c\beta_2^{Sc}$. Slight modifications of the pH's of some chromatographic steps were introduced due to the difference in charge between HbS and HbA_o. Flow sheets of the various chromatographic steps are shown in Figs. 1 and 2.

The reaction with cystamine. The SH groups of HbS were protected (3) by reaction with cystamine at pH 8.5 for 1 hour

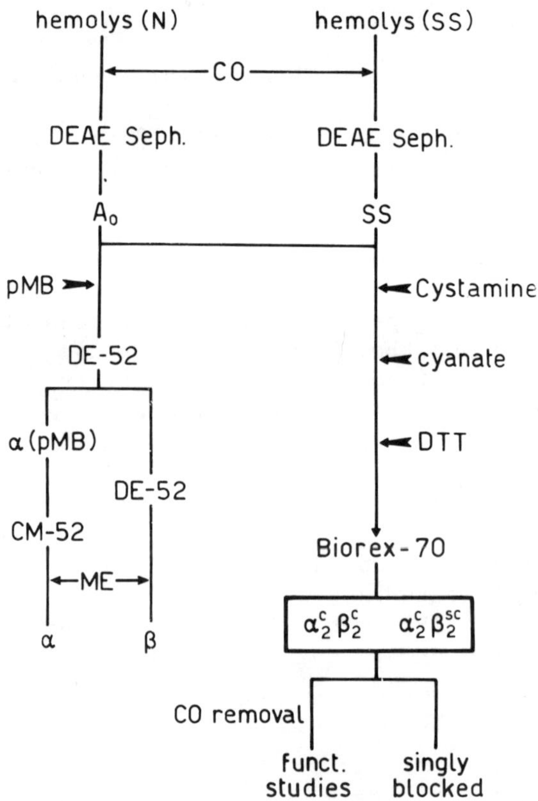

Fig. 1. Schematic diagram for the preparation of the doubly blocked derivatives of $\alpha_2\beta_2$ and $\alpha_2\beta_2^S$, and for the preparation of α and β chains of HbA_o.

at 0° under CO. The hemoglobin sample was equilibrated with 25 mM Na_2HPO_4 by gel-filtration; and after addition of 109 mg cystamine hydrochloride per gram of hemoglobin, the pH was adjusted to 8.5 with 1 M TRIS.

The reaction with cyanate. The cystamine treated protein was equilibrated with 0.2 M sodium phosphate, pH 6.0,

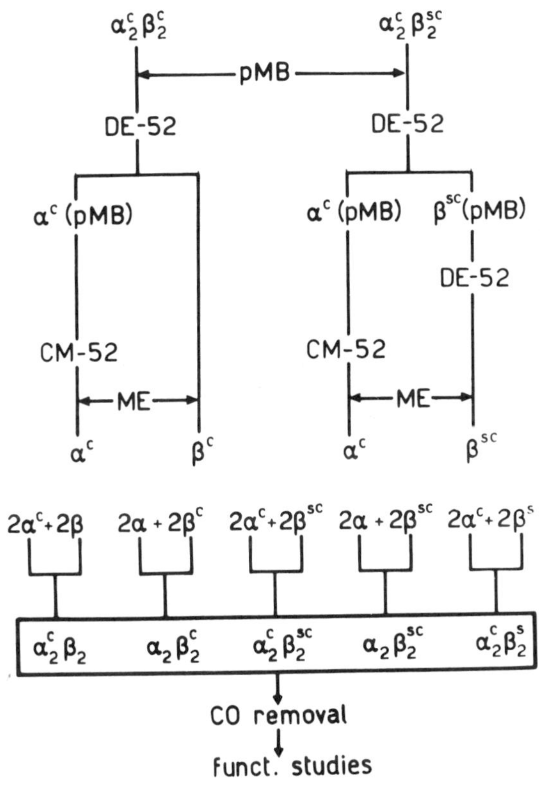

Fig. 2. The preparation of α and β chains of normal and HbS reacted with cyanate at the terminal α-amino group, and the preparation of the singly blocked derivatives of HbA_o and HbS_o.

and diluted to *ca* 20 mg/ml with buffer. Freshly recrystallized KCNO at 200 mg per gram of HbS was then added and the reaction was allowed to proceed for 2 hours at 25° under CO. The excess cyanate was at the same time removed and the solution equilibrated with 25 mM Na_2HPO_4 by gel-filtration on a G25 Sephadex column.

The removal of cystamine. The SH-protecting cystamine was removed by adding to the hemoglobin solution, 4% (w/v) dithiothreitol solution in 25 mM Na_2HPO_4 (265 mg DTT per g HbS). Following adjustment of pH to 8.5 with 1 M TRIS, the solution was left at 4° for 12 hours under CO. Excess DTT was then removed and the hemoglobin solution equilibrated with 50 mM sodium phosphate, pH 7.1, by gel-filtration.

Separation of the double-blocked derivative of HbS ($\alpha_2^c\beta_2^{sc}$). A column of Biorex 70 equilibrated with 50 mM sodium phosphate, pH 7.1, was used. Column size (for *ca* 1 g of protein) was 3 x 50 cm. For larger quantities the column diameter was increased proportionally.

At pH 7.1 the products of reaction between the ε-amino groups of lysine and cyanate have the fastest mobility, while the double-blocked derivative follows more slowly and is seen as the main band in the column. The single-blocked derivatives, $\alpha_2\beta_2^{sc}$ and $\alpha_2^c\beta_2^s$, move more slowly and trail behind. The unreacted protein is more firmly bound to the resin.

To avoid excessive spreading of the $\alpha_2^c\beta_2^{sc}$ band, the buffer molarity was increased to 0.1 when the peak position was at approximately 2/3 of the column. The yield in $\alpha_2^c\beta_2^{sc}$ was usually 30 to 35%. Fig. 3 shows a typical elution pattern.

Preparation of α and β Chains Reacted at the Terminal α-Amino Groups

The procedure previously described (3) was followed except for a few modifications.

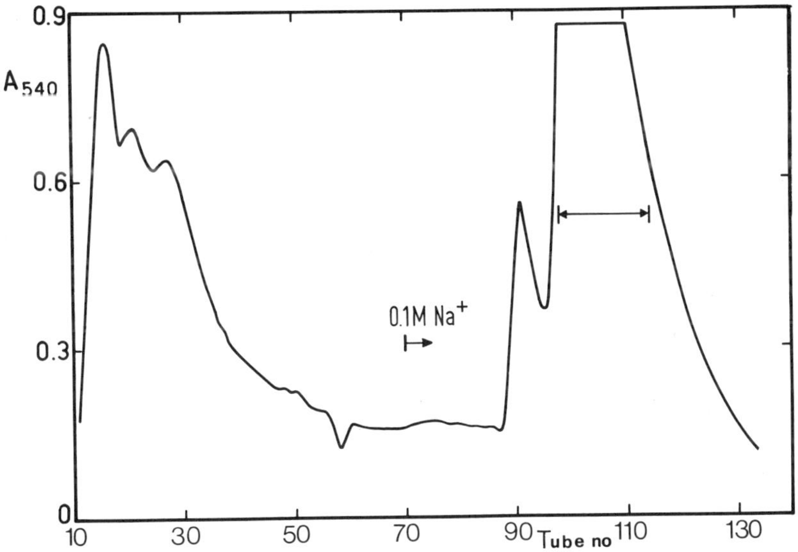

Fig. 3. Chromatography on a Biorex 70 column (4 x 50 cm) of 1.74 g of carbamylated HbS. The flow rate was *ca* 100 ml/hr. The fractions collected were *ca* 26 ml each. The first three peaks on the chromatogram (eluted from 790 to 1000 ml) contain mostly products of carbamylation of the ε-amino group of lysines. The molarity of the eluting buffer, 50 mM phosphate, pH 7.1, was changed to 0.1 M after *ca* 1800 ml of effluent. The double arrow shows the fractions containing the double-blocked derivative $\alpha_2^c\beta_2^{sc}$ (*ca* 570 mg, representing an approximate 33% yield).

Reaction with pMB. The $\alpha_2^c\beta_2^{sc}$ solution was equilibrated with 50 mM sodium phosphate, pH 6.0, by gel-filtration. Solid NaCl was added to a final concentration of 0.2 M, and the protein reacted with p-hydroxymercuribenzoate (64 mg of pMB per gram of derivative). pMB was added as a 2% solution in 2 M glycine-KOH, pH 8.0. The pH of the solution was adjusted to 5.8 with 0.1 M H_3PO_4 and left at 4° for 12 hours under CO.

Separation of the pMB chains. The reaction mixture was centrifuged at 10.000 x *g* x 15 min to remove insoluble matter and equilibrated with 10 mM potassium phosphate, pH 7.8. The sample was applied to a DE-52 column (1 x 30 cm was found adequate for 1 to 1.5 g of starting material) equilibrated with the same buffer. At pH 7.8 the α^{c}-pMB chains are not retained by the column, while the β^{sc}-pMB chains move slowly.

The effluent containing the α^{c}-pMB chains was carefully acidified to pH 6.6 using 0.4 M H_3PO_4; mercaptoethanol (ME) was then added (final concentration 0.05 M) and the solution stored at 4° for 30 min under CO. In order to remove any remaining pMB, the α^{c} chain solution was loaded on a CM-52 column (1 x 8 cm) equilibrated with 10 mM sodium phosphate, pH 6.6: at this pH the chains are firmly bound to the resin. The chains bound to the resin were washed with 50 to 100 ml of 0.4% ME in buffer and then with buffer only to remove excess ME. Finally, the free α^{c} chains were eluted using 33 mM TRIS-HCl buffer, pH 8.5.

To elute the β^{sc}-pMB chains from the DE-52 column, a linear gradient (250 ml/250 ml) of 10 mM K phosphate, pH 7.8, to 60 mM K phosphate, pH 7.4, was applied to the column. The gradient allows a better separation between β^{sc}-pMB chains and any unreacted $\alpha_2^{c}\beta_2^{sc}$ (Fig. 4).

Removal of pMB from the β^{sc}-pMB chains was accomplished by the use of another DE-52 column equilibrated with 50 mM TRIS-HCl, pH 8.9: under such chromatographic conditions the β^{sc} chains are firmly bound to the resin. The β^{sc}-pMB chains were washed with 150 ml of 0.5% ME over a period of 4 hours while bound to the resin, and then eluted with 60 mM K phosphate, pH 7.4. Excess ME was removed by gel-filtration using 25 mM Na_2HPO_4.

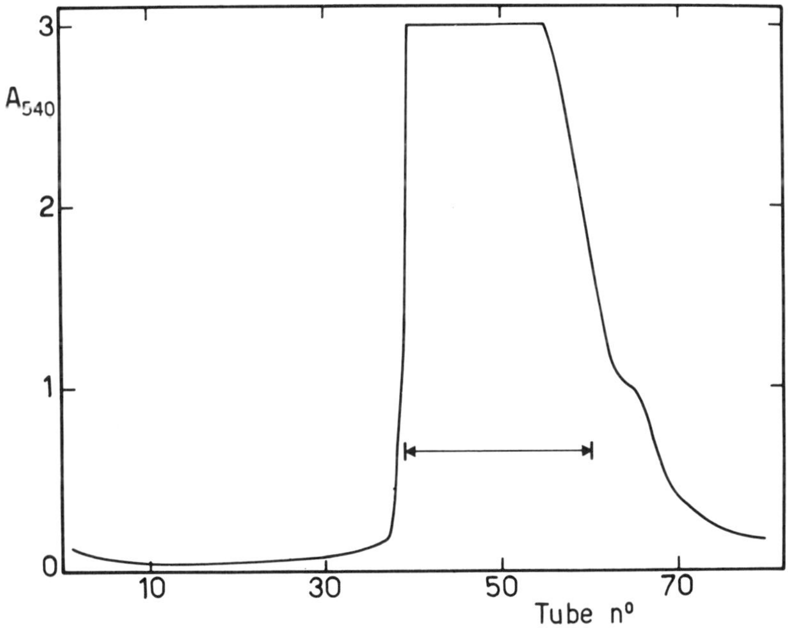

Fig. 4. Chromatogram of the β^S-pMB chains eluted from a DE-52 column (1.3 x 27 cm) with a gradient from 10 mM K phosphate, pH 7.8, to 60 mM K phosphate, pH 7.4. The flow rate was not critical and the fastest possible rate under a pressure *ca* 150 cm H_2O was used. Fractions of 2.5 ml each were collected. The β^S-pMB chains were obtained by reacting 866 mg of HbS with 54 mg pMB as described in the text. The α-pMB chains were eluted from the same column by the 10 mM K phosphate, pH 7.1. The α chain recovery, following removal of pMB, was practically quantitative (430 mg). The recovery of the β^S chains was 43% (185 mg).

Preparation of the Single-Blocked Derivatives, $\alpha_2^C\beta_2^S$ and $\alpha_2\beta_2^{SC}$

The free chains of HbS were prepared using the same conditions described for the chain separation of $\alpha_2^C\beta_2^{SC}$. By mixing the chains in a 1:1 ratio, the hybrids $\alpha_2^C\beta_2^S$ and $\alpha_2\beta_2^{SC}$ were prepared. Concentration of dilute chain solutions was carried out in the presence of DTT (1 ml 4% DTT per 200 mg

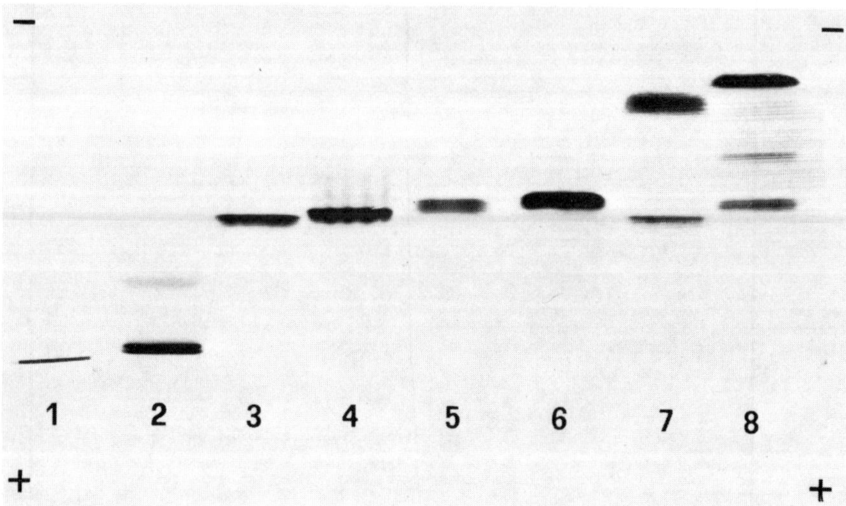

Fig. 5. Isoelectric focusing of HbS and its carbamylated derivatives. The isoelectric focusing was performed in a 5% acrylamide gel slab, containing 2% Ampholine in the pH range 6 to 9, according to Righetti and Bianchi-Bosisio=Righetti (6). The apparatus used was an LKB 2127 Multiphor. Runs were terminated in 90 min, at a final voltage of 1200 V, at 4°. Sample 1 - carbamylated β^{SC} chains; 2 - free β^{S} chains; 3 - $\alpha_2^{C}\beta_2^{SC}$ (reconstituted from free α^{C} and β^{SC}); 4 - $\alpha_2^{C}\beta_2^{S}$; 5 - $\alpha_2\beta_2^{SC}$; 6 - $\alpha_2\beta_2^{S}$; 7 - α_2^{C}; 8 - α_2. Sample 7 contains traces of HbS carbamylated at the α and β chains, whereas sample 8 is contaminated by HbS and met-HbS. All samples contain traces of the met-Hb which can be seen as faint bands also in samples 2 and 3.

of derivative), at pH 8.5, under CO. DTT was allowed to react for one hour at 4° in order to remove any pMB left and to reduce any oxidized SH group of hemoglobin. The absorbances of the free chains at 540 mm have to be carefully matched before mixing to avoid contamination of the hybrids with free chains.

TABLE I

Isoelectric Points* of HbS and Its Carbamylated Derivatives

Species	pI at 4°
β^{sc}-chains	6.90
β^{s}-chains	7.08
$\alpha_2^c\beta_2^{sc}$	7.52
$\alpha_2^c\beta_2^s$	7.57
$\alpha_2\beta_2^{sc}$	7.58
$\alpha_2\beta_2^s$	7.62
α^c-chains	8.04
α-chains	8.12

* The pI's have been determined by cutting a 2 mm slice containing the band of interest and eluting it with 10 mM NaCl (0.2 ml). These samples were kept under nitrogen and shaken for 3 hours. The pH readings were obtained at 4° using a combination micro-electrode. The values reported represent an average of three determinations. Each value was reproducible within ± 0.02 pH units.

Isoelectric Focusing of HbS and Its Carbamylated Derivatives

The purity of HbS and its carbamylated derivatives has been checked by isoelectric focusing. The results are shown in Fig. 5 and in Table I.

ACKNOWLEDGEMENTS

This study was supported by U. S. Public Health Service Grant No. HL-15613.

BIBLIOGRAPHY

1. Kilmartin, J. V., and Rossi-Bernardi, L., *In:* CO_2: Chemical, Biochemical and Physiological Aspects, edited by R. E. Forster, J. T. Edsall, A. B. Otis, and F. J. W. Roughton. Washington, U. S. Government Printing Office, NASA No. SP-188, 73, 1969.

2. Kilmartin, J. V., and Rossi-Bernardi, L. *Nature*, 222: 1243, 1969.

3. Kilmartin, J. V., and Rossi-Bernardi, L. *Biochem. J.*, 124: 31, 1971.

4. Adair, G. S., and Adair, M. E., *Biochem. J.*, 28: 1230, 1934.

5. Huisman, T. H. J., and Dozy, A. M., *J. Chromatogr.*, 19: 160, 1965.

6. Righetti, P. G., and Bianchi-Bosisio-Righetti, A., *In:* Isoelectric Focusing of Proteins and Related Substances, J. P. Arbuthnott and Beeley J. A., eds. Butterworths, London, in press.

Appendix

The location of the cyanate in $\alpha_2{}^c\beta_2{}^{cs}$ was found by reaction of $\alpha_2\beta_2{}^s$ with ^{14}C-cyanate. After chromatography on Bio-Rex 70, 1.8 moles of cyanate per moles of $\alpha\beta$ were present in the $\alpha_2{}^c\beta_2{}^{cs}$ peak. This radioactivity was found to be located at the α-amino groups of the α and β chains by tryptic digestion and fingerprinting, since only the N-terminal tryptic peptides were found to be radioactive. This was confirmed by isolation of 85% of the radioactivity present in $\alpha_2{}^c\beta_2{}^{cs}$ as valine hydantoin (Stark, G. R. and Smyth, D. G. (1963) J. Biol. Chem. 238 214) showing that 90% of the radioactivity was present as carbamylated valine at the N-Termini of the α and β chain.

DISCUSSION

Dr. Perutz: This raises another point which I have been flagging for years. Again on the principle of Ockham's razor, you do not need to postulate anything to explain the low oxygen affinity of sickle cell blood, except that on oxygenation the lattice energy of the precipitate has to be overcome. The oxygen affinity of normal Hb is low because the energy of the salt bridges between the subunits of the same molecule has to be overcome before the molecule can click to the oxy form. In sickle cell Hb, additional constraints between molecules have to be broken on oxygenation. Dr. Rossi's results have shown that this postulate is sufficient.

Dr. Rossi-Bernardi: What we have to do now is to look more carefully at the oxygen equilibrium at constant pH of sickle cell hemoglobin in concentrated solutions. We should have then the possibility of further probing into the mechanism of the lowered affinity of Hb S molecule upon sickling.

Dr. Conley: Your observations on the functional adequacy of sickle cell blood in oxygen transport correspond very well to the clinical situation. Patients with sickle cell anemia are not much troubled by the anemia; in fact, many are capable of vigorous activity. If they had only anemia, they wouldn't be so sick.

FACTORS LEADING TO VASCULAR OCCLUSION IN SICKLE CELL ANEMIA

Samuel Charache, M.D. and C. L. Conley, M.D.

Johns Hopkins University School of Medicine

Baltimore, Maryland 21205

INTRODUCTION

In 1934, Diggs and Ching suggested that "elongated and spiked (sickle) cells interlock and pass with more difficulty through narrow spaces than do normal cells" (1). Six years later, Ham and Castle observed that deoxygenated sickle cells could not be packed as tightly as oxygenated cells during centrifugation, and then demonstrated that the viscosity of deoxygenated sickle cell (SS) blood was increased. They postulated a "viscious cycle of erythrostasis", in which increased blood viscosity led to increased deoxygenation, further sickling, and eventual infarction (2). Bauer, working from a different point of view, came to essentially the same conclusion (3), and increased blood viscosity has played a central role in theories of the pathogenesis of sickle cell crises since that time (4-10).

The cause of increased blood viscosity in sickle cell anemia is not only the irregular and assymetric shape of sickled cells, but their rigidity, first noted by Murphy and Shapiro in 1944 (11), and expanded upon by others since that time (8, 10, 12-14). Even oxygenated SS blood exhibits increased viscosity, related largely to its content of irreversibly sickled cells (4).

Although the fine details of the sickling process are nearly worked out, at the molecular level, we still do not know why patients develop vaso-occlusive sickle cell crises one day, but not the next. Aside from a few unusual situations (mostly involving hypoxemia), red cells and cardiopulmonary dynamics remain unchanged, but something happens to produce vascular occlusion, ischemia, and infarction. Suggested precipitating agents have ranged from atmospheric disturbances (15-17) to acidosis (18). The latter is typical of suggestions which have led to attempts at therapy; subsequent studies showed that most patients in crisis are not acidotic (19, 20), and treatment of crises with alkali was unsuccessful (21). Possible exceptions are the instances in which a crisis follows an infection (22, 23), or occurs for the first time in pregnancy (24), particularly in hemoglobin SC disease (25-27). Plasma fibrinogen rises in both situations (28-30), is known to increase during (and sometimes before) sickle cell crises (17, 31), and it is known to be an important determinant of the non-Newtonian viscosity of blood (32, 33).

Thirty-four years ago, Ham and Castle pointed out that "when any condition, such as an infection, causes a primary increase of the plasma viscosity or of rouleaux formation in the blood of these patients, any resulting delay in the passage of the erythrocytes through the capillaries will decrease their oxygen content" (2), enhance sickling, and lead to further erythrostasis. The present study was initiated to try to measure changes in the non-Newtonian viscosity of blood from patients with sickle cell anemia (hereafter called SS blood) under 3 sets of conditions: (I) in association with sickle cell crises; (II) after transfusion; and (III) after treatment of blood, in vitro, with chemicals known to inhibit sickling. We made these 3 sets of measurements to try to distinguish between factors that determine when a crisis occurs and those that determine whether a crisis will occur at all. We did this, obviously, to try to find some feature of the process which could be manipulated or exploited as a means of treatment.

Non-Newtonian viscosity was measured, for reasons given above; this sticky subject is made even stickier by its peculiar vocabulary and units of measurement, and it seemed wise to insert a preliminary discussion of rheologic terminology.

Measurement of Blood Viscosity

Blood is a non-Newtonian fluid; the faster it flows, the less viscous it becomes (14). Before flow starts, red cells are randomly oriented, and bound together in loose aggregates, primarily by fibrinogen (32-34). As flow begins, the aggregates break up, a lubricating layer of plasma forms at the periphery of the vessel, the red cells orient themselves and may become deformed; as a result less force is required to maintain flow (35, 36). The relative importance of cell-plasma and cell-cell interaction is a function of both hematocrit value and shear rate (35). The process of orientation and deformation takes time, and these time dependent decreases in viscosity are called "thixotropy".

Blood viscosity, as measured in viscometers, rather than in much more complicated patients, is determined by at least 4 factors, each of which is abnormal in sickle cell anemia. It depends on the particle fraction, the axial ratio of the particles, the plasticity of the particles, and interactions between particles and suspending medium.

In sickle cell anemia, the particle fraction, or hematocrit, is low -- this tends to reduce viscosity. The axial ratio of elongated sickled cells is high -- this increases viscosity. The plasticity is low -- this also increases viscosity. Finally, interaction between particles and plasma is probably abnormally high, because of plasma protein abnormalities in SS patients. Both

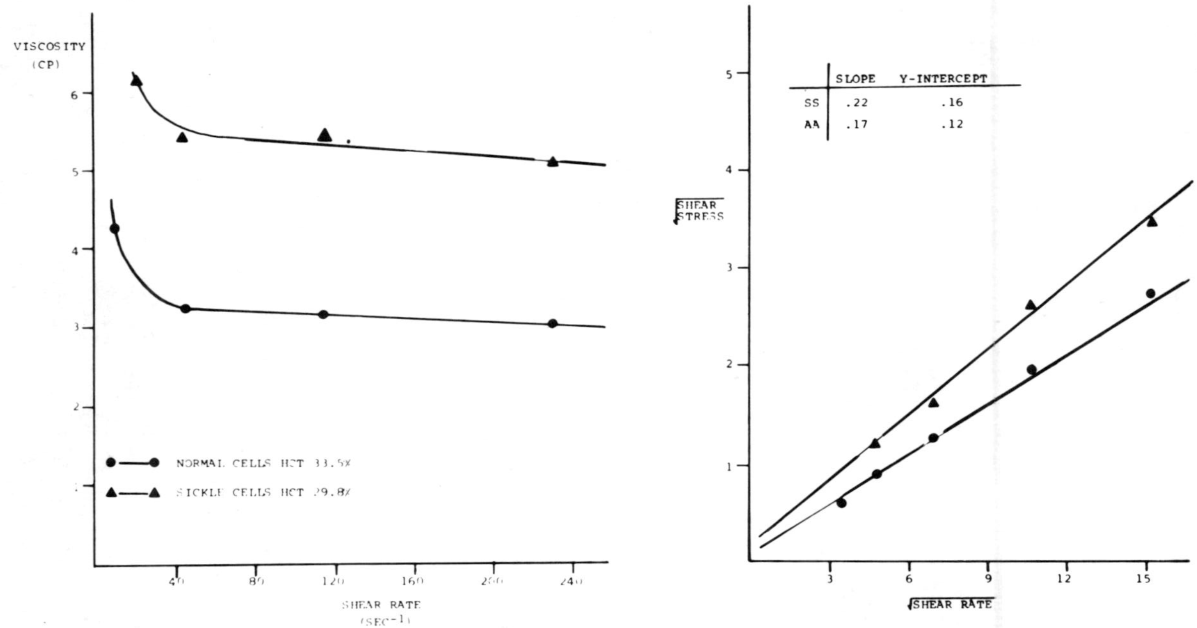

Figure 1: Viscosity of partially deoxygenated SS blood compared with that of an anemic patient with normal hemoglobin. Left viscosity as a function of shear rate; right, Casson plot.

decreased plasticity of sickled cells, and increased particle solvent interaction, would tend to exaggerate the non-Newtonian properties of blood.

The speed at which a cell flows (measured in cm/sec) divided by its distance from the stationary wall of its conduit (measured in cm) is called "shear rate" ($\dot{\gamma}$), and it is measured in inverse sections (sec^{-1}). Shear rates for Newtonian fluids in steady flow depend upon flow rate and vessel diameter. The situation for blood, a non-Newtonian fluid in pulsatile flow, is much more complicated. The average shear rate in the aorta is 100-200 sec^{-1}, while that in capillaries may be high (35, 37) or low (32, 38) (see Discussion).

Capillary viscometers of the Ostwald type make measurements at high shear rates. Our measurements were made in a modified cone-plate viscometer, in which shear rates are defined by the geometry of the instrument and the speed of its motor (39, 40). The device measures the force (shear stress) (τ) necessary to maintain a fixed shear rate; viscosity is defined as shear stress divided by shear rate, and is conviently measured in a unit called the "centipoise" (for Poiseiulle) (Fig. 1).

All measurements are subject to experimental error, and we have plotted our data according to Casson's equation

$$\tau^{1/2} = \tau_y^{1/2} + (b\dot{\gamma})^{1/2}$$

to minimize those errors and provide a more-or-less convenient mode of expression. Casson's model is based on the behavior of pigment particles in printer's ink (41); it has little relevance to blood flow, but can be used as an empirical description (much as Hill's equation is used in studies of hemoglobin function).

If the square root of shear stress ($(\tau)^{1/2}$) is plotted against the square root of shear rate ($(\dot{\gamma})^{1/2}$) a straight line (see Figure 1) is obtained with slope "b" and y-intercept $\tau_y^{1/2}$; experimental data can be fit to such a line by linear regression techniques. In the graphs which follow, neither symbols nor units are used on the axes: $\sqrt{\text{shear stress}}$ and $\sqrt{\text{shear rate}}$ refer to experimental data, and "y-intercept" and "slope" are derived from Casson plots. The physical and biological significance of these parameters is unclear, but they do measure departures from Newtonian flow. In Figure 2, for instance, plasma behaves as a nearly Newtonian fluid; blood does not, and its anomalous behavior becomes more marked as fibrinogen content rises. In many instances, an example of the experimental data is presented alongside the derived data (see Figure 7), to try to maintain the reader's touch with reality.

METHODS

Viscosity was measured with a modified Brookfield LVT cone-plate viscometer (39, 40). Blood samples always exceeded 3 ml in volume. Although the device was fitted with special gas inlets to maintain a desired pO_2 within the viscometer, these proved to be unncesary, probably because the blood sample and the cone acted as an effective seal for the thin film of fluid between the cone and plate (see Reference 40).

Plasma fibrinogen levels in patients with sickle cell anemia may exceed 800 mgm/dl; the viscometer easily detected differences between samples with fibrinogen levels of 400 to 800 mgm/dl (Figure 2). These were prepared by dissolving human fibrinogen* in plasma which had been collected in 1/10 volume of 7.6% sodium citrate Fibrinogen concentrations were assayed by the method of Dacie and Lewis (42). Blood samples for studies of patients during and after crisis were collected in Vacutainers(R) containing K_3EDTA (1.5 mgm/ml blood).

*Fibrinogen (Human), Dried; Hyland Division, Travenol Laboratories, Inc., Los Angeles, Calif. 90039

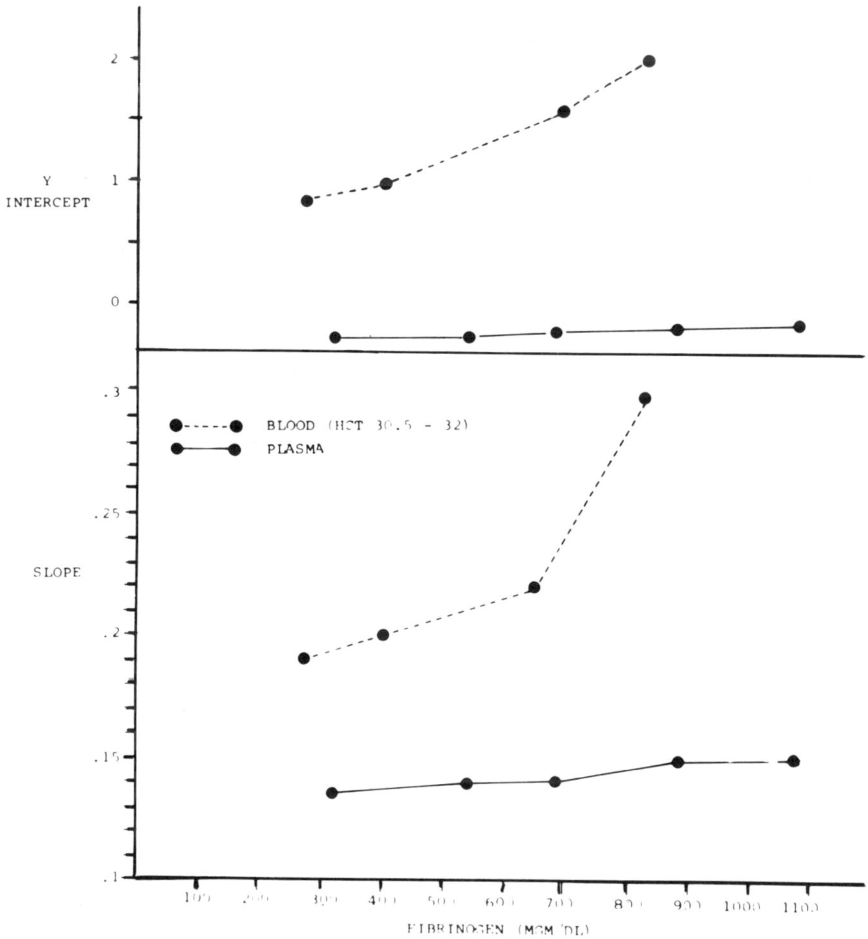

Figure 2: Parameters from Casson plots of partially de-oxygenated SS blood containing added human fibrinogen. Parameters for plasma are included, indicating that its behavior is nearly that of a Newtonian fluid.

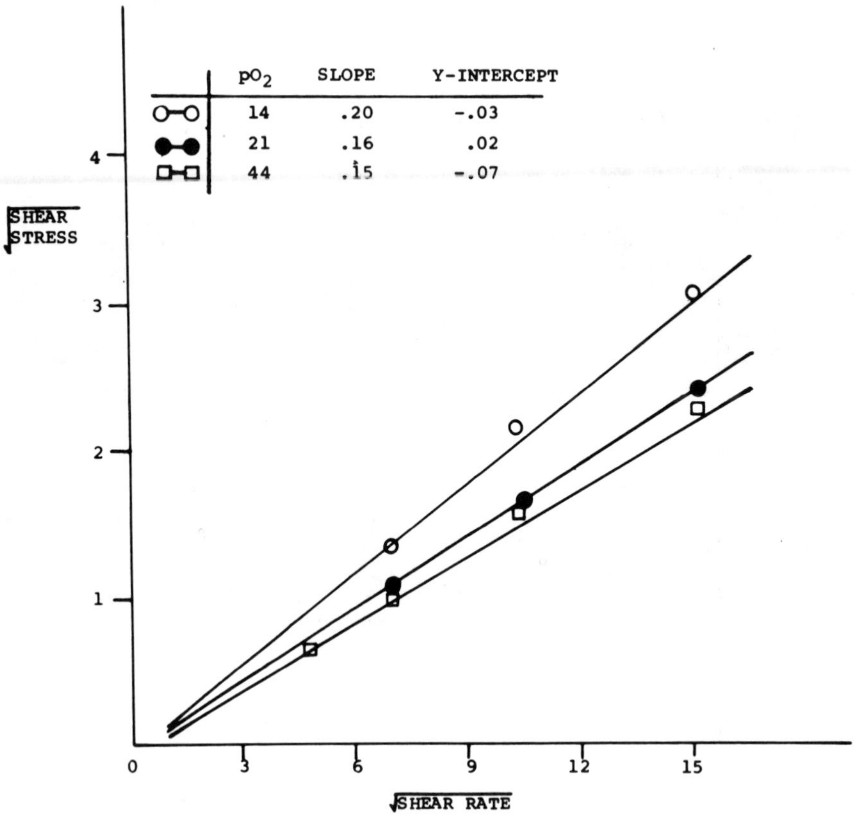

Figure 3: Casson plots of SS blood studied after equilibration with 3 different gas mixtures.

Comparison of samples collected in heparin (10 units/ml) with those collected in EDTA showed no consistent difference at hematocrit values of 30-70%.

Samples were partially deoxygenated by equilibrating 5 ml of blood in a Kugeltonometer* with 3% O_2, 5% CO_2, 92% N_2 at 37°C for 40 minutes; when barometric pressure was 760 mm Hg, the pO_2 of the blood was 21 mm Hg. Oxygen saturation of samples with hematocrits of 20-35%, measured with a CoOximeter** after viscometry, was 30-40%, with occasional lower values in patients with very low oxygen affinity. When blood samples were equilibrated with gas mixtures containing more or less than 3% O_2, the anticipated changes in viscosity were observed (Figure 3).

It became evident that simply measuring the viscosity of patients' blood would not be profitable, for many SS patients were so anemic that the viscosity of their partially deoxygenated blood was <u>less</u> than that of normal controls (Figure 4). If one measures viscosity at a series of hematocrits (Figure 5), differences between AA and SS blood are evident, being more marked the higher the hematocrit. It seems likely that sickled cells differ from normal ones most markedly in their internal viscosity, and this can be crudely approximated by measurements of the viscosity of packed red cells (13, 43). We could not make such determinations, for patients objected to the repeated removal of the relatively large volumes of blood required to prepare such samples. A hematocrit value of 50% was chosen as a compromise, but no significance is attached to the choice other than that of expediency; the effect of fibrinogen would be expected to be near maximal in this situation (44), and it was hoped that measurements would reflect both intracellular viscosity and cell-cell interaction. Measurements were also made at the patients own hematocrit, since no manipulation was needed to prepare these samples. In

---

*Eschweiler & Co., Kiel, Germany
**Model 182, Instrumentation Laboratory, Lexington, Mass. 02173

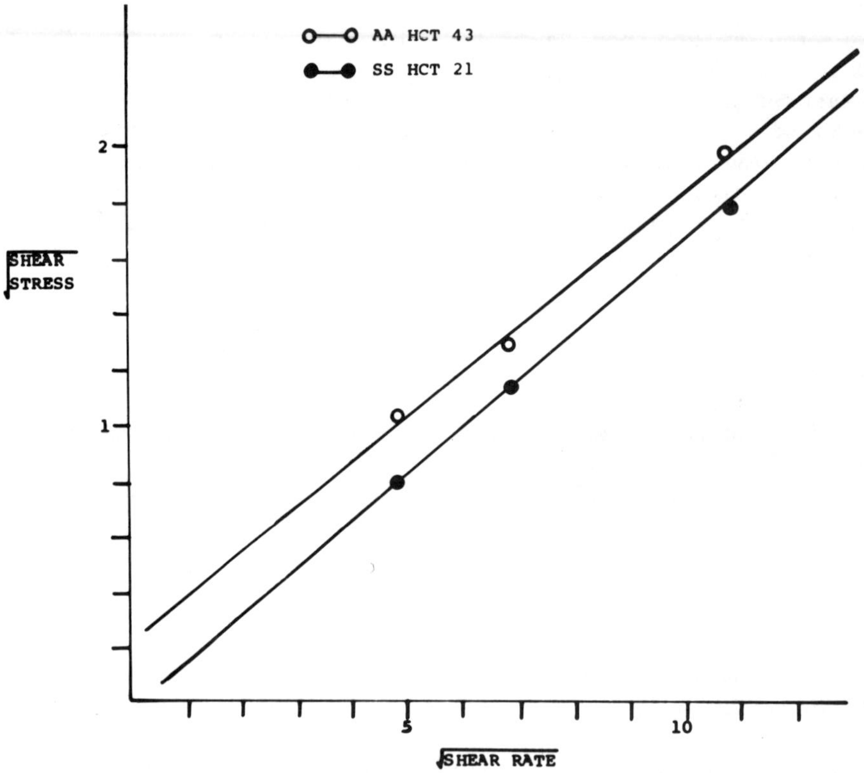

Figure 4: Casson plots comparing partially deoxygenated SS and normal blood.

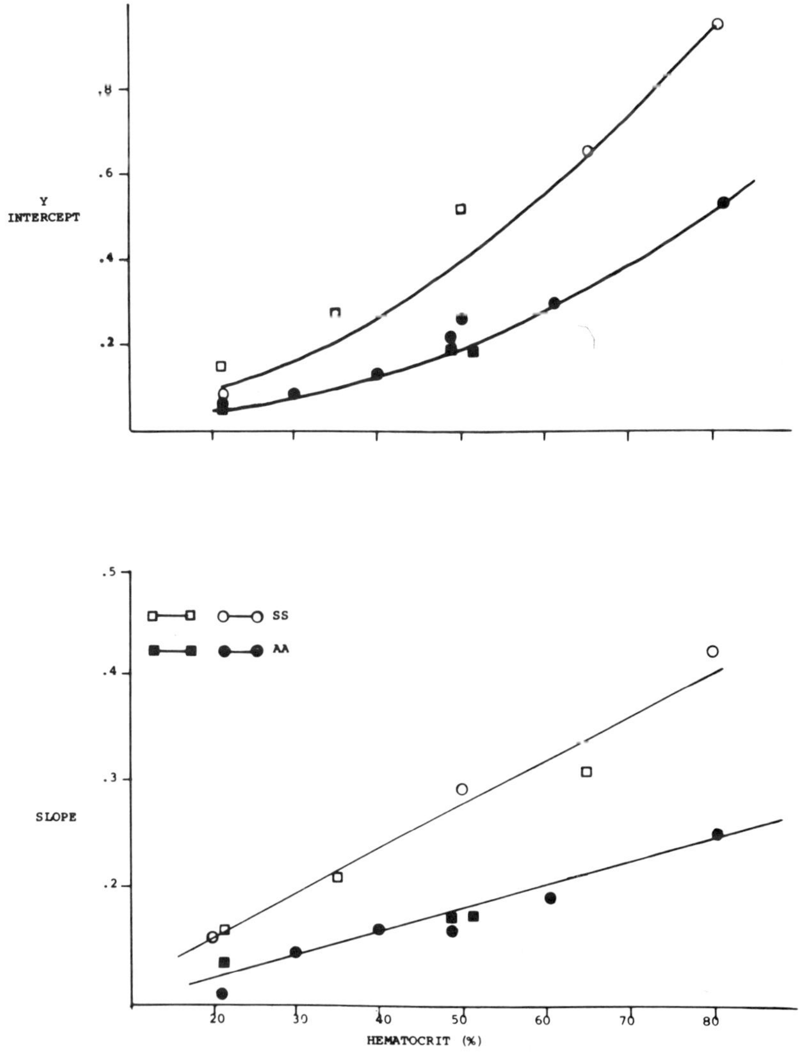

Figure 5: Parameters from Casson plots as a function of hematocrit, comparing partially deoxygenated SS and normal blood.

every case, hematocrits were measured on oxygenated blood, before viscometry, in a micro hematocrit centrifuge*. Hematocrits were adjusted by addition of the patient's leukocyte poor plasma to his own packed red cells after removal of as much of the buffy coat as possible.

In studies of the effect of chemicals on sickling, packed unwashed red cells (Hct 65-70%), which had been collected in heparin, were incubated for 1 hour at 37°C with .15 M recrystallized and charcoal absorbed NaNCO; Mustargen(R)** solution (20 mgm/ml distilled water, containing 2 mgm of nitrogen mustard (HN2)/ml; nor-nitrogen mustard (nor-HN2)*** (20 mgm/ml .1 M NaOH); propranolol**** hydrochloride (1 mgm/ml .15 M NaCl solution); "compound x"***** (1 mgm/ml .15 M NaCl solution) or procaine hydrochloride****** (250 mgm/ml of tris buffered saline (45)). The incubated cells were then added to .1 M phosphate pH 7 buffered (.05 ml/3 ml buffer). Half of this suspension was completely deoxygenated with 95% N_2 5% CO_2 for 15 minutes at 37°, and then fixed: the other half was fixed before deoxygenation.

For studies of the viscosity of treated cells, blood samples were collected in 1/10 volume of 7.6% sodium citrate (heparin was used in the study of propranolol, since calcium is known to be needed for its effect on membrane function in erythrocytes (46). Plasma was removed, the chemical under study was added, and sample was incubated at 37°C for 1 hour (samples containing procaine

---

*International Micro-Capillary Centrifuge Model MB.

**Merck Sharp and Dohme, West Point, Pa. 19486.

***Aldrich Chemical Company, Milwaukee, Wis. 53233. The pH of the solution was 8.6; when added to whole blood, it raised pH by about .4 pH unit.

****Ayerst Laboratories, New York, N. Y. 10017.

*****"Compound x" is now the subject of a patent as a treatment for sickle cell anemia. Its structure cannot be divulged until the Patent Office of the manufacturer gives approval.

******Procaine Base (J. P. Baker) neutralized with HCl.

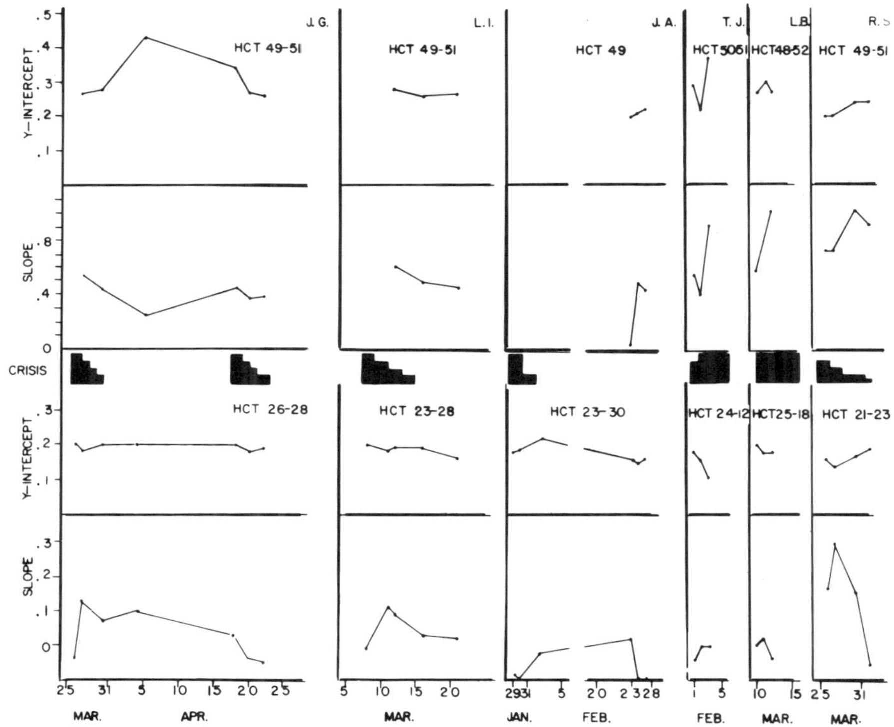

Figure 6: Parameters from Casson plots of partially deoxygenated blood from 6 SS patients, during and after crises. Studies at the patient's own hematocrit are shown in the lower 2 panels, and studies at hematocrits about 50% are shown in the upper 2. Crisis severity is diagrammed in the middle panel.

hydrochloride were kept in the refrigerator for 3 hours (45)). Supernatant fluid was removed after centrifugation, and the patients' plasma was added back to his red cells to give desired hematocrit values. These samples were partially deoxygenated with 3% O_2, as in studies of untreated blood. Portions were fixed for estimation of sickling after viscometry was completed. Since incubation alone can alter cell rigidity (47) control cells were always incubated at the same time as treated cells, in phosphate buffered saline.

Blood samples were fixed for microscopic examination by adding .5-1.0 ml of red cell suspension to 3 ml of 10% formalin (4% formaldehyde solution) in phosphate buffered saline. The proportion of sickled cells was estimated after the samples were coded; only cells with sharp points or an axial ratio of more than 3:1 were considered to have sickled.

RESULTS

I. Serial Studies of Patients During Crises

Summaries of studies from some of the patients studied are shown in Figure 6. Viscosity of the patients' blood at their own hematocrit values showed no consistent change during crisis, after crisis, or in a few patients, before the next crisis. Changes were seen in samples with hematocrits about 50%, but again these were not consistent (compare patient J.G. in March and April, or with patient R.S., or with J.A. in late February when he was not in crisis). In a few instances, decreases in viscosity during crisis were associated with decreases in the proportion of irreversibly sickled cells, with a subsequent rise, but this also was not a consistent observation.

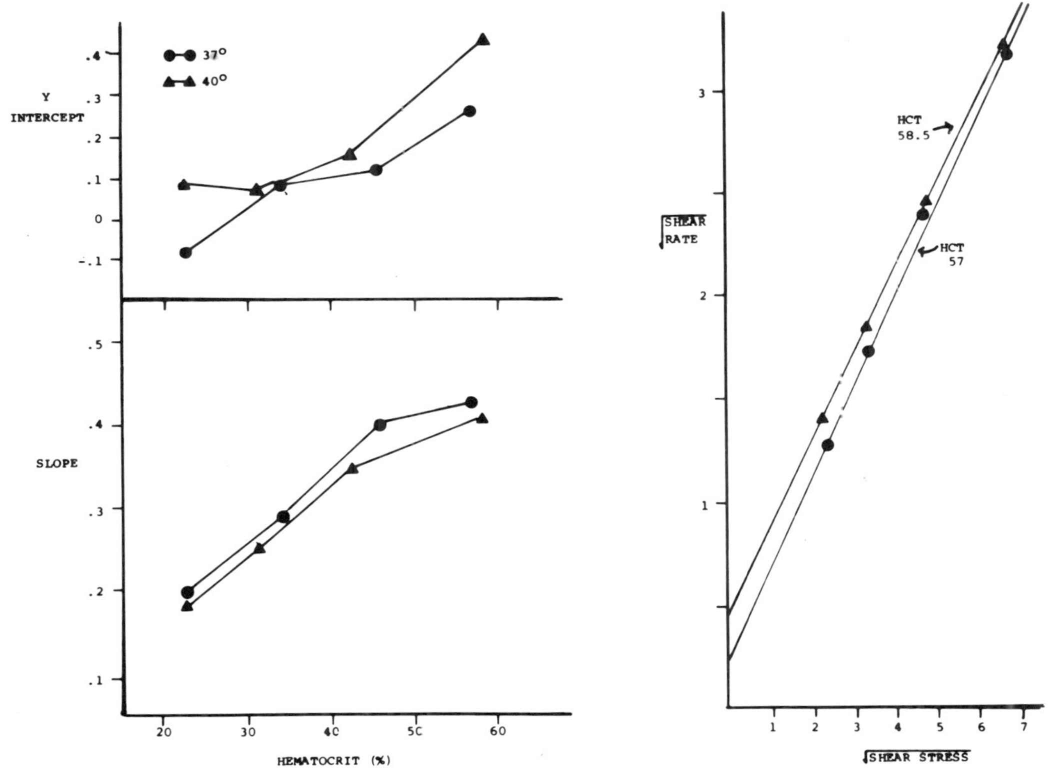

Figure 7: Left, parameters from Casson plots of SS blood, partialled deoxygenated and measured at 37° or 40°C, as a function of hematocrit. Right, Casson plot at hematocrits about 58%.

Infections are usually associated with fever, and fever alone has been implicated in the precipitation of sickle cell crises (17, 48). Oxygen consumption increases during pyrexia, and mixed venous pO_2 may decrease, particularly in a patient with pre-exisiting cardio-pulmonary disease (49, 50). Oxygen affinity decreases (51), and it seemed possible that viscosity of SS blood might increase in vitro, as well as in vivo, if studied at a higher temperature than usual. Blood was equilibrated with 3% oxygen at 37° and 40°, and viscosity was measured at the same temperatures. Blood viscosity was lower at the higher temperature, but the viscosity of the suspending plasma decreased only minimally (Figure 7).

II. Studies During Exchange Transfusion

We have maintained a few patients on chronic transfusion programs for some years, and in general they remain symtom-free if the proportion of sickle cells in their blood is kept below 50%. Patients are usually started on the program with a partial exchange transfusion (9, 52), and sometimes partial exchange is carried out later (if the patients' veins are large enough for a phlebotomy). Measurements of the viscosity of patient's blood during the initial exchange, without adjusting the hematocrit, showed a consistent increase after transfusion (Figure 8), particularly when hematocrit values rose from the low 20's to 40%. Measurements during a subsequent exchange, in which hematocrit value was maintained at about 40%, showed little change if the proportion of sickle cells was initially less than 50%.

Measurements were made on samples prepared with hematocrit values of 20-50%, using cells obtained from a patient during transfusion (Figure 9). There was little difference between samples with hematocrits of 20-40%, but there were differences in the slope of the Casson plot at a hematocrit about 50%. At higher hematocrits (Figure 10), these differences were more marked, but there was no pattern to the location of Y-intercept.

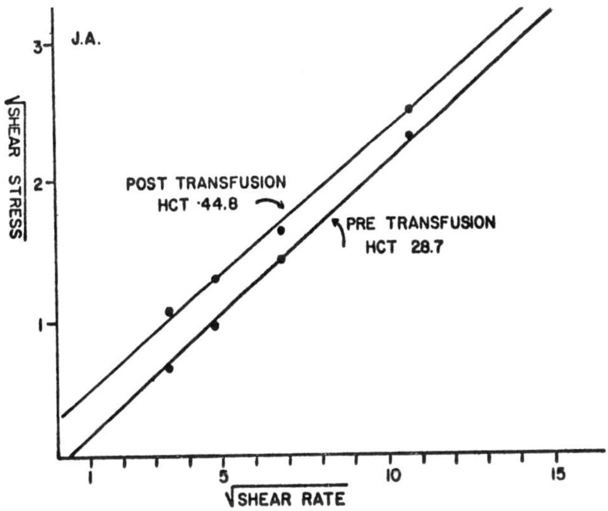

Figure 8: Casson plot of partially deoxygenated blood before and after partial exchange transfusion. There were 40% normal cells in the post-transfusion sample.

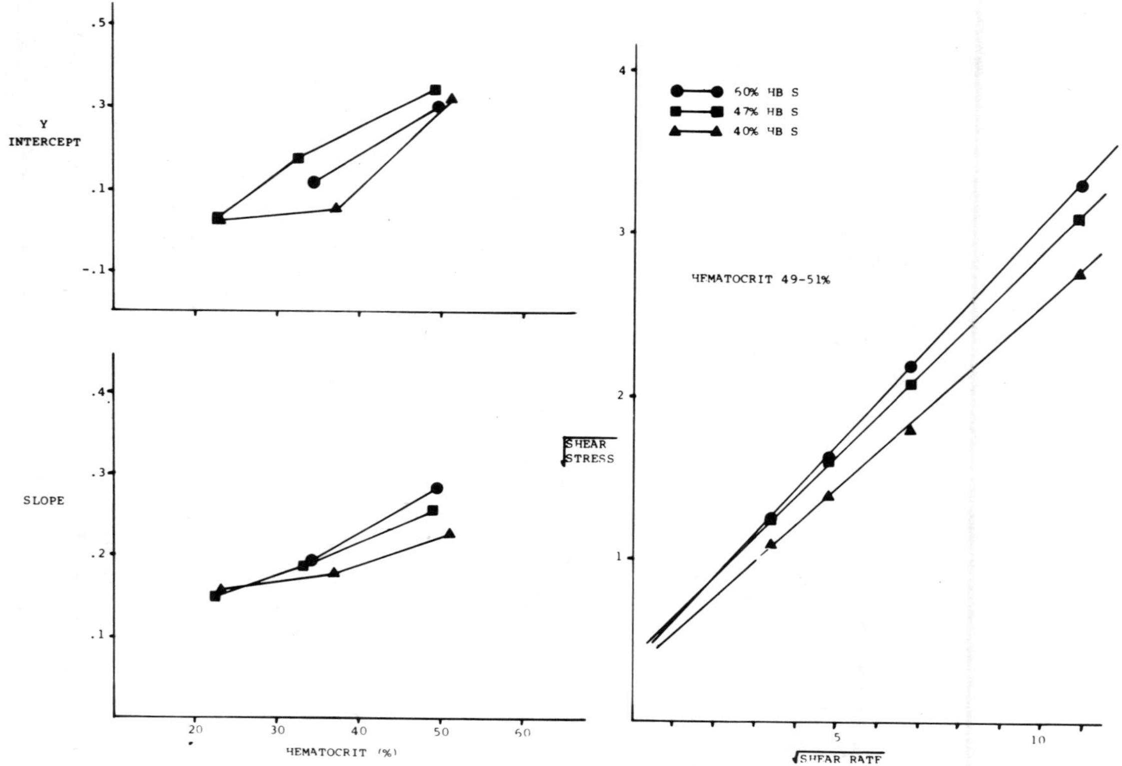

Figure 9: Left, parameters from Casson plot of partially deoxygenated blood from a patient during exchange transfusion, as a function of hematocrit. Right, Casson plot at hematocrit about 50%.

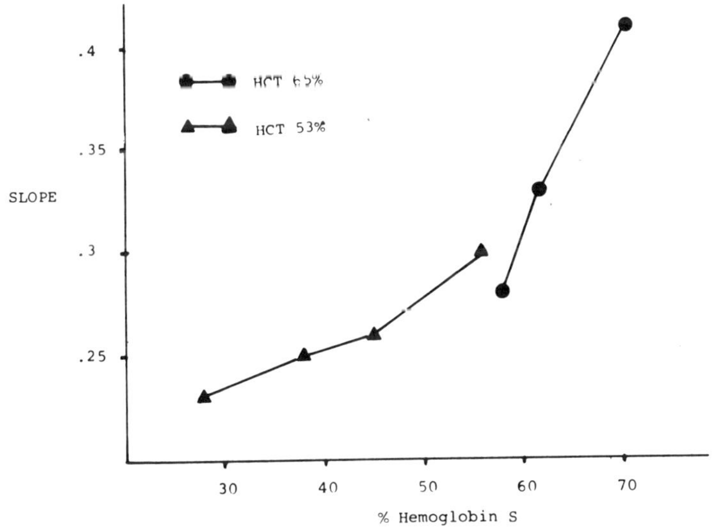

Figure 10: Slope of Casson plots as a function of the proportion of normal cells in a mixture of AA and SS cells, at hematocrits of 53 and 65%.

Studies in patient J.P were of particular interest (Figure 11). After an initial transfusion, he did not keep appointments for subsequent transfusions, and was admitted for painful crises 3 times between June and September (having kept his appointments during July and August). In each instance, the proportion of circulating sickle cells was above 50%. With transfusion, the slope of the Casson plot fell, but the Y-intercept increased.

III. Studies of Anti-sickling Agents

Sodium cyanate, nitrogen mustard, nor-nitrogen mustard, procaine hydrochloride, propranolol, and "compound x" all inhibited sickling (Table 1). Red cells incubated with the latter 2 compounds showed easily vis-

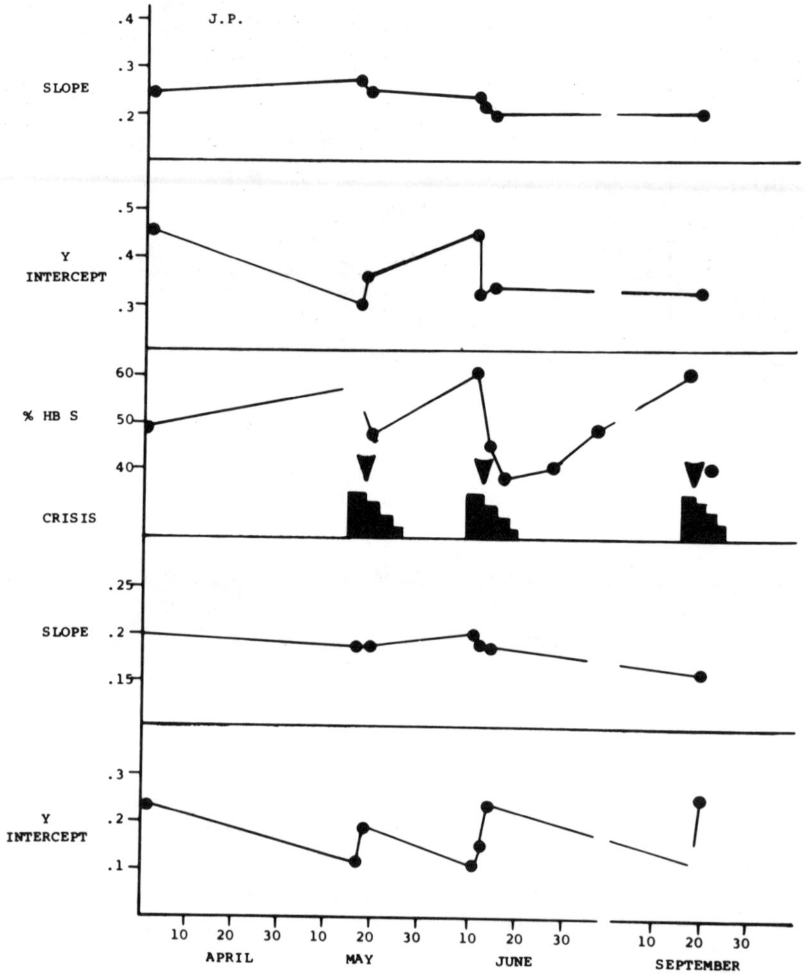

Figure 11: Serial studies at the patient's own hematocrit (35-40%); upper 2 panels, studies at hematocrits about 50%. Middle panels, proportion of sickle cells, and severity of crises. Transfusions were administered at the arrows (▼).

Table 1. Anti-Sickling Effect of Selected Compounds

Compound	Concentration	% Sickled Cells		Remarks
		Oxy	Deoxy	
Nitrogen Mustard	.2 mgm/ml	3	39	
	.4 " "	3	8	
Nor-Nitrogen Mustard	2 mgm/ml	2	56	
	4 " "	1	14	
NaNCO	.01 M	0	24	
	.015 M	1	26	
Procaine HCl	.007 M	0	65	
	.09 M	0	0	Budding spheres
	.13 M	-	-	Hemolyzed
RMI-6792	.3 mgm/ml	0	12	
	.4 " "	1	8	Spheres
Propranolol	.1 mgm/ml	10	13	? Crystals
	.2 " "	12	14	
Control-NaCl	.15 M	0	60	
.1M PO_4 pH 7.4	.1 M	2	72	
No Addition		1	66	

ible hemolysis in the supernatant fluid after incubation, and microscopic examination of deoxygenated suspensions showed the presence of many spherocytes. In the concentrations originally reported to affect irreversibly sickled cells (.09M), procaine hydrochloride produced spherocytes; at lower concentrations (.001M), it had no effect on sickling.

As with samples from transfused patients, there was little difference between the viscosity of treated and control red cells when studied at hematocrits of 20-30% (Figure 12). When a range of hematocrit values was studied, cells which had been incubated with .01M NaNCO showed a variable difference in viscosity from control cells, sometimes being a bit more and sometimes a bit less viscous. Fixed preparations contained almost nc sickled cells, although the viscosity of the blood remained high (Figure 13).

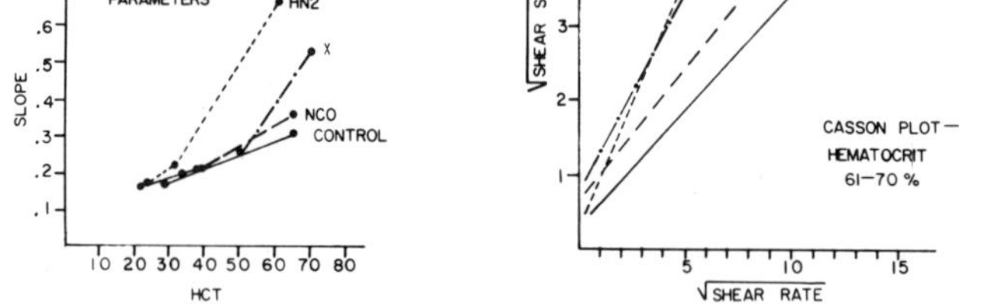

Figure 12: Left, parameters from Casson plots for partially deoxygenated SS blood, after treatment with nitrogen mustard (HN2), "compound x" and sodium cyanate (NCO). Sickling was inhibited by each of these agents (see text). Right Casson plots at hematocrits about 65%.

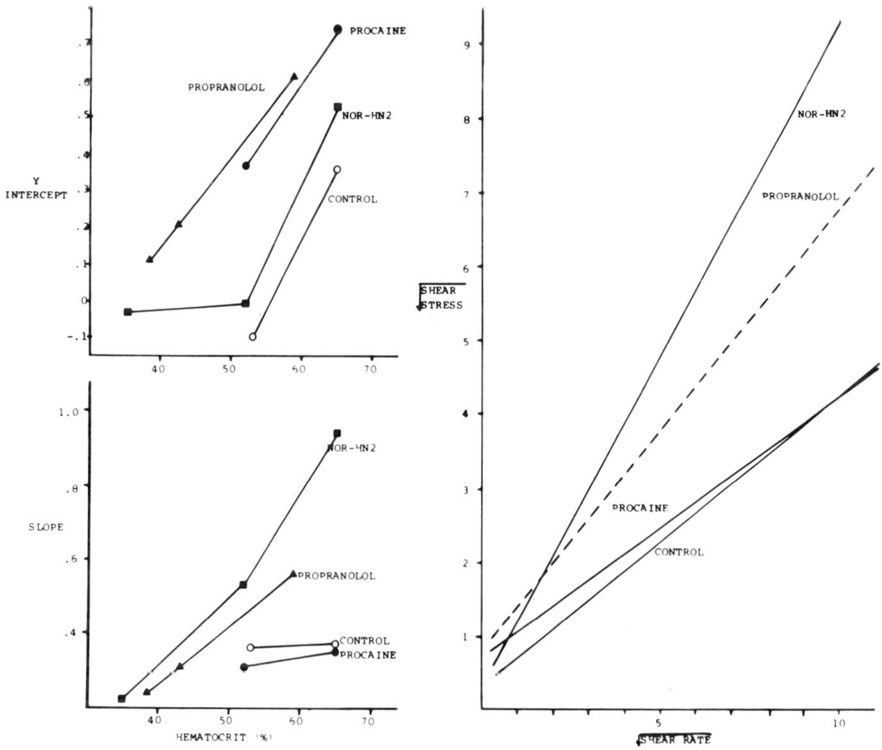

Figure 13: Left, parameters from Casson plots for partially deoxygenated SS blood, after treatment with nor-nitrogen mustard (nor-HN2), .09M procaine hydrochloride (procaine), and propranolol. Sickling was inhibited by each of these agents (see text). Right, Casson plots at hematocrit about 65%. The line for propranolol was constructed by extrapolation of slope and y-intercept lines to the higher hematocrit.

The effects of nitrogen mustard, nor-nitrogen mustard, propranolol, and "compound x" were impressive, for treated cells were more viscous than control cells in every instance (Figure 12, 13). The mustard treated cells were difficult to resuspend after centrifugation, suggesting that their surfaces had become "sticky". Red cells were sphered by "compound x", and deformed by propranolol. Increased hemolysis was noted in supernatant plasma after viscometry, in samples which had been treated with the former compound.

DISCUSSION

Our initial expectation was that we would find exaggerations of the non-Newtonian nature of blood flow in temporal relation to vaso-occlusive sickle cell crises. We found changes, but they were minor at low hematocrit values and inconsistent at high ones. Since our viscometer is a much less expensive piece of apparatus than those used by others (18, 32, 38), one must ask if it was sensitive enough to measure what we sought.

Blood flow through capillaries is intermittent (8, 53), and shear rates *in vivo* must vary from high to low or zero, as transient conditions (35). The thixotropic behavior of blood makes measurement of viscosity particularly difficult, and flow through cylindrical tubes adds yet another degree of complexity. The hypothesis, that crises are precipitated by a preceding exaggeration of non-Newtonian flow, would best be tested with an instrument which is sensitive to time-dependent variations in flow. The LVT viscometer is poorly suited for that purpose, but no consistent pattern of transient changes in shear stress was noted in passing from high to low shear rates (34). The question cannot be considered as closed, but our data suggest that whatever it is that triggers a sickle cell crisis, it *is not intrinsic to the blood*.

The effects of blood transfusion are perlexing, for although most clinicians agree that they are beneficial in sickle cell anemia, they *increase* the viscosity of patient's blood (Figure 8). Although our data are not conclusive, they suggest that transfused cells decrease non-Newtonian viscosity at very high hematocrit values (Figure 10). That observation is consistent with the view that the microvasculature is the site at which vaso-occlusive crises begin (8), for as red cells squeeze through narrow capillaries their deformability becomes of critical imporance (14), and this is mirrored by measurements of the viscosity of packed cells (40).

Reemphasis of the role of the microvasculature probably provides an answer to the precipitation of vaso-occlusive crises, for it is not difficult to envision changes there which could lead to vascular occlusion. Endothelium could become sticky, and vessels could close down enough to stop blood flow entirely, or they could become so narrow that blood flow slowed significantly. Since sickling is a time-dependent process (54-57), that slowing or interruption of flow could provide enough time for sickle cells to become rigid while passing through a region of low pO_2.

When our data suggested that viscosity measurements at high hematocrits bore a relation to whether crises would occur, but not when they could, investigation of anti-sickling agents seemed a logical next step, and we proceeded to study a number of them.

Sodium cyanate was of greatest interest, for it is currently being evaluated in a controlled clinical trial (58). The concentration of NaNCO used in our incubation mixture (.01M) can be expected to yield .6 moles of carbamylated N-terminal groups per mole of hemoglobin, a level similar to that found in treated patients. Continuously carbamylated cells in the blood of patients taking daily oral doses of cyanate must be different from those carbamylated by a "one-shot" incubation in vitro, but the equivocal changes we observed in the laboratory are similar to the equivocal (at best) changes we have seen in the clinic, and those reported in clinical trials (58). Sickling was effectively inhibited, but viscosity did not change.

Nitrogen mustard (59), and nor-nitrogen mustard (60), probably inhibit sickling in a different manner from NaNCO (61). They produce an increase in viscosity of red cells, perhaps by alkylating the cell membrane, and our findings would suggest that the survial of nitrogen-mustard treated sickle cells will not be increased. Those measurements have not yet been made in man, but surely will be of great interest.

Procaine hydrochloride has recently been reported to "unsickle" irreversibly sickled cells, and improve their filterability (45). It is one of a group of cationic surface-active substances which includes phenothiazines, antihistamines, and reserpine (62). Depending upon drug concentration and the pH of the medium, these compounds inhibit osmotic lysis of red cells, but can also sphere and lyse them under other conditions, perhaps by internalization of cell membranes (62). Incubation of red cells with chlorpromazine is known to increase their viscosity, when studies are carried out at hematocrits above 50% (63). In our studies, incubation of sickle cells with .09M procaine caused sphering, which is known to inhibit sickling (64). Lower concentrations had no effect. Viscosity was not significantly altered by high or low concentrations, but hemolysis was produced by the shearing stress within the viscometer when the procaine concentration was .09M (65).

"Compound x" is one of several compounds we have studied recently, which also inhibit sickling by producing spherocytes. Its mode of action may be similar to that of procaine, but it produced a distinct increase in viscosity. It seems unlikely that any chemical which has its primary effect on the red cell membrane will significantly improve red cell survival in sickling disorders. Polymerization of molecules of hemoglobin is the initial step in the pathogenesis of sickle cell crises, and we must search for an agent which interrupts that process without altering the integrity of the cell membrane. Nitrogen mustard and nor-nitrogen mustard meet the first criterion, but may not meet the second.

Our studies of patients during and after crises led to no suggestion of a therapeutic maneuver, for we could detect no consistent alteration in blood viscosity. Blood transfusion remains a mainstay of therapy, if one must do something, but its mode of action is still far from clear. Perhaps a direct attack on the microcirculation should be considered: vasodilators have not been a success (66), but with current activity in the field of thrombosis research, maybe an agent could be found which alters endothelial charge or adhesiveness. The search for such an agent must necessarily be difficult, since it implies investigation at a much more complex level of integration than measurements of blood viscosity.

SUMMARY

Pregnancy and infection have been reported to precipitate sickle cell crises, and both are known to produce elevations in plasma fibrinogen, which is an important determinant of the non-Newtonian viscosity of blood. Viscosity was measured before and after crises, but no consistant pattern of alteration was observed in shear stress/ shear rate relationships. A pattern was observed in blood from transfused patients, for the slope of Casson plots was related to the proportion of normal red cells when studies were carried out at high hematocrits. When a number of potential therapeutic agents were studied, none decreased blood viscosity, and most of them increased it, although sickling was inhibited by all. The correlation between proportion of transfused cells and viscosity at high hematocrits suggests, once again, that the rigidity of red cells traversing the microcirculation is an important determinant of <u>whether</u> sickle cell crises will occur. The status of the microvasculature may determine <u>when</u> crises occur, and the search for a therapeutic agent for sickle cell anemia should continue to include that field of approach.

ACKNOWLEDGEMENTS

These studies were supported by National Heart and Lung Institute grant HL-02799 and contract 72-2930-B, Clinical Research Center grant 5-MO-IRR3511 from the National Institutes of Health, and a gift from the Women's Club of Towson. Miss Carolyn Gould did the initial studies of the viscosity of deoxygenated blood. All patients studied gave informed consent to chronic transfusion therapy, and for obtaining blood samples.

REFERENCES

1. Diggs, L.W. and Ching, R.E. (1934) South Med. J. 27:839-844.

2. Ham, T.H. and Castle, W.B. (1940) Trans. Assn. Am. Phys. 50:127-132.

3. Bauer, J. (1940) Arch. Surg. 41:1344-1362.

4. Chien, S., Usami, S. and Bertles, J.F. (1970) J. Clin. Invest. 49:623-634.

5. Harris, J.W., Brewster, H.A., Ham, T.H. and Castle, W.B. (1956) Arch. Int. Intern. Med. 97:145-168.

6. Griggs, R.C. and Harris, J.W. (1956) Arch. Intern. Med. 97:315-326.

7. Milner, P.F. (1974) Clinics in Haematology 3:289-331.

8. Murphy, J.R. (1973) in The Microcirculation in Clinical Medicine, Academic Press, New York, p. 227-252.

9. Anderson, R., Cassell, M., Mullinax, G.L. and Chaplin, H. Jr. (1963) Arch. Intern. Med. 111:286-294.

10. Klug, P.P., Lessin, L.S. and Radice, P. (1974) Arch. Intern. Med. 133:577-590.

11. Murphy, R.C., Jr. and Shapiro, S. (1944) Arch. Intern. Med. 74:28-35.

12. Jandl, J.H., Simmons, R.L. and Castle, W.B. (1961) Blood 18:133-148.

13. Dintenfass, L. (1964) J. Lab. Clin. Med. 64:594-600.

14. LaCelle, P.L. and Weed, R.I. (1971) Progr. Hemat. 7:1-31.

15. Konotey-Ahulu, F.I. (1965) Lancet 1:1003-1004.

16. Diggs, L.W. and Flowers, E. (1971) Clin. Pediat. 10:697-700.

17. Diggs, L.W. (1965) Am. J. Clin. Path. 44:1-19.

18. Greenberg, M.S. and Kass, E.H. (1958) Arch. Intern. Med. 101:355-363.

19. Ringelhann, B., Konotey-Ahulu, F.I. (1971) Clin. Chim. Acta 34:63-66.

20. Ho Ping Kong, H. and Alleyne, G.A.O. (1969) Brit. Med. J. 3:271-273.

21. Cooperative Urea Trials Group (1974) JAMA 228:1129-1131.

22. Wright, C-S and Gardner, E., Jr. (1960) Ann. Intern. Med. 52:530-537.

23. Konotey-Ahulu, F.I. (1971) Ghana Med. J. 10:241-260.

24. Hendrickse, J.P. de V., Harrison, K.A., Watson-Williams, E.J., Luzzatto, L. and Ajabor, L.N. (1972) J. Obst. Gynec. Brit. Comm. 79:396-409.

25. Smith, E.W. and Conley, C.L. (1954) Bull. Johns Hopkins Hosp. 94:289.

26. Perkins, R.P. (1971) Am. J. Obst. Gynecol. 111:120-159.

27. Freeman, M.G. and Ruth, G.J. (1969) Clin. Obst. Gynecol. 121:134-156.

28. Fahraeus, R. (1929) Physiol. Rev. 9:241-274.

29. Ham, T.H. and Curtis, F. (1938) Medicine 17:447-483.

30. Gilligan, D.R. and Ernstene, A.C. (1934) Am. J. Med. Sci. 187:552-556.

31. Chaplin, H., Jr. Alkjaersig, N., and Fletcher, A.P. (1974) DHEW Pub. No (NIH)74:704.

32. Wells, R.E., Jr., Gawronski, T.H., Cox, P.J. and Perera, R.D. (1964) Am. J. Physiol. 207:1035-1040.

33. Chien, S. (1973) Bibliotheca Anat. 11:244-250.

34. Schmid-Schönbein, H., Gehtgens, P. and Hirsch, H. (1968) J. Clin. Invest. 47:1447-1454.

35. Chien, S. (1969) Adv. Microcirc. 2:89-103.

36. Goldsmith, H.L. (1968) J. Gen. Physiol. 52:5s-28s.

37. Whitmore, R.L. (1967) Nature 215:123-126.

38. Chien, S., Usami, S., Taylor, H.M. Lundber, J.L., and Gregersen, M.I. (1966) J. Appl. Physiol. 21:81-87.

39. Wells, R.E., Jr., Denton, R., and Merrill, E.W. (1961) J. Lab. Clin. Med. 57:646-656.

40. Charache, S., Conley, C.L., Waugh, D.F., Vgoretz, R.J. and Spurrell, J.R. (1967) J. Clin. Invest. 46:1795-1811.

41. Casson, N. (1959) Rheology of Disperse Systems, C.C. Mill, ed., London, Pergamon Press, p. 84-104.

42. Dacie, J.V. and Lewis, S.M. (1968) Practical Hematology, New York, Grune & Stratton.

43. Dintenfass, L. (1962) Angiology 13:333-344.

44. Usami, S., Chien, S., and Gregersen, M.I. (1969) Am. J. Physiol. 217:884-890.

45. Baker, R., Powars, D. and Haywood, L.J. (1974) Biochem. Biophys. Res. Comm. 59:548-556.

46. Glynn, I.M. and Warner, A.E. (1972) Brit. J. Pharmacol. 44:271-278.

47. Braasch, D. (1971) Physiol. Rev. 51:679-701.

48. Basu, A.K. and Woodruff, A.W. (1963) Lancet IV:1088-1090.

49. Bay, J., Nunn, J.F. and Prys-Roberts, C. (1968) Brit. J. Anaesth. 40:398-406.

50. Graettinger, J.S. Parson, R.L. and Campbell, J.A. (1963) Ann. Intern. Med. 58:617-626.

51. Severinghaus, J.W. (1966) J. Appl. Physiol 21:1108-1116.

52. Charache, S. (1974) Arch. Int. Med. 133:698-705.

53. Fulton, G. and Lutz, B.R. (1957) Med. Biol. Illust. 7:26-32.

54. Messer, M.J. and Harris, J.W. (1970) J. Lab. Clin. Med. 76:537-547.

55. Hofrichter, J., Ross, P.D. and Eaton, W.A. (1974) DHEW Pub. No. (NIH) 74:704.

56. Messer, M.J., Woodruff, H.K. and Bradley, T.B. (1974) DHEW Pub. No. (NIH)74:704.

57. Rampling, M.W. and Sirs, J.A. (1973) Clin. Sci. Mol. Med. 45:655-664.

58. Harkness, D., Meta, L., Sheedy, B., Lebos, H., and Tovat, M. (1974) Abstracts, XV Congr. Int. Soc. Hemat., p. 379.

60. Roth, E.F., Jr., Nagel, R.L., Bookchin, R.M. and Grayzel, A.I. (1972) Biochem. Biophys. Res. Comm. 48:612-618.

61. Nagel, R.L. (1974) This conference.

62. Seeman, P. (1966) Chin. Pharm. 15:1753-1766.

63. Braasch, D. (1967) Arch. Ges. Physiol. 300:185-188.

64. Raper, A.B. (1969) Ghana Med. J. 8:29-34.

65. Nevaril, C.G., Lynch, E.C., Alfrey, C.P., Jr.,and Hellums, J.D. (1968) J. Lab. Clin. Med. 71:784-790.

66. Smith, E., Rosenblatt, P., and Bedo, A.V. (1953) J. Pediat. 43:655-660.

DISCUSSION

Dr. Nagel: Eugene Roth, in our laboratory, has studied the survival of nor-nitrogen mustard treated red cells in rabbits and found a normal life span. Do you have any data on red cell survival with these compounds?

Dr. Charache: Survival was decreased at higher doses than the minimum inhibition for sickling; we're still studying cells treated with lower concentrations of both nitrogen mustard and nor nitrogen mustard.

Dr. Henderson: You mentioned the effect of fibrinogen, but I never did quite find out what effect you meant.

Dr. Charache: It's the same kind of thing that causes red cells to form rouleaux. Fibrinogen in blood at rest forms bonds between adjacent red cells, and those bonds must be broken before flow can start. We expected to see exaggerations of normal non-Newtonian viscosity.

Dr. Henderson: Did you utilize globulins for the same studies?

Dr. Charache: No, sir. We did not.

Dr. Henderson: A number of studies made me realize that there was something else that would cause vaso-occlusive phenomena, and one of these was the fact that patients could form, not only rouleaux, but large clumps, and clumping of blood cells going through small vascular radicals could inhibit blood flow and cause vaso-occlusive phenomena.

Dr. Bunn: Sam, one practical aspect of your studies: If we decide that a sickle patient would be benefited by a term of transfusion therapy, for example, to get her through pregnancy or surgery, are we to gather that we are not doing the patient much good unless we transfuse to at least 50% AA red cells?

Dr. Charache: I think so. In a few patients with frequent objectively verifiable crises, it seems that crises occur when the proportion of sickle cells gets above 50%.

Dr. Diederich: Yes, a question along that same line, Sam. Are we not dealing with two things? Deoxygenation itself increases viscosity, so that you have benefit in the anemic individual from the low hematocrit in terms of blood viscosity. You have another disadvantage, at least theoretically, and that would be enhanced oxygen release from the cells when you reach a low level. I'm speaking of a hemoglobin in the six gm % range or thereabouts. There would be increased oxygen extraction which would seemingly largely balance the hematocrit. Now in transfusion, would you not likewise have the opposite side of the coin? You would be increasing circulating red cell mass; you'd have less deoxygenation of your cells, and, I'm troubled a little about the amount of A you'd have to have. It seems to me that if you had a way of looking at the deoxygenation of the circulating S cell in both situations, then one might be able to get a little closer.

Dr. Charache: Yes, I wish there were some way you could make a little window and take a look inside, but I haven't thought of it yet.

Dr. Woodson: I was unable to read some of the shear rates. How low were the shear rates at which you measured viscosity?

Dr. Charache: With the viscometer we used, how low the shear rate·gets depends on how viscous the solution is. With normal blood, we really don't even try to make measurements below a shear rate of about 23 Sec^{-1}. With the very thick viscous materials, you're working 1½ Sec^{-1} sometimes, usually a little bit more than that.

Dr. Woodson: What were the oxygen saturations and fibrinogen concentrations of the bloods with hematocrits in the 50's and 60's in which you detected differences in viscosity as a function of the SS cell fraction?

Dr. Charache: The oxygen saturation was about 30 or 40%. I don't know the fibrinogen concentration. Most patients like this, but not necessarily the one from whom those measurements came, run 300 mg %.

Dr. Orringer: Dr. Charache, is it reasonable to study whole blood viscosity at hematocrit levels of 50-65% when most of the sicklers have hematocrit values which are far lower, even after transfusion?

Dr. Charache: That's higher than what you'll get out of their veins, but the key thing is what's happening in the microvasculature, where the red cells are either going through single file, or maybe going through two at a time. The hematocrit is effectively very high there.

Dr. Orringer: I see. Could I ask one other thing? You mentioned that for calculation of particle number, you used hematocrit. Is there a difference in whole blood viscosity between two blood samples of the same hematocrit in which one sample has twice as many RBC which are hypochromic microcytes?

Dr. Charache: I think that the number of particles as well as the volume of particles makes a difference, but I don't really know.

Dr. Orringer: Another possible example would be a patient with polycythemia who has been phlebotomized and made iron deficient.

Dr. Charache: That's actually where we've made such measurements, because they are very hypochromic microcytic.

Dr. Orringer: Yes, occasionally, ten million red cells or more.

Unidentified Speaker: In animal blood with red cells of very differing sizes, my recollection is that the particle's size is much less important than the particle fraction.

Dr. Charache: I remember the paper; I don't remember the answer.

Dr. Fuller: Could we imply from what you said that if you infuse the sickle cell anemia patient with a large amount of fibrinogen you might induce a crisis?

Dr. Charache: We, that's what I would have guessed. Our data don't suggest that that happens.

Dr. Woodson: It seems to me that we need to keep clear in our minds the distinction between vessels where viscometry data might apply to some degree and vessels where it certainly does not apply at all. Those vessels in which shear rate is probably the lowest are post-capillary venules and small veins. Since shear rates are quite high throughout the rest of the circulation, and since blood is non-Newtonian, one would expect that if there is a propensity toward sickling detectable by viscometric measurements, it would be in vessels where the shear rate is lowest. When you speak of two sickle cells jamming in a capillary, I don't think viscometry measurements apply at all. If any physical measurement would correlate at the capillary level it would probably be deformability of the red cell.

Dr. Charache: That was one of my points, that whatever we're measuring may not be the right thing to measure. Regarding shear rates in capillaries, they're anything you'd like them to be depending on your model. If flow is continuing through a narrow tube, then shear rates are probably high--300 Sec^{-1}. But, is this appropriate? Supposedly about a fifth of the capillary bed is either perfused or nonperfused at any given point in time. They open and close so that shear rates can go from zero to high in capillaries.

IN VITRO CARBAMYLATION IN SICKLE CELL ANEMIA

Dennis Diederich, Paul Gill, Robert Trueworthy, and William Larsen
Department of Medicine
University of Kansas Medical Center
Kansas City, Kansas 66103

INTRODUCTION

The intracellular aggregation of S Hb which occurs coincident with deoxygenation of the sickle erythrocyte is the basic pathophysiological defect in sickle cell anemia. The sickling phenomenon occurs only with S Hb in the deoxygenated form. The in vivo sickling of erythrocytes produces diverse manifestations. Two of the major clinical sequellae of the in vivo sickling phenomenon are red cell destruction and microcirculatory vaso-occlusive phenomena. The inability of either reversibly (RSC) or irreversibly sickled cells (ISC) to transgress the capillary circulation gives rise to ischemia and or infarction of tissue as well as to the vaso-occlusive painful crises.

The observations that hemoglobin carbamylation inhibits in vitro (Cerami and Manning, 1971; Kraus and Kraus, 1971) as well as in vivo sickling (Gillette et al. 1971) led to the initiation of a number of studies designed to explore the use of carbamylation as a therapeutic measure in sickle cell anemia. Pilot studies employing in vitro red cell carbamylation with NaCNO were undertaken in a select group of symptomatic sicklemic patients at our institution in early 1973.

Two objectives of these studies to be discussed in this presentation were: (1) to determine the effects of repeated in vitro red cell carbamylation upon in vivo sickling, and (2) to determine if repeated in vitro carbamylation altered the in vivo sickling propensity of cells.

METHODS

Patient Selection: Fifteen patients homozygous for S Hb, ranging in age from 17 to 40 years were entered in the study for one of the following indications: a) two or more painful crises requiring hospitalization in the previous six month period (12 patients,) b) severe anemia with high output cardiac failure (1 patient,) c) chronic refractory malleolar ulcers (2 patients.)

Protocol: At weekly intervals, ∿20% of the circulating red cell mass was incubated with sufficient NaCNO to achieve 1.5 ± 0.4 moles of CNO incorporation/tetrameric mole of Hb. Plasma was reinfused without carbamylation; carbamylated red cells were washed once prior to reinfusion.

At each visit the Hb, hematocrit, reticulocyte count, ISC count, P_{50} with sickle curve, red cell pH, 2,3-DPG and ATP were determined. Mean red cell lifespan of carbamylated and untreated cells were determined simultaneously utilizing two isotopes of diisopropylfluorophosphate (^{3}H-DFP, ^{32}P-DFP or ^{14}C-DFP) to label the different cell populations.

Assays: Whole blood P_{50} (oxygen tension at which $\frac{HbO_2}{Hb}$ = 1 at 37°, pH 7.40) was measured using the 1L 217 Blood Gas Laboratory. Oxygen tensions were selected to achieve 80, 60, 40 and 20% HbO_2 saturations. At each equilibration during the curve, red cells were placed in buffered formalin saline and subsequently analyzed for % sickling (Figure 1). The total sickled cells present at each point were then corrected for the % ISC present in the patient sample (% RSC). The in vitro sickling propensity was characterized by plotting the % reversibly sickled cells against % HbO_2 as shown in Figure 2. For convenience, the

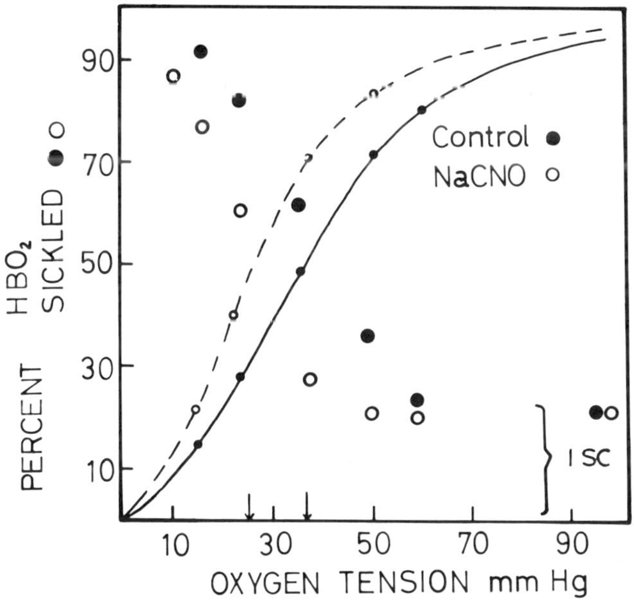

Figure 1. Effects of NaCNO preincubation on the oxygen dissociation and sickling curve of a sample of SS blood. ● Control SS blood; O SS blood with 1.3 moles ^{14}CNO/mole Hb.

position of the curve so obtained was characterized by the term S_{50}, which represents the % HbO_2 at which 50% reversible sickling occurs at 37°, pH 7.40 ± .04. ISC counts were determined on blood equilibrated with 95% O_2 - 5% CO_2 using criteria previously described (Bertles and Milner, 1969.) To measure red cell pH, blood at pH 7.40 ± .04, equilibrated with 20% O_2 - 5.3% CO_2, was drawn into a 1 ml gas-equilibrated syringe and centrifuged plunger-down;

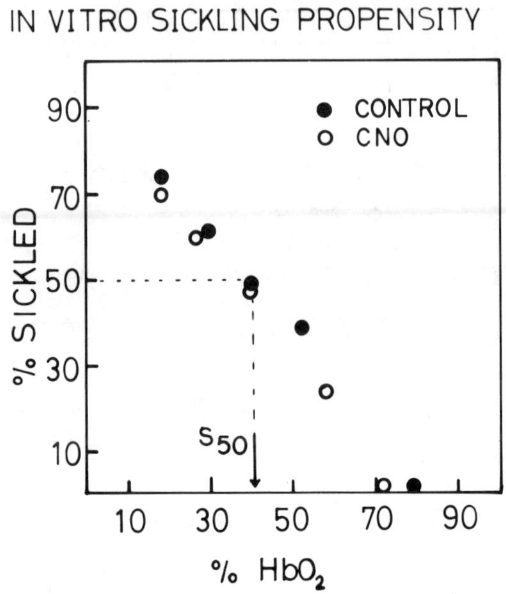

Figure 2. The data for % Hb O_2 and % reversibly sickled cells (%RSC) from Figure 1 are plotted in this figure. S_{50} reversible sickling occurs at pH 7.4, 37°.

plasma was expressed and red cell pH was measured after freeze-thaw lysis. 2,3-DPG was measured enzymatically and ATP by the luciferase method. Red cell Ca, Mg, K, and Zn were measured by atomic absorption.

Selection of degree and frequency of carbamylation: The decision to aim for 1.5 ± 0.4 moles of CNO/mole of Hb at each carbamylation visit was based upon both the anti-sickling properties of CNO and triple labelled red cell survival studies of untreated cells and of cells carbamylated at two levels, 0.8 - 1.0 and 1.5 - 2.0 moles of CNO/mole Hb. The pertinent antisickling properties of CNO are depicted in Figures 1 and 2. Incorporation of 1.3 moles of CNO/mole Hb reduced blood P_{50} in this sample of SS blood from 36 to 26 mm Hg. Figure 2 demonstrates that the major antisickling effect of CNO is due to the increased oxygen affinity of the carbamylated Hb; the oxygenation-independent sickling propensity of treated and untreated cells was not appreciably altered. Cell survival curves demonstrated greater prolongation of the survival of cells with high level Hb carbamylation than with low level. Thus the major factor determining the degree of Hb carbamylation desirable was the resultant blood P_{50}. We elected not to decrease the patient P_{50} below 24 mm Hg.

The second objective was to achieve a stable state wherein 30-40% of the circulating red cell mass had previously been carbamylated. This objective was realized by carbamylating ca 20% of the red cell mass at weekly intervals.

RESULTS

Effects of carbamylation upon in vivo sickling:
Ten patients underwent repeated carbamylation for 4 to 18 months, 7 patients for over 12 months. The total duration of carbamylation for the group was 120 months.

The hematologic responses observed for these ten patients is summarized in Figure 3. During the 2 month pretreatment period, the mean P_{50}, reticulocyte, ISC and Hb values remained stable. With initiation of carbamylation there was a progressive decrease in blood P_{50}, in reticulocytosis, and in the circulating ISC levels, and a gradual rise in circulating Hb levels. All values tend to stabilize at new levels after the third month. The mean P_{50} decreased from 34 to 26.8 mm Hg, the Hb rose from a mean of 6.1 to 8.6 g%. Pretreatment, a mean of 20% of the circulating erythrocytes were irreversibly sickled. After 3 months of carbamylation this value was less than 5%, an

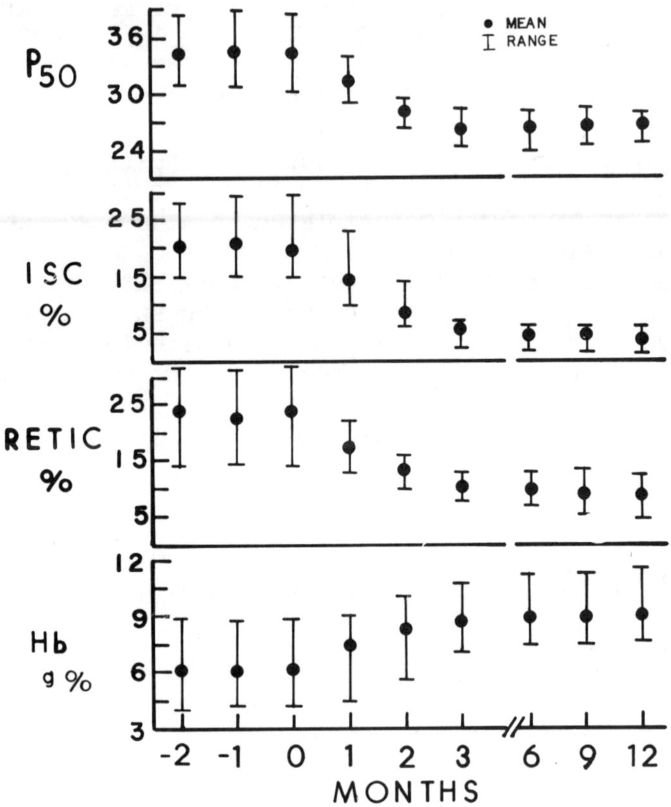

Figure 3. Hematological responses of 10 patients undergoing weekly in vitro red cell carbamylation; carbamylation began at time 0.

impressive drop. The absolute number of circulating ISC and reticulocytes decreased by 65% and 40% respectively. Untreated red cell lifespan increased from a mean of 13 days pretreatment to 21.6 days after 3 months of carbamylation.

The frequency of severe painful crises is decreased thus far during the treatment period. Crises were defined as severe painful episodes of greater than 12 hours duration requiring hospitalization. Crises were classified as idiopathic when no underlying precipitating event was detectable or as induced when such events were present. An average of 0.25 crises/month occurred during the 12 month period prior to treatment. Sixty % of these crises were precipitated by concurrent illness, a febrile respiratory illness in the vast majority. During the

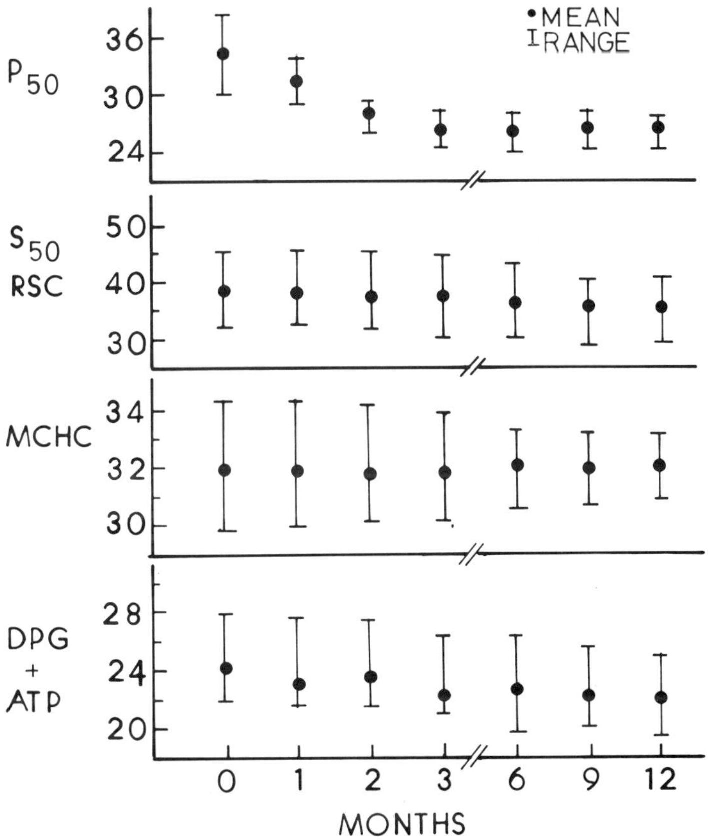

Figure 4. Factors influencing in vitro sickling propensity. See text for details.

first 120 cumulative months of carbamylation in the 10 patients, the average frequency was 0.08 crises/month. The proportion of idiopathic crises was unchanged.

Effects of In Vitro Carbamylation upon Sickling Propensity. The mean sickling propensity, S_{50}, for reversible sickling for the 10 patients is shown in Figure 4 along with mean corpuscular Hb concentration (MCHC), red cell 2,3-DPG + ATP and P_{50}. The mean S_{50} value decreased from 38% to 36%. The mean MCHC remained unchanged during carbamylation; there was less variability for the group after several months of carbamylation. The mean DPG + ATP decreased only minimally from 24.2 to 22 μ moles/g Hb during carbamylation.

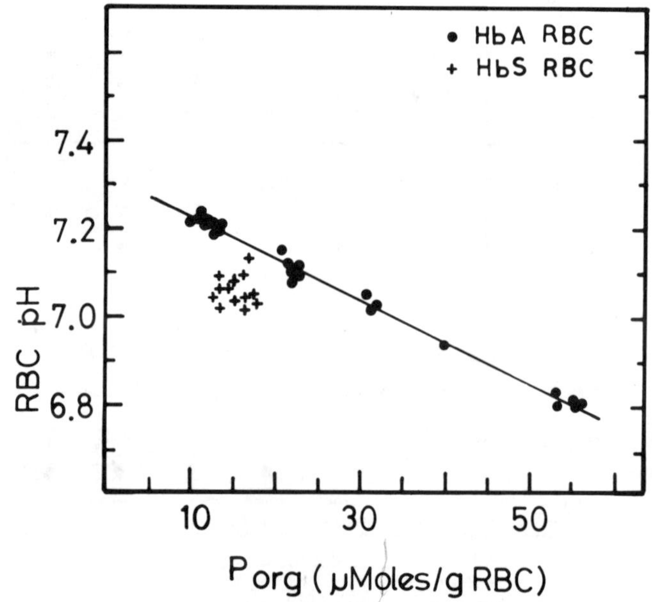

Figure 5. Relationship between intracellular pH and intracellular organic phosphate concentrations of Hb AA and SS erythrocytes at whole blood pH 7.4, 37°.

A finding of paramount importance noted in analyzing in vivo factors which influence sickling propensity was the abnormally low pH of SS red cells. The erythrolysate pH in patients undergoing carbamylation remained abnormally low. Representative values for red cell pH for these patients and for AA red cells are shown in Figure 5 as a function of red cell organic phosphate content as described by Duhm and Gerlach (1973). Elevations of Hb A red cell organic phosphates were achieved by preincubation with phosphate, pyruvate and inosine as described by Duhm (1971).

Red cell Ca concentrations in normal subjects and in the patients being maintained on carbamylation are presented in the following table.

Table 1. ERYTHROCYTE CALCIUM CONCENTRATIONS IN NORMAL SUBJECTS AND PATIENTS WITH HEMOGLOBIN SS UNDERGOING CARBAMYLATION

SUBJECTS	N	MEAN	RANGE
NORMAL	10	28.	13.-48.
Hb SS DISEASE	10	55.	32.-91.

VALUES EXPRESSED IN μMOLE Ca/LITER PACKED RED CELLS

For comparison, Eaton et al. (1973) reported mean calcium concentrations of 24.9 ± 8.2 and 188.8 ± 68.8 μ moles of Ca^{++}/liter packed red cells for normal and SS erythrocytes respectively.

DISCUSSION

Effect of Carbamylation on In Vivo Sickling:

Repeated in vitro carbamylation decreased the in vivo sickling of erythrocytes, lessening the severity of the hemolytic process. This statement is based upon the observations that an increase in hemoglobin occurred coincident with a decrease in reticulocytosis, a decrease in ISC levels, and a prolongation of erythrocyte lifespan. Thus, decreased destruction rather than increased production of erythrocytes is responsible for the observed hematologic improvements.

The number of painful crises during carbamylation was less than during the pretreatment year for the group of patients. The patients by necessity were followed at frequent intervals during carbamylation and received immediate attention for superimposed illnesses by an identifiable group of physicians. The decrease in induced crises during carbamylation attests to this fact. Prompt recognition and treatment of febrile superimposed illnesses, in particular respiratory infections, is more important than carbamylation in averting induced painful crises. These studies were not controlled studies designed to test the effect of in vitro carbamylation on painful crises; thus the decreased crises observed must be taken merely as an observation.

Effects of Carbamylation on Sickling Propensity:
No overall change in the sickling propensity was observed in the data presented. In analyzing data such as MCHC, the organic phosphate content, or red cell pH, it is important to keep in mind we are dealing with a heterogenous population of cells from two standpoints. First we have a spectrum of S erythrocytes which extends from the immature new cells, reflected in the reticulocytosis, to the markedly abnormal ISC, the culmination of sickle-induced red cell injury stemming from repeated sickle events (Bertles and Milner, 1968). Between these two extremes are the remaining circulating S erythrocytes. Second, in these studies we have additional heterogeneity by virtue of the fact there are carbamylated and non-carbamylated cells circulating.

In the pretreatment period, the compositional alterations of the ISC fraction (decreased red cell organic phosphates and red cell pH, elevated MCHC) are somewhat balanced by alterations of the reticulocyte population in the opposite direction. The percent ISC and of reticulocytes were quite similar. As the ISC levels decreased during carbamylation, there was also a decrease in magnitude of reticulocytosis. Thus when analyzing whole blood, abnormalities due to the presence of ISC (i.e. elevated MCHC) were obscured by the presence of reticulocytosis.

The existence of heterogenous red cell populations thus makes interpretation of changes in S_{50} tenuous at best. The only salient factor capable of diminishing in vivo sickling demonstrable during these studies was the decrease in P_{50}. This decrease in P_{50} appears due in large part to the carbamylation of Hb. The alterations noted in MCHC, 2,3-DPG + ATP and in the red cell pH during carbamylation were inadequate to explain the observed decrease in P_{50}. The circulating P_{50} was kept above 24 mm Hg by decreasing the degree or frequency of red cell carbamylation. Inordinate Hb carbamylation would provide a population of cells incapable of releasing oxygen at physiological oxygen tensions. Increased oxygen release from non-carbamylated would be necessitated, thus subjecting these cells to exaggerated deoxygenation, sickling, and ultimate destruction. The increased lifespan of circulating erythrocytes, the decrease in reticulocytes and increase in Hb during carbamylation all suggest that such premature destruction of untreated cells is not occurring in these patients.

The relative intracellular acidosis of the sickle erythrocyte has important implications. Acidosis enhances the sickling of S erythrocytes both by oxygenation-dependent (P_{50}) and oxygenation-independent (S_{50}) mechanisms. In analyzing data from individual patients there appears to be a relationship between red cell pH and MCHC as recently suggested by Murphy et al (1974). In recent studies in our laboratory most clear relationship between red cell pH and MCHC was noted in the ISC rich fraction of red cells separated by centrifugation. A marked intracellular acidosis (pH 6.9-7.0), an elevated MCHC and low organic phosphate content was noted in this fraction. Since the ISC is commonly viewed as the end result of sickle-induced membrane alterations, it seems reasonable to suggest that the abnormally low red cell pH we have observed in these studies is a reflection of less advanced alterations in membrane integrity.

The increased permeability of the S red cell to Ca during sickling described by Eaton et al (1973) may well be an additional important in vivo factor influencing the sickling propensity. It is tempting to speculate that the decreased red cell Ca concentrations observed in the patients reported herein when compared to those reported by Eaton et al (1974) is a reflection of decreased in vivo sickling and hence decreased membrane alterations. The striking decrease in ISC levels during carbamylation supports this notion.

CONCLUSION

Repeated in vitro carbamylation of erythrocytes of sicklemic patients diminished in vivo sickling and destruction of erythrocytes. We were unable to demonstrate a significant decrease in in vivo sickling propensity (oxygenation-independent) during in vitro carbamylation. Relative intracellular acidosis noted in all patients was not totally corrected during carbamylation.

In view of the potential and reported toxicity of oral cyanate at doses sufficient to obtain significant Hb carbamylation (Peterson et al, 1974), alternate methods of Hb carbamylation will be necessary. We do not envision weekly carbamylation as done in this study to be such a method. Information obtained from this study however, can be applied to a technique wherein the entire circulating red cell mass is carbamylated in a short period of time without exposing the patient to free cyanate or carbamyl phosphate systemically. This procedure could be repeated at less frequent intervals. It is apparent such an approach would be practical only for patients with severe, symptomatic sicklemia. The goal of such an approach would be to ameliorate the severity of the symptoms and organ destruction.

ACKNOWLEDGEMENTS

The work reported in this paper was supported by USPHS, contract N01-HL-2-2919-B and grants 1R01 HL15228-01 and HL13701. We wish to acknowledge the contributions of B. Lawson, A. Odenbaugh, M. Curran and A. Diederich who carried out the studies reported herein, and to thank L. Carrigan for assistance in preparation of this manuscript.

REFERENCES

Bertles, J. F., and Milner, P. F. A. (1968). Irreversibly sickled erythrocytes: A consequence of the heterogenous distribution of hemoglobin types in sickle-cell anemia. J. Clin. Invet. 47: 1731.

Cerami, A., and Manning, J. M. (1971). Potassium cyanate as an inhibitor of the sickling of red blood cells in vitro. Proc.Nat. Acad. Sci. (U.S.) 68:1180.

Duhm, J. (1971). Effects of 2,3-phosphoglycerate and other organic phosphate on oxygen affinity and intracellular pH of human erythrocytes. Pflugers Arch. 336: 341.

Duhm, J.,and Gerlach, E. (1973). Metabolism and function of 2,3-diphosphoglycerate in red blood cells. The Human Red Cell In Vitro ed. T. J. Greenwalt and G. A. Jamieson, Grune & Stratton, New York pp. 111-152.

Eaton, J. W. et. al (1973). Elevated erythrocyte calcium in sickle cell disease. Nature 246:105.

Gillette, P. N., Manning, J. M. and Cerami, A. (1971). Increased survival of sickle-cell erythrocytes after treatment in vitro with sodium cyanate. Proc. Nat. Acad. Sci. (U.S.) 68:2791.

Kraus, L. M., and Kraus, A. P. (1971). Carbamyl phosphate mediated inhibition of the sickling of erythrocytes in vitro. Biochem. Biophys. Res. Comm. 44:1381.

Murphy, J. R., Wengerd, M., and Kellermeyer, R. W. (1974). Erythrocyte O_2 affinity: Influence of cell density and in vitro changes in hemoglobin concentration. J. Lab. and Clin. Med. 84:218.

Peterson, C. M., et. al. (1974). Sodium cyanate induced polyneuropathy in patients with sickle-cell disease. Ann. Int. Med. 81:152.

DISCUSSION

Dr. Meyers: Could you tell me by what method you measured irreversibly sickle cells? Also, at what temperatures some of these pH measurements were taken?

Dr. Diederich: The last question first. All of our blood studies are done in heparinized blood at 37° just as soon after collecting as possible. It's tonometered blood in an IL system, and the red cell pH measurements were taken at 37°. They are spun at 37°, frozen, thawed, and then measured at 37°. Regarding the first question--what is an irreversibly sickled cell, we can consider two criteria--the overall morphology, i.e., elongation of the cell (we usually like to see a threefold ratio between long dimension and diameter) and the appearance of the membrane under phase. The definition of an irreversibly sickled cell is somewhat arbitrary, but I think it is one that's very easy to appreciate when you're looking at the cells before and after on a patient.

Dr. Brewer: Did you say that with treatment you were able to lower the red cell calcium, or not?

Dr. Diederich: We have not yet measured calcium with the same technique before and after treatment in the same patients. We have measured calcium, but we have made many changes in the assay along the way. We have more elevated calcium values in untreated patients than treated patients but we do not have good data for carbamylated patients before and after treatment.

Dr. Brewer: You seemed very hesitant to suggest that you might be preventing crisis.

Dr. Diederich: I don't have any question that the patients have many less crises during this period of time than they had before. I think that's indisputable by anyone who has been near the patients. The point is, what caused that decrease in crises? I'm sure they have gotten more antibiotics and physician time than before.

Dr. Salhany: I was wondering, Dr. Diederich, if you or if anyone else has tried raising the pH *in vitro* to see if the number of irreversibly sickled cells goes down?

Dr. Diederich: I haven't found anything that will change the morphology of the banana, or whatever you want to call it. You can lyse it, but I haven't been able to really change it.

Dr. Salhany: I'd like to share an experience that I had quite a while ago which was never published, but which was reproducible. When I added isomolar Tris buffer to sickle blood and deoxygenated it, I didn't see any morphological evidence of sickling. Now, it's well known that Tris buffer raises the intracellular pH. It changes the gradient. And when I saw that your sickle cells had a decreased intracellular pH, I wondered whether there might be a connection, and whether it might be worth looking at?

Dr. Diederich: I appreciate your comments. There are a couple of agents that will elevate red cell pH. Tris is one, but we get a lot of pseudopods from the cell. It looks like echinocyte transformation, which makes it awfully difficult to evaluate an antisickling agent. Specifically, however, we have not tried to unsickle the ISC with Tris.

Dr. Woodson: I am interested that you observed a larger ΔpH in sickle cells and I believe you also noted an increased ΔpH in the irreversibly sickled cell fraction, where the p50 is higher. Does the relatively lower intracellular pH, at a given DPG level, largely account for the higher p50 of the sickle cell?

Dr. Diederich: No, unfortunately, it doesn't work quite as you would like it to. I might mention a recent paper in the Jour. of Lab. and Clin. Med., "The Function of Mean Corpuscular Hb Concentration and pH inside the Cell," by Murphy. There is a very nice relationship in a patient between the hemoglobin concentration and red cell pH. It breaks down in other areas, but in the sickle erythrocytes that we've looked at, one could predict the red cell pH by looking at the hemoglobin concentration in the cell. This is an area of which we were not aware prior to reading his paper, and I think it's pertinent.

Dr. Orringer: One possible explanation for the lower than predicted intracellular pH is related to cell water content, perhaps as you have just alluded to. Gary-Bobo and Solomon have shown that the net negative charge on the hemoglobin molecule is greatly influenced by the status of hydration within the cell. As the cells shrink, the hemoglobin molecule becomes less negatively charged and vice versa. Do you have any cell water measurements?

Dr. Diederich: I can't answer the question definitively. The sickle erythrocytes that we're talking about have a large range in cell potassium, although generally low. The cells with the markedly low pH have a very low potassium content, and an elevated mean corpuscular hemoglobin, so there are trends. I'm not prepared to say what the explanation for this is.

Dr. Duhm: Another factor is that the hemoglobin concentration is very high in some of the sickle cells. This should lead to a considerable increase of the osmotic coefficient of hemoglobin and, consequently, to a corresponding increase in the osmotic pressure of hemoglobin which is involved in establishing the Donnan equilibrium. The second point I would like to raise is that in your shrunken cells you have a higher DPG concentration on a water basis although the ratio of DPG to hemoglobin might be normal. Since the concentration of free DPG in the cell water is the parameter which affects the oxygen affinity of hemoglobin, this factor should be considered in explaining the unexpected high p50 in the sickle cells.

Dr. Diederich: If you will notice the in vitro experiments where we separate the cell, the cells that had the delta pH of 0.4 had distinctly low organic phosphates. They are depleted.

Dr. Glader: We have performed similar studies in separated

ISC's that have been formed in vivo. Indeed these ISCs have the cation composition you describe, a marked decrease in potassium which is quantitatively much more than sodium gain. They are dehydrated cells; the cell water is significantly decreased. The chloride distribution ratio in those cells is markedly reduced, and the calculated intracellular pH is similar to what you are seeing. I believe this pH change is due to K and water loss, resulting in an increase in the impermeable anion concentration (total organic phosphates, plus hemoglobin concentration).

Dr. Diederich: I'm troubled on that last point, Bert. I didn't show it on the slide, but we did the total organic phosphate.

Dr. Glader: What about the concentration of hemoglobin added to that of the organic phosphates?

Dr. Diederich: Yes, I'd have to do that, but DPG, ATP and total organic phosphate are down. I believe we're dealing with a leaky membrane, more so than a membrane that's holding impermeant anions. The organic phosphate of the ISC is so diminished that I fail to see how that could still be a mechanism of...

Unidentified Speaker: But is it diminished when you calculate their concentration on the basis of cell water?

Dr. Diederich: Well, I don't have good enough data to say.

Unidentified speaker: I'd be surprised if it were.

Dr. Brewer: I'd like to comment on Dr. Orringer's comment about the Gary-Bobo studies. We reported at the last conference on similar studies--i.e., an increase in hemoglobin concentration causing the release of protons and a fall in pH. However, we found that the effect disappeared at physiological salt concentrations with hemoglobin A. However, with sickle hemoglobin we do detect such an effect, we think, in the following manner. During deoxygenation, we find less Bohr effect with hemoglobin S than with hemoglobin A. We believe that this is because during deoxygenation the hemoglobin S molecules polymerize, decreasing their intermolecular spacing so much that this intermolecular release of protons occurs in spite of the screening out effect of salt.

Dr. Perutz: What would you say would be the minimum interval between transfusions needed on a long-term basis to keep sickle cell patients well?

Dr. Diederich: That's a very difficult question to answer. If we're dealing with cyanate, the cyanate treated cell will sickle. We came up with our schedule on the measured red cell survival, and aiming for 30-35% circulating treated cells, which was our initial goal. I would have a bias that if one could carbamylate the entire red cell mass in a less extensive fashion than we're doing now, that it would be theoretically possible to use two to three week intervals.

Dr. Perutz: For how long is it practical to do this to the patient?

Dr. Diederich: It's hard to say. I appreciate your point, because I think to ask a patient to come into the center for four to five hours each week, he has to have a fair amount of disability, and you have to be competing with pretty severe disease before you have something to offer the patient.

Dr. Perutz: And there are no complications setting in because you puncture these veins once a month?

Dr. Diederich: The venipuncture vein is an emotional vein that no one violates except the person doing the venipuncture. I think the potential complications are those of taking blood out of the body and either contaminating it or in some way damaging the cells.

Dr. Conley: Doctor Diederich has performed a complex biologic experiment with therapeutic implications. He has been appropriately and admirably cautious in his interpretations. The intermittent extracorporeal carbamylation of blood of patients with sickle cell anemia leaves the patient with three populations of red cells. Those erythrocytes produced after the last treatment are uncarbamylated and are susceptible to sickling in the usual fashion. Another population of cells has been carbamylated after sickling-unsickling cycles have already occurred, presumably producing variable but irreversible damage to the cells. Still another group of red cells is carbamylated before sickling has occurred and these cells are maximally protected. In answer to Doctor Perutz' question on the minimum frequency of treatment, it is clearly impossible to predict, as Doctor Diederich has indicated. The experiment is meritorious, but careful clinical observations will be required to evaluate therapeutic effects at various frequencies and degrees of carbamylation.

IN VIVO EFFECTS OF CARBAMYL PHOSPHATE IN DOGS

L. M. Kraus, H. M. Jernigan, C. M. Blatteis
and A. P. Kraus
The University of Tennessee Center for Health Sciences and the Comprehensive Center for Research and Service in Sickle Cell Disease, Memphis, Tennessee

It is now 25 years since Pauling and coworkers first discovered that the erythrocytes from patients whose red cells changed from the pliable biconcave disc to a rigid sickled cell in the presence of decreased oxygen contained a different hemoglobin (Pauling, et al., 1949). However the challenge that faced us then still remains, that is, how to alleviate a molecular disease by chemically altering this abnormal molecule. In hemoglobin S, the sixth amino acid from the amino-terminal end of the β chain is valine (Ingram, 1957) instead of glutamic acid found in hemoglobin A. This single difference changes the molecular interaction of deoxyhemoglobin S so that it assembles into a fibrous tubule made up of six filaments. Each filament is a linear formation of single hemoglobin molecules. A planar transection through the tubule show six hemoglobin molecules forming a hexagon. These molecules make contact with four neighboring molecules at any one level in the fibrous tubule due to the longitudinal register of the six hemoglobin filaments. This helical tubule repeats itself about every eight rings (Finch, et al., 1973). This arrangement of deoxyhemoglobin S molecules therefore allows multiple points for intermolecular interaction while its rigid nature causes the distortion of the erythrocyte into its sickled cell appearance. This sickling phenomenon can be changed by chemically tailoring hemoglobin S so as to cause a conformational change that would prevent the aggregation of deoxyhemoglobin S molecules into microtubules. A chemical modification of hemoglobin S can also change the oxygen affinity so that it may be increased or it can result in a combination of both structural and functional changes. Ideally the chemical chosen to modify hemoglobin S should be specific for the target molecule, or if not, a mechanism should exist in the body to prevent the reagent from reacting with and altering the functions of proteins other than hemoglobin. There should also be a method for specific quantitation of the reagent in vivo in order to be able to evaluate the bioavailability of the reagent as it is being utilized.

One such agent is carbamyl phosphate (carbamyl P). Carbamyl P has advantages over other antisickling agents because it is a normally occurring molecule in man with mechanisms available for both its synthesis and destruction. It is used in the biosynthesis of urea, arginine and the pyrimidines. Its enzymatic destruction results in production of NH_4, CO_2, and PO_4. When degradating enzymes are present in tissue, the effectiveness of carbamyl P as a carbamylating agent should be altered and different from that of cyanate. To become a carbamylating agent, carbamyl P undergoes a monomolecular elimination to form cyanate and phosphate at physiological pH, 37°, in aqueous solutions with a half life of 40 minutes (Eq 1).

Eq 1
Spontaneous

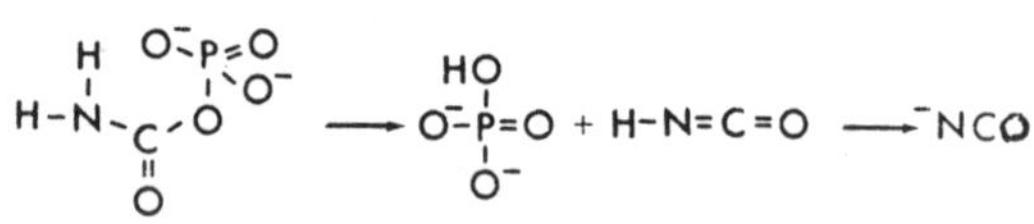

Eq 2
Enzymatic

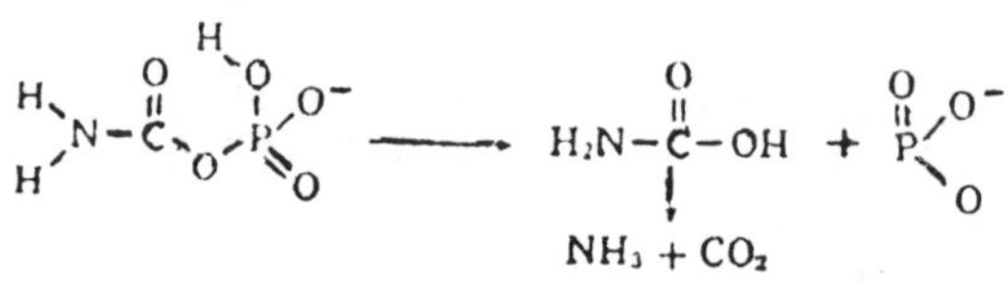

The antisickling activity of carbamyl P was established by Kraus and Kraus in 1971. This laboratory subsequently showed that extracorporeal treatment of blood with carbamyl P results in an extended survival time of erythrocytes that are returned into the patient with sickle cell anemia. Enzyme activity in the treated erythrocyte is within the normal range and red blood cell antigens are unchanged. Carbamyl P-induced carbamylation occurs preferentially on the α chain while cyanate under the same conditions preferentially carbamylates the β chain. Competitive studies using labeled either carbamyl P or cyanate in combination with nonlabeled cyanate or carbamyl P, respectively, indicate that the activity of carbamyl P additionally may involve a change in the conformation of the hemoglobin molecule. Instead of the expected dilution of ^{14}C cyanate labeling of hemoglobin, it enhances the amount of label and changes the labeling pattern of the hemoglobin peptides from that seen when ^{14}C cyanate alone is reacted with blood from patients with sickle cell anemia (Kraus, et al., 1972).

The present report deals with the results of in-progress long term studies to determine the physiological, pharmacological, hematologic and biochemical effects of the regimen of administration of carbamyl P to experimental dogs. Intravenous, rectal and oral routes of administration are being compared.

METHODS

Chronic Administration of Carbamyl P

Intravenous route. One adult male conditioned mongrel dog weighing 9.5 kg at the initiation of the study is receiving a single injection of carbamyl P in sterile physiological saline each day for 4 days, followed by 3 days without injections. This cycle has continued for a year. The amount of carbamyl P has remained fixed at 1.276 g in 34 ml of saline, a dose of 7.46 millimoles per day. Because the dog has gained weight, the dose has ranged from 150 to 125 mg/kg of body weight per injection. Food and water are presented ad lib.

Rectal route. One adult male beagle dog is being given a single suppository daily for 5 days followed by a 2 day rest, in a cycle that has continued for 11 months. This dog is receiving 3.5 millimoles of carbamyl P per day, equal to 50 mg/k body weight in a cocoa butter suppository containing 600 mg carbamyl P. The dog has access to food and water ad lib.

Oral route. Beginning at age 6-months, 4 male beagle pups are fed enteric-coated capsules in a divided dose approximately 8 hours apart. The first aliquot is given 1 hour preprandially, then food is made available for 1 hour, and thereafter only water remains available ad lib. The dogs have received 100 mg of carbamyl P per kg of body weight daily for 6 months. The dose of carbamyl P has ranged from 3.8 to 6.9 milli moles per day due to dose adjustment for weight gain with growth

Biochemical Studies

The dogs are bled weekly and the following serum parameters are measured: Cl^-, HCO_3^-, K^+, Na^+, B.U.N., glucose, total protein, albumin, Ca^{++}, Pi, cholesterol, uric acid, creatinine, total bilirubin, alkaline phosphatase, CPK, LDH, and SGOT. Valine hydantoin, as moles per mole of hemoglobin is being measured by the method of Manning, et al., 1973, in order to determine the progressive degree of carbamylation of the amino-terminal valines of hemoglobin. Any carbamylation of the ε amino group of lysine was determined by amino acid analysis with examination for homocritrulline using a Technicon TSM Amino Acid Autoanalyzer. The levels of carbamyl P recovered in blood in vivo are being measured by a specific enzymatic method using the conversion of carbamyl P to citrulline by ornithine carbamyl transferase (OCT) (Jernigan and Kraus, 1974).

Hematologic Studies

Hemoglobin, hematocrit, red cell morphology and reticulocytes are being determined weekly.

Physiological Studies

Hemoglobin affinity for oxygen is measured weekly using an IL 217 Blood Gas Laboratory. The blood is equilibrated for 30 minutes at 37° with gas mixtures containing 7 per cent, 4 per cent, or 2 per cent oxygen in 5.6 per cent CO_2, balance N_2 and the oxyhemoglobin dissociation curve constructed.

The dogs are examined daily for any changes in appearance, activity, body temperature, heart and respiration rates, food and water intake, and weight.

RESULTS

The regimen of daily, single intravenous injections of carbamyl P successively for 4 days followed by a 3 day rest has been well tolerated by the recipient dog. As the dog gained weight, and the dose of carbamyl P remained constant at 7.46 millimoles per day, the ratio of carbamyl P to hemoglobin decreased from 4.9 to 3.9 millimoles of carbamyl P per millimole of hemoglobin tetramer. Relating this to the available number of amino-terminal reaction sites on hemoglobin chains, the ratio of carbamyl P per chain was 1.25:1 during the first month of treatment and gradually changed to a 1:1 ratio at the end of a year. The degree of hemoglobin carbamylation, measured as moles of valine hydantoin per mole of hemoglobin tetramer, increased in 1 month of injections so that one chain was carbamylated in every 10 molecules of hemoglobin. After 5 months of this regimen, approximately 2

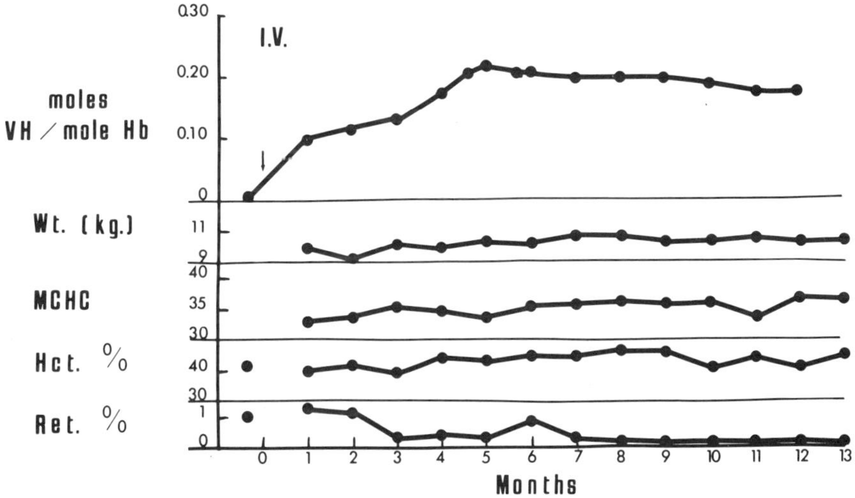

Figure 1. The effect of intravenous injections of carbamyl P for 1 year upon hemoglobin carbamylation, body weight, mean cell hemoglobin concentration (MCHC), hematocrit and reticulocyte production in an adult male mongrel dog.

chains in 10 molecules of hemoglobin were carbamylated (i.e., measured as 0.2 moles valine hydantoin per mole hemoglobin tetramer). From 5 months on, the carbamylation of hemoglobin has plateaued at this level (Figure 1). There has been no evidence of carbamylation of the ε amino group of lysine as determined by amino acid analysis for homocitrulline.

The increase in carbamylation has been accompanied by an increase in oxygen affinity, reflected by a shift to the left of the P_{50} from 32 to 24 mm Hg (Figure 2). No anorexia, nausea or vomiting have occurred during the injections (administered in less than 2 minutes) or thereafter. There have been no demonstrable signs of stress and the dog has gained approximately 1 kg over the year of treatment. All the hematologic parameters have stayed within the normal range with

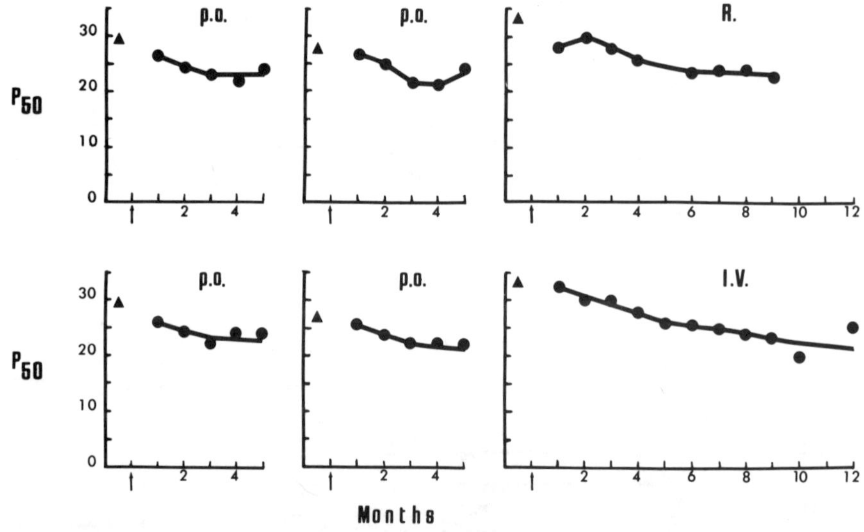

Figure 2. Effect of the administration of carbamyl P upon the oxygen affinity of hemoglobin measured as changes in P_{50} during the course of treatment. The carbamyl P was given orally (p.o.) in enteric coated capsules; rectally (R.) in cocoa butter suppositories; or by intravenous injection (I.V.). The doses and regimen of treatment are reported in METHODS. The control value is designated by ▲.

Table 1. Blood chemistry of a dog receiving intravenous injections of carbamyl P for 1 year reported as mean and standard error of weekly values. The control values were measured before treatment was started.

	Control	Treated Mean	Treated SE		Control	Treated Mean	Treated SE
Cl^- (mEq/L)	110	109.7	± 0.5	Inorg. Phos. (mg%P)	4.90	3.81	± 0.09
HCO_3^- (mEq/L)	26	24.0	± 0.3	Cholesterol (mg%)	155	146.3	± 3.1
K^+ (mEq/L)	4.3	4.6	± 0.1	Uric Acid (mg%)	0.78	0.62	± 0.02
Na^+ (mEq/L)	151	148.4	± 0.5	Creatinine (mg%)	1.13	1.20	± 0.04
B.U.N. (mg%)	16	16.7	± 0.6	T. Bilirubin (mg%)	0.10	0.25	± 0.03
Glucose (mg%)	100	89.5	± 1.4	Alk. Phos. (mU/ml)	57	45.5	± 6.4
Total Protein (gm%)	7.2	7.20	± 0.06	CPK (mU/ml)	260	137.6	±18.3
Albumin (gm%)	1.58	1.78	± 0.05	LDH (mU/ml)	269	155.8	±20.8
Ca^{++} (mg%)	9.79	10.34	± 0.16	SGOT (mU/ml)	60	39.5	± 2.8

little variation, and the reticulocyte count has not been greater than 1 per cent (Figure 1). The blood chemistry evaluated weekly is reported in Table 1. There have been no significant changes from control values.

The administration of carbamyl P via the rectal route in cocoa butter suppositories (600 mg per dose) approximately 50 mg per kg of body weight for 11 months has caused no detectable difficulties in the male beagle dog who was 1 year old at the start of treatment. The carbamylation of hemoglobin reached a peak of 0.39 moles of valine hydantoin per mole of hemoglobin tetramer within 4 months of treatment (Figure 3). At this degree of carbamylation, the amino-terminus of any 4 chains have been carbamylated from the 40 available chains in 10 molecules of hemoglobin. The decrease in carbamylation started when a different mechanical method of preparing the suppositories was used. Although the dose of carbamyl P remained the same, the suppositories made by the second method were not as dense or firm. Also the var-

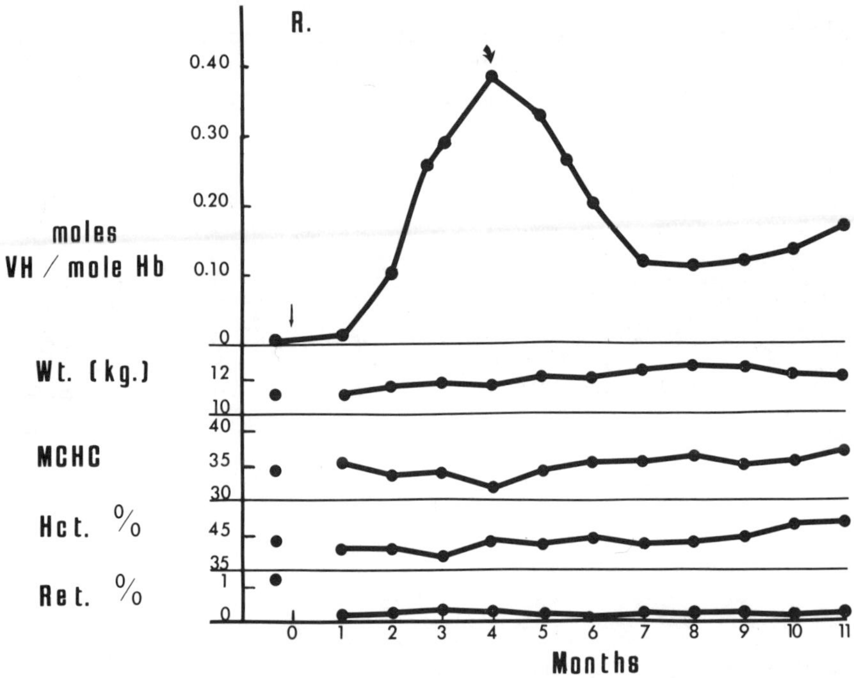

Figure 3. The effect of rectal administration of carbamyl P suppositories for 11 months upon hemoglobin carbamylation, body weight, mean cell hemoglobin concentration (MCHC), hematocrit and reticulocyte production in an adult male beagle dog. The heavy arrow indicates the time that the mechanical way of preparing suppositories was changed. The gradual decrease in carbamylation can be related to the life span of the red cell.

iability in retention of the suppository in a dog may have some bearing on these findings. However, there is a measurable change in the oxygen affinity of this dog's hemoglobin (Figure 2) with a shift to the left of 9 mm Hg. The increase in oxygen affinity appears to reach a steady state at 6 months of treatment when hemoglobin carbamylation has decreased to between 0.2 to 0.1 moles of valine hydantoin per mole of hem-

Table 2. Blood chemistry of a dog receiving carbamyl P by the rectal route for 11 months reported as mean and standard error of weekly values. The control values were measured before treatment was started.

	Control Mean	Control SE	Treated Mean	Treated SE		Control Mean	Control SE	Treated Mean	Treated SE
Cl^- (mEq/L)	106.0	± 1.5	112.3	± 0.5	Inorg. Phos. (mg%P)	6.49	± 0.42	5.45	± 0.12
HCO_3^- (mEq/L)	22.3	± 1.3	21.8	± 0.2	Cholesterol (mg%)	173.7	±16.8	143.6	± 2.1
K^+ (mEq/L)	5.0	± 0.1	4.86	± 0.03	Uric Acid (mg%)	0.65	± 0.09	0.51	± 0.02
Na^+ (mEq/L)	150.0	± 1.5	149.3	± 0.4	Creatinine (mg%)	0.90	± 0.10	1.04	± 0.02
B.U.N. (mg%)	12.0	± 1.5	12.4	± 0.4	T. Bilirubin (mg%)	0.10	± 0.01	0.21	± 0.02
Glucose (mg%)	120.7	± 8.8	100.7	± 1.2	Alk. Phos. (mU/ml)	120		64.6	± 7.3
Total Protein (gm%)	6.25	± 0.24	6.35	± 0.05	CPK (mU/ml)	298		161.2	±16.4
Albumin (gm%)	1.73	± 0.12	1.76	± 0.05	LDH (mU/ml)	230		136.6	±14.9
Ca^{++} (mg%)	10.79	± 0.19	10.65	± 0.09	SGOT (mU/ml)	55		44.1	± 2.5

Table 3. Blood chemistry of 4 beagle pups started on oral administration of carbamyl P when 6 months old. Reported are the mean and standard error of weekly values during 6 months of treatment. The control values were measured before treatment was started.

	Control Mean	Control SE	Treated Mean	Treated SE		Control Mean	Control SE	Treated Mean	Treated SE
Cl^- (mEq/L)	108.2	± 1.2	110.0	± 0.7	Inorg. Phos. (mg%P)	7.0	± 0.1	5.5	± 0.1
HCO_3^- (mEq/L)	23.8	± 0.2	20.8	± 0.5	Cholesterol (mg%)	189.8	± 7.1	184.5	± 4.5
K^+ (mEq/L)	5.3	± 0.2	5.00	± 0.05	Uric Acid (mg%)	0.61	± 0.04	0.55	± 0.01
Na^+ (mEq/L)	143.2	± 0.6	144.20	± 0.25	Creatinine (mg%)	0.72	± 0.08	0.89	± 0.02
B.U.N. (mg%)	11.0	± 0.9	11.5	± 0.3	T. Bilirubin (mg%)	0.14	± 0.02	0.28	± 0.02
Glucose (mg%)	104.8	± 6.0	92.2	± 1.0	Alk. Phos. (mU/ml)	168.5	±14.2	106.8	±26.2
Total Protein (gm%)	5.5	± 0.2	6.50	± 0.04	CPK (mU/ml)	230.2	±28.4	192.2	±11.0
Albumin (gm%)	1.30	± 0.04	1.40	± 0.02	LDH (mU/ml)	138.3	±12.1	157.0	±26.8
Ca^{++} (mg%)	9.90	± 0.09	10.50	± 0.06	SGOT (mU/ml)	46.5	± 7.4	59.2	± 6.3

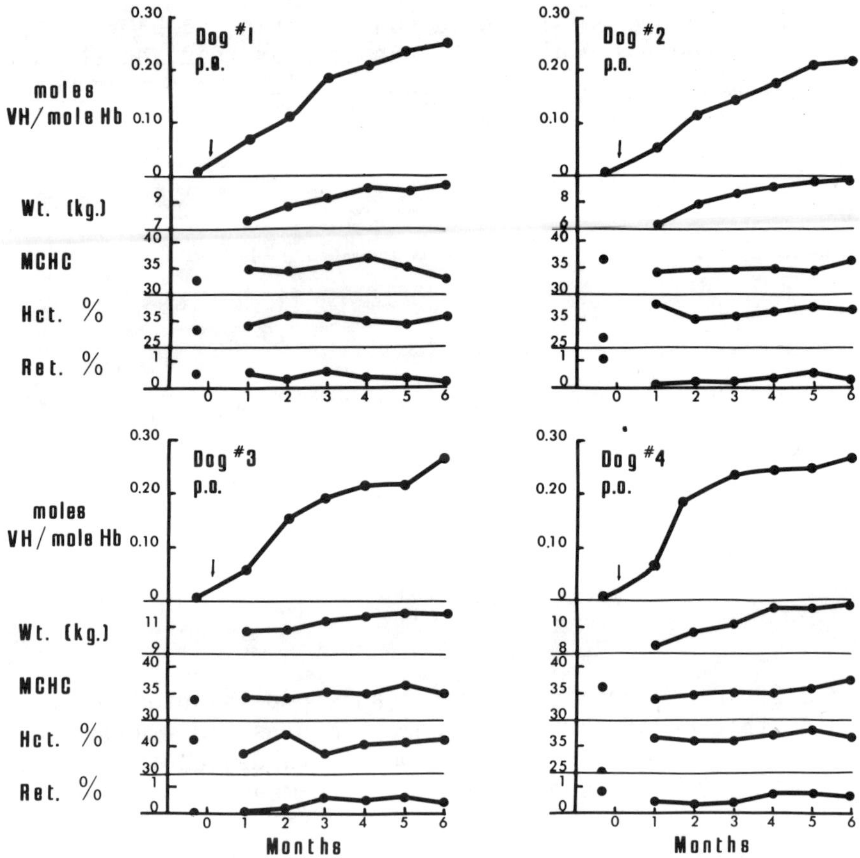

Figure 4. The effect of oral administration of carbamyl P for 6 months to 4 beagle pups started on treatment at 6 months of age. Hemoglobin carbamylation, body weight, mean cell hemoglobin concentration (MCHC), hematocrit and reticulocyte production are reported for each dog.

oglobin tetramer. The dog has gained weight and the hematologic values have remained within the normal range (Figure 3). The blood chemistry has also remained in the normal range (Table 2).

Oral administration of enteric coated capsules of carbamyl P to 4 beagle pups was started when the pups were 6 month old. This continuing study is reviewed after 6 months of treatment. The dose of carbamyl P was increased as the dogs increased in body weight and is being maintained at 100 mg per kg. This has resulted in a steady linear increase in hemoglobin carbamylation to almost 0.3 moles valine hydantoin per hemoglobin tetramer in each dog (Figure 4). The mole per mole ratio of carbamyl P to hemoglobin chain has remained essentially the same for each dog. There is slightly less than 1 mole of carbamyl P for each available mole of hemoglobin chain ranging from 0.96:1 to 0.76:1. Associated with carbamylation is an increase in hemoglobin oxygen affinity with a shift to the left of the P_{50} from 29 to 24 mm Hg (Figure 2). There have been no demonstrable changes from normal in these dogs. They have steadily grown in size and weight and all hematologic parameters are normal (Figure 4). The only change in blood chemistry is related to the age of the dogs, i.e. alkaline phosphatase is higher in pups and decreases as the dogs become adults (Table 3).

DISCUSSION

The administration of carbamyl P to dogs by 3 routes, namely, intravenous, rectal and oral, has resulted in hemoglobin carbamylation with a concomitant increase in hemoglobin oxygen affinity. The P_{50} shifts to the left are moderate, from 5 to 9 mm Hg, thereby permitting sufficient oxygen exchange to other tissues so that no physiological changes from normal have been observed. The 6 months of normal growth and weight gain attest to this in the pups given carbamyl P orally. There have been no biochemical or hematologic changes from normal in any of the dogs. All routes of administration are equally well tolerated. For obvious practical reasons, the oral route seems to be the route of choice. There has been no evidence of toxicity in the animals under study.

The bioavailability of carbamyl P can be determined by a specific enzymatic assay using the enzyme ornithine carbamyl transferase (Jernigan and Kraus, 1974). In the assay carbamyl P is converted quantitatively to citrulline and the citrulline is measured. With this method, we have shown that the monomolecular elimination of carbamyl P to cyanate (Eq 1) has a $T_{1/2}$ of 40 minutes in whole blood *in vitro*. This is consistent with the report of Rakitzis and Mills, (1969), that an acyl phosphatase purified from human erythrocytes does not hydrolyze carbamyl P. Acyl phosphatases capable of dephosphorylating carbamyl P, however, have been reported to be widely distributed in a variety of tissues including muscle (Lipmann, 1946; Grisolia, *et al*., 1954; and Harary, 1963) and brain (Grisolia, *et al*., 1954; Grisolia, *et al*., 1958; and Raijman, *et al*., 1960) from a number of species, including dog and rat. Therefore in tissues other than erythrocytic tissue, carbamyl P's role as a carbamylating agent should be altered where carbamyl P might be subjected to enzymatic hydrolysis (Eq 2) before it could undergo monomolecular elimination to form cyanate. Thus it appears that nature may have provided a means of protection from undesirable carbamylation of proteins when carbamyl P is administered *in vivo*. This mechanism would not be in operation when cyanate is the drug used as a carbamylating agent.

Application of this enzymatic method to determine bioavailability of carbamyl P (Jernigan and Kraus, 1974) following intravenous injections in dogs has shown that the clearance of carbamyl P from the circulation has a $T_{1/2}$ of 2.2 minutes. Therefore half of the injected dose was no longer measurable in 2 - 3 minutes. However, in this *in vivo* dog study the injected dose of carbamyl P,provided an availability of carbamyl P to hemoglobin chain on a mole per mole basis that is 1:1 or slightly less than 1:1. From the present observations of the short *in vivo* clearance time of carbamyl P from dog blood and of carbamylation occurring in 1 of every 20 available hemoglobin chains when carbamyl P was given intravenously (and in 1 of every 15 chains when given orally), the conclusion may be drawn that carbamyl P is an effective carbamylating agent *in vivo*. These features, the moderately increased hemoglobin oxygen affinity induced by carbamyl P and the established antisickling action of carbamyl P *in vitro* (Kraus and Kraus, 1971) all suggest that carbamyl P appears to have the properties desired in an effective therapeutic antisickling agent.

SUMMARY

1. Carbamyl P administered to dogs orally, intravenously, or rectally carbamylated the N-terminal valine residues of hemoglobin chains and concomitantly increased the oxygen affinity of the dogs' hemoglobin.

2. Carbamyl P did not cause any biochemical, physiological or hematologic changes from normal.

3. No toxic effects were found using carbamyl P after intravenous administration for 1 year, after rectal administration for 11 months, or after oral administration for 6 months.

ACKNOWLEDGEMENTS

This work was supported in part by USPHS Grants AM13248 and HL15169.

The authors wish to thank Dr. B. B. Sheth for his help in formulating the oral dose; and Ms. Stephanie Bryan, Mr. L. E. Bryan, Ms. Clare Ralston and Ms. Michelle Pawlick for the excellent technical assistance; Mr. Jon Garcia for his constant vigilance over the dogs; and Ms. Anita Rogers for her careful and excellent organization of data.

REFERENCES

Allen, C. M. and Jones, M. E. (1964). Decomposition of carbamyl phosphate in aqueous solutions. Biochemistry 3: 1238.

Finch, J. T., Perutz, M. F., Bertles, J. F., and Dobler, J. (1973). Structure of sickled erythrocytes and of sickle-cell hemoglobin fibers. Proc. Nat. Acad. Sci. 70: 718.

Grisolia, S., and Marshall, R. O. (1954). Enzymatic decomposition of the active intermediate in citrulline synthesis. Biochim. Biophys. Acta 14: 446.

Grisolia, S., Caravaca, J., and Joyce, B. K. (1958). Purifications and properties of brain carbamyl and acyl phosphatase. Biochim. Biophys. Acta 29: 432.

Harary, I. (1963). Acyl phosphatase from skeletal muscle. In "Methods in Enzymology, VI" (Colowick, S. P., and Kaplan, N. O., eds.) pp 557-566, Academic Press, New York.

Ingram, V. M. (1957). Gene mutations in human haemoglobin: the chemical difference between normal and sickle-cell haemoglobin. Nature 180: 326.

Jernigan, H.M., Jr. and Kraus, L.M. (1974) Determination of carbamyl phosphate in blood. ABS. PAP. A.C.S.1974 34. (J. Lab. Clin. Med. in review).

Kraus, L. M. and Kraus, A. P. (1971). Carbamyl phosphate mediated inhibition of the sickling of erythrocytes in vitro. Biochem. Biophys. Res. Commun. 44: 1381.

Kraus, L. M., Rasad, A. and Kraus, A. P. (1972). Carbamyl phosphate modification of hemoglobin S structure resulting in altered sickling. Adv. Exper. Med. Biol. 28: 279.

Lipmann, F. (1946). Acetyl phosphate. Adv. Enzymol. 6: 231.

Manning, J. M., Lee, C. K., Cerami, A., and Gillette, P. N. (1973). Gas chromatographic determination of the carbamylation of hemoglobin S by cyanate J. Lab. Clin, Med. 81: 941.

Pauling, L.,Itano, H. A., Singer, S. J. and Wells, I. C. (1949) Sickle cell anemia, a molecular disease. Sciences 110: 543.

Raijman, L., Grisolia, S., and Edelhock, H. (1960). Purification and properties of brain acyl phosphatase. J. Biol. Che 235: 2340.

Rakitzis, E. T., and Mills, G. C. (1969). Purification and properties of acyl phosphatase from human erythrocytes. Arc Biochem. Biophys. 134: 372.

DISCUSSION

Dr. Nagel: It is clear, from the work of the Rockefeller group, that cyanate-induced blood parameter changes are directly related to the extent of carbamylation. Don't you think that the levels of carbamylation you are achieving in your animals (0.2-0.3 carbamyl/tetramer) are rather low? We have to recognize that if carbamyl phosphate is going to have any advantage over cyanate for per os administration it will have to be non toxic at levels in which carbamylation of Hb is atleast in the range associated with modification of blood parameters.

Dr. Kraus: Hemoglobin carbamylation is measured as moles of valine hydantoin per mole of hemoglobin tetramer. In other terms, when the valine hydantoin level is 0.3 moles/mole hemoglobin tetramer then 3 chains in 10 molecules of hemoglobin have been carbamylated or 3 chains out of 40 chains have been carbamylated. I think that what we are forgetting is that carbamyl phosphate is a molecule that is not cyanate. It does carbamylate. But it does have the phosphate binding end, the phosphate anion and we have results which show, and I reported them here two years ago, that carbamyl phosphate will, we think, do more than carbamylation. For instance, if you use radioactive cyanate and cold carbamyl phosphate in equal molar amounts, and measure this at a time where you have evolution of cold cyanate from the cold carbamyl phosphate, one would expect that there would be a decrease in radioactivity because after all, you are diluting radioactivity with the non-labeled carbamylating compound and this is what we are measuring. However, instead of there being a decrease in radioactivity, there is a marked increase in radioactivity in the Hb molecule. The distribution of the radioactivity is changed and there are more peptides that are carbamylated than when using cyanate alone. I propose from this and other bits of work that we have done that carbamyl phosphate does change, in some way, the conformation of the molecule so that we are getting a difference, in effect more than we are getting with cyanate itself. Furthermore, it's not the carbamylation of the Hb that has gotten the cyanate into trouble. It's the carbamylation of proteins other than Hb. We feel that we certainly do not want to do anything that is going to cause any patient any difficulties. We are moving very slowly and very carefully. But we also feel that with carbamyl phosphate, with the parameters that we can measure, and with the enzymes that are present in other tissues, we may find that carbamyl phosphate is destroyed before it can carbamylate in tissues other than blood. Here we have an agent that has potential advantages over cyanate.

Unidentified Speaker: Have you measured the degree of carbamyl phosphorylation in other proteins like albumin or some peptides

Dr. Kraus: We know that in the plasma proteins the albumin mobility is modified, but we have not seen any other modifications.

Dr. Nagel: I don't doubt that there might be differences in the rates of reaction of carbamyl phosphate as compared to cyanate. But it is clear in my mind that in order to be careful, precisely one should study these agents at doses two or three fold above the effective level. By studying toxicity with doses that achieve only 0.2 carbamyl/tetramer I think we are on the low side.

Dr. Stern: I would characterize your study as a safety study rather than a toxicologic study since we really don't know, from what I have seen, what toxicologic effects overdoses or susceptible systems might display from excessive carbamyl phosphate. The first question I would like to ask is whether you have increased the dosage of carbamyl phosphate to the point of seeing development of toxicity of one form or another and how would you characterize that toxicity?

Dr. Kraus: We have not in the dog. In the mouse the LD_{50} for carbamyl phosphate given intravenously or intraperitoneall is 1,250 mg. per kg. Whereas the LD_{50} in mice using cyanate are something like 300 or 320 mg. per kg. So, this may answer your question partially.

Dr. Stern: The second point I'd like to inquire about is the absorption of intact carbamyl phosphate from the GI tract; just on general inspection as a highly charged compound, it might be absorbed rather slowly or perhaps not at all. Is there any interference in your detection reaction with cyanate per se or would it be possible to do a combined ^{32}P,^{14}C, experiment where you look at the absorption of both of those materials at the same time.?

Dr. Kraus: This would be a nice experiment to do, thank you for the suggestion.

Dr. Salhany: My question is related to one of the points just made. I was wondering how the carbamylation was occurring, that is, how the carbamyl phosphate was being transported into the red cell to do its thing. Is it being transported as carbamyl phosphate or is it being transported as cyanate or what? Do you know?

Dr. Kraus: We think from the radioactivity experiments that we have done that it is being transported as carbamyl phosphate, otherwise we wouldn't see the effects we have seen. We have done other experiments. After all, carbamyl phosphate does cross mitchrondrial membrane and.......

Dr. Salhany: The question is the rate. I mean if carbamyl phosphate goes in slower than it goes to cyanate, then the question is, which is the faster rate?

Dr. Kraus: We don't have evidence to show that it does this. We have evidence to the opposite.

ZINC IN SICKLE CELL ANEMIA

George J. Brewer, Fred J. Oelshlegel, Jr., and Ananda S. Prasad
Department of Human Genetics, University of Michigan, Ann Arbor, and Department of Medicine, Wayne State University, Detroit

INTRODUCTION

Our work has led us to believe that zinc may play an important clinical role in sickle cell anemia. First, as reported by Prasad et al. in this volume, we have found that a significant proportion of adult patients with sickle cell anemia are zinc deficient. Zinc deficiency may be an explanation for puzzling features of the disease which occur in certain patients, such as retarded growth and hypogonadism (Schoomaker et al., 1973; Prasad et al., 1974).

In addition to zinc deficiency we have observed a pharmacological action of zinc on hemoglobin, as discussed by Gilman et al. in this volume. This is the direct binding of zinc to hemoglobin which increases oxygen affinity, thereby giving zinc one type of antisickling potential (Oelshlegel et al., 1973; Oelshlegel et al., 1974). As with cyanate, the increased oxygen affinity produced by zinc could have an antisickling effect provided high enough blood levels of zinc can be obtained. Our early observations with oral zinc therapy suggested that this might be the case. When we administered zinc to sickle cell anemia patients, primarily for indications of zinc deficiency, we observed an apparent symptomatic response in terms of reduced pain. However, we were unable to detect a change in oxygen affinity in these patients as a result of zinc administration, and our assays revealed that the amount of additional zinc present in the red cells was not sufficient to produce a change in oxygen affinity (Brewer et al., 1974a). The combination of apparent symptomatic effects of zinc administration and red cell zinc concentrations too low to be affecting oxygen affinity has led us to investigations centering on the red cell membrane. We will now briefly review our membrane related studies.

ZINC AND RED CELL MEMBRANES

We have previously reported that incubation of sickle cells with zinc improves their filterability through 3.0 micron Nuclepore filters at intermediate oxygen tensions (Brewer et al, 1974b). Some of our studies have had as their objective an effort to understand the mechanisms by which zinc improves filterability and most important how it may be acting to prevent pain *in vivo*.

One of our early studies revealed that zinc decreased hemoglobin binding by single stage ghosts (Dash et al., 1974). During hypotonic lysis, aliquots of the cells were suspended in control media, in 1.5 mM zinc, in 1.0 mM calcium, and in 1.0 mM calcium plus 1.5 mM zinc. The ghosts were resealed with isotonic saline and washed three times with resealing solution. Ghosts which had been exposed to zinc retained much less hemoglobin than controls. Ghosts exposed to calcium, as was already known, had an increased hemoglobin retention. The presence of zinc in such calcium exposed preparations had a marked effect on reducing hemoglobin retention.

Eaton and colleagues (1973) have suggested that calcium accumulation in sickle cells may be intimately involved with the formation of irreversibly sickled cells. They have shown that calcium accumulates during sickling and that irreversibly sickled cells in the circulation contain more calcium than do normal appearing cells. It is well known that calcium in red cells adversely affects their deformability, although the mechanism is not clear (Weed and La Celle, 1969).

To evaluate the possibility that zinc might be improving sickle cell deformability through an effect on calcium, we have studied the effect of zinc on ^{45}Ca incorporation into red cell ghosts (Brewer et al., 1974b). In these studies, which have been previously reported, both single stage ghosts and ghosts which were prepared to minimize hemoglobin retention by multiple washes during lysis had significantly less ^{45}Ca accumulation in the presence of zinc. In summary, then, it appears that zinc not only reduces hemoglobin retention by membranes, but also decreases calcium retention of red cell membranes, and this effect on calcium is not dependent on the hemoglobin effect.

We have made some preliminary observations on the effect of zinc on the morphologic appearance of red cell membranes as observed by scanning electron microscopy (Figure 1). In the experiment shown in Figure 1, four preparations of single stage ghosts were made. One was a control, the second was treated with zinc during hypotonic exposure, the third was treated with calcium during hypotonic exposure, and the fourth was exposed to both zinc and calcium. After exposure to the agents the ghosts were resealed and washed prior to fixation. From Figure 1 it can be seen that a substantial proportion of the control membranes are echinocytes although some smooth membranes are also present. The echinocytic change is markedly protected against by zinc. Calcium is a strong inducer of these changes but the effect of calcium is partially protected against by zinc. Counts of echinocytes taken from these and other photos by a blinded technician (the technician did not know which preparation was which during the observations) bear out the qualitative observations that zinc does indeed seem to protect against this membrane change.

We would like now to speculate briefly on the sickling process. Lessin (1973) has shown by freeze-fracture techniques that sickling is associated with accumulation of particles, presumably polymerized hemoglobin on the inner surface of the red cell membrane. We would like to propose: 1) That hemoglobin binding to the inside of the sickled red cell membrane is an important feature of the development of

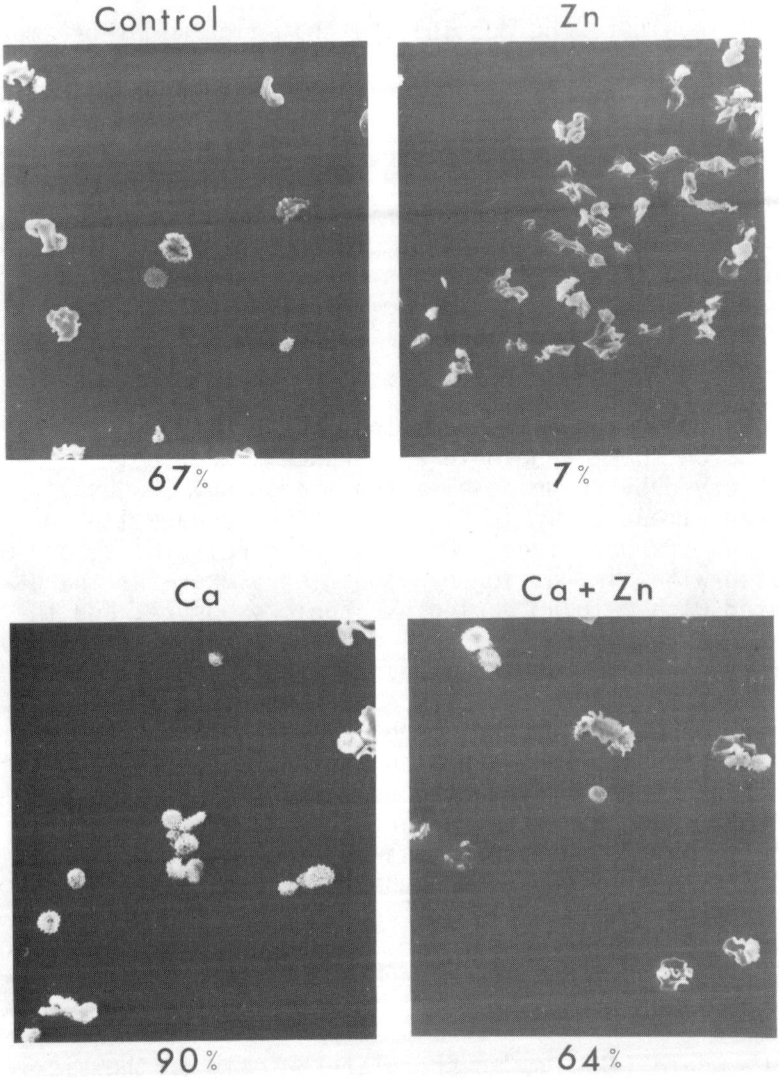

Figure 1. Single stage ghosts prepared by hypotonic lysis in the presence of cations as indicated, presented for comparison of echinocytic changes. Zinc markedly reduced echinocytic changes in zinc vs. control, and zinc/calcium vs. calcium. Counts of echinocytes are shown below each type photo. Concentrations of cations were: zinc - 1.5 mM, calcium - 1.0 mM.

the so-called irreversibly sickled cell; 2) that calcium facilitates the binding of hemoglobin particles; 3) that binding of hemoglobin particles to the membrane increases its stiffness and rigidity, perhaps by crosslinking mechanisms; and 4) that zinc protects against these changes by partially blocking the binding of hemoglobin to the membrane either directly or by an interaction with calcium, and as a result, less hemoglobin is bound to the membrane in the presence of zinc, and the deformability of the cell is thereby protected. In addition, calcium may have deleterious effects on the deformability of the membrane not related to hemoglobin binding, and zinc may partially block these effects.

CLINICAL STUDIES

Our clinical studies with oral zinc administration have been carried out, with informed consent, on homozygous sickle cell anemia patients over the age of 16. The effect of zinc on zinc deficiency-related symptomatology in these patients is discussed by Prasad et al. in this volume.

In terms of hematologic response, we have data on nine patients given zinc from periods of time varying from 6 to 19 months (Table 1). The hemoglobin values in Table 1 (and the plasma zinc values in Table 2) are the means of three determinations before zinc treatment and the means of the three most recent determinations after zinc therapy. As shown, the hemoglobin levels increased an average of 0.5 grams % (Table 1). Six of nine patients showed an increased hemoglobin, two showed lower levels, and one showed no change. Three male patients accounted for the greatest proportion of the total increase in hemoglobin. This increase in hemoglobin may be related to improved erythropoiesis as a result of the androgenic stimulation, or to a reduction in hemolysis, or both. Many male sickle cell anemia patients are hypogonadal and this state can be dramatically improved by zinc administration (Prasad et al, this volume).

Table I

Pt.	Sex	Months of Rx.	Hb (gm.%) Before Zn	After Zn	ΔHb
LS	M	16	7.8	9.5	+1.6
IC	M	15	8.4	8.9	+0.5
BJ	F	12	7.5	8.0	+0.5
RG	M	19	8.1	8.1	0
RC	M	14	9.6	9.4	-0.2
MM	M	6	8.9	10.1	+1.2
JM	M	7	9.3	11.1	+1.8
DM	F	7	5.8	5.9	+0.1
BP	M	7	10.8	10.3	-0.5
		Means	8.47	9.03	+0.5

Data on ^{51}chromium red cell half time survival (^{51}Cr $t_{1/2}$) and red cell volume before and after approximately a year of zinc therapy are available on four patients (Tables II and III). There was an average increase of 1.25 days in the ^{51}Cr $t_{1/2}$ in the four patients with three of the four showing an increased and one a decreased survival. It should be noted that we have had difficulty sustaining a high level of plasma zinc in the patient (RG) who did not show an improvement in ^{51}Cr red cell survival (Table II--each value is the average of three plasma zinc determinations). Red blood cell mass increased an average of 207 ml. in these four patients (Table III), with the same three who had increased red cell survival showing an increase in red cell volume. Two of these patients (LS and RC) had growth retardation and responded to zinc by an increase in body mass, increasing expected red cell mass. Nonetheless, when the data were calculated on the basis of the observed red cell mass in relation to the expected red cell mass for the new

Table II

Pt.	Sex	^{51}Cr RBC Survival ($T_{1/2}$ Days) Before Zn	After Zn	$\Delta T_{1/2}$	Plasma Zn (μcg %) Before Zn	After Zn	ΔZn
LS	M	13	16	+3	119	193	+74
IC	M	5	6.5	+1.5	135	228	+93
RG	M	7	5	-2	99	145	+46
RC	M	9	11.5	+2.5	128	163	+35
	Means	8.5	9.75	+1.25	120	182	+62

Table III

Pt.	RBC Mass (ml RBC) Before Zn	After Zn	ΔRBC Mass	% Expected RBC Mass Before Zn	After Zn	Δ% Expected
LS	491	720	+229	56	62	+ 6
IC	1259	1351	+ 92	65	69	+ 4
RG	952	913	- 39	59	56	- 3
RC	766	1312	+546	55	83	+28
Means	867	1074	+207	58.7	67.5	+ 8.8

body weight, these three patients still revealed an increase, with two being modest and the other rather impressive (Table III). The patient (RG) with no increase in red cell mass is the same one who had a decreased red cell survival on zinc (Table II), and no improvement in hemoglobin (Table I).

In summary of the hematologic data then, the Cr^{51} red cell survival data suggest, but so far do not prove, some decrease in hemolytic rate with zinc therapy. A substantial improvement in red cell mass occurs in some patients in response to zinc along with a modest increase in hemoglobin levels. These improvements may be partly due to a decrease in hemolysis, but may also be due in part to an androgenic effect on the bone marrow.

Turning now to the symptomatic response to oral zinc therapy in sickle cell anemia, we are quite enthusiastic. We are only at the stage of very limited, uncontrolled trials, but the results so far are encouraging. Positive results in uncontrolled trials are, of course, part of the justification for the expense and trouble, both to patients and investigators, of double blind, controlled therapeutic trials. A positive therapeutic response in uncontrolled trials, plus laboratory findings supportive of a therapeutic rationale, plus low toxicity, all are part of the necessary preliminary development for a new therapeutic agent, and zinc is successfully meeting these criteria so far. The uncontrolled observations on symptoms which follow should be viewed as part of the preliminary assessment of oral zinc as a therapy in sickle cell anemia.

For evaluating the symptomatic response to zinc therapy, we arbitrarily divided pain symptoms into two types. One was painful sickling crises requiring hospital admission or a trip to the emergency room, such visits giving us something specific to count. Other pain potentially related to sickling but not requiring admission or emergency room visit has been graded by the patient and evaluated separately.

Six of the nine patients had recurring episodes of this latter type pain. Severity of pain at the various sites prior to zinc was graded one to three by the patient, with grade one being mild pain not requiring drugs, grade two being pain requiring soft drugs such as Darvon or aspirin, and grade three requiring narcotics. A similar evaluation after zinc therapy was then made. Certain types of pain such as headache and chronic joint pains tended to be unchanged in frequency and severity. However, a number of types of pains, particularly migratory pains, chest and back pains, were graded as improved by many patients, some of them disappearing, and others with a decreased frequency and/or severity.

Turning now to the effect of zinc on the prophylaxis of crisis, four of the nine patients had sickle cell crises requiring admission or emergency room visit at varying frequencies before zinc. Their crisis histories before and after zinc are shown in Figures 2 and 3. The first patient (Figure 2) had six crises over a four year period prior to zinc administration, and has had no crises during 12 months of zinc therapy. The second patient had four crises in the two year period prior to zinc administration. He has had two crises during one and a half years of zinc therapy. The crisis data on this patient are not especially encouraging, but it might be noted that this is RG, the patient in whom we have had the greatest difficulty obtaining a high blood zinc level and who has had no increase in red cell survival and red cell mass with zinc.

The third patient (Figure 2) has had a good symptomatic response to zinc. He had 14 admissions over a three and a quarter year period prior to zinc therapy, or a rate of about four crises a year. In 13 months of therapy he has had two crises, both mild compared to his earlier ones, and both related to specific incidents, one a street fight in which he was badly beaten up, and the second an episode of heavy physical exertion shoveling snow for several hours. Even more encouraging to us is that he has had a very good year, and was able to attend school regularly, something he had not been able to do in the past. In fact, his being in a fight and out at all during the snow storm attests to a changed attitude and life style.

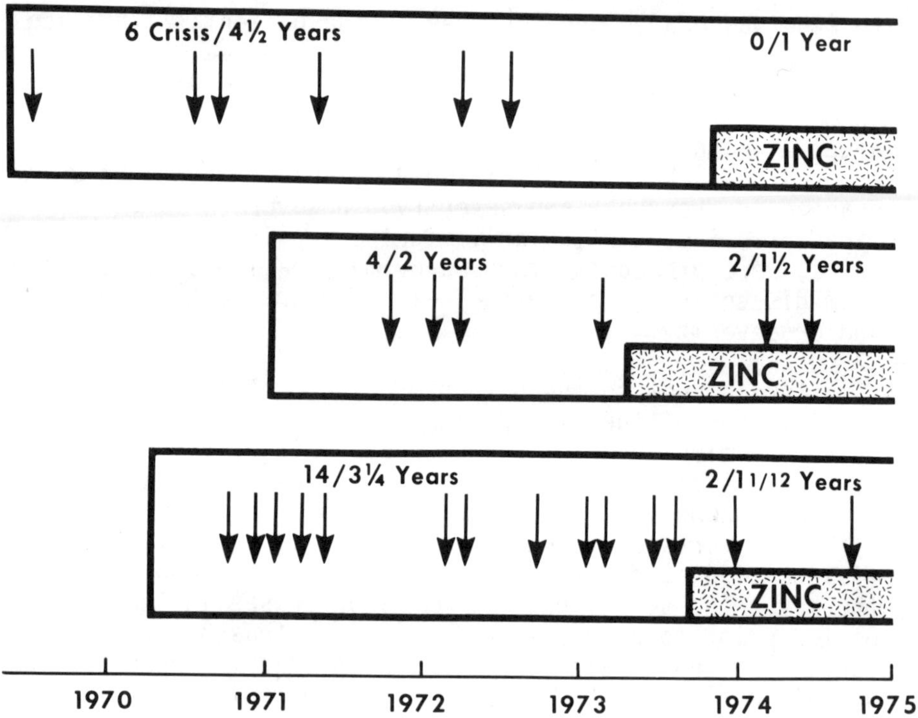

Figure 2. The crisis histories of three patients with sickle cell anemia before and after zinc therapy. Each arrow represents an admission or emergency room visit for pain crisis. The patients from top to bottom are BJ, RG, and RC.

The fourth patient (Figure 3) has had the most impressive response of all to zinc. This is a patient who has been literally crippled by crises over the last several years. His history prior to zinc includes seven admissions to Grace Hospital over six months for severe, generalized, painful sickle cell crises. With zinc we have interrupted this situation. He has been admitted twice during a six month period for painful episodes, both quite mild. Subsequent to these episodes we have altered his diet based upon new data on dietary factors affecting zinc absorption, to be discussed in a moment, and he has had no crises during the last three months

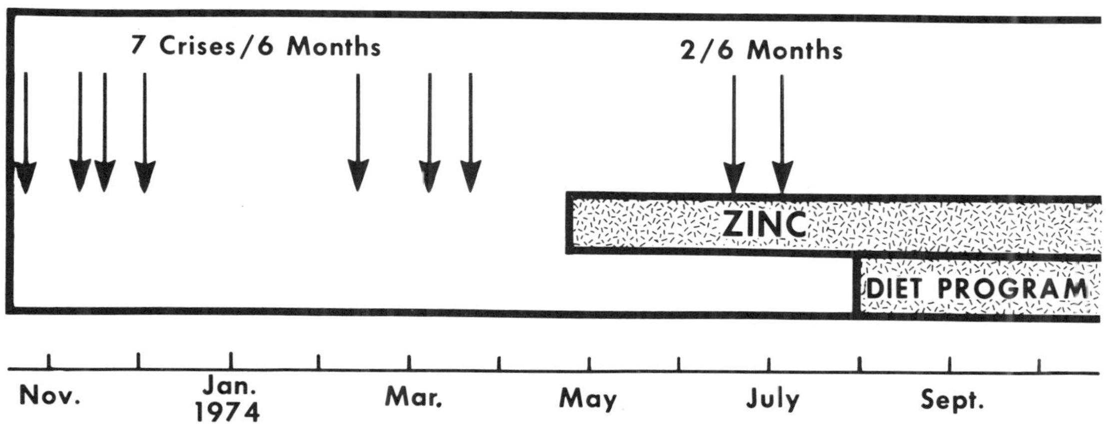

Figure 3. The crisis history in a fourth patient with sickle cell anemia before and after zinc therapy. This is patient MM.

As with the third patient, the most impressive feature is his changed life style. Previously, he was badly crippled by his disease, spending much of his time in the hospital and most of his other time in pain. His physicians feared for his life during a protracted crisis last spring. He now has a job and a greatly expanded social life.

Both types of data just reviewed--that on pain not requiring admission and that on crises--may be strongly influenced by psychological factors. The obvious answer to this problem is a controlled double-blind clinical trial, and this is the direction in which we would like to proceed. There are some problems regarding needs for improving zinc absorption with a better pharmacological preparation which probably

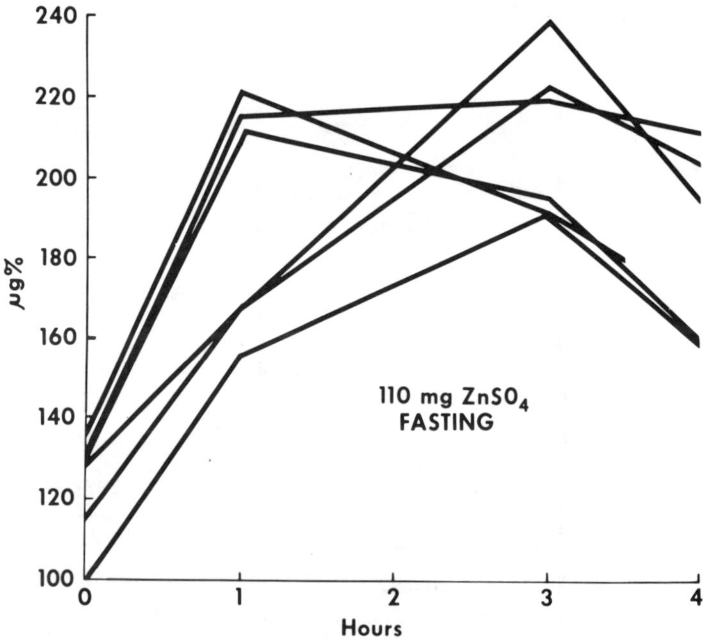

Figure 4. These are zinc tolerance curves in which six normal subjects took 110 mg zinc sulfate while in a fasting condition. Plasma zinc levels are shown on the ordinate.

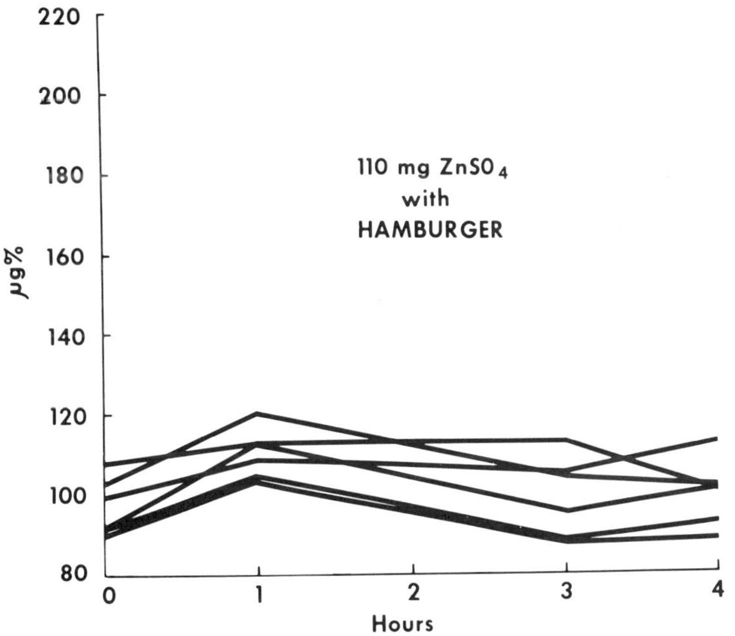

Figure 5. Zinc tolerance curves in the same subjects as Figure 4, but the subjects ingested a hamburger simultaneously with the zinc.

should be solved before such trials are undertaken. We will now discuss some oral zinc absorption studies which will highlight that need.

Oral Zinc Absorption Studies

Figures 4, 5, and 6 are zinc tolerance curves in six normal subjects. The abscissa is time and the ordinate is plasma zinc in micrograms %. The first value reflects plasma zinc levels prior to administration of a single dose of zinc, and the other values are at various subsequent times. In the experiment in Figure 4, 110 mg. of zinc sulfate was taken fasting. Plasma zinc increases to some 200 micrograms % in one to two hours and after four hours declines, in some cases more drastically than in others. From these preliminary data, we have reasoned that our best protection against sickling with oral zinc sulfate might be with a dose every four hours. Therefore, our current treatment program is 110 mg of zinc sulfate six times daily. Parenthetically it might be noted that it was at the time that we switched to six times versus three times a day administration that two of our symptomatic patients began to notice improvement in various types of recurrent pain.

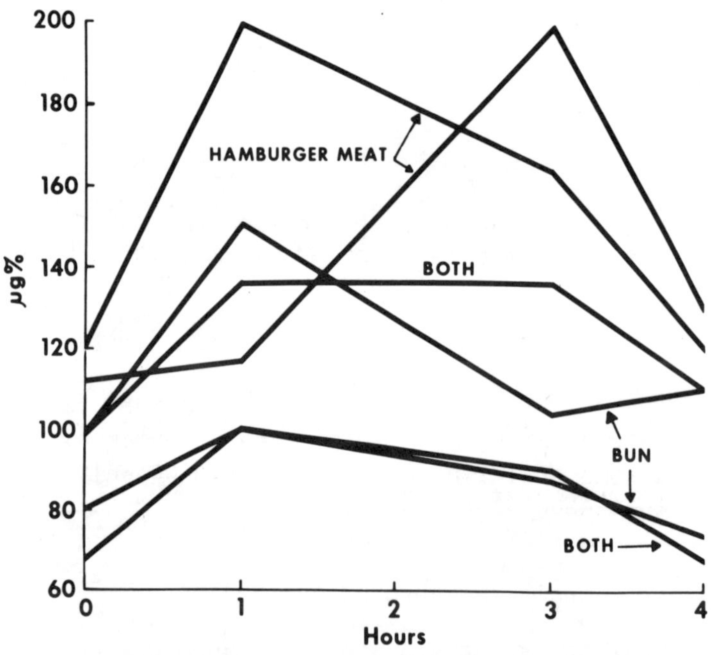

Figure 6. Zinc tolerance curves (110 mg zinc sulfate) in the same subjects, but two subjects ingested hamburger meat, two a hamburger bun, and two both meat and bun.

Zinc sulfate causes gastric irritation in some patients, and we wanted to establish which foods maximized zinc absorption, or at least did not block it, and therefore could be safely taken with zinc. To our surprise, the old American standby, the hamburger, completely blocked zinc absorption in all subjects (Figure 5). Subsequent studies revealed that the meat itself did not adversely affect zinc absorption, and that the primary culprit was the bun (Figure 6). Actually, it is well known that breads contain phytate which chelate zinc and prevent its absorption. Our studies have revealed other substances in foods, and still other substances are known from work elsewhere, which adversely affect zinc absorption. Thus our current zinc therapeutic regime for crisis and pain symptom prophylaxis involves zinc administration every four hours, and dietary coordination with zinc ingestion, and is rather complicated and unwieldy for any large scale study requiring a high degree of compliance.

In summary then, zinc is non-toxic, has been effective in decreasing symptoms and crisis in limited uncontrolled studies, and appears to have a therapeutic rationale. The latter is based on effects of zinc on the red cell membrane by which it decreases hemoglobin and calcium binding and improves deformability. We think this results in lessened trapping of sickle cells in capillaries where pain is normally produced. Zinc deserves thorough evaluation as a treatment for sickle cell anemia.

ACKNOWLEDGEMENTS

This work was supported in part by Contract NHLI 72-2918-B of the National Institutes of Health. We would also like to express our appreciation to the Clinical Research Unit of University Hospital which is supported by USPHS Grant 5M01-FR-42.

REFERENCES

Brewer, G.J., Oelshlegel, F.J., Jr., Prasad, A.S. Knutsen, C.A., and Meyers, N. (1974a). Antisickling effects of zinc. Proceedings of 1st National Symposium on Sickle Cell Disease, Bethesda, Md., 27-28 June 1974. In press.

Brewer, G.J., and Oelshlegel, F.J., (1974b). Antisickling effects of zinc. Biochem. Biophys. Res. Commun. 58:854.

Dash, S., Brewer, G.J., and Oelshlegel, F.J., Jr. (1974). Effect of zinc on haemoglobin binding by red blood cell membranes. Nature 250:251.

Eaton, J.W., Skelton, T.D., Swofford, H.S., Kolpin, C.E., and Jacob, H.S. (1973). Elevated erythrocyte calcium in sickle cell disease. Nature 246:105.

Lessin, L.S. (1973). Membrane ultrastructure of normal, sickled and Heinz-body erythrocytes by freeze-etching. In Red Cell Shape (M. Bessis, R.I. Weed, and P.F. Leblond, eds.). Springer-Verlag, New York, pp. 151-168.

Oelshlegel, F.J., Jr., Brewer, G.J., Prasad, A.S., Knutsen, C., and Schoomaker, E.B. (1973). Effect of zinc on increasing oxygen affinity of sickle and normal red blood cells. Biochem. Biophys. Res. Commun. 53:560.

Oelshlegel, F.J., Jr., Brewer, G.J., Knutsen, C., Prasad, A.S., and Schoomaker, E.B. (1974) Studies on the interaction of zinc with human hemoglobin. Arch. Biochem. Biophys. 163:742.

Prasad, A.S., Schoomaker, E.B., Ortega, J., Brewer, G.J., Oberleas, D., and Oelshlegel, F.J., Jr. (1974). Deficiency of zinc in sickle cell disease patients. Proceedings of 1st National Symposium on Sickle Cell Disease, Bethesda, Md., 27-28 June 1974. In press.

Schoomaker, E.B., Prasad, A., Oelshlegel, F.J., Jr., Ortega, J., and Brewer, G.J. (1973). Clin. Res. 21:834.

Weed, R.I., and La Celle, P.L. (1969). ATP Dependence of erythrocyte membrane deformability. In Red Cell Membrane Structure and Function (G.A. Jamieson and T.J. Greenwalt, eds.) J.B. Lippincott Co., Philadelphia. pp. 318-338.

DISCUSSION

Dr. Nagel: Does zinc inhibit morphologic sickling?

Dr. Brewer: Do you mean *in vitro*? We haven't studied it exhaustively, but as far as we can determine, no. There's a limit of about 1.5 mM zinc in incubations, since it's a protein precipitant. At that level we haven't seen a morphologic effect. We're just beginning to study irreversibly sickled cells in patients on a longitutinal basis and we really have no data on that yet.

Dr. Nagel: Siegmund Fischer, in our laboratory, has shown that the increase in Hb associated with ghosts prepared from sickle cell anemia blood can be almost entirely accounted by the contribution of the irreversibly sickled cells. I was wondering how much of the effect you are seeing with zinc might be due to the effect of this metal on the irreversibly sickled cells.

Dr. Brewer: Our working hypothesis is that might very well be the point of action of zinc.

Dr. Greenquist: Have you looked at *in vitro* uptake of zinc by intact red cells? Do they take up zinc?

Dr. Brewer: Yes, they do. They take it up at a slow temperature dependent rate. But even at 4° they will take up some zinc; at 37° the uptake is fairly good. You get equilibration with the suspending media, probably, I think, in 10 or 12 hours.

Dr. Greenquist: Does zinc reverse deformability in intact cells? Increase deformability in, say, depleted cells?

Dr. Brewer: We don't know.

Dr. Woosley: What was the concentration of zinc in the *in vitro* studies?

Dr. Brewer: 1.5 mM is what we've used mostly, but we have found an effect on filterability down to about 0.3 mM. Nothing below that. This is in a 2 hour incubation with these concentrations.

Dr. Woosley: What about the ghost studies?

Dr. Brewer: The ghost studies were carried out with 1.5 mM zinc, as well, and 1.0 mM calcium.

Dr. Diederich: Dr. Brewer, I thought I understood when you started your discussion that a zinc deficient patient has a double defect in his cell, that is zinc deficiency enhances the sickling of the cell. But what you're really suggesting is that one does not need to screen for zinc deficient patients to enlist patients into a zinc protocol, but it can be used on patients, no matter what the red cell zinc is. Is that correct, now?

Dr. Brewer: Yes. We think they're independent. Dr. Prasad and I initiated our work because of zinc deficiency, and it was as a result of this interest that we began to look into other things that zinc might be doing and discovered its possible antisickling effects. So the two, I believe, are independent. We don't think that the zinc deficient patient has more pain symptoms as a result of zinc deficiency as compared to a non-deficient patient. As a matter of fact, one of the dwarfed sickle cell patients, the most severely growth retarded, has tended to be relatively asymptomatic in terms of pain.

Dr. Diederich: O.K., now, two more quick questions. The obvious is that the patients with the chronic ulcers are more likely to be zinc deficient, or, is there any correlation at all?

Dr. Brewer: The four patients with leg ulcers that we have studied all have been zinc deficient. I should mention that Sargent has previously used zinc in Jamaica for leg ulcers in sickle cell anemia patients and has reported a beneficial effect. We have had a good response in one patient who had a small ulcer, which healed up; a fair response in two patients with intermediate-sized ulcers that decreased in size, but they were also getting much better medical care; and no response in the fourth patient, an elderly lady with some cardiac failure. I think zinc is playing a role in healing these ulcers. Zinc deficiency is one factor that reduces the healing, but I don't think that it's the only factor in leg ulcers.

Dr. Diederich: Have you had the opportunity to look at calcium content of cells during zinc therapy?

Dr. Brewer: No, we haven't. It's something that John Eaton and I have talked about, but we haven't done such studies.

Dr. Glader: Is there any qualitative difference between the zinc effect versus that which you might see with chlorpromazine, vinblastine or other agents which displace calcium from the membrane? They all seem to do the same thing. Is there a difference?

Dr. Brewer: I would be speculating, but my own hunch is that agents such as procaine and zinc, and possibly some of those you mentioned, are doing the same thing, at least in terms of calcium displacement. This may be the way to go for sickle cell therapy.

ALTERATION OF THE DEFORMABILITY OF SICKLE CELLS BY PROCAINE HYDROCHLORIDE

Richard Baker, Darleen Powars, and
L. Julian Haywood
Departments of Microbiology, Pediatrics
and Medicine, University of Southern California
School of Medicine, Los Angeles, California

INTRODUCTION

Since the discovery of the hemoglobin defect in sickle cell anemia by Pauling and co-workers (Pauling et al, 1949) and the elucidation of the nature of this defect by Ingram (1956), it has been a basic assumption that deoxygenation-induced hemoglobin gelling distorted the red cell into the sickled shape thereby causing the 'cryptogenic sickle cell crisis'. Even though no clear correlation can be made between the numbers of irreversibly sickled cells (ISC) observed in any given patient and the presence of clinical symptomatology, many investigators still consider the end stage ISC to be the important factor in the pathogenesis of the disorder.

Irreversibly sickled cells which remain distorted even after reoxygenation were recognized at an early date (Diggs and Bibb, 1939, Shen et al 1949). However, Serjeant (Serjeant et al 1969) has shown a correlation between the percentage of irreversibly sickled cells in adult SS patients and a decrease in the red cell survival time (Cr^{51}). Since oxygenated ISC show no evidence of hemoglobin polymerization (Bertles and Dobler 1969) attention has recently shifted to the role of the membrane in the formation of ISC's. Fragmentation as a result of repeated sickling-unsickling episodes has been suggested

(Padilla et al 1973) as an important factor in the origin of ISC's. Red cell energy metabolism, especially the ATP level is believed (Jensen, Shohet and Nathan 1973) to be more important than fragmentation in the formation of ISC's. These workers demonstrated a correlation between numbers of ISC formed and erythrocyte ATP levels after deoxygenated SS cells were incubated for 24 hours at 37°C. Lessin and Wallas (1974) found that in vitro incubation of deoxygenated SS cells at 37°C results in increased amounts of membrane-bound hemoglobin; also, they demonstrated by the freeze-etching method microaggregates of hemoglobin attached to the membrane. They concluded that ISC formation was independent of ATP concentration. Elevated calcium levels in both SS cells and ISC have been reported (Eaton et al 1973). Oxygenated SS cells (non-ISC cells) contained 8 times the calcium of normal AA cells. Oxygenated ISC were 16 times richer in calcium than normal AA cells. It is known that excess membrane-bound calcium is responsible for the deformability loss suffered by normal red cells which have been metabolically depleted by 24 hour 37°C incubation (Weed, LaCelle and Merrill, 1969). Some calcium was bound to ATP but was freed to diffuse to the membrane on depletion of the ATP. Extracellular calcium then accumulated in the cell due to the non-functioning calcium pump. Accordingly, these workers (Eaton et al, 1973) suggest that ISC formation may be due to excess calcium binding to the red cell membrane in vivo.

It has been demonstrated (Kwant and Seeman, 1969) that the cationic anesthetics compete with calcium for binding sites on the intracellular side of cell membrane. Binding of these agents to normal red cell membranes also increases the membrane area, protects against osmotic hemolysis, and increases the membrane fluidity (Seeman 1972). A reversible change in shape from biconcave to cup-shaped is caused by the positively charged agents, while anionic agents cause crenation (Deuticke, 1968). It has been recently reported that procaine hydrochloride, a cationic anesthetic, added before or after incubation of SS cells in the deoxygenated state, will induce a shape change with increased deformability when such cells are reoxygenated (Baker, Powars, and Haywood 1974).

Without the additive the cells remain rigid and permanently deformed.

It is the purpose of this report to demonstrate that the generation of ISC's in vitro is accompanied by an increase in rigidity which is proportional to the time spent in the deoxygenated state and that the rate of formation of ISC's may be decreased by the addition of optimum amounts of procaine hydrochloride, p-aminobenzoic acid (PABA), or diethylaminoethanol (DAE).

MATERIALS AND METHODS

Blood Collection

Blood samples were drawn intravenously from patients with sickle cell anemia, into EDTA anticoagulant. Diagnosis of sickle cell anemia was based on the hematological parameters of a hemolytic anemia, hemoglobin electrophoresis, and demonstration of the sickling phenomenon. Hemoglobin F, as determined by the Singer alkali denaturation method, was less than 10% in all patients studied. Percentages of irreversibly sickled cells were estimated by phase microscopy of wet mounts of oxygenated whole blood. Samples of adult AA blood were obtained by venipuncture from volunteers.

In Vitro ISC Formation

Deoxygenation was carried out by mixing 1 volume of blood with 2 volumes of 2% sodium metabisulfite (in distilled water). Milliosmolarity of this mixture was 252 mOsm as measured on a freezing point osmometer (Precision Systems, Newton, Mass.). Final extracellular pH was 6.6. Incubation of the blood-bisulfite mixture was carried out at 37°C for varying periods of time, following which reoxygenation of aliquots was done by dilution and washing in fresh tris (147mM NaCl; 2mM $CaCl_2$; 12mM tris; pH 7.4) or phosphate (70mM NaCl; 11mM KH_2PO_4; 60mM Na_2HPO_4; pH 7.4) buffer which had been saturated with 95% O_2-5% N_2.

Deformability Assay

Deformability was assayed by measuring flow rates through Nuclepore polycarbonate filters (Nuclepore Corp., Pleasanton, Calif.) with 3μm pore size. Fifty μl of whole blood was diluted to 0.25% v/v with tris or phosphate buffer and 3 ml was filtered via gravity feed through a Nuclepore filter (N300, 3.0μm, 25 mm diameter). After collection of the first 0.5 ml of suspension, times were recorded for the next 0.2, 0.3, 0.5, and 1 ml to pass the filter. Initially, individual filters were used for each measurement, with the attendant variability (~10%) inherent in the manufacture of the filters with respect to pore density and diameter. It was found that 3 minutes ultrasonication (L+R Mfg. Co., Kearny, N.J.) in distilled water, followed by 3 minutes ultrasonication in tris or phosphate buffer allowed re-use of the same filter. The flow rate of 1 ml of buffer solution was measured prior to each blood filtration. The blood dilution factor was monitored by cell counts with a Coulter counter Model B.

Metabolic Depletion

Metabolic depletion of normal AA blood was done by incubating AA cells in plasma at a 10% hematocrit for 20-48 hours at 37°C, or alternatively, in tris buffer containing 2mM $CaCl_2$ at the same hematocrit.

Drugs

Procaine hydrochloride (FW 272.78), para-aminobenzoic acid (PABA, FW 137.1) and 2-diethylaminoethanol (DAE, FW 117.2) were obtained from Matheson, Coleman, and Bell. Stated concentrations of procaine and p-aminobenzoic acid were prepared on a w/v basis with serial dilutions to achieve the desired concentrations. 2-diethylaminoethanol was prepared on a v/v basis. Dilutions were done in tris buffer. The drugs were added to the blood samples and equilibrated at room temperature for 30 minutes prior to incubation.

Red Cell Ghosts

Three 0.4 ml samples of normal AA blood were washed twice with 5 ml tris buffer. After discarding the supernatant, the cells were hemolyzed as follows: #1 in 15 ml of 30 mOsm phosphate buffer with no calcium; #2 in 15 ml of 30 mOsm tris buffer containing 2 mM Ca; #3 in 15 ml of 30 mOsm tris containing 2 mM Ca and 6 mM procaine hydrochloride. The ghosts were spun down re-suspended in 300 mOsm phosphate buffer to a concentration equivalent to 0.25% v/v intact red cells, before Nuclepore filtration.

Scanning Microscopy

Red cells were processed for scanning microscopy by fixation in 2% buffered glutaraldehyde for 1 hour, followed by 4 washes in distilled water. Drops of the suspension were air dried on aluminum specimen stubs, following which the stubs were coated by evaporation with 200AU of 60:40 gold-palladium alloy. Scanning and photography were done on an AMR 1000 scanning microscope at 20 KV, with 45° specimen tilt.

RESULTS

Figures 1, 2, and 3 are graphs of flow rates versus incubation time at 37°C for blood samples containing various concentrations of procaine HCL, PABA, and DAE. The data in each figure represent a self-contained experiment and therefore direct comparison of flow rates between different figures is invalid. The family of curves representing different experiments in general were displaced horizontally on the incubation time scale. The amount of the displacement will depend on the source of the blood, storage time of the sample at 4°C, average percentage of Hb F, percentage of in vivo-formed ISC's etc. Stated differently, the incubation time associated with a given deformability will vary with the above factors, as will the time needed to achieve non-reversibility on reoxygenation. It is clear from Fig. 1 that deformability is changing at a minimum rate for a procaine hydrochloride concentration between 10^{-3}M and 10^{-5}M.

Fig. 1

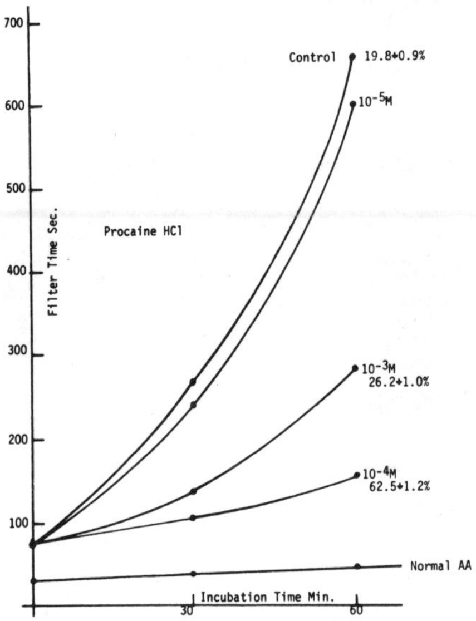

Figs. 1,2,3 Filtration vs incubation times for 1 ml of 0.25% SS blood treated with stated concentrations of procaine, PABA, and DAE. Percentages of cells passing through filter at 90 min. incubation are shown in Fig. 1 which also includes data for normal AA blood.

Fig. 2

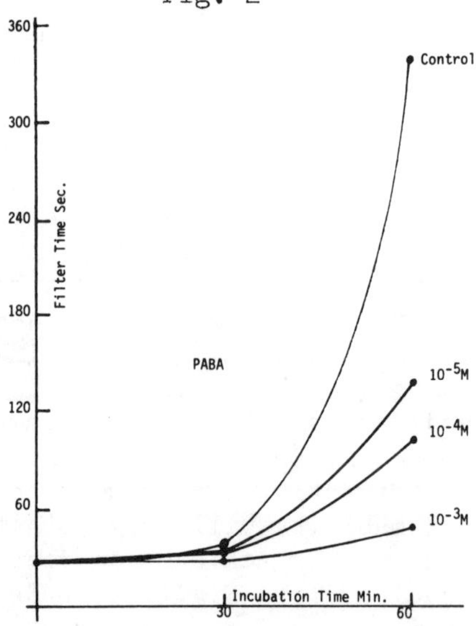

Fig. 3

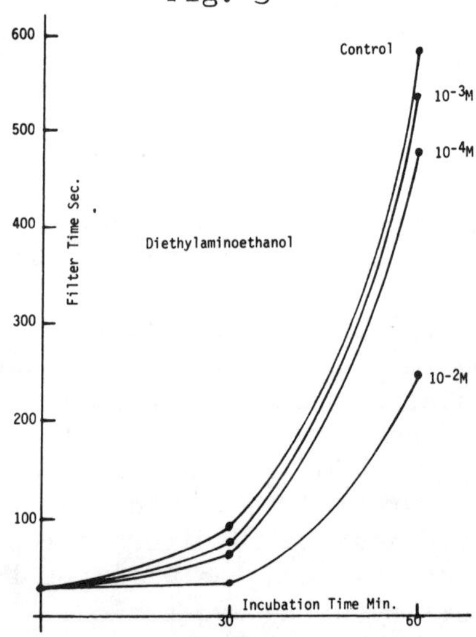

Although flow rates for PABA and DAE at higher concentrations have not been plotted, the optimum concentration for PABA lies between 10^{-2}M and 10^{-4}M, while for DAE it lies between 10^{-1}M and 10^{-3}M. The flow rate measurements were terminated when the filtration times became unduly long. This occurred after 60 min. incubation in the experiments plotted in Figures 1, 2, and 3. After 90 min. incubation, cell counts from the suspension above and below the filter were measured with a Coulter counter. The ratio of the hematocrits above and below the filter expressed as a percentage is shown on Fig. 1. Thus, even after filter times through 3 µm pores were impractically long, the procaine-treated cells were more flexible than the untreated cells. Shape reversal after re-oxygenation of cells treated with optimum drug concentrations did not occur.

Table 1 summarizes the changes in the numbers of cells undergoing shape alterations as a function of time after re-oxygenation. In this experiment, 1 volume of whole blood was incubated for 4 hours at 37°C, with and without 0.09M procaine hydrochloride, after addition of 2 volumes of sodium metabisulfite. After 4 hours incubation, the cells were centrifuged and washed three times in tris buffer. Wet mounts were prepared at hourly intervals and examined for visual evidence of shape changes. The control cells remained over 90% sickled, while 55% of the procaine-treated cells within 3 hours reverted to spheres.

Table 2 illustrates the protection which is afforded by 6 mM procaine hydrochloride against the stiffening induced by metabolic depletion at 37°C of normal AA cells. The cells were suspended in tris buffer containing 2 mM $CaCl_2$ during the incubation period. Individual filters were used for each determination.

Table 3 shows the increased membrane rigidity of ghosts caused by the presence of 2 mM calcium in the hemolyzing solution, and the cancellation of this increase in rigidity when both calcium and 6 mM procaine were present at the time of hemolysis. Individual filters were used and 1 ml filter times were corrected to the same buffer time.

TABLE 1

Reversal of sickle cell shape with time after start of oxygenation

t hr.	Percentage of sickled cells 0.09M procaine	control
0	88	95
1	45	95
2	40	96
3	33	95
20	30	92

Time course of reversal of in vitro-formed ISC by procaine hydrochloride in a typical experiment. Percentage of remaining deformed cells is tabulated as a function of time in hours after removal of reducing agent and exposure to room air. $p < 0.001$ Courtesy of Academic Press

Scanning micrographs of normal red cells treated with procaine HCl, PABA, and DAE are shown in Figs. 4 and 5. Figure 4 illustrates the effect on cell shape of treatment with 4 concentrations of procaine HCl. The cell shape is unaltered by 10^{-4}M procaine, while cupping and invagination become more pronounced as the concentration increases to 0.1M (Fig. 4d). Cell shape in the presence of 10^{-3}M PABA is normal biconcave, but 10^{-2}M PABA (Fig. 5b) induces sphering and invagination. Cell shape is unaffected by 10^{-2}M DAE (Fig. 5c).

TABLE 2

Effect of procaine hydrochloride on normal erythrocyte deformability

Blood Sample	Incub. time, hr.	Volume Collected, ml 0.1	0.2	0.3	0.5	1.0	t/t_0 for 1 ml
Control	0	3	5	9	16	39	1.0
Control	20	15	36	79	300	900	23
Control	48	1020	-	-	-	-	-
Procaine	20	3	7	12	21	54	1.4
Procaine	48	8	9	15	32	103	2.6

Normal red cell deformability before and after metabolic depletion with and without .006M procaine. Filtration time in seconds as a function of incubation time and volume collected. Filter flow rate reproducibility 10.8%, based on 133 determinations, 3 μm pore size. t/t_0=sample flow time/ fresh blood flow time for 1 ml. Courtesy of Academic Press

TABLE 3

Tube #	Time	Buffer Time	Corr. Time
1	75	35.5	75
2	378	28.5	470
3	50	27.0	66

Filtration time for AA ghosts prepared in: 1-phosphate buffer no calcium; 2-tris buffer + 2 mM calcium; 3-tris buffer + 2mM calcium + 6 mM procaine hydrochloride. Filter times corrected to buffer time of 35.5 sec.

DISCUSSION

It is probable that loss of deformability of the red cell is responsible for much of the clinical pathology of sickle cell anemia. Since calcium accumulation is a likely factor in the loss of deformability associated with the generation of ISC's and since excessive inward calcium flow occurs during deoxygenation, the rate of ISC formation should be a function of the total time spent in the deoxygenated state. Thus, any agent which interferes with membrane calcium binding should improve the function and increase the life span of the SS cells. Evidence for competition between procaine or its by-products and calcium for membrane binding sites is clearly shown by the deformability data on normal red cell ghosts (Table 3). The addition of procaine and calcium to the hemolyzing medium insured their rapid entry into the ghost and contact with the membrane. Hydrolysis of the procaine by membrane cholinesterase of course cannot be ruled out even though in this experiment short interaction times are involved.

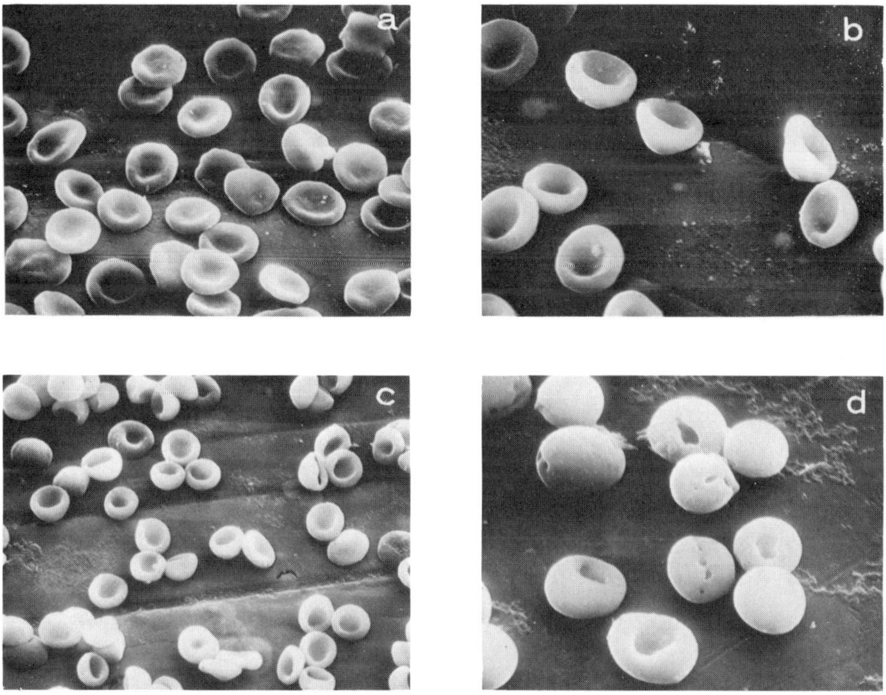

Fig. 4 Scanning micrographs of normal human red cells treated 1 hour in phosphate buffer (10% Hct) with various concentrations of procaine hydrochloride.
(a) 10^{-4}M (b) 10^{-3}M (c) 10^{-2}M (d) 10^{-1}M

Further evidence for involvement of procaine or its by-products in membrane-calcium interaction is furnished by the data in Table 2. It has been clearly established (Weed, LaCelle and Merrill, 1969) that calcium is a prime determinant in the deformability loss associated with metabolic depletion. If the calcium is omitted from the incubation medium, deformability loss is greatly reduced. In the experi-

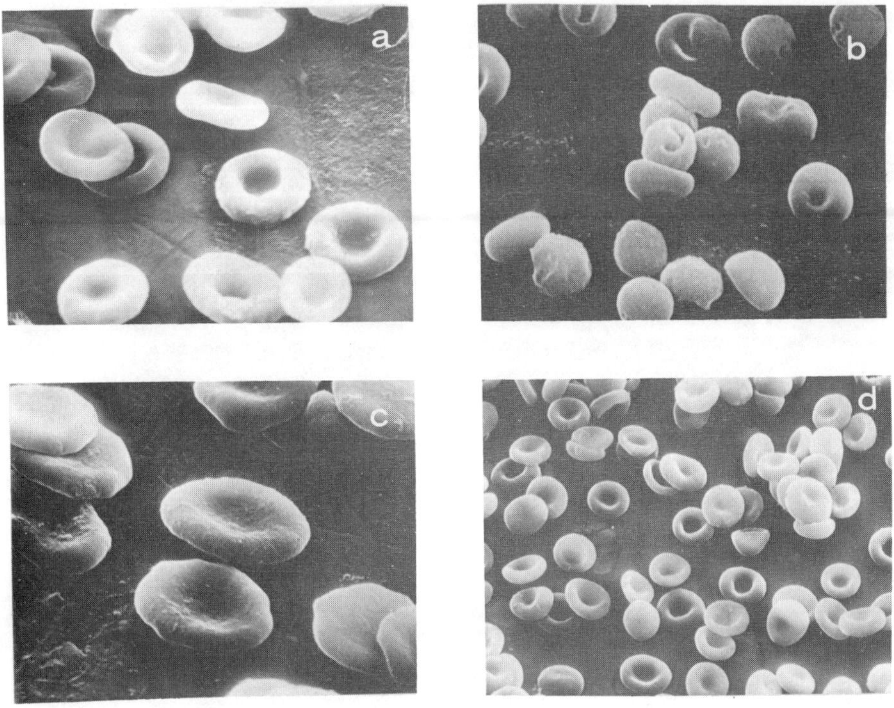

Fig. 5 Scanning micrographs of normal human red cells treated 1 hour in phosphate buffer (10% Hct) with (a) 10^{-3}M PABA (b) 10^{-2}M PABA (c) 10^{-2}M DAE (d) Control

ments reported by us, procaine, PABA or DAE must be replacing calcium or else reducing membrane-bound calcium by some indirect mechanism.

We have shown that treatment of SS erythrocytes with optimum concentrations of procaine, PABA or DAE will delay the formation of ISC in vitro by altering the deformability. Little is known concerning the specific mechanism by which procaine, PABA, or DAE influence red cell deformability. The positively charged anesthetics are known to compete with and displace membrane-bound calcium (Kwant and Seeman, 1969) and such calcium apparently plays an important role in determining membrane deformability (Weed, LaCelle and Merrill, 1969). It is not clear whether the calcium binding sites involve the protein moiety or the lipid moiety or both. Negatively charged molecules (anions) on the other hand, may increase the amount of membrane-bound calcium to phospholipids (Blaustein 1967; Blaustein and Goldman, 1966). The filtration data of Fig. 2 indicate that in the presence of paraaminobenzoic acid at a concentration of 10^{-3}M, deoxygenated SS cells lose deformability at a slower rate than otherwise would occur during 37°C incubation. It may be concluded either that PABA influences the amount of membrane-bound calcium by competing for negatively charged sites, or that PABA is having an effect on deformability by some mechanism which does not directly involve calcium.

In all of the experiments reported here, involving SS cells, procaine HCl was added to whole blood, where it was presumably hydrolyzed to PABA and DAE by plasma and membrane cholinesterase. The hydrolysis of the procaine could be avoided by the use of a cholinesterase inhibitor. Inhibitors were not used in this preliminary study. Therefore, the interpretation of the data pertaining to added procaine must take into account the fact that the effects observed were probably due to a mixture of procaine, PABA and DAE in unknown proportions.

The use of a reducing agent to induce the deoxygenation state merits discussion. Many workers use nitrogen for this purpose. Mixtures of 95%N_2-5%CO_2 (Jensen, Shohet and Nathan, 1973; Bertles and Dobler, 1969) have been most frequently employed. A reducing agent such as sodium metabisulfite will sickle 90-100% of SS cells in contrast to the lower efficiency of nitrogen deoxygenation. However, the effects of this chemical are not confined to its reducing properties. Additional effects include a drop in pH from 7.4 to 6.6 for a 2:1 mixture of bisulfite-blood. The enzyme 2, 3DPG phosphatase is optimally active at pH 6.5 (de Verdier, 1964). Also Parker, (1969) has shown a reversible increase in passive permeability to K and Na ions as a result of bisulfite treatment. The data on normal deoxygenated red cells shown in

Fig. 1 indicate that within an incubation period of 1 hour the bisulfite is having no effect on cell deformability.

Since Serjeant (1969) has shown that the numbers of ISC's observed do correlate with red cell survival, a demonstration of decreased numbers of ISC in vitro could be a useful monitor of therapeutic effectiveness of agents such as procaine, PABA or DAE. Even more significant would be a finding of greater cell deformability throughout the life span of the SS cells, which might well modify the clinical course of the disease.

SUMMARY

Changes in deformability of sickle cells and normal red cells induced by procaine hydrochloride, p-aminobenzoic acid and diethylaminoethanol have been measured by Nuclepore filtration. The rate of formation of irreversibly sickled cells in vitro was decreased by treatment of SS cells with 10^{-4}M procaine HCl, 10^{-3}M p-aminobenzoic acid, or 10^{-2}M diethylaminoethanol. 6mM procaine HCl protected normal red cells against deformability loss associated with metabolic depletion. Normal red cell ghosts produced by hemolysis in 2mM $CaCl_2$ plus 6mM procaine HCl were as deformable as ghosts prepared in calcium-free medium; in contrast to the 7-fold longer filter time of ghosts prepared in 2mM $CaCl_2$.

ACKNOWLEDGEMENTS

It is a pleasure to acknowledge the excellent technical assistance of Meredith Cox and Sylvia Lee. This work was supported in part by NIH grant HL 15162 and grants from the Robert E. and Mary R. Wright Foundation and the Professional Staff Association of the Los Angeles County-USC Medical Center.

REFERENCES

Baker, Richard, Powars, Darleen and L. Julian Haywood (1974) Restoration of the Deformability of "Irreversibly" Sickled Cells by Procaine Hydrochloride. Biochem. Biophys. Res. Comm. 59:548.

Bertles, J.F. and Dobler, J. (1969) Reversible and Irreversible Sickling: A Distinction by Electron Microscopy. Blood 33:884.

Blaustein (1967) Phospholipids an Ion Exchangers: Implications for a Possible Role in Biological Membrane Excitability and Anesthesia. Biochim Biophys Acta 135:653.

Blaustein, M.P. and Goldman, D.E. (1966) Competitive Action of Calcium and Procaine on Lobster. Axon. 49:1043.

Deuticke, B. (1968) Transformation and Restoration of Biconcave Shape of Human Erythrocytes Induced by Amphilic Agents and Changes of Ionic Environment. Biochim Biophys Acta 163:494.

de Verdier, C.H. (1964) Purification of 2, 3-Diphosphoglycerate Phosphatase from Human Erythrocytes. Biochem J. 92:38.

Diggs, L.W. and Bibb, J. (1939) The Erythrocyte in Sickle Cell Anemia. J.M.S. 112:695.

Eaton, J.W., Skelton, T.D., Swofford, H.S., Kolpin, C.E., and Jacob, H.S. (1973) Elevated Erythrocyte Calcium in Sickle Cell Disease. Nature 246:105

Ingram, V.M. (1956) A Specific Chemical Difference Between the Globins of Normal Human and Sickle Cell Anemia Haemoglobins. Nature 178:792.

Jensen, M., Shohet, S.B., and Nathan, D.G. (1973) The Role of Red Cell Energy Metabolism in the Generation of Irreversibly Sickled Cells in Vitro. Blood 42:835.

Kwant, W.O. and Seeman, P. (1969) The Displacement of Membrane Calcium by a Local Anesthetic (Chlorpromazine). Biochim Biophys Acta 193:338.

Lessin, L.S. and Wallas, G.H. (1974) Biochemical Basis for Membrane Alterations in Irreversibly Sickled Cells (ISC).First National Symposium on Sickle Cell Disease, Washington, D.C., June 27-29, 1974.

Padilla, F., Bromberg, P.A., and Jensen, W.N. (1973) The Sickle-Unsickle Cycle: A Cause of Cell Fragmentation

Leading to Permanently Deformed Cells. Blood 41:653.
Parker, J.C. (1969) Influence of 2, 3-Diphosphoglycerate Metabolism on Sodium Potassium Permability in Human Red Blood Cells: Studies with Bisulfite and Other Redox Reagents. J. Clin. Invest. 48:117.
Pauling, L., Itano, H.A., Singer, S.J., and Wells, I.C. (1949) Sickle Cell Anemia, a Molecular Disease. Science 110:543.
Seeman, P. (1972) The Membrane Actions of Anesthetics and Tranquilizers in Pharmacological Reviews. Williams and Wilkins Press 24, #4:583.
Serjeant, G.R., Serjeant, B.E., and Milner, P.F. (1969) The Irreversibly Sickled Cell: A Determinant of Hemolysis in Sickle Cell Anemia. Br. J. Haem. 17:527.
Shen, S.C., Fleming, E.M., and Castle, W.B. (1949) Studies on the Destruction of Red Blood Cells Irreversibly Sickled Erythrocytes: Their Experimental Production in Vitro. Blood 4:498.
Weed, R.I., LaCelle, P.L., and Merrill, E.W. (1969) The Metabolic Dependence of Red Cell Deformability. J. Clin. Invest. 48:795.

DISCUSSION

Dr. Minakami: Did you check for a change in the oxygen dissocation curve after treatment with Procaine?

Dr. Baker: That is one of the many things we haven't done. We badly need to do ATP and 2,3-DPG levels and dissociation curves as well, but we just haven't had time to do these things yet.

Dr. Minakami: I'd like to point to one experiment we did, not on sickle cells but on normal cells, with procaine and other local anesthetics in regard to the effect on membranes. We did not measure the oxygen dissociation curve, simply because the effect on the membrane might not necessarily show on the dissociation curve. Instead we measured the kinetics of oxygen dissociation from the red cells after incubation in these local anesthetics. Interestingly, the concentration range we worked on was pretty much the same as yours. We found out, that the kinetics doubled after two hours of incubation in Novacaine, in this case, about 10^{-3} to 10^{-5} M. Therefore, this may also be added evidence that these local anesthetics can really modify the structure of membranes at the molecular level.

Dr. LaCelle: Dr. Seeman spoke of anesthetics expanding membranes to increase the area to volume ratio. I wonder if you looked at volumes or if you think this is a mechanism. I raise this question because when people filter cyanate cells they feel they've improved filtration by cyanate treatment, but actually they may have reduced the volume substantially and so the improved filtration is a function of the volume decrease.

Dr. Baker: We have not made detailed studies of volume. However, the filtration time of cells with the added agent was the same as the cells without the agent, which we took to mean that the volume hadn't changed appreciably at zero time.

HUMAN SICKLE CELLS IN A HETEROLOGOUS SPECIES: A MODEL FOR THE SCREENING OF ANTI-SICKLING AGENTS

Oswaldo Castro, Richard Roth, Jerome Orlin
and Stuart C. Finch
Yale University School of Medicine
Department of Internal Medicine
333 Cedar Street, New Haven, Ct. 06510

Erythrocyte (RBC) sickling is thought to be an important cause of the decreased RBC life-span and of the recurrent vaso-occlusive episodes in patients with sickle cell anemia. Compounds that interfere with RBC sickling such as urea (1), cyanate (1), carbamyl phosphate (2), nitrogen mustard (3) and zinc (4) have been recently the subject of extensive *in vitro* investigation. Understanding the mechanisms of their anti-sickling effect could lead to the development of agents that may be useful in the treatment of sickle cell anemia. The toxicity of these compounds can be estimated by examining their effects on human RBCs *in vitro* and their systemic effects in animals. Assessment of the effectiveness of an anti-sickling compound has been largely dependent on human studies. A heterologous transfusion technique that allows study of the behavior of abnormal human RBCs after transfusion into rats has been developed recently. In this model, the behavior of erythrocytes from patients with sickle cell anemia (SS RBCs) is different from that of human RBCs from subjects without hemoglobin abnormalities in two important respects: (a) The ^{51}Cr T 1/2 survival of SS RBCs transfused into rats is shorter than that of control RBCs (5), and (b) the total number of SS RBCs circulating in the animal at a given time is dependent on the amount of oxygen the rats breathe (6). This phenomenon-- not observed with control RBCs-- is due presumably to the presence among human SS RBCs of a population of cells that is readily removed from the rats' circulation by lowering oxygen tension and released back into circulation by increasing pO_2. In this communication we report the use of the above characteristics of SS RBCs to study the effectiveness of anti-sickling compounds *in vivo*.

METHODS

The general design of our experiments involved *in vitro* treatment of SS RBCs and of control human RBCs with either sodium cyanate, zinc chloride or nitrogen mustard, labeling the human RBCs with ^{51}Cr and tranfusing them into ethyl palmitate and cobra venom factor treated rats. The post transfusion survival characteristics of the labeled human RBCs was then determined by radioassay of sequential blood samples from rats kept in room air or exposed to varying oxygen concentrations.

Erythrocytes from 9 patients (2 children and 7 adults) were studied. All had sickle cell anemia as determined by a characteristic clinical picture and Hb electrophoresis. Their ages varied between 1 and 37 years. The RBCs from 7 adult volunteers without hematologic abnormalities were used as controls. All blood samples were collected in acid-citrate-dextrose solution and either studied immediately or after storage for 1 to 4 days in ACD at $4^{o}C$ under sterile conditions.

The treatment of RBCs with cyanate has been previously described (7). Briefly, the RBCs were incubated with 50 mM sodium cyanate at $37^{o}C$ for 90 min. and then washed three times with isotonic saline before transfusion. This treatment resulted in the carbamylation of the amino terminal valine by 2.0 cyanate residues per mole of hemoglobin tetramer.

The zinc study was carried out as follows: equal volumes of blood and a $ZnCl_2$ solution in phosphate buffered saline (PBS), pH 7.4 were mixed so that the final $ZnCl_2$

concentration was 1.5 mM. The mixture was incubated for 2 hours at 37°C with occasional shaking. Non-treated SS- and control RBCs were incubated under the same conditions except that zinc chloride was not added to the PBS solution. The RBCs were washed x 3 with isotonic saline and adjusted to a final suspension of 50% with isotonic saline before transfusion.

Nitrogen mustard (mechlorethamine, USP) was dissolved in PBS solution, pH 7.4 to a concentration of 2.0 mg/ml. This solution was immediately added to an equal volume of whole blood. This was then followed by incubation and RBC washing as described above for zinc chloride.

Labeling of the human RBCs with ^{51}Cr (sodium chromate, 50 µCi per ml of whole blood) took place during the last 30 min. of incubation of the above mixtures. The final ^{51}Cr RBC suspension in saline was injected intravenously at a dose of 1-2.5 ml of packed RBCs/kg rat wt into rats that had been pretreated with 0.5 to 3.0 g/kg of ethyl palmitate, a blocker of RES phagocytic function, and with 10 units of cobra venom factor, an inhibitor of the 3rd component of complement. Fifteen minutes after transfusion and at sequential intervals thereafter, 10 to 20 microliter capillary blood samples were obtained from the cut surface of the rats' tails and their radioactivity plotted in semilogarithmic paper to determine the ^{51}Cr blood T 1/2 of the transfused human erythrocytes. A minimum of 2 rats was used for each patient and control study. Studies were carried out both in room air and during exposure of the recipient rats to alternating 30 min. periods during which they breathed either 100% O_2 or 7.5% O_2.

RESULTS:

In room air, the mean ^{51}Cr T 1/2 survival of untreated SS RBCs was 9.09 hours (±4.30 hours SD) while the mean survival of control human RBCs was 22.25 hours (range: 15.6 to 31.6 hours). Table I shows the effect of the *in vitro* treatment of SS- and control RBCs with anti-sickling agents on their room air ^{51}Cr survival. Sodium cyanate,

TABLE I: EFFECT OF *IN VITRO* TREATMENT OF SICKLE CELLS WITH CYANATE, ZINC AND NITROGEN MUSTARD ON THEIR ^{51}Cr SURVIVAL AFTER TRANSFUSION INTO RATS

RBCs	Anti-Sickling Agent (concentration)		% change in RBC survival after treatment
Patient 1	Sodium Cyanate (50 mM)		+ 60
2	"		+ 50
3	"		+375
4	"		+120
		Mean	+152 ($P < 0.1$)*
Control human RBCs		Mean of 3 subjects	-20
Patient 4	Zinc Chloride (1.5 mM)		+ 46
5	"		+ 19
6	"		+ 45
		Mean	+ 36.6 ($P < 0.05$)*
Control human RBCs		Mean of 2 subjects	-3.5
Patient 4	Nitrogen Mustard (1 mg/ml)		+ 28.1
5	"		+ 5.1
7	"		+ 10.5
8	"		+ 16.8
9	"		+ 8.6
		Mean	+ 13.82 ($P < 0.05$)*
Control human RBCs		Mean of 2 subjects	-15

*t test on paired samples

zinc chloride and nitrogen mustard each resulted in a statistically significant increase in the survival of SS RBCs expressed as percent change from the value for untreated SS RBCs from the same patients. Although there was a great deal of patient variability, the most marked increases were observed with cyanate treatment, the smallest changes with nitrogen mustard and intermediate values with zinc chloride. Only one patient was studied with all three drugs and the degree of improvement in the ^{51}Cr survival with cyanate (+120%), zinc (+46%) and nitrogen mustard (+28%) paralleled that for each drug in the patient groups. When rats transfused with SS RBCs were exposed to alternating hyperoxia and hypoxia periods an oxygen "sensitive" population of SS RBCs was detected in each patient: Blood ^{51}Cr activity rose and fell by 20 to 40% during exposure of the animals to 100% O_2 and 7.5% O_2, respectively. This phenomenon was not affected by previous *in vitro* treatment of the SS RBCs with any of the drugs tested.

The ^{51}Cr survival of control AA RBCs was not increased by the *in vitro* treatment with cyanate, zinc or nitrogen mustard. There was evidence of a modest shortening of the ^{51}Cr survival after *in vitro* treatment with the drugs but the small number of studies carried out with each individual agent did not allow statistical analysis.

DISCUSSION:

We have shown that chemical agents that inhibit sickling *in vitro* also prolong the intravascular survival of human sickle cells transfused into rats. This effect was not observed with transfused human RBCs not containing hemoglobin S, suggesting that the improved survival of sickle cells was due to decreased sickling *in vivo*. The anti-sickling action of sodium cyanate is due largely to increase in hemoglobin oxygen affinity as a result of specific carbamylation of the N-terminal groups of hemoglobin by cyanate. The survival of cyanate-treated erythrocytes from patients with sickle cell anemia in autologous human recipients is prolonged. With degrees of hemoglobin carbamylation comparable to those used in the present study, the mean ^{51}Cr T 1/2 of cyanate-treated SS RBCs increased by 109% (8) and mean life span of carbamylated SS RBCs increased by 92% (9). The degree of improvement in the survival of sickle cells in humans following in vitro carbamylation is similar to that observed in rat recipients. This similarity suggests that the animal model may be useful in predicting the survival of human sickle cells treated in vitro with anti-sickling compounds. Zinc chloride probably inhibits sickling by two mechanisms: the oxygen affinity of hemoglobin S is increased by zinc at high doses (4); in addition, at low doses, zinc may interfere with the binding of hemoglobin to the erythrocyte membrane (10). The improvement in ^{51}Cr survival of zinc treated sickle cells in the rats could be due to both of these zinc effects. Nitrogen mustard inhibits hemoglobin S gelation but the precise mechanism of this "anti-sickling" action has not been identified. A direct alteration of the β6 valine region that interferes with hemoglobin S polymerization may be responsible for the anti-sickling effect (11).

The prolongation of the ^{51}Cr survival of sickle cells with zinc and with nitrogen mustard was considerably less than that observed with cyanate treatment. Therefore, of the three drugs tested, cyanate appears to be the most effective agent for enhancement of the post-transfusion life span of extracorporeally treated sickle cells.

It is important to emphasize that the hemolytic process in sickle cell anemia, although severe, is not as important in determining morbidity and mortality as are the recurrent, painful vaso-occlusive episodes. The clinical experience with patients who have, in addition to homozygous sickle cell anemia, the "Memphis" abnormality on their α chains, illustrates this point. These patients, although severely anemic, are largely asymptomatic because they do not have vaso-occlusive crisis (12).

None of the drugs tested in the present study affected the reversible loss of a proportion of sickle cells from the animals' blood during severe hypoxia. Preliminary experiments in our laboratory indicate that this loss is largely due to the trapping of oxygen-sensitive (presumably sickled) erythrocytes in the livers and spleens of the hypoxic animals. The precise significance of this phenomenon in terms of human physiopathology is presently under investigation. If the trapping of human SS RBCs in the liver and spleen of hypoxic rats were a model for human vaso-occlusive or sequestration crises, our findings would indicate that the anti-sickling agents studied, while effective in decreasing <u>in vivo</u> hemolysis, may not be helpful in preventing or treating vaso-occlusive episodes in sickle cell anemia. Further experiments will have to determine whether the systemic administration of the same anti-sickling compounds to rats transfused with human sickle cells is a more effective way of preventing their sequestration in the microvasculature of hypoxic animals.

Our studies suggest that this animal model can be helpful in investigating the <u>in vivo</u> effectiveness of chemical agents that inhibit erythrocyte sickling, thus avoiding the risks associated with human experimentation.

SUMMARY:

The ^{51}Cr survival of human sickle erythrocytes treated <u>in vitro</u> with either sodium cyanate, zinc chloride or nitrogen mustard was determined after transfusion into RES-blocked and complement depleted rats. Each drug resulted in significant enhancement of the survival of treated sickle cells when compared to that of untreated cells. The greatest effect was observed with cyanate. The proportion of human sickle cells that was reversibly sequestered from the rats' circulation during severe hypoxia was not decreased by treatment with any of the drugs studied. This heterologous transfusion system appears to be a workable model for the screening of anti-sickling drugs.

REFERENCES:

1) Segel, G.B., Feig, S.A., Mentzer, W.C., McCaffrey, R.P., et al. (1972). Effects of urea and cyanate on sickling *in vitro*. *New Engl. J. Med.* *287*:59.

2) Kraus, L.M., Rasad, A., Friedman, B.I., Avis, K.E., et al. (1972). Sickle cell anemia: carbamyl phosphate an affinity labeling agent prolongs red cell survival. *Blood* *40*:928 (abstr.).

3) Roth, E.F. Jr., Nagel, R.L., Bookchin, R.M. and Grayzel, A.I. (1972). Nitrogen mustard: an "in vitro" inhibitor of erythrocyte sickling. *Biochem. Biophys. Res. Commun.* *48*:612.

4) Oelshlegel, F.J. Jr., Brewer, G.J., Prasad, A.S., Knutsen, C., et al. (1973). Effect of zinc on increasing oxygen affinity of sickle and normal red blood cells. *Biochem. Biophys. Res. Commun.* *53*:560.

5) Castro, O., Orlin, J., Rosen, M.W. and Finch, S.C. (1973). Survival of human sickle-cell erythrocytes in heterologous species: response to variations in oxygen tension. *Proc. Nat. Acad. Sci. USA* *70*:2356.

6) Castro, O., Orlin, J., Rosen, M.W. and Finch, S.C. (1974). Oxygen dependent circulation of sickle cells. *Clin. Res.* *22*:386A (abstr.).

7) Castro, O., Orlin, J., and Finch, S.C. (1974). The effect of hemoglobin carbamylation on the survival of human sickle cell erythrocytes in rats. *Yale J. Biol. Med.* *47*:55.

8) Gillette, P.N., Manning, J.M., and Cerami, A. (1971). Increased survival of sickle-cell erythrocytes after treatment *in vitro* with sodium cyanate. *Proc. Nat. Acad. Sci. USA* *68*:2791.

9) Milner, P.F. and Charache, S. (1973). Life span of

carbamylated red cells in sickle cell anemia. J. Clin. Invest. 52:3161.

10) Brewer, G.J., Dash, S., and Oelshlegel, F.J. Jr. (1974). The effect of zinc on hemoglobin binding by red blood cell membranes. J. Clin. Invest. 53:11a (abstr.).

11) Roth, E.F. Jr., Nagel, R.L., Bookchin, R.M. and Jaffe, E. (1974). The effects of nitrogen and sulfur mustards on hemoglobin S and on intact red cells. Abstracts of the First National Symposium on Sickle Cell Disease, DHEW Pub. No. (NIH) 74-704.

12) Cooper, M.R., Kraus, A.P., Felts, J.H., Ramseur, W.L., et al. (1973). A third case of hemoglobin Memphis/ sickle cell disease: whole blood viscosity used as a screening test. Am. J. Med. 55:535.

DISCUSSION

Dr. Brewer: How did you do the zinc experiments?

Dr. Castro: We mixed whole blood with a solution of zinc chloride so that the final concentration was 1.5 mM. Phosphate buffered saline was used in order to obtain a pH of 7.4. Blood and zinc were incubated for 2 hours at 37° C. following which the red cells were labeled with 51 chromium, washed three times and then suspended in normal saline.

Dr. Diederich: In patient studies sequential chromium studies are fraught with great difficulty. Do you not have that problem in your model? My question would be: Have you done dual labels of treated and untreated cells in the same animal simultaneously?

Dr. Castro: No, we have not. We have tried to label red cells with technetium and chromium at the same time and found that technetium is a very good way of damaging human red cells. I suspect that a better approach might be to label non-treated cells with iodine and treated cells with chromium before injection into the same animal. Obviously this would be the ideal experiment but we haven't done this yet.

Dr. Glader: May I ask a question which is not related directly to your paper, Dr. Castro, but relative to all the sickle papers and may tie in with the membrane papers which we're going to hear this afternoon. Whenever we look at irreversibly sickled cells separated from patients or when we generate them *in vitro*, invariably there is cellular dehydration and marked potassium loss. I think this is fairly characteristic of ISC's. One of our questions is whether cellular dehydration, which might lead to a viscous intracellular milieu, may in any way be responsible for ISC formation or is it merely an effect of this cellular distortion? Although we all think in terms of ISC formation being primarily a membrane phenomenon, the question we are asking is whether or not the viscous intracellular medium could be partially responsible. Basically what we have done is generated irreversibly sickled cells *in vitro*, either by prolonged incubation in nitrogen or with short exposures to propanolol and calcium. We then compared ISC formation in a potassium buffer versus a sodium buffer. In the presence of sodium there is marked K and water loss and increased ISC production. Under the same conditions, in the cells incubated in a potassium buffer, we observed no K or water loss and there was no ISC formation. Preliminary evidence suggests there is an increased calcium content in both of these membranes. So what we are left with is the concept that the increased intracellular viscosity is partially responsible for the morphologic alterations resulting in the irreversibly sickled cell. The changes in the membrane *per se* seem to be of secondary importance. I'd appreciate any feedback on this.

Dr. Nagel: I don't intend to answer the question, but to point out one fact. When you prepare ghosts from irreversibly sickled cells, they have properties that are different from ghosts prepared from other layers of the same blood. So if the membrane changes are not the whole story, they are at least a good part of it.

PROGRESS IN UNDERSTANDING CELL MEMBRANES

Chairman: P. L. La Celle

VASOACTIVE HORMONES AND THE HUMAN ERYTHROCYTE

Howard Rasmussen, William Lake, Greg Gasic, and James Allen

University of Pennsylvania
Department of Biochemistry, School of Medicine
Philadelphia, Pennsylvania 19174

The human red blood cell has been one of the most intensively studied of human tissues, both because of its ready availability, its relatively simple metabolic properties, and because, in particular, it has been a source of a relatively uncontaminated plasma membrane preparation. Studies of these red cell membranes have been of central importance in developing concepts of membrane structure and function (Bretscher, 1973; Hanahan, 1973; Reynolds, 1973; Singer and Nicolson, 1972; Steck, 1974; Zwaal, _et al_., 1974).

In spite of this intensive study, additional properties of these membranes continue to be discovered. For example, these cells have not generally been considered target cells for mammalian hormone action. Yet recently, Roth (1973) has described the presence of peptide hormone receptors on their surfaces, indicating that they share an additional feature in common with many fixed tissue cells. However, the receptors discovered by Roth (1973) have not yet been shown to have a functional significance. Hence, it can be argued that, at best, they represent the remnant of an earlier evolutionary function.

In this report we wish to discuss another type of receptor on the human red blood cell - a receptor for the vasoactive hormones, catecholamines and prostaglandins, and for exogenous cyclic adenosine monophosphate (cAMP), which are functional in the sense that hormone (or nucleotide) receptor-interaction leads to a change in cell properties and cell volume.

These hormonal effects are of interest on three accounts. First, they open up a new possibility for exploring the mechanisms underlying the control of cell membrane properties; second, they offer a simpler cell model in which to explore the mode of action of these hormones; and, third, they raise the possibility that hormonal control of red cell properties may be a component of a system underlying the control of the microcirculation.

Our studies to date (Allen and Rasmussen, 1971, 1972) have been concerned solely with the first two of these areas, and we have yet to address the third. These studies have concentrated first on establishing the basic fact that human red cells do, in fact, respond to the hormones with a change in structure and function, and, second, on attempts to establish the mechanism underlying these responses.

Although the first task appeared relatively easy, it was not. Considerable difficulties in obtaining reproducible results were encountered until we realized that the responsiveness of cells from female donors to these hormones varied with the menstrual cycle (Allen and Rasmussen, 1972). All of the subsequent studies have been carried out on washed red cells obtained from healthy young male donors. The results have been highly reproducible.

A major aspect of the second part of our studies concerning mechanism has centered around the possible role of cyclic AMP (Guthrow, et al., 1972; Guthrow, et al.,1973), and,to a lesser extent, calcium ion in these responses. In spite of considerable progress in these studies, we cannot as yet clearly define the mechanism of these changes nor the precise role of cAMP in them.

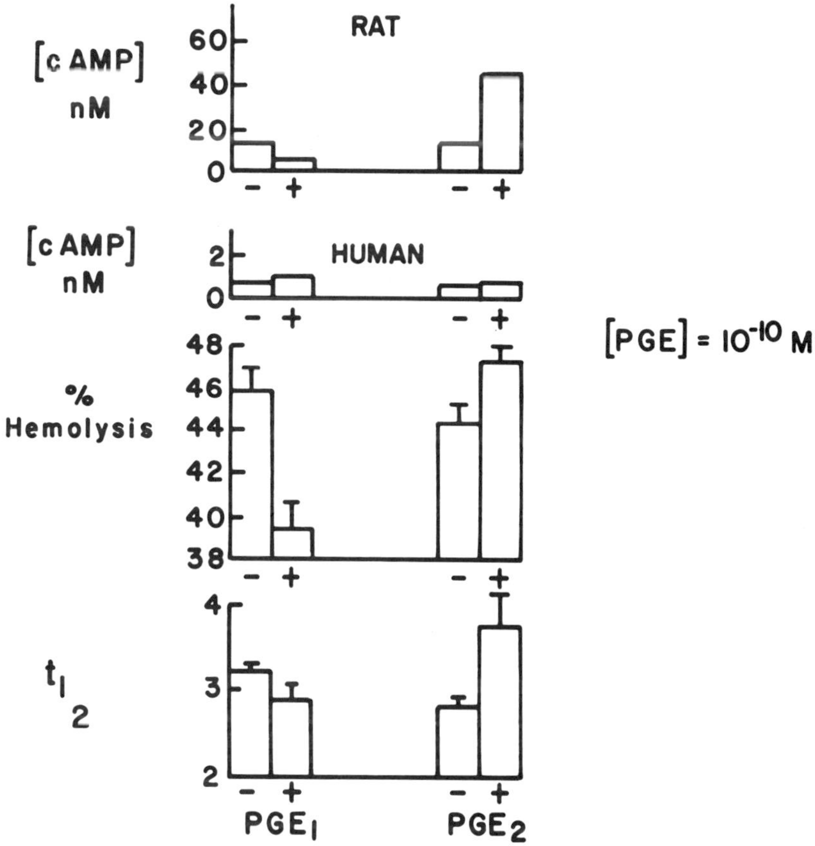

Figure 1. The effect of the addition of 10^{-10} M PGE_1 (left) and PGE_2 (right) to washed human erythrocytes upon cyclic adenosine 3'5'-monophosphate (cAMP) content, percent hemolysis under standard conditions, and the halftime ($t\frac{1}{2}$) of filterability of packed cells. Also shown are the effects of PGE_1 and PGE_2 upon cAMP content of washed rat erythrocytes.

PROSTAGLANDIN E_2 AND E_1 EFFECTS

Initial hormonal effects were observed using as the index of response the filterability of cells through standard paper filters (Allen and Rasmussen, 1971, 1972). The initial observations were that addition of catecholamines or prostaglandin E_2 in appropriate concentrations to washed human cells led to a decrease in their filterability (Fig. 1), and that PGE_1 addition led to an increase (Allen and Rasmussen, 1971, 1972). However, it is difficult to measure graded responses with this technique, so other means were sought. It was then found that the addition of catecholamines or prostaglandin E_2 led to an increase, and PGE_1 to a decrease in osmotic fragility (Fig. 1).

Similar effects of these two prostaglandins and catecholamines were found when washed red cells from young rats were employed. Because of these facts, and the fact that both PGE_2 and epinephrine had been shown to stimulate an adenylate cyclase in rodent erythrocyte ghosts (Sheppard and Burghardt, 1969), the effect of the prostaglandins on the content of cyclic adenosine monophosphate (cAMP) in human red cells was examined. Neither PGE_1 nor PGE_2, in concentrations sufficient to induce maximal changes in either filterability or hypotonic hemolysis, altered the cAMP concentration, either within the human red cells (Fig. 1) or in the incubation medium of these cells. In contrast, addition of PGE_1 to washed rat red cells caused a fall, and addition of PGE_2 a rise, in the cAMP content (Fig. 1). Thus, in the rat cell cAMP appeared to be a second messenger in hormone action, but in human cells this evidence suggested it was not. (This point will be more fully explored below.)

Further exploration of the dose-response characteristic of prostaglandin action revealed that the dose-response curve with either PGE_1 or PGE_2, as measured by change in hypotonic hemolysis, was biphasic (Fig. 2). Addition of 10^{-11} to 10^{-9} M PGE_1 led to a significant decrease in hypotonic hemolysis, but at 10^{-9} and 10^{-8} M hypotonic hemolysis was equal to or greater than in control cells. Conversely, 10^{-11} to 10^{-10} M PGE_2 led to a significant increase in

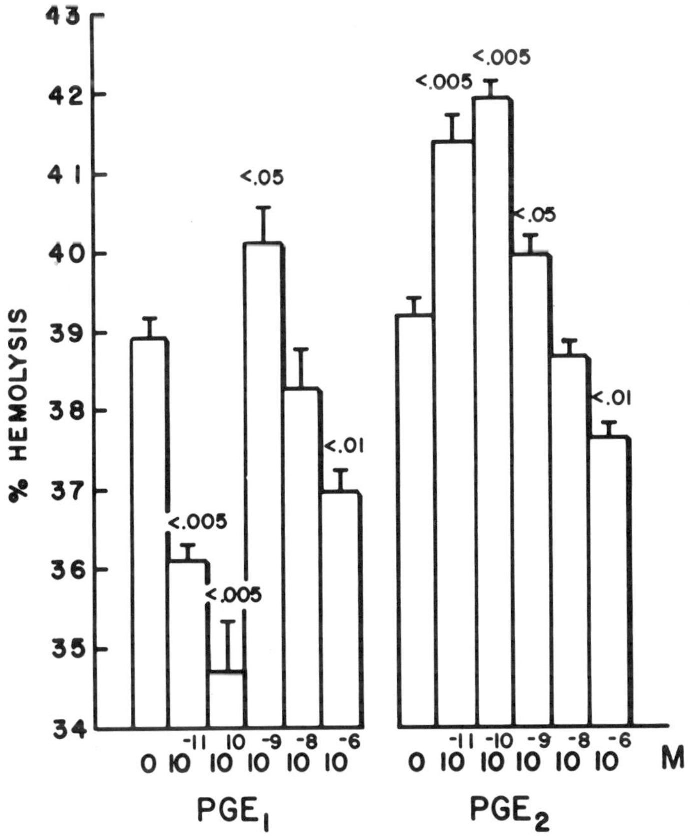

Fig. 2. The percent hemolysis of washed human red cells add to 0.46% NaCl in the absence (0) and presence of increasing concentrations of PGE_1 (left) and PGE_2(right). The results are recorded as mean±SEM. The numbers(e.g.,<.005)above the bars indicate the values which were significantly different from the values seen in absence of prostaglandin addition.

hypotonic hemolysis, whereas high doses were either less effective, ineffective, or caused a slight decrease in hemolysis.

The effective doses of these agents are particularly noteworthy. Our calculations indicate that 1 molecule per cell is sufficient to initiate a response, and 10-100 molecules per cell are needed to produce a maximal response. The effective concentrations of catecholamines (see below) are approximately one order of magnitude higher (100-1000 molecules per cell).

The hormonally-induced changes in filterability and hypotonic hemolysis could result from one of two general mechanisms: either a change in cell volume, or a change in the intrinsic deformability of the cell membrane. In an effort to determine if the former were a factor, two types of experiments were carried out. One was to measure the ion content of the incubation medium after hormone addition, and the other to measure cell size using a Coulter counter.

In the studies of ion content, washed red cells were incubated at 50% hematocrit, then exposed to either PGE_1 or PGE_2, and the cells then separated from the medium by centrifugation, following which the Na^+ and K^+ content of the medium was measured. As shown in Fig.3, the prostaglandins caused changes in medium electrolyte content: PGE_2 caused an increase in the concentrations of both Na^+ and K^+, whereas PGE_1 caused a decrease. The dose-response characteristics were identical to the dose-response characteristics of the hormone-induced changes in hypotonic hemolysis (Fig.2). These results argue that a change in volume occurred after PGE_2 and PGE_1, with PGE_2 causing an increase and PGE_1 a decrease in cell volume.

Results with the Coulter counter confirm this conclusion (Fig.4). Addition of PGE_2 led to a significant increase in mean red cell size within 4 minutes after PGE_2 addition. These experiments were carried out at very low hematocrits (0.0004%), so the conditions were quite different than those of the ion experiments (50% Hct). Of

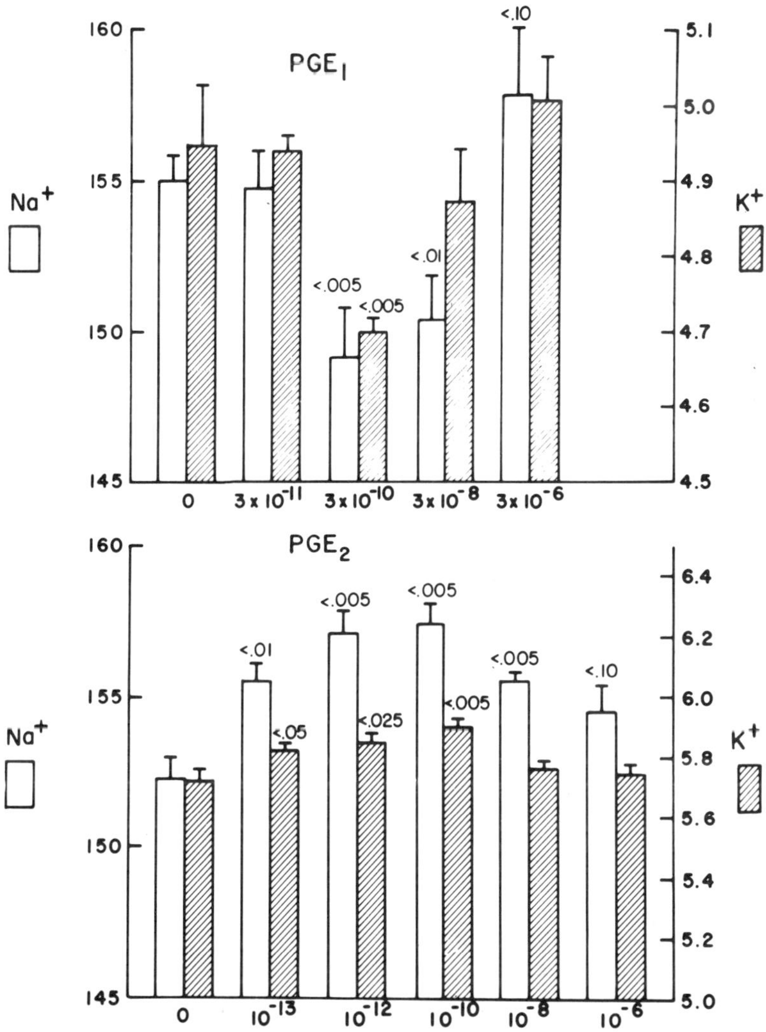

Fig.3. The Na^+ and K^+ contents of the incubation medium of washed human red cells treated with increasing concentrations of PGE_2 and PGE_1. Note that the dose-response pattern seen with this index is similar to that seen when percentage of hemolysis was measured (Fig. 2).

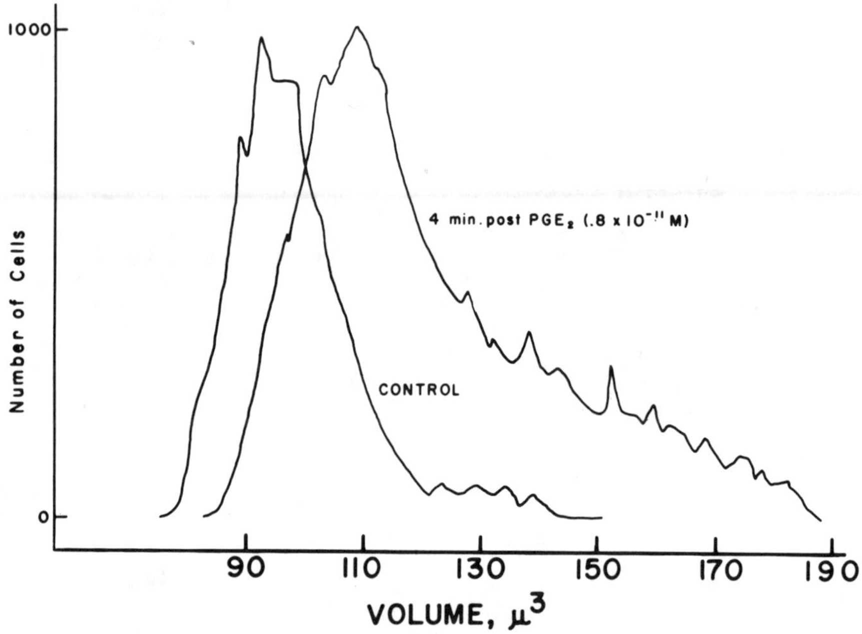

Fig.4. The effect of 8 x 10^{-12} M PGE_2 upon mean cell size as measured in the Coulter counter. Note that 4 min after PGE_2 addition there is a significant shift in the distribution of cell volumes and an increase in mean cell volume.

particular importance is that lower concentrations of PGE_2 were effective with very low red cell counts as used in the Coulter counter experiments, so that the ratio of hormone molecules to red cell were similar to those in the other studies.

The results shown in Fig.4 are of significance in another way. The results of the studies in which hormone effects were monitored, either by a change in filterability or hypotonic hemolysis, could have been explained by an effect of the hormones on a small subpopulation of the total cell population. The data in Fig. 4 show quite clearly this was not the case. The mean size of the entire cell population increased.

Our initial attempts to demonstrate an effect of PGE_1 on cell volume using the Coulter counter method were

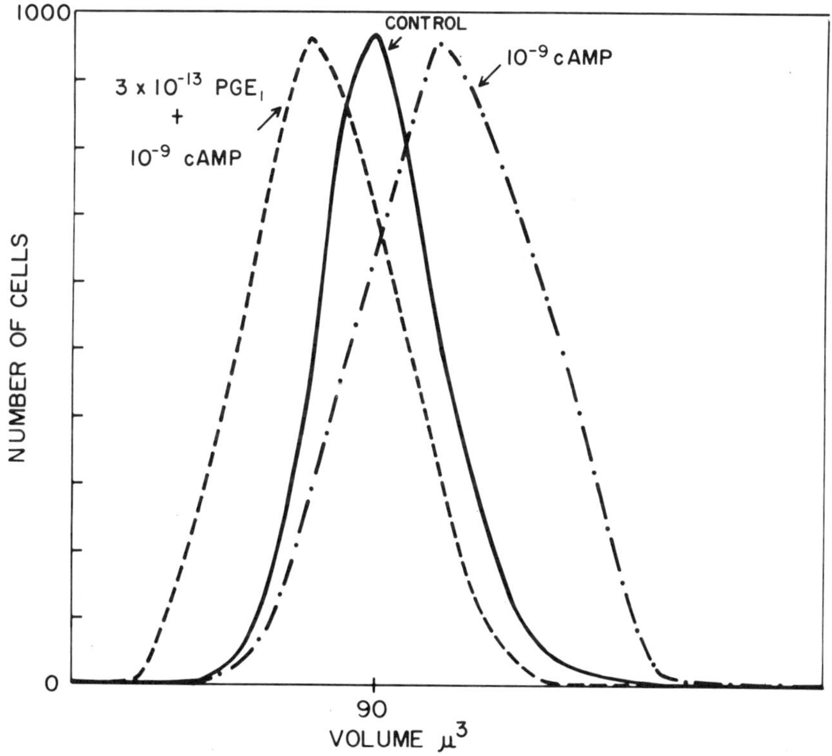

Fig. 5. The effect of exogenous cAMP and PGE_1 upon mean cell volume of washed human erythrocytes as measured in a Coulter counter.

unsuccessful. However, more recently we have been succesful (Fig. 5). When cells were first treated with exogenous cAMP, there was an increase in cell size (Fig.5). Subsequent addition of PGE_1 caused a very marked decrease in mean cell size to a size well below that of the control cells (Fig.5).

These data suggest that PGE_2 caused an increase and PGE_1 a decrease in mean cell size. If this were the case, these changes in cell size could account for the changes in filterability and in hypotonic hemolysis. However, our results do not rule out the possibility that the prostaglandins also alter intrinsic membrane properties. Recently, Kury, McConnell, and Ramwell (1974) have reported that PGE_2 and PGE_1 alter the membrane environment of spin-labeled fatty acids. The effects of the two prostaglandins differ: PGE_1 causes a decrease and PGE_2 an increase in the $t_{1/2}$ for time of relaxation of shear-oriented fatty acid spin-labeled erythrocytes to the disoriented state. Also, PGE_1 decreases and PGE_2 increases the order parameter in the electron spin resonance spectra. This implies that the fatty acid chains are less flexible in the presence of PGE_2 and more flexible in the presence of PGE_1. These results have been interpreted as indicative of a change in membrane structure with PGE_2 causing a decrease and PGE_1 an increase in membrane deformability. These results might simply be a consequence of an altered cell volume and thus be secondary to a PGE-induced change in cell volume.

The results of Kury, _et al._ (1974), were obtained with doses of PGE_1 and PGE_2 similar to those which we employed, and these authors noted a similar biphasic response curve (e.g., Fig. 2). Their experiments represent independent confirmation of our basic observations by a completely different measurement of cell response.

ROLE OF CYCLIC AMP IN CELL RESPONSE

Because of the large body of knowledge linking cAMP to the action of epinephrine and other catecholamines (Sutherland and Rall, 1960; Robison, _et al._, 1971), considerable attention has been devoted to an analysis of

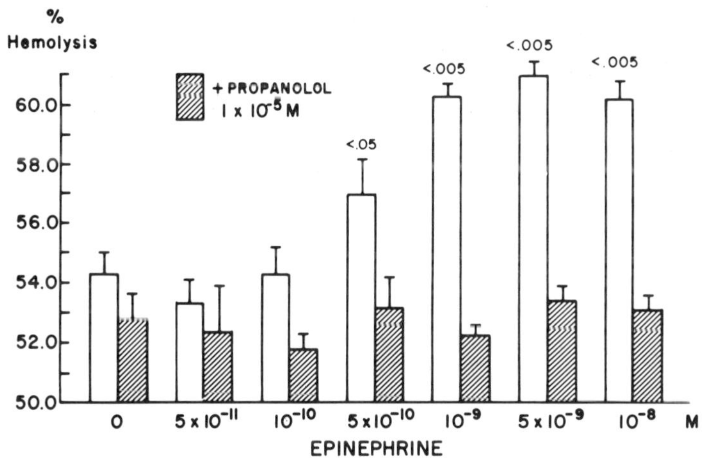

Fig.6. The effect of increasing doses of L-epinephrine upon percent hemolysis of washed human erythrocytes in the presence and absence of 10^{-5} M propranolol.

the possible role of cAMP in the response of the human red cell to catecholamines and PGE_2. In the ensuing discussion attention will be focused upon the catecholamines. Isoproterenol or epinephrine, at a concentration of 10^{-9} M, produced an increase in both the halftime of filterability (decreased filterability)and in hypotonic hemolysis, both in rat and human cells. These effects were similar to those produced by PGE_2(Fig.1). The only difference being that with increasing doses of isoproterenol or epinephrine(Fig.6) there is a monophasic dose response curve: 10^{-8} to 10^{-6} M epinephrine produces the same change in susceptibility to hypotonic hemolysis as does 10^{-9} M,i.e.,there was no inhibition of response with high agonist concentrations as was the case with PGE_2(Fig.2). Just as with PGE_2(Fig.1), so with the catecholamines there was a difference in the response of the rat and human cell to hormone. The addition of isoproterenol to rat but not to human cells caused a rise in cellular cAMP content. These data suggest that cAMP was not a second messenger in the action of catecholamines on the human red cell. However, it remained possible that small undetectable changes in cAMP concentration did occur and were involved in hormone action. To examine this possibility more fully three other types of experiments were conducted: 1)pharmacological characterization of the catecholamine receptor upon the cell surface was carried out; 2)the effect of low concentrations of exogenous cAMP on cell response was examined; and 3)a search was made for cAMP receptor proteins and cAMP-dependent protein kinases in membrane ghosts prepared from human red cells.

The rationale for the first approach was based on the fact that two types of receptors for catecholamines can be identified on the cell surface of mammalian cells(Alhquist, 1959;Himms-Hagen,1967). These are classified as alpha or beta in type, primarily on the ability of certain antagonists to block one or the other type, and on the basis of their agonist specificity toward a variety of natural and synthetic catecholamines. From a great deal of work the generalization has been made that a close coupling exists between β-receptors and adenylate cyclase(Robison,*et al*., 1971).

Isoproterenol and epinephrine were found to be considerably more effective agonists than nor-epinephrine when hypotonic hemolysis was assessed. This result is consistent with the presence of a beta receptor. This conclusion was supported by the results obtained with a beta receptor blocker, propranolol, and an alpha receptor blocker, phentolamine. As shown in Fig. 6, propranolol blocked the effect of isoproterenol, whereas phentolamine had very little effect (not shown). Also, when the hormonal activation of the rat red cell adenylate cyclase was examined, as expected, propranolol blocked and phentolamine did not block the effect of epinephrine on this enzyme.Thus, one is left in the paradoxical situation of identifying in the human red cell a catecholamine receptor having many of the properties of a beta receptor but having no evident coupling to a membrane-bound adenylate cyclase. To be certain of this conclusion, the effect of theophylline upon the response to epinephrine was examined, because this compound blocks the enzyme which catalyzes the hydrolysis of cAMP to 5'-AMP(Sutherland and Rall,1960). Even in the presence of 10mM theophylline, epinephrine did not cause an increase in the cAMP content of the human red cell.

As already indicated(Fig.5), the addition of exogenous cAMP at a concentration of 10^{-9}M led to a significant increase in mean size of human red cells. Also, when its effects upon hypotonic hemolysis and medium ion content were examined, positive effects were observed.

One of the major sites of action of cAMP within cells is thought to be a class of enzymes, protein kinases (Kuo and Greengard,1969;Robison,*et al.*,1971)which catalyze the ATP-dependent phosphorylation of specific proteins. It was found that the addition of cAMP at a concentration of 10^{-6}M led to an activation of a membrane-bound protein kinase and the phosphorylation of specific membrane proteins: increased incorporation of label in band I and a protein between bands IV and V - Fairbank's Notation(Guthrow,*et al.*, 1972). Similar results have also been reported by Ruben and Rosen(1973)and Ruben,*et al.*(1972).Likewise, specific cAMP-binding sites were identified on human red cell ghosts and by employing [^{3}H]N^6-(Ethyl 2-diazomalonyl)-adenosine 3':5'-cyclic monophosphate and photolysis at 253.7nm, it was possible to identify a single cAMP-binding protein(in the same region on the gel as the ^{32}P-labeled product)when the labeled membrane was solubilized and subjected to disc gel electrophoresis in sodium dodecyl sulfate(Guthrow,*etal*,1973).

From all of our evidence in the human red cell we must conclude that a cAMP-responsive biochemical system exists in the membrane, that exogenous cAMP in low concentrations alters membrane structure in a manner qualitatively similar to that induced by catecholamines, and that the catecholamine receptor linked to catecholamine-induced change in cell size has many of the properties of a beta receptor. This evidence argues strongly for a second messenger function of cAMP in catecholamine action on the red cell. However, direct measurement of cell cAMP content after catecholamines have shown no change even in the presence of theophylline. Thus, in spite of all the circumstantial evidence, direct evidence for cAMP as second messenger is lacking.

ROLE OF CALCIUM ION IN CELL RESPONSE

An attractive alternative candidate for a second messenger is calcium ion. Evidence accumulated over the past six years has established that Ca^{2+} does play a critical and general role in cell activation, and that cellular calcium metabolism is regulated in part by cAMP (Rasmussen, 1970; Rasmussen, et al., 1972). Many of the phosphoprotein products of cAMP-dependent protein kinase are calcium-binding proteins, some are enzymes which are Ca^{2+} activated, and some of these enzymes are specific protein kinases. Thus, not only cAMP-dependent but Ca^{2+}-dependent protein kinases are involved in cell regulation.

In addition to this background, there is considerable evidence indicating that the intracellular content of Ca^{2+} in the red cell is low, is maintained low by the expenditure of metabolic energy, and is involved in regulating red cell size and shape (Weed, et al., 1969; LeBlond, et al., 1971; Dunn, 1974). Changes in calcium ion concentration play a critical role in the changes in red cell size and deformability which occur in metabolically-depleted erythrocytes (Weed, et al., 1969; LaCelle, 1970). More recently, Dunn (1974) has shown that increases in cell calcium cause a decrease in mean cell size. Also, ghosts prepared in the presence of calcium had a smaller mean volume than ghosts prepared in its absence (Palek, et al., 1971). Thus, a Ca^{2+}-induced change in membrane structure may underlie the effects of the catecholamines and the prostaglandins on the human erythrocytes. When calcium was removed from the incubation medium the extent of hypotonic hemolysis was greater in the absence of Ca^{2+} than in its presence, and the addition of isoproterenol did not alter the extent of hemolysis. Similar results were obtained with PGE_2 and PGE_1, i.e., no effect in the absence of Ca^{2+}. Likewise, when cells were examined in the Coulter counter in the absence of Ca^{2+}, mean cell size was slightly increased, and PGE_2 addition had no effect. Kury, et al. (1974), using electron spin resonance spectroscopy and spin-labeled fatty acids to assess membrane lipid structure (see above), also showed that the effects of both PGE_1 and PGE_2 were abolished when cells were preincubated in a calcium-free medium. To obtain direct evidence for a hormone-induced change in cell calcium, studies of [^{45}Ca] exchange in isolated cells were undertaken. By incubating cells in a medium containing [^{45}Ca], then delivering aliquots into cold buffer without [^{45}Ca] but containing 2 x 10^{-5}M $LaCl_3$, and washing in this solution several times, it was possible to develop a method for measuring uptake of Ca^{2+} by these cells. Nonetheless, no matter how the experiments were carried out, a significant time-dependent variation in cell [^{45}Ca] content was seen. The content changed with a period of oscillation of 15 seconds, hence it was extremely difficult to obtain accurate information without very large numbers of measurement. However, as shown in Fig. 7, addition of 10^{-9}M isoproterenol caused a decrease in the mean size of this exchangeable pool of calcium and a significant decrease in the amplitude of its oscillation. The size of this exchangeable calcium pool was approximately 1/10 of the size of the total cellular calcium pool. Preliminary results with PGE_2 showed that this hormone also decreased the size of the exchangeable calcium pool. However, the

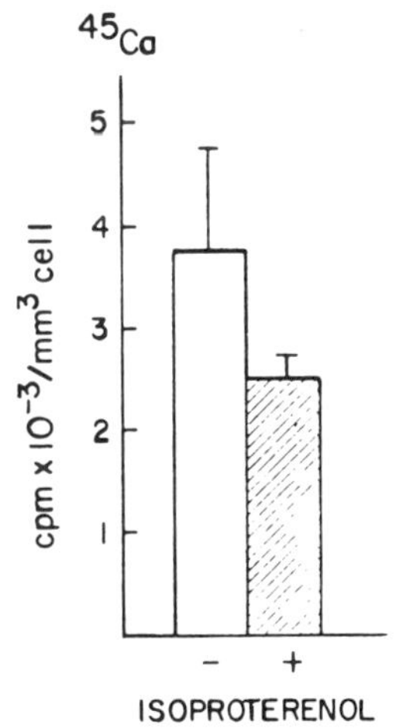

Fig. 7. The effect of isoproterenol upon the mean size of an exchangeable calcium pool in the washed human erythrocyte.

difficulties of making these measurements are such that different ways of measuring calcium exchange are being sought.

On the basis of our present evidence it seems safe to conclude that catecholamines do decrease the size of an exchangeable calcium pool in the red cell (or red cell membrane), that this is associated with an increase in mean red cell size, an increase in red cell deformability, a change in gross lipid structure (Kury, et al., 1974), and a decrease in red cell filterability. In the light of the evidence relating cell calcium to cell size (see above), these data are consistent with a model in which an increase in cell Ca^{2+} is the second messenger in PGE_1 action, and a decrease in cell calcium is the second messenger in PGE_2 and epinephrine action. The means by which such hormone-induced changes in cell calcium alter red cell size and deformability remain to be worked out, but an attractive possibility is that calcium ions regulate the state of aggregation of the proteins of the spectrin complex, which have been located just beneath but coupled to the erythrocyte membrane (Marchesi, et al., 1970; Nicolson, et al., 1971; Steck, 1974) and have been shown to undergo a Ca^{2+}-dependent change in aggregation (Rosenthal, et al., 1970). It has been proposed (Steck, 1974) that protein bands 1, 2, and 5 found in the gel electrophoresis pattern of Triton-X-100-treated red cell membranes constitute a self-associated reticulum of microfilaments adherent to the cytoplasmic surface of the cell membrane. It has also been proposed (Steck, 1974) that this filamentous system could control cell shape and size and, perhaps, respond to extracellular signals (see also Durham, 1974). It is our working hypothesis that this is indeed the subcellular system which is under hormonal control in the human red cell, and that Ca^{2+} plays a role in coupling hormone-receptor interaction to a change in microfilament orientation(Fig.8). It is also possible that a calcium-dependent protein kinase is a component of this sub-membrane reticular system, and that the state of phosphorylation of one or more components of this system controls its state of aggregation. (See Greenquist and Shohet - this volume.)

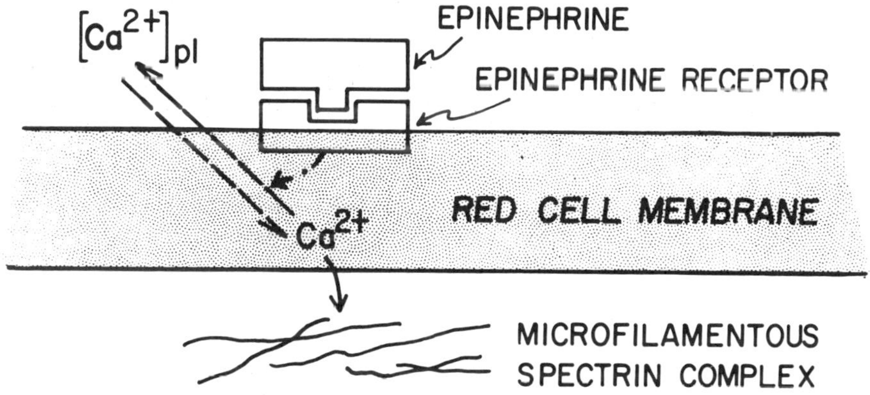

Fig. 8. A proposed model for the action of epinephrine upon the human red blood cell. See text for discussion.

SUMMARY

The vasoactive hormones, epinephrine, prostaglandin E_2, and E_1 alter the deformability, osmotic fragility, gross membrane structure, and size of washed human red blood cells. These changes do not appear to be mediated by changes in the adenylate cyclase-cAMP control system, but may involve a calcium-mediated change in a sub-membrane-surface cytoskeleton in the red cell. The effects of PGE_1 and PGE_2 are highly specific and opposite: PGE_1 causes a decrease and PGE_2 an increase in cell size. These effects are of interest on three counts: 1) they represent an ideal system in which to analyze hormone-membrane interaction; 2) they represent a means of helping define the role of the spectrin complex in maintenance of red cell size and shape; and 3) they raise the possibility that hormonally-induced changes in red cell shape, size, and/or deformability play a role in the control of the microcirculation.

ACKNOWLEDGEMENTS

This work was initiated by Dr. James Allen. It was his insight and his dedication which brought it to its present state. Tragically, Dr. Allen became ill during this work. In spite of a chronic and progressive illness, he devoted his energies and imagination to the furtherance of these studies. His death a few months ago deprived him of the opportunity to participate in this meeting, but it also deprived us of a most unique and valued colleague. On the occasion of our presentation of this work, we wish to acknowledge our debt to him.

These studies were supported partially by a grant from the Office of Naval Research (NR 202-005) and partially by a grant (AM09650) from the National Institute of Arthritis, Metabolism, and Digestive Diseases. Dr. Lake is supported by a research fellowship award (6 F22 AM00369-01) from the National Institute of Arthritis, Metabolism, and Digestive Diseases.

REFERENCES

Alhquist, R.P.(1967). The receptors for epinephrine and norepinephrine. Pharmacol.Rev. 11: 441.

Allen, J.E., and Rasmussen, H.(1971). Human red blood cells: Prostaglandin E_2, epinephrine, and isoproterenol alter deformability. Science 174: 512.

Allen, J.E., and Rasmussen, H.(1972). Some effects of vasoactive hormones on the mammalian red blood cell. In Prostaglandins in Cellular Biology. Ramwell, P.W., and Pharriss, B.B., Editors, Plenum Publishing Corp., New York, pp. 27-51.

Bretscher, M.(1973). Membrane structure: Some general principles. Science 181: 622.

Dunn, M.J.(1974). Red blood cell calcium and magnesium: Effects upon sodium and potassium transport and cellular morphology. Biochim.Biophys.Acta 352: 97.

Durham, A.C.H.(1974). A unified theory of the control of actin and myosin in non-muscle movements. Cell 2: 123.

Guthrow, C.E., Allen, J.E., and Rasmussen, H.(1972). Phosphorylation of an endogenous membrane protein by an endogenous membrane-associated cyclic adenosine 3',5'-monophosphate-dependent protein kinase in human erythrocyte ghosts. J.Biol.Chem. 247: 8145.

Guthrow, C.E., Rasmussen, H., Brunswick, D.J., and Cooperman, B.S.(1973). Specific photoaffinity labeling of the adenosine 3':5'-cyclic monophosphate receptor in intact ghosts from human erythrocytes. Proc.Nat. Acad. Sci.USA 70: 3344.

Hanahan, D.J.(1973). The erythrocyte membrane: Variability and membrane enzyme activity. Biochim.Biophys.Acta 300: 319.

Himms-Hagen, J.(1967). Sympathetic regulation of metabolism. Pharmacol.Rev. 19: 367.

Kuo, J.F., and Greengard, P.(1969). Cyclic nucleotide-dependent protein kinases. IV. Widespread occurrence of adenosine 3'5'-monophosphate protein kinase in various tissues and phyla of the animal kingdom. Proc.Nat.Acad. Sci.USA 64: 1349.

Kury, P.G., Ramwell, P.W., and McConnell, H.M.(1974). The effect of prostaglandin E_1 and E_2 on the human erythrocyte as monitored by spin labels. Biochem. Biophys.Res.Commun. 56: 478.

LaCelle, P.L.(1970). Alterations of membrane deformability in hemolytic anemias. Seminars Hematol. 7: 355.

LeBlond, P.F., LaCelle, P.L., and Weed, R.I.(1971). Cellular deformability: A possible determinant of the normal release of maturing erythrocytes from the bone marrow. Blood 37: 40.

Marchesi, S.L., Steers, E., Marchesi, V.T., and Tillack, T.W.(1970). Physical and chemical properties of a protein isolated from red cell membranes. Biochemistry 9: 50.

Nicolson, G.L., Marchesi, V.T., and Singer, S.J.(1971). The localization of spectrin on the inner surface of human red blood cell membranes by ferritin-conjugated antibodies. J.CellBiol. 51: 265.

Palek, J., Curby, W.A., and Leonetti, F.J.(1971). Effects of calcium and adenosine triphosphate on volume of human red cell ghosts. Am.J.Physiol. 220: 19.

Rasmussen, H.(1970). Cell communication, calcium ion, and cyclic adenosine monophosphate. Science 170: 404.

Rasmussen, H., Goodman, D.B.P., and Tenenhouse, A.(1972). The role of cyclic AMP and calcium in cell activation. CRC Crit.Rev.Biochem. 1: 95.

Reynolds, J.A.(1973). Red cell membranes: Fact and fancy. Fed.Proc. 32: 2034.

Robison, G.A., Butcher, R.W., and Sutherland, E.W.(1971). Cyclic AMP. Academic Press, New York.

Rosenthal, A.S., Kregenow, F.M., and Moses, H.L.(1970). Some characteristics of a Ca^{2+}-dependent ATPase activity associated with a group of erythrocyte membrane proteins which form fibrils. Biochim.Biophys. Acta 196: 254.

Roth, J.(1973). Peptide hormone binding to receptors. A review of direct studies in vitro. Metabolism 22: 1059.

Ruben, C.S., Erlichman, J., and Rosen, O.M.(1972). Cyclic adenosine 3',5'-monophosphate-dependent protein kinase of human erythrocyte membranes. J.Biol.Chem. 247: 6135.

Ruben, C.S., and Rosen, O.M.(1973). The role of cyclic AMP in the phosphorylation of proteins in erythrocyte membranes. Biochem.Biophys.Res.Commun. 50: 421.

Sheppard, H., and Burghardt, C.R.(1969). Adenyl cyclase in non-nucleated erythrocytes of several mammalian species. Biochem.Pharmacol. 18: 2576.

Singer, S.J., and Nicolson, G.L.(1972). The fluid mosaic model of the structure of cell membranes. Science 175: 720.

Steck, T.L.(1974). The organization of proteins in the human red blood cell membrane. J.Cell Biol. 62: 1

Sutherland, E.W., and Rall, T.W.(1960). The relation of adenosine 3',5'-phosphate and phosphorylase to the actions of catecholamines and other hormones. Pharmacol. Rev. 12: 265.

Weed, R.I., LaCelle, P.L., and Merrill, E.W.(1969). Metabolic dependence of red cell deformability. J.Clin. Invest. 48: 795.

Zwaal, R.F., Roelofsen, B., and Colley, C.M.(1973). Localization of red cell membrane constituents. Biochim.Biophys.Acta 300: 159.

DISCUSSION

Dr. Salhany: I have two questions. I think I missed the comment as to how big a volume change you were seeing and I wasn't quite sure whether I caught how fast the volume change was occurring. Do you have that information?

Dr. Rasmussen: If we use the Coulter Counter, one can begin to see a change within one minute, and if you'll recall that slide, at four minutes there was a very significant change. Now as to the size of the change, with a 50% hematocrit the change in sodium ion concentration is approximately 5 mM. So if you assume as we do that water is moving into the cell without electrolyte that gives you an estimate of the magnitude of the volume change.

Dr. Charache: Your initial slide had prostaglandin F_2 alpha on it also. How does that fit into this scheme?

Dr. Rasmussen: It turns out that in cells from females obtained in mid-cycle, prostaglandin F_2 alpha has a very dramatic effect on decreasing deformability and decreasing the sensitivity to hypertonic hemolysis. When I say mid-menstrual cycle, what I'm really talking about is females on the pill. The day before they start their next cycle F_2 alpha does nothing to their cells.

Dr. Jacob: Dr. Rasmussen, may I congratulate you on not buying that Coulter Counter. You have shown us two slides with Coulter sizing. In one the control mean cell volume (MCV) was 60, and in the other it was 90. Most of us would recognize that an MCV of 60 is abnormally low. The increase with prostaglandin to 80 would, in fact, reflect a normal MCV. I therefore wonder whether a technical artifact is involved. Be that as it may, a shift from 60 to 80 is a huge volume change and I would think that you would be able to detect this by hematocrit determinations of these cells. That is, an approximate 33% increase in hematocrit would be expected. I wonder if you've looked for that.

Dr. Rasmussen: May I say that there was an error on the first slide; the MCV in both cases before prostaglandin addition was 90. We've looked at that but I think you have to understand you're under quite different conditions when you're doing a Coulter Counter experiment and when you're doing an experiment at 50% hematocrit. If, in fact, water is moving into a cell at 50% hematocrit then there is a significant change in the ion content of the extracellular fluid which will restrict any continuing increase in volume, whereas data from the Coulter Counter which I did not show indicate that with time the cell continues to increase in volume after PGE_2. The hematocrit in the Coulter Counter experiments is less than .05% or something of that order. So it's quite a different experimental circumstance and I don't think you can extrapolate from one to the other.

Dr. Jacob: The precision of your percent hemolysis values is extraordinary. Could you tell us how these data are gathered? I assume you use a tonicity of salt solutions which yields hemolysis of roughly 50%.

Dr. Rasmussen: That's right.

Dr. Jacob: Most of us would recognize that the osmotic fragility curve is extremely steep at tonicities yielding 50% lysis; that is, the tiniest alteration in tonicity would lead to marked differences in % hemolysis. I think most of your results with prostaglandins demonstrated only 3-4% changes in lysis. How do you keep your tonicity so constant and the reproducibility of % lysis assays so exact as to assure that 3-4% differences are significant?

Dr. Rasmussen: Well, you come to Philadelphia and we'll be happy to show you.

Dr. La Celle: I'd like to ask one final question. How do you interpret McConnell's studies where the probe is in the lipid? Do you believe that this reflects a very gross membrane change, that is, one with hormone on a protein constituent which in turn affects the lipid, or what do you think is happening there?

Dr. Rasmussen: The experiment which McConnell has promised to do is to take some cells and swell them and shrink them by 5% or so and see if that will change the way his spin labels orient and whether they relax or not. That is the critical experiment. If that's negative then his data suggest that there is, independent of whatever happens to volume, a change in the gross lipid structure so that in the PGE_2 treated cell there is less fluid lipid matrix than in the normal cell. Until he has done that experiment I don't see how we know where to go.

Dr. Duhm: May I ask you to speculate about what the stimulus is for the water to move?

Dr. Rasmussen: Well, there are two obvious mechanisms: One is that somehow you generate osmotically active particles in the cell that were bound to something, e.g., you release potassium from hemoglobin. The other is that there is some sort of contractile system in the cell membrane which relaxes or contracts. However, both mechanisms are impossible on the basis of the data in the literature. In order to have a contractile system, for example, that would relax and lead to a change in volume, the pressure gradient across the membrane to account for this change in volume would have to be enormous. Yet everybody who has tried to measure it indirectly comes to the conclusion that there is practically none. There is a debate in that some people consider there is a significant amount of potassium bound in the cell and not osmotically active, but then you're left with the problem of how a few molecules of prostaglandin magically cause this bound potassium to be released suddenly in amounts sufficient to cause cell swelling. So at the present time neither one of those explanations is satisfactory.

Dr. Brewer: Your last remark at the close of your talk implied that you might be able to explain the mystery of the missing cyclic AMP with much of the rest of the system being there. Did you have something to add to that?

Dr. Rasmussen: No, only that what we're working on at the present time is the role of calcium in this system and we have a fair amount of data that argues that that may well be the link and not cyclic AMP.

Dr. Woosley: Because of some work that has been done in smooth muscle cells. I wondered if anyone has looked at cyclic GMP especially in light of its relationship to calcium binding to membranes?

Dr. Rasmussen: We aren't able to measure any cyclic GMP even in the rat cell, much less the human cell. Also, we're not certain that we can get any consistent effect of added cyclic GMP. If we add it in the same concentrations at which we add cyclic AMP or lower, there is no effect. If we add it in very high concentrations, if we get any effects, and it is very sporadic, it's like cyclic AMP.

Unidentified Speaker: Will dibutyryl cAMP get into cells better and maybe have a better effect?

Dr. Rasmussen: As a matter of fact, I don't think we've done anything with dibutyryl cAMP.

COMPOSITE MATERIAL STRUCTURE OF RED CELL MEMBRANES

Evan A. Evans

Departments of Biomedical Engineering and
Surgery, Duke University
Durham, North Carolina 27706

INTRODUCTION

The significance of the plasma membrane barrier surrounding cells in transport of ions and larger molecules to the cell interior has long been recognized and has received much attention. However, the structural characteristics of the membrane, which provide security for the interior cytoplasm, have only recently been under investigation. The importance of membrane physical properties in cell viability is obvious and defects or breakdowns in these properties can be disastrous to the cell. Nowhere is the mechanical deformability of cells more in evidence than in the circulation, especially the microcirculation. In the microcirculation, red blood cells are pushed through capillaries that are of the same size or smaller in cross-section, forcing the cells to alter their shape greatly. Therefore, the red cell membrane has to be strong enough to sustain large deformations, recovering its original shape, and yet possess sufficient flexibility to undergo the deformations easily. Questions that arise are: what type of material structure is responsible for this "hyperelastic" behavior; what are the failure mechanisms that limit membrane viability; and what determines the mechano-chemical equilibrium of the membrane?

In order to answer these questions, mechanical experiments are required to obtain the intrinsic material properties of the membrane; i.e., properties of the material itself, independent of the extrinsic shape of the red cell membrane. Three types of single cell experiments have been used: 1) osmotic swelling; 2) fluid shear deformation of red cells attached to glass surfaces; and 3) micropipette aspiration of red cells. Osmotic swelling experiments cannot give direct measurement of material constants of the membrane because there is no way to ascertain the transmembrane pressure difference; however, a very important observation was recorded in the swelling test: no surface area change could be detected (1,2). This established that the red cell membrane behaves essentially as a two-dimensional incompressible material (maintaining constant area when deformed); the constant area (2-D incompressibility) does not imply inextensibility.[1] Indeed, the equatorial belt of the red cell disk shrinks by 20% during the swelling into a spheroid at constant surface area. Furthermore, the other two types of mechanical experiments demonstrate very large deformations under the action of small forces. Guided by these observations, the mechanics of a two-dimensional, hyperelastic, solid material with large resistance to area dilation (or compression) were developed (2,4) and applied to the analysis of fluid shear deformed cells and micropipette aspiration of red cell disks (3,5). The analyses for these two experiments yielded the same result for the material constant characterizing the hyperdeformability, i.e., the membrane "shear" modulus. The material relation correlated the general behavior between the applied forces and deformations (surface strains).

[1]As examples of two-dimensional incompressibility, a square element of membrane surface can be deformed into a rectangle under simple extension and a rhombus under pure shear, maintaining constant surface area. Figure 1 illustrates the material deformations discussed here. In the illustration, T's are forces per unit length on the element sides (tensions); λ_x and λ_y are the extension ratios in the x and y directions, respectively (ratio of deformed to the undeformed lengths; e.g., $\lambda_x = \Delta x/\Delta x_o$).

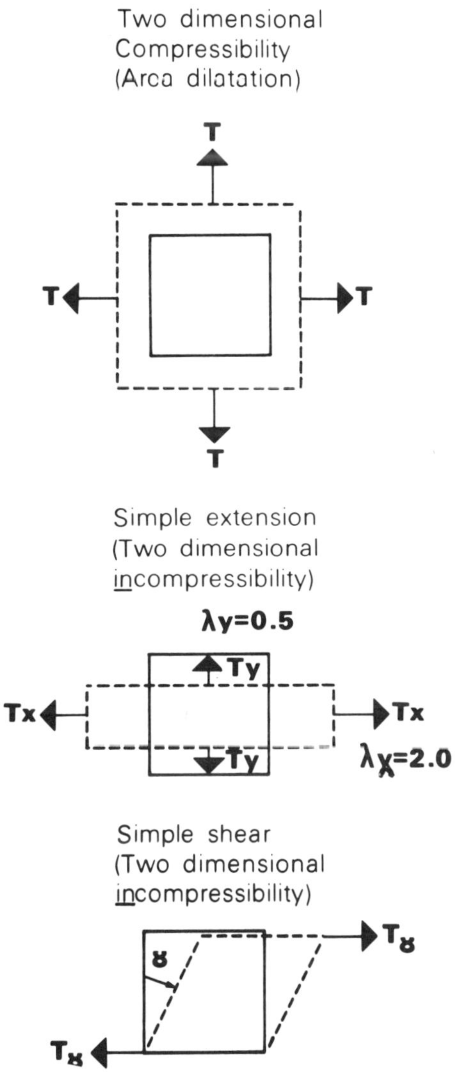

Figure 1. Material deformations of a membrane surface element under the action of isotropic tension (top) yielding uniform dilation, in uniaxial extension at constant area (middle), and in simple shear at constant area (bottom).

In addition to the two-dimensional "shear" modulus which represents the resistance to deformation in a specific direction without constraining the other surface direction (e.g., deformation of a square surface segment into a rectangular segment at constant area), there is a second modulus, referred to as a two-dimensional "bulk" or area modulus; the "area" modulus is inversely proportional to the area compressibility (e.g., uniform dilation or compression of a surface segment). Both fluid and solid materials possess "bulk" moduli; likewise a two-dimensional fluid membrane and an elastic solid membrane have "area" moduli. A perfect fluid membrane would not resist deformation (only the time rate of deformation through viscosity) and would not elastically resume its original shape in the absence of applied forces. However, as already discussed, the red cell membrane exhibits elastic solid character distinguished by a non-zero "shear" modulus. This appears to lead to a conflict with the large amount of experimental evidence indicating a "fluid mosaic" arrangement in the membrane (6). Both sets of experimental observations are well founded and, on the contrary, are complementary. The result is a composite membrane model: a structural "network" or matrix covered by (or perhaps immersed in) a two-dimensional liquid "sealer". The two-dimensional "network" provides the structural rigidity required to keep the membrane intact under deformation and measured as the "shear" modulus. The lipid bilayer forms a "sealer" insulating the cytoplasmic chemistry from the extracellular environment (additional "floating" intramembranous particles can exist without contributing to the material properties directly).

MEMBRANE MATERIAL COMPOSITE AND ELASTIC FREE ENERGY CONTENT

The membrane composite proposed is a trilamellar system: layer one, cytoplasmic surface, is a loose "network" of linear flexible molecules (perhaps spectrin [7,8]) held tightly against layers two and three, a lipid bilayer. Figure 2 illustrates the concept. The "network" is forced against the underface of the lipid bilayer by its immisci-

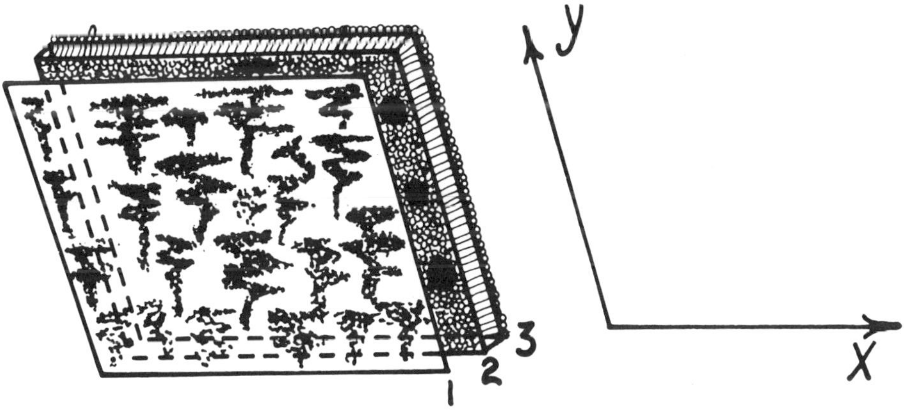

Figure 2. Schematic of Trilamellar Membrane Composite

bility in the cytoplasm. The "network" may or may not be cross-linked; micropipette aspiration studies (5) indicate only weak connections, if at all, because the "shear" modulus is constant for large deformations (finite strains of the order 400%). Layers two and three are unconnected lipid monolayers containing "floating" intramembranous particles (9,10).

Three physico-chemical phenomena contribute to the elastic free energy of the composite: 1) surface constriction due to the chemical interaction with the adjacent environment (represented by the interfacial surface tension, γ); 2) surface pressure resisting constriction of the surface or cohesive forces resisting dilation (represented by the "area" modulus of compressibility, and 3) surface rigidity opposing extension and shear at constant surface area (represented by the "shear" modulus, μ). The constants (γ, K, μ) all have units of dynes/cm. The first two phenomena are possessed by all three layers, i.e., by both two-dimensional liquids and solids; in the absence of external forces, the constrictive effect of interfacial surface tension, γ, is balanced by the compression resistance ("packing") of the molecules in the surface. (Interfacial surface tension is acting to minimize the surface area whereas the surface pressure is attempting to expand the surface.)

In general, the resistance to compression is different from the resistance to dilation of the surface, which results from cohesive forces. For example, consider packed billiard balls held together with an elastic rubber band. The elastic rubber band is analogous to interfacial surface tension, and the solid character of each billiard ball represents the compression resistance (modulus of compressibility). However, if one pulls the rubber band uniformly outward to put the "billiard ball surface" into tension, there will be no resistance to dilation (the billiard balls will simply roll away from each other) unless the billiard balls are "sticky", i.e., are cohesively bonded.

The interfacial surface tension and surface pressure (resistance to uniform compression or dilation) contributions are not altered with shape changes at constant area. On the other hand, the "network" resists extension at constant area because perhaps either the configurational entropy decreases with alignment of the molecules in the direction of extension (requiring addition of free energy) or interconnections exist between molecules of the "network" resisting deformation. Because of the hyperelastic behavior previously discussed, it appears that the entropy mechanism is likely (a two-dimensional analog of an "elastomer"). Table 1 summarizes the elastic free energy components for each layer. For a thin membrane, the area A of each layer is approximately the same (areas with superscript zero are the hypothetical unconstricted areas, without the effect of surface tension; i.e., the "reference" areas). The extension ratios λ_x, λ_y, are the "degree" of stretch in the x and y directions, respectively (ratio of deformed to the undeformed length, e.g., $\lambda_x = \Delta x/\Delta x_o$); λ_x, λ_y equal one in the undeformed condition.

Table 1

FREE ENERGY COMPOSITION FOR EACH LAYER

	Surface Free Energy Density (Interfacial Surface Tension)	Surface Compressibility (Eq'n. of State)	Surface Rigidity (Shear Resistance)
Layer 1	$\gamma_1 A_1$	$\frac{1}{2} K_1 (A_1 - A_1^\circ)^2 / A_1^\circ$	$\frac{\mu}{4}(\lambda_x^2 + \lambda_y^2 - 2) A_1$
Layer 2	$\gamma_2 A_2$	$\frac{1}{2} K_2 (A_2 - A_2^\circ)^2 / A_2^\circ$	0
Layer 3	$\gamma_3 A_3$	$\frac{1}{2} K_3 (A_3 - A_3^\circ)^2 / A_3^\circ$	0

For Thin Membrane (also requires $A_1^\circ = A_2^\circ = A_3^\circ$)

$$F_{TOTAL} = \gamma_T A + K_T \frac{(A - A^\circ)^2}{2 A^\circ} + \frac{\mu}{4}(\lambda_x^2 + \lambda_y^2 - 2) A$$

Comparing osmotic swelling experiments with micropipette aspiration and fluid-shear deformation of red cells, it is observed that the total interfacial surface tension and area compressibility modulus are much larger than the shear modulus (5) and that the membrane essentially undergoes deformation at constant area (except at the final lysis point of osmotic swelling). The surface is tightly "packed" with the area compression given by:

$$\frac{\Delta A}{A} = -\frac{\gamma_T}{K_T}$$

The "shear" modulus, μ, is of the order 10^{-2} dynes/cm; the area modulus is not well established, but an estimate of at least 10^2 dynes/cm is reasonable (11); interfacial surface tension is of the order of 1 dyne/cm.

MEMBRANE FAILURE MECHANISMS: LYSIS VERSUS FRAGMENTATION

For the composite structure proposed, there will be two modes of material failure: lysis and fragmentation. Lysis results from failure of the surface in isotropic tension, dilation of the surface (see Figure 1); this mode is fatal. The tension must be greater than the sum of the interfacial surface tension and the cohesive forces in the membrane.

$$T_L \geq \gamma_T + \underbrace{K_T \frac{\Delta A}{A}}_{\text{cohesion}}$$

For lipid bilayers, cohesive forces are negligible; therefore, only the "network" contributes to cohesion. The yield tension T_n for the "network" can be inserted in the above criterion for lysis:

$$T_L \geq \gamma_T + T_n$$

From micropipette measurements on swollen cells, the tension at lysis, T_L, is at least 10 dynes/cm. The corresponding free energy required for each cell would be:

$$\Delta F_L \sim 10^{-5} \text{ dynes-cm/RBC}$$

The second type of material failure, fragmentation, is not immediately fatal for the red cell but results in eventual removal of the cell remnants by the reticulo endothelial system. Fragmentation does not require surface area of the membrane to change; therefore, the interfacial surface tension and surface cohesive forces are not involved. The membrane fragments by plastic extension failure of the "network" (similar to pulling off a small piece of chewing gum). The surface lipid bilayer reseals, leaving remnants with more "spherical" shapes than the original cell, thereby becoming susceptible to removal by the spleen. At the large extension ratios (stretch) for failure, the tension is approximately given by:

$$T_F \simeq \frac{\mu}{2} \lambda_F^2$$

The value of the extension ratio λ_F at failure (yield point) depends on the rate of deformation and, as yet, is not well defined. It is greater than 4:1, but probably less than 10:1. Using the upper bound ($\lambda_F \simeq 10$), the tension for fragmentation failure would be:

$$T_F \simeq 50\mu \simeq 0.5 \text{ dynes/cm}$$

The tension for fragmentation is one to two orders of magnitude less than that required for lysis, *but* the free energy required is considerably less because *only* a small region of the membrane is involved in fragmentation failure (at the "neck" or "pinch-off" location). The free energy change for fragmentation of a single cell is:

$$\Delta F_F \sim 10^{-8} \text{ dynes-cm/RBC}$$

Therefore, the free energy change for fragmentation is three orders of magnitude less than that required by hemolysis, even though in both cases the cells are eventually removed from the circulation. From this discussion, it is apparent that fragmentation mechanisms present the major threat to red cell viability in the circulation and that the higher energy failure mechanism of hemolysis is less likely to occur. However, if *in vivo* or *in vitro* surface chemical effects take place to reduce significantly the interfacial surface tension, γ, and cohesive forces of the "network", then hemolysis can become a major failure mechanism. In the study of anemia and hemolytic disorders, the intrinsic material properties can provide the inherent mechanisms involved.

MECHANO-CHEMICAL EQUILIBRIUM OF THE MEMBRANE

It is generally accepted that the equilibrium or "natural" state of the mature red cell is a biconcave disk.

This implies that each layer of the composite is in turn in equilibrium determined by the balance of interfacial surface tension against surface compressibility (pressure). If, however, the chemical equilibrium of one layer is altered (by changing the interfacial surface tension or area compressibility modulus), then the surface area of that particular layer would adjust accordingly. When one layer attempts to either constrict or dilate relative to the others, a bending moment is created, and curvature is induced to accommodate the relative area changes (since the layers held tightly against each other).

There have been extensive observations of induced curvature in red cell membranes resulting from alterations in chemical environment (12). The red cell shape spectrum ranges from a normal biconcave disk to a tightly crenated sphere; the intermediate states are spiculated shapes called echinocytes of different degrees. The reversible shape change from a biconcave disk into a crenated sphere still remains an unsolved puzzle for many a hematologist and cell physiologist. A vast amount of information has been accumulated concerning the multiplicity of agents and conditions that produce this transformation, but the underlying mechanism has not been established (13). The possibility that the spiculation or curvature can be produced by chemically induced bending moments in the lipid bilayer was recently investigated (14). In this case, crenation would be the result of expansion of the outer surface relative to the inner survace. Such conditions would arise either when the outer interfacial free energy density (γ^u) decreased (e.g., the addition of electrical charges to the outer layer) or when inner interfacial free energy (γ^ℓ) increased (e.g., Ca^{++} binding between negatively charged amphiphilic molecules of the inner surface).

The analysis of mechano-chemical equilibrium of two layers shows that the average curvature per spicule must increase as the interfacial free energy density of the outer surface decreases:

$$-\langle C \rangle_{\text{Spicule}} = ([\delta\gamma^u/K^u] - [\delta\gamma^\ell/K^\ell])\ 1/h.$$

where $\delta\gamma$ is the variation in interfacial surface tension; K is the area compressibility modulus; h is the separation distance between the two layers. (The superscripts u,ℓ designate the two layers.) The average curvature is obtained by integrating the total curvature (determined by the principal radii of curvature R_1, R_2) over the surface.

$$\langle C \rangle = \frac{1}{A_m} \int \left(\frac{1}{R_1} + \frac{1}{R_2} \right) ds$$

For a fixed surface like the red cell membrane, the average curvature per spicule increases with increasing number of spicules. Therefore, the number of spicules progressively increases with the interfacial free energy change. In addition, it is apparent that reducing the surface compressibility amplifies the effect (e.g., by incorporating material in the membrane like cholesterol).

Implicit in the preceding discussion has been the assumption that the structural rigidity possessed by the red cell membrane can be neglected. In order to evaluate this assumption, the elastic free energy of the structural component must be compared with the alteration in interfacial surface tension. The "network" will elastically store the chemically induced free energy change. When the induced curvature of the surface is very small, the interfacial free energy change must be greater than the membrane shear modulus in order to initiate bending,

$$\delta\gamma \sim \mu .$$

However, when the curvature is not small, the interfacial free energy change will be proportional to the ratio of "network" deformation to the relative area change between layers.

$$\delta\gamma \sim \frac{\mu(\lambda_x{}^2 + \lambda_y{}^{-2} - 2)}{h\langle C \rangle}$$

In this case $\delta\gamma$ can be of the order of 100 times the shear modulus. The red cell membrane shear modulus has been measured to be about 10^{-2} dyn/cm; therefore, the interfacial free energy change would have to be between 10^{-2} and 1 dyn/cm for the progressive crenation of red cells.

Only the crenation of red cells has been discussed; but, the concept is also compatible with the red cell disk to cup shape transformation (12). In this case, the opposite situation exists: the inner surface is expanding relative to the outer surface (in other words, the cell is trying to turn "inside-out"). Here, either the inner surface interfacial free energy density (γ^{ℓ}) decreases, or the outer surface interfacial free energy density (γ^{u}) increases.

SUMMARY

The intrinsic material properties of the red cell membrane (e.g., hyperelasticity) obtained by direct mechanical experiments indicate a composite structure that provides separation between red cell cytoplasm and the extracellular medium. The composite proposed is a trilamellar system: layer one, (cytoplasmic surface), is a loose "network" of linear flexible molecules (perhaps spectrin) held tightly against a lipid bilayer, (layers two and three), by its immiscibility in the cytoplasm. The "network" provides the structural rigidity required by the membrane and measured as the membrane 2-D "shear modulus" (elastic constant for extension at constant area). The "network" may or may not be cross-linked; preliminary information indicates it is only weakly connected, if at all. The lipid bilayer forms a "sealer" insulating the cytoplasmic chemistry from the extracellular environment (with additional "floating" intramembranous particles that do not necessarily contribute to the material properties directly).

The free energy content of the red cell membrane is examined when undergoing deformation. Three physico-chemical phenomena contribute to the free energy: 1) surface constriction due to the chemical interaction with the adjacent environment (interfacial surface tension); 2) surface pressure resisting constriction or cohesive forces resisting expansion (two-dimensional liquid characteristics); 3) surface rigidity opposing extension and shear at constant surface area (a solid property). The relative importance of each phenomenon is discussed for the two membrane failure mechanisms: lysis and fragmentation. Fragmentation requires less than 10^{-3} times the free energy change that lysis does and will, therefore, be of primary importance in the circulation. However, in vivo and in vitro surface chemical effects can greatly reduce the resistance to lysis.

Finally, the stability of the red cell shape is discussed for changes in the membrane chemical equilibrium. Such changes can induce surface curvature and are considered as a possible mechanism for red cell shape changes (e.g., echinocytes).

REFERENCES

1. Evans, E.A., and Leblond, P.F., Geometric Properties of Individual Red Blood Cell Discocyte-Spherocyte Transformations. Biorheol. 10:393, 1973.

2. Evans, E.A., A New Material Concept for the Red Cell Membrane, Biophys. J. 13:926, 1973.

3. Evans, E.A., New Membrane Concept Applied to the Analysis of Fluid-Shear and Micropipette Deformed Red Blood Cells. Biophys.J. 13:941, 1973.

4. Skalak, R., Tozeren, A., Zarda, R.P., and Chien, S., Strain Energy Function of Red Blood Cell Membranes. Biophys. J. 13:245, 1973.

5. Evans, E.A., and LaCelle, P.L., Intrinsic Material Properties of the Erythrocyte Membrane Indicated by Mechanical Analysis of Deformation, Blood, (in press).

6. Singer, S.J., and Nicolson, G.L., The Fluid Mosaic Model of the Structure of Cell Membranes. Science 175:720, 1972.

7. Marchesi, V.T., Steers, E., Tillack, T.W., and Marchesi, S.L., Some Properties of Spectrin: A Fibrous Protein Isolated from Red Cell Membranes. In Jamieson and Greenwalt, editors, Red Cell Membrane (Lippincott, Philadelphia) 1969, 117.

8. Steck, T.L., The Organization of Proteins in the Human Red Blood Cell Membrane. J.Cell.Biol. 62:1, 1974.

9. Mateu, L., Luzzati, V., London, Y., Gould, R.M., Vossberg, F.G.A., and Olive, J., X-Ray Diffraction and Electron Microscope Study of the Interactions of Myelin Components. J.Mol.Biol. 75:697, 1973.

10. Tardieu, A., Luzzati, V., and Remau, F.C., Structure and Polymorphism of the Hydrocarbon Chains of Lipids: A Study of Lecithin-Water Phases. J.Mol.Biol. 75:711, 1973.

11. Rand, R.P., Mechanical Properties of the Red Cell Membrane II. Biophys.J. 4:303, 1964.

12. Bessis, M., Living Blood Cells and Their Ultrastructure. (Springer-Verlag, New York), 1973.

13. Ponder, E., Hemolysis and Related Phenomena, (Grune and Stratton, New York) 1971.

14. Evans, E.A., Bending Resistance and Chemically Induced Moments in Membrane Bilayers. Biophys.J. 14 (in press) 1974.

DISCUSSION

Dr. Jacob: Could you tell us from your model what would happen if the membrane is capable of contraction? Good morphologic evidence exists that some agents--for instance, vinblastine, cause red cell sphering due to endocytosis which, in turn, reflects contraction of the membrane. Such contraction occurs only in the presence of ATP. Thus, there is evidently an active process in the red cell membrane which allows it to contract and invaginate. Can you comment?

Dr. Evans: I would like to. I'm glad you asked that question actually because my concept here is that when you talk about an active mechanism what you're really talking about is something that interferes with the chemical equilibrium of some system. Let's take, for instance, the example that you've given and look at what you would call a contractile type of mechanism on the cytoplasmic membrane face--let's say in the spectrin network as a thesis. In this particular case what is essentially changing is the surface free energy density of that spectrin network. This is exactly what we're talking about. When you say contractile mechanism, in general people confuse this with muscular systems with organized structures. I prefer not to do that because I don't think there is any evidence that a truly organized structure exists here. On the contrary, a contractile mechanism via uniform constriction (resulting from condensation of the spectrin network, i.e., changing the area specific volume of that spectrin network) can indeed produce exactly what we're talking about. So it is compatible and I think there are a number of things that can happen. Also, don't forget that you can do exactly the same thing by adding calcium ion to the phosphatidyl serine of the underface of the bilayer, the lipid bilayer, causing it to contract by condensing the inner surface. I think that's not to be confused with an overall area change because this is very difficult to show. I don't know of any evidence that would show very large area changes, especially for lipids. One thing about lipids is that if you try to compress them their resistance to compression in the condensed state is tremendous. It's like a liquid, indeed like a two dimensional liquid so it takes atmospheres of pressure change to get small area changes.

My feeling is that unless you do something to change the amount of substance in the membrane (in other words, by releasing lipid from one layer relative to the other or both layers or by incorporating lipid on some other substance) it is very difficult to make area changes; but as far as contraction I think that is quite compatible with the overall chemistry of the type of processes we're talking about here. I think you can deal with contraction from physical chemistry as well as from a physiological viewpoint.

Dr. Mizukami: Your experiment somehow seems to be related to Dr. Rasmussen's. In the figure showing the effect of PGE and PGE_2, one of them shows single phase hemolysis and the other bi-phase. Do you think you could speculate on some correlation with what you have said?

Dr. Evans: I really don't feel competent enough to comment on his experiments because I really don't know that much about them. I witnessed the same presentation you did but I'm not sure I really understand the mechanisms there. What is hard for me to understand is the effect of a small number of molecules on a surface that contains 10^{10} molecules. One of the things you learn in statistical physics is that in order to measurably affect a property of a substance, you have to involve numbers of particles greater than 1 over the square root of the total number of particles that you deal with. So if you take 100 particles out of 10^{10} that is a ratio of 10^8, you get 1 over the square root of 10^8 which is 1 part in 10^4. You find it very difficult to accept that 100 particles are able to interfere with properties of the surface. If we assume that it does interfere with the surface free energy density, for instance reduces the total surface free energy density, in this case you can increase the propensity to lyse but here we're talking about thesis rather than necessarily experimental proof. You have to do the mechanical experiments to prove or disprove the free energy change. The other effect is possible reduction of cohesive forces that might exist in the surface. Perhaps the prostaglandins interfere with the cohesive aspects of some surface element. I really don't know. That's all I can say.

X-RAY DIFFRACTION STUDIES OF THE HUMAN ERYTHROCYTE MEMBRANE

James B. Stamatoff, Samuel Krimm, and Nancy R. Harvie
Biophysics Research Division and Department of Physics
University of Michigan, Ann Arbor, Michigan 48104

INTRODUCTION

Although the electron microscopic technique can provide information on the morphology and external structural characteristics of membranes, it is less suitable for determining the distribution of constituents within membranes. This is particularly true if such structural features in the native state are of interest, primarily because of the drastic physical and chemical methods used to prepare a specimen for electron microscopic examination. On the other hand, the technique of x-ray diffraction, if it can be applied appropriately, furnishes an electron density distribution directly, thus providing an important starting point for elaborating the structure of the membrane.

The crux of applying the x-ray diffraction method to the study of red cell membranes is the ability to obtain well-ordered arrays of erythrocyte ghosts, since the more perfect is the periodic organization of the membranes, the more extensive will be the x-ray diffraction pattern obtained. An analysis of the pattern, however, depends not only on having a large number of diffraction spectra but on the possibility of determining their phases. Nevertheless, these two factors are not totally unrelated, since swelling techniques for phase determination (1) require a reasonable number of diffraction spectra in order to succeed.

Previous x-ray diffraction studies of erythrocyte membranes (2-8) have reported three or four orders of a ~110A periodicity for membranes containing large amounts of hemoglobin and two orders of a ~70A periodicity for hemoglobin-free erythrocyte membranes. These data are insufficient for phase determination by swelling techniques (1).

We have concentrated our initial studies on hemoglobin-free erythrocyte membranes, since this system is simpler and easier to analyze, and provides a necessary foundation for studying hemoglobin-bound membranes. Using improved preparative methods, we have been able to obtain x-ray patterns of hemoglobin-free ghosts which exhibit six or seven orders of diffraction. Phase angles have been deduced for these reflections, and we have thus been able to derive a projected electron density for the hemoglobin-free erythrocyte membrane of the human red cell.

METHODS AND ANALYSIS

Details of the experimental techniques will not be given here, since they are presented elsewhere (9,10). Hemoglobin-free membranes were prepared by the method of Dodge, et al (11), and characterized biochemically for total protein and for hemoglobin content (10). Samples for x-ray diffraction (preserved from bacterial action by adding 5×10^{-4}M NaN_3 to the buffer) were prepared by ultracentrifugation at 10^5g for 24 hours. X-ray diffraction patterns with the beam parallel to the membrane surface were obtained with the sample at 4°C and equilibrated at relative humidities of 75% to 100%. A mirror-monochromator Guinier camera system was used with a rotating anode generator, and exposures were of the order of 48 hours.

Variation of the relative humidity in the range of 75% to 100% was used to obtain seven patterns whose basic periodicity varied from 55.5A to 69.6A. In addition to the observed sharp reflections, which are higher orders of this spacing, weak diffuse scattering was recorded between the beam stop and the first order reflection. A plot of the integrated intensities of the reflections in the above seven sets of data produced an intensity transform, from the periodicity of which phase angles of 0 or π for each reflection could be deduced using the minimum wavelength principle (12). (The phase angles are limited to the above two values since the membrane vescicles are intact, and should therefore maintain a center of symmetry in projection.) Since this principle does not rigorously provide phases, we have used an electron density comparison method (9,13) to obtain the phases independently and with greater confidence. This method leads to the same phase assignment, and suggests that we have correctly phased the observed reflections. Using these phases, a one-dimensional Fourier transform of the scattering amplitude was calculated, which gives the electron density within the unit cell projected on a line perpendicular to the membrane surface.

RESULTS AND DISCUSSION

The projected electron densities for two values of the unit cell periodicity, viz., 56.5A and 64.2A, are shown in Figure 1. The basic repeating structure is about 55A wide. Since variation in humidity effectively alters only the separation between the high density peaks, we interpret this distribution as representing a single symmetric membrane 55A wide. (While it would be consistent with a centrosymmetric arrangement of asymmetric membranes of 27.5A width, the swelling characteristics, as well as the unreasonableness of a 27.5A wide lipid bilayer (14) or membrane (15), argue against such an interpretation.) The observed symmetry of course applies only within the resolution of our data, about 9A, and to the projected structure. These, as well as other factors such as heterogeneity of cell population, may well hide at this stage small asymmetries which have been indicated by biochemical studies (16).

Our analyses suggest that Figure 1 represents the projected electron density distribution of an intact membrane,

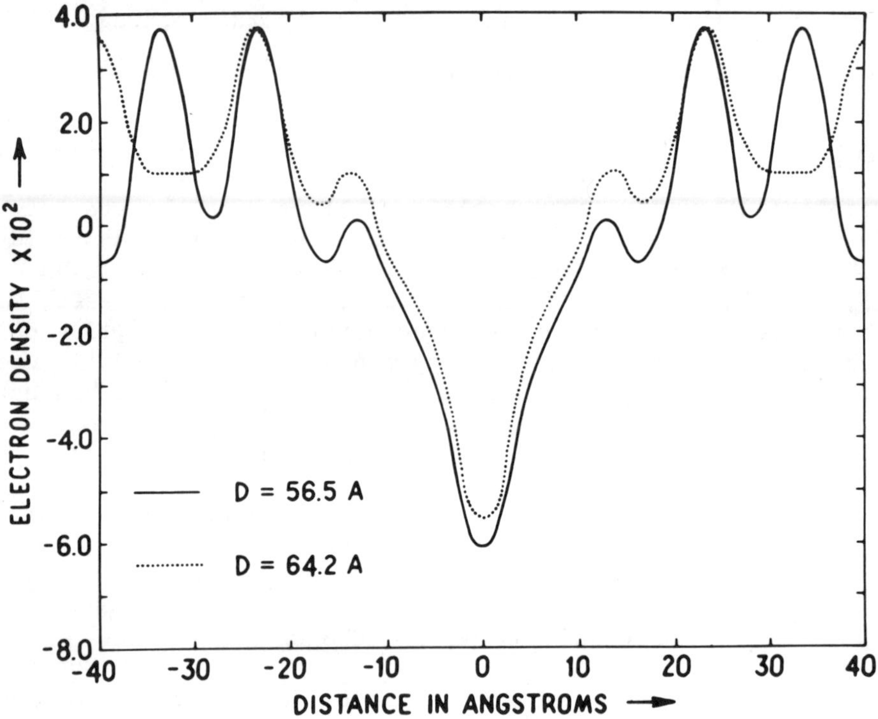

Fig. 1. Projected electron density distributions of hemoglobin-free human erythrocyte membranes for unit cell periodicities of 56.5A and 64.2A.

despite claims (6) that membrane components can separate as a result of dehydration. A wide range of phenomena support this conclusion (9,10,17): 1) We find that the diffuse scattering, which had previously been associated with a residual lipoprotein phase (6), can be accounted for by assuming that the electron density distribution of Figure 1 occurs in distorted lattices in addition to the well-ordered lattices which produce the sharp reflections. 2) The continuous scattered intensity curve computed for a single membrane from the distribution of Figure 1 agrees well with the experimental scattering from dispersions of isolated membranes (obviously not dehydrated) observed by ourselves and others (18). 3) We have recorded good x-ray diffraction patterns in buffer of neuraminidase-treated hemoglobin-free erythrocytes to which poly-L-lysine was bound; the observed periodicity of 67A is consistent with our proposed 55A wide membranes separated by monolayers of the polypeptide. We therefore conclude that in our preparations we are observing intact hemoglobin-free erythrocyte membranes.

It had been concluded from earlier work (4) that the thickness of the erythrocyte membrane is 112A, in contrast to our proposed value of 55A. It should be noted that the figure of 112A is derived from a study of partially dehydrated samples which were bound with large quantities of hemoglobin (4). Our results on poly-L-lysine bound membranes in buffer show that the thickness must be much less than 112A. Similar experiments involving re-binding of hemoglobin (9,17) give a periodicity of about 112A, showing that this value is characteristic of the membrane-hemoglobin complex. It is interesting to note that our width of 55A compares well with that obtained by the use of energy transfer techniques (19).

A detailed interpretation of the electron density distributions of Figure 1 is probably not warranted at the present time, although their general appearance is consistent with the phospholipid bilayer arrangement present in the fluid mosaic model of membrane structure (20). It is clear that the distribution differs significantly from that obtained from the total extracted lipids of human erythrocyte membranes (21). This is one of the many structural features which we hope can be elucidated now that the basic membrane profile is known.

This research was supported by a Macromolecular Research Center Fellowship (J.B.S.) and by National Science Foundation Grant GB-15682 (S.K.).

REFERENCES

1. Worthington, C.R., King, G.I., and McIntosh, T.J., Biophys. J. 13, 480 (1973)
2. Finean, J.B., Coleman, R., Green, W.G., and Limbrick, A.R., J. Cell Sci. 1, 287 (1966)
3. Finean, J.B., Coleman, R., Knutton, S., Limbrick, A.R., and Thompson, J.E., J. Gen. Physiol. 51, 195 (1968)
4. Finean, J.B., Quart. Revs. Biophys. 2, 1 (1969)
5. Coleman, R., Finean, J.B., Knutton, S., and Limbrick, A.R., Biochim. Biophys. Acta 219, 81 (1970)
6. Knutton, S., Finean, J.B., Coleman, R., and Limbrick, A.R., J. Cell Sci. 7, 357 (1970)
7. Finean, J.B., Chem. Phys. Lipids 8,279 (1972)
8. Finean, J.B., Biochem. Soc. Trans. 1, 327 (1973)
9. Stamatoff, J.B., Ph.D. Thesis, University of Michigan 1974
10. Stamatoff, J.B., Krimm, S., and Harvie, N.R., Proc. Natl. Acad. Sci., in press
11. Dodge, J.J., Mitchell, C., and Hanahan, D.J., Arch. Biochem. Biophys. 100, 119 (1963)
12. Bragg, W.L. and Perutz, M.F., Proc. Roy. Soc. Lond. A213, 425 (1952)
13. Stamatoff, J.B. and Krimm, S., to be published
14. Lesslauer, W., Cain, J.E., and Blaisie, J.K., Proc. Natl. Acad. Sci. 69, 1499 (1972)
15. McIntosh, T.J. and Worthington, C.R., Biophys. J. 14, 363 (1974)
16. Bretscher, M.S., Science 181, 622 (1973)
17. Stamatoff, J.B. and Krimm, S., to be published
18. Wilkins, M.H.F., Blaurock, A.E., and Engleman, D.M., Nature New Biol. 230, 72 (1971)
19. Peters, R., Biochim. Biophys. Acta 330, 53 (1973)
20. Singer, S.J. and Nicolson, G.L., Science 175, 720 (1972)
21. Rand, R.P. and Luzzati, V., Biophys. J. 8, 125 (1968)

DISCUSSION

Dr. Perutz: I should like to congratulate Dr. Stamatoff and Dr. Krimm on their fantastic technical feat of extending the diffraction pattern from red cell membranes from two orders to seven. I wondered whether you have thought of taking your specimens to Brookhaven and doing neutron diffraction on them. Preparation of your specimen in H_2O and D_2O would give you a ready method of checking your phases.

Dr. Krimm: This is one of the many things on our list of things to do. Indeed that makes imminent sense and we hope that we will have an opportunity of doing that, as well as other methods such as we were talking about yesterday for independent phase determination.

Dr. Perutz: This might be better than the introduction of CsCl I suggested yesterday because you would not introduce anything into the membrane that might falsify the results.

Dr. Krimm: If we can get Brookhaven to agree with us on this ....

Dr. Perutz: I think Schoenborn might be quite keen.

Unidentified Speaker: A number of laboratories have been studying membranes with phospholipases and have indications that there are different phospholipids on different sides. Does this change your interpretation in any way?

Dr. Krimm: No. You have to realize the following. First of all we can't see anything, at the moment, to better than 10 angstroms resolution. So, there could well be biochemical asymmetries inherent in the membranes which are not showing up at this resolution. Secondly, the population may have, probably does have, heterogeneities which we don't control at the moment. For example, perhaps there are differences between cells of different ages. We have used just whole human blood, taken and worked up. We have hopes of looking at the structure as a function of the age of the cell. So there could well be heterogeneities that hide any inherent biochemical asymmetry. Certainly what is suggested here is that at 10 angstroms resolution there is not dramatic asymmetry in the membrane. I think there are other things that still have to be done and so there is no contradiction, as yet, between our work and the work of Bretscher and others who have suggested certain kinds of asymmetry in the membrane.

Dr. La Celle: Is it known by any technique what the actual hydration of the original membrane is and how this would correspond to the degree of hydration you acheive when you're doing your studies?

Dr. Krimm: By the original membrane what do you mean?

Dr. La Celle: The natural state.

Dr. Krimm: Oh, in the natural state. I don't know the answer to what the hydration is in the natural state. Perhaps someone else does and can help me out. But, certainly when we talk about relative humidity we're talking here about the relative humidity established in the chamber, that is, in the x-ray chamber, in which the experiment is done and that may not even have a one to one correlation with what is present around the membranes themselves. So, it's merely a way of varying the distance between membranes, and that's all we're interested in because as soon as you do that you begin sampling the membrane transform at different points.

PHOSPHORYLATION AND DEPHOSPHORYLATION IN THE ERYTHROCYTE MEMBRANE

Alfred C. Greenquist and Stephen B. Shohet

Division of Hematology, University of California
Medical Center, San Francisco, Ca. 94143

A membrane-bound cyclic AMP dependent protein kinase was studied in normal erythrocyte membrane and in membrane from erythrocytes with hereditary defects in cell shape. Pronounced reductions in the level of phosphorylation of several membrane protein substrates were found in hereditary spherocytosis (6 patients), hereditary stomatocytosis (1 patient) but not in hereditary elliptocytosis (2 patients). The deficiency persisted in the presence of cyclic AMP. The extent of incorporation was not dependent upon reticulocyte count in hereditary spherocytosis. Ruthenium red caused negligible inhibition at concentrations which inhibit Ca++, Mg++-ATPase. The reaction showed a time and concentration dependent inhibition by sevéral sulfhydryl reagents under conditions which generate spherocytes in intact cells. The membrane was shown to possess a Mg++ dependent protein phosphatase which reverses the phosphorylation reaction. Intact cells, incubated with ^{32}Pi, incorporate label into the same polypeptide substrates labeled in isolated membrane. The incorporation was energy dependent and dephosphorylation occurred with reincubation after the addition of sodium fluoride or removal of glucose under conditions which lead to spherocytosis.

INTRODUCTION

Modification of enzymes by alternative phosphorylation or dephosphorylation reaction has been established as one of the regulatory mechanisms which modulate the expression of enzyme activities. A number of these reactions have been characterized which involve soluble protein kinases and their substrates (1). The presence of membrane-bound protein kinases and their substrates has been recognized more recently in a number of membranes (2-6). Several studies have demonstrated protein phosphorylation reactions in the erythrocyte membrane (7-11). Other studies have shown a reduced storage stability for this reaction in erythrocyte membrane from patients with myotonic muscular dystrophy (12). We have reported on a protein kinase dependent reduced phosphorylation in erythrocyte membrane from patients with hereditary spherocytosis (13-15). This study deals with the relationship of the phosphorylation reaction to erythrocyte cell shape control in normal and pathological cells.

METHODS

Membrane Isolation and Electrophoresis. Erythrocyte membrane was obtained basically according to Dodge, et al. (16) using an 0.01 M Tris-Cl buffer, pH 7.4. Electrophoresis was performed in a 5% polyacrylamide gel (PAGE) containing 0.1% sodium dodecyl sulfate (SDS) as described by Weber and Osborn (17). The membrane was incubated in 1% SDS and 40 mM dithiothreitol for one hour prior to electrophoresis. When required, gels were fixed and stained with the first staining solution described by Fairbanks, et al. (18). The numbering of polypeptides follow the designations previously described (18). Bands I and II have been collectively described as spectrin. Gels containing radiolabeled polypeptides were generally sliced in 2 mm sections, the gel segments were transferred to scintillation vials and dissolved in 0.2 ml of 30% H_2O_2. Counting was performed by Cerenkov radiation in a Packard Model 3341 liquid scintillation spectrophotometer

Phosphorylation of Membrane Protein. The phosphorylation conditions are similar to those previously described (15) using a 0.5 ml reaction mixture containing 0.25 mg of freeze-thawed membrane protein, 0.15 mM [γ-^{32}P] ATP (~20 cpm/pmole), 2.5 mM Mg++ and 0.01 M Tris-Cl at pH 7.4. Incubations were at 37° for one hour, then the reaction was stopped with 2.0 ml of cold 0.01 M Tris-Cl, 0.05 M NaCl, 1 mM EDTA at pH 7.4. The suspension was centrifuged at 20,000 x g for 10 minutes and the membranes washed two times prior to analysis by SDS-PAGE.

Sulfhydryl Inhibition. Membrane was preincubated generally with 1 mM sulfhydryl agent for up to one hour prior to initiation of the phosphorylation reaction by addition of Mg++ and ATP. A portion of the incubated samples were electrophoresed in gels for staining with coomasie blue. Controls and sulfhydryl-treated membrane yielded equivalent gel patterns.

Breakdown of Membrane Phosphoprotein. Membrane polypeptides were phosphorylated as described above and the labeled membrane was washed at 0° without EDTA. The membrane was then reincubated in a 0.5 ml reaction mixture containing 0.01 M Tris-Cl and further additions as noted in Table V.

Labeling of Intact Cells. Cells from freshly obtained blood were washed three times with normal saline and suspended to a 50% hematocrit. The reaction had a 0.5 ml final volume containing 0.1 ml cell suspension, 50 mM imadazole · HCl, pH 7.4, 10 mM glucose and 1-2 · 10^6 cpm of carrier free ^{32}Pi. Isotonicity was maintained with NaCl. The preparations were incubated at 37° for 20 hours. Cells for reincubation were prepared by washing two times in N saline, and resuspending with 10 mM glucose, without glucose, or with glucose and 10 mM sodium fluoride. These cells were reincubated for 20 hours. Membrane was isolated from these cells and analyzed for incorporated label as described above.

RESULTS

Identification of Labeled Polypeptides. The polypeptides labeled during the protein kinase catalyzed phosphorylation reaction are shown in Fig. 1. The label was incorporated from [γ-^{32}P] ATP into each component of the spectrin doublet (Bands I and II) and into a component in the 90,000 molecular weight position on the gel. The specific polypeptides labeled in the Band III position has not been determined. An additional polypeptide with a molecular weight of about 50,000 was labeled only in the presence of cyclic AMP as has been previously described (8,11). The final peak to the right contained residual ATP and labeled polyphosphoinositides (19).

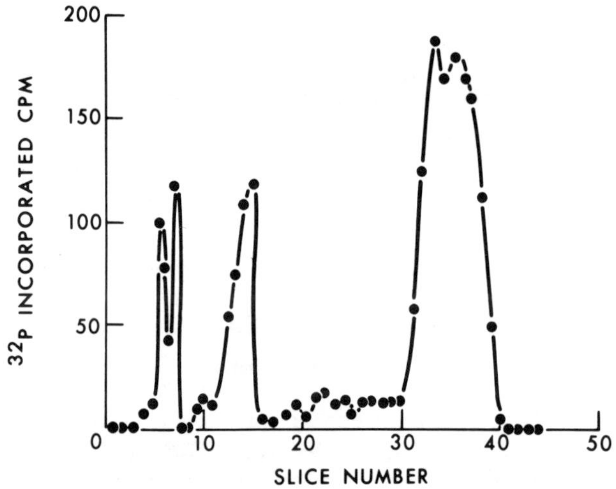

Figure 1. ^{32}P labeling profile of erythrocyte membrane protein phosphorylation without cyclic AMP as described in the text and resolved by SDS PAGE. A 50 µg sample was applied to the gel. Gel segments of 1 mM were obtained through peaks 1 and 2 and 2 mm segments thereafter. A coomassie blue stained gel run with 75 µg of protein is shown below.

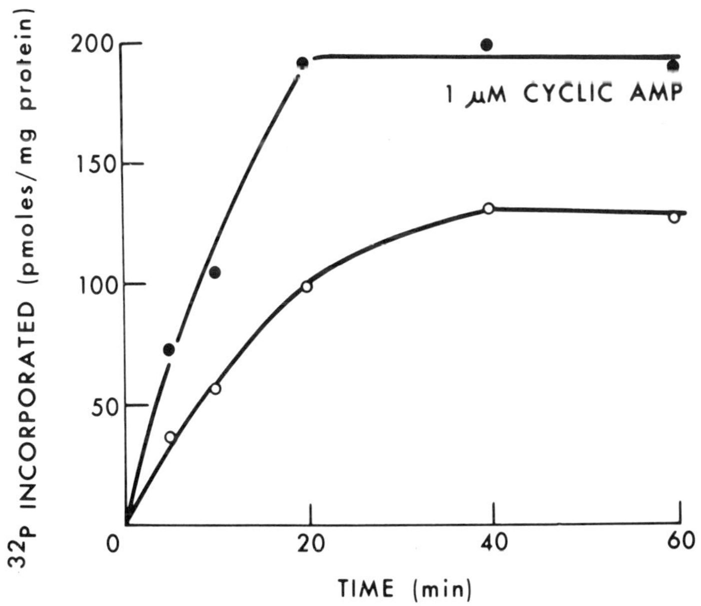

Figure 2. Kinetics of spectrin (Bands I and II) phosphorylation. Membrane protein was obtained from out-dated blood bank blood and incubated with .05 mM ATP.

The kinetics of label incorporation into the spectrin component is shown in Fig. 2. As noted by others (8,11), the reaction was non-linear and approached an equilibrium value after about 20 minutes. Both the rate and the extent of incorporation were enhanced by 1 µM cyclic AMP.

Modification of Protein Kinase Activity. The effects of several agents which have potential relationships to cell shape and deformability were studied to determine their effects on the protein kinase activity as shown in Table I. Addition of the chelator, ethyleneglycol-bis (β-aminoethyl-ether) N, N'-tetraacetic acid, (EGTA), enhanced incorporation of label. The addition of Ca++ resulted in a concentration dependent inhibition of the reaction. No effect was observed

Table I. Modification of Membrane Protein Phosphorylation

Additions	^{32}P Incorporation (% control)	
	Spectrin	Band III
EGTA, 1mM	109	103
Ca++, 0.5mM	70	55
Ca++, 3.0mM	0	0
Na+, K+, 50mM ea.	102	95
Ruthenium Red, 60µM	94	101
Ruthenium Red, 1.2mM	62	77

with Na+ or K+ indicating the absence of specific ion effects and also the insensitivity of the reaction to changes in ionic strength.

Ruthenium Red was studied because the agent is reported to selectively inhibit the Ca++, Mg++ stimulated component of the red cell adenosine triphosphatase (ATPase) activities (20). At concentrations (60 µM) that severely reduce the ATPase activity, the effect on phosphorylation was negligible. At higher concentrations, some inhibition was observed. Vinblastin and vincristin were examined because of their spherocytogenic effect and previous reports suggesting a selective interaction with structural protein in the red cell membrane (21). Under conditions of incubation with vinblastin which produce spherocytosis in intact cells, this agent had no effect upon the phosphorylation reaction after exposure up to one hour prior to initiation of the reaction (Table II). Vincristin also failed to inhibit the incorporation at .2 mM and slightly increased incorporation at 1 mM.

Examination of Membranes from Abnormal Cells. The membrane polypeptide patterns obtained by SDS-PAGE are shown in Fig. 3 for normal and hereditary spherocytosis (HS) membrane. The patterns obtained for the abnormal membrane polypeptides appeared equivalent in both the mobility and relative quantity of each component. The pattern

Table II. Effect of Vinblastin and Vincristin

Agent	Preincubation Time	^{32}P Incorporation (% control)	
		Spectrin	Band III
Vinblastin			
0.2mM	30 min.	100	102
	1 h.	98	102
Vincristin			
0.2mM	1 h.	103	97
1.0mM	1 h.	106	107

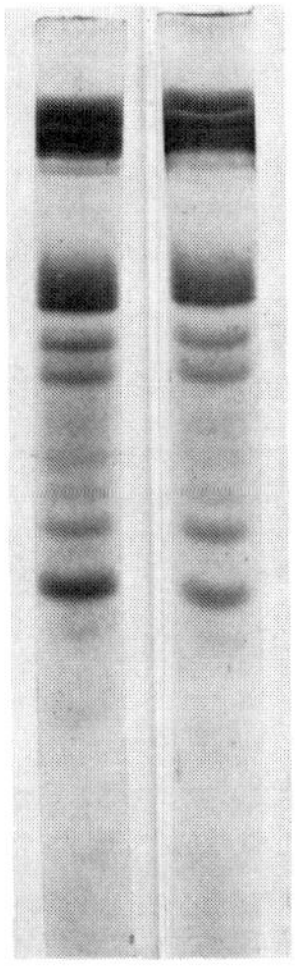

Figure 3. SDS polyacrylamide gel electrophoresis of hereditary spherocytosis membrane (on left) and a normal membrane run simultaneously. Gels were stained with coomassie blue.

Table III. Membrane Protein Phosphorylation in Abnormal Cell Membranes

Sample	^{32}P Incorporation (% of normal)			
	Spectrin		Band III	
	-cAMP	+cAMP	-cAMP	+cAMP
Hereditary Spherocytosis				
JS	39	30	38	27
FT	31	31	31	26
NB	32	--	--	--
AT	34	44	68	63
JE	40	66	45	42
CA	43	70	74	75
Hereditary Stomatocytosis				
WD	23	37	27	40
Hereditary Elliptocytosis				
HF	105	--	100	--
DS	98	--	90	--
Controls	100 (±11)	100 (±13)	100 (±11)	100 (±11)

Values in parenthesis for controls are ±S.D. for 10 normal membranes. The patient values are averages of quadruplicate determinations whose absolute value has a standard error of less than 10%. Cyclic AMP was 1 μM.

obtained with hereditary stomatocyte and hereditary elliptocyte membrane also appeared equivalent to normals (not shown).

The phosphorylation of membrane polypeptides in isolated membrane from abnormal cells is compared to normals in Table III. Phosphorylation was reduced in the membrane polypeptides of 6 patients with HS. The reduced incorporation was found in both the spectrin and Band III polypeptides. Although label incorporation into membrane polypeptides was stimulated about 1.3 times by cyclic AMP the deficiency with respect to normal membrane persisted.

Two other types of inherited erythrocyte membrane abnormalities have been studied. The hereditary stomatocyte (cup-shaped) membrane (Table III) has been studied in one case and also showed deficient label incorporation into spectrin and Band III polypeptides. In contrast, hereditary elliptocyte membranes from two patients showed normal levels of incorporation.

Effects of Sulfhydryl Agents. Several sulfhydryl agents were examined for their effects on the protein kinase (Table IV). Inhibition of activity was observed in each case although the extent of inhibition depended upon the particular agent utilized; the most effective was p-hydroxymercuribenzoate (p-HMB). The inhibition was sensitive to both the concentration of the sulfhydryl agent, as noted in the case of 5,5'-dithiobis-(2-nitrobenzoic acid), (DTNB), and to the time of incubation as shown in N-ethylmaleimide (NEM).

Table IV. Sulfhydryl Reagent Effects on Membrane Protein Phosphorylation

Additions	^{32}P Incorporation (% control)	
	Spectrin	Band III
PHMB	10	31
DTNB		
0.2mM	35	49
1.0mM	15	36
NEM		
15 min.	89	93
30 min.	64	65
60 min.	30	50

Incubations are with 1mM sulfhydryl agent for 1 h. at 37° prior to initiation of the phosphorylation reaction unless otherwise specified.

Table V. Dephosphorylation of Membrane Phosphoprotein

	^{32}P Remaining (% control)	
	Spectrin	Band III
Unreincubated Control	100 (±7)	100 (+7)
Additions at Reincubation (30',37°)		
Buffer	85 (±5)	92 (±7)
Buffer + EDTA, 1mM	98 (±3)	96 (±7)
Ca++, 2.5mM	87 (±7)	85 (±6)
Mg++, 2.5mM; 15'	62 (±3)	72 (±2)
Mg++, 2.5mM; 30'	44 (±4)	45 (±4)

Breakdown of the Phosphorylated Protein. The stability of preformed labeled polypeptides was studied by reincubation of membranes after removal of labeled ATP (Table V). The addition of 1 mM EDTA stabilized the labeled proteins which show some turnover in buffer alone. The addition of calcium ion at low or high concentrations did not effect the breakdown of the phosphoprotein. In contrast, the addition of magnesium resulted in a time dependent loss of label from spectrin and a Band III phosphoprotein.

Labeling of Intact Cells. Incubation of intact cells with ^{32}Pi resulted in labeling of the Band II and a Band III

Table VI. Phosphorylation -- Dephosphorylation of Membrane Protein in Intact Erythrocytes

Additions at 20 h.	Reincubation Time	cpm/ml of RBC	
		Spectrin	Band III
ATP Depleted Cells	0 h.	85	0
None	0	5360	2120
+Glucose	20	6300	5490
+NaF (10mM)	20	2460	1350
-Glucose	20	3000	1820

polypeptide. The incorporation was energy dependent since red cells, depleted by prior incubation without glucose, did not incorporate label into membrane polypeptides (Table VI). Cells reincubated with glucose were predominantly biconcave discs with less than 5% spherocytes. Cells reincubated without glucose or with glucose and sodium fluoride were uniformly present as spherocytes, analogous to results originally reported by Nakao, et al. (22) and by Weed, et al. (23). In the absence of glucose or with sodium fluoride, the labeling of membrane protein was reversed. These results demonstrated the presence of a protein phosphatase in the intact cell which leads to dephosphorylation of membrane polypeptides under condition of energy depletion.

DISCUSSION

Modification of protein by phosphorylation and dephosphorylation is a well-established regulatory mechanism for controlling enzyme reactivity (1). Several studies have demonstrated the presence of protein kinases and their polypeptide substrates in membranes from synaptic vesicles (2), rat liver plasma membrane (24), adenohypophyseal granules (25), rat skeletal muscle plasma membrane (6) and rod outer segments (4). The function of these reactions are not yet known. We have presented evidence which suggests the possible importance of a membrane bound protein kinase and a protein phosphatase in effecting the control of the erythrocyte biconcave shape and in the etiology of hereditary spherocytosis (13-15,26).

The phosphorylation reaction, as noted in Fig. 2, is non-linear. Interestingly, the addition of cyclic AMP, which stimulates the rate of the reaction 1.3 to 1.4 fold, also effects the final level of label incorporated. The shift in the level of incorporation suggests that the measured value for phosphorylation depends on two reactions involving initially phosphorylation while subsequently including the dephosphorylation of membrane protein which produces an equilibrium value within one hour.

An understanding of the etiology of abnormally shaped erythrocytes should be instructive in appreciating the normal mechanisms which control cell shape. A number of observations support the conclusion that hereditary spherocytosis (HS) involves a membrane defect including the enhanced passive Na+ premeability (27), a tendency to lose lipid (28) and release vesicles *in vitro* (29) and a reduced deformability of isolated HS membrane (30). The reduced deformability in HS is reversible upon addition of adenosine (30). The abnormal shape and apparent sensitivity to metabolic changes readily presents this cell as a useful subject for study of phosphorylation (13). The phosphorylation was reduced both with or without splenectomy and no correlation was apparent to the reticulocyte count (15). Because reduced incorporation was found in distinct polypeptide substrates, resolved in polyacrylamide gels, it is unlikely that the defect involves an alteration in these polypeptides since these presumably represent separate gene products. Rather, the primary deficiency appears to reside in the protein kinase itself. The deficiency may result from altered kinetic parameters of the enzyme or possibly from reduced production of the enzyme. The incorporation into hereditary stomatocyte membrane is also deficient and, in fact, shows the lowest level of incorporation in the spectrin component found for any sample. Additional studies are necessary to determine if the differences between spherocytosis and stomatocytosis can be attributed to quantitative differences in the level of membrane protein phosphorylation. The normal phosphorylation in each case of hereditary elliptocytosis suggests that a different mechanism produces the shape deficiency in these cells.

The phosphorylation reaction was studied in normal membrane to obtain further evidence for the role of this reaction in normal cell physiology. Ruthenium red is reported to selectively inhibit the ATPase activity stimulated by Ca++ and Mg++ (20). Since the erythrocyte membrane also shows an ATP dependent increase in Ca++ binding (31), the possible involvement of the membrane protein kinase deserves consideration. However, the protein kinase reaction is negligibly affected by ruthenium red (Table I) under conditions which markedly inhibit the ATPase activity. Moreover, cAMP does not affect Ca++ uptake while ruthenium red does (32). The data presented here does not support a relationship between the phosphorylation reaction and Ca++, Mg++-ATPase activity or ATP dependent Ca++ uptake by the membrane.

The effects of the alkaloid, vinblastin, were of interest because of its capacity to produce spherocytes and the suggestion that vinblastin may produce this effect by specific interaction with membrane microfilamentous protein resulting in altered cell shape (21). Incubation of membrane with vinblastin or vincristin under conditions which produce shape changes did not inhibit the phosphorylation reaction (Table II). The effect of vinblastin on cell shape does not appear to involve the phosphorylation reaction. An alternative explanation for the shape effects of vinblastin has been suggested by Seeman et al. (33) who suggested that the agent behaves like many other cationic drugs which have a membrane expanding effect. Such a process might behave independently of direct protein dependent shape changes in the membrane.

The effects of sulfhydryl agents on the membrane were examined because normal erythrocytes are perturbed by these agents causing altered ion permeability, lipid loss and shape change (34). The effective inhibition of the protein kinase by these agents demonstrate the importance of a sulfhydryl group in the catalytic activity and are also consistent with the possible interdependence of protein phosphorylation and cell shape control.

Reduced levels of ATP resulting from metabolic depletion on inhibition occur with the reversible transition from a biconcave disc to a spherocyte (22,23) and with a loss of membrane deformability (23). These results suggested that some reversible ATP dependent mechanism controls erythrocyte shape and deformability.

If the protein phosphorylation mechanism is important in rationalizing the ATP dependent deformability and shape changes, it is necessary to demonstrate a capacity to alter protein phosphorylation with changes in available ATP. It was apparent that the cell must have the capacity to dephosphorylate membrane protein. The stabilization by EDTA and the increased breakdown of each polypeptide in the presence of Mg++ demonstrated that the membrane possesses a Mg++-dependent protein phosphatase. The presence of a phosphorylation-dephosphorylation mechanism is analogous to such systems as the pyruvate dehydrogenase complex which contains a protein kinase and a Mg++-dependent protein phosphatase which regulates the activity of the dehydrogenase (35).

A study of membrane protein phosphorylation in intact cells is important in demonstrating the response of the reaction to conditions which alter deformability and shape of the intact cell. These studies required the use of ^{32}Pi since [γ-^{32}P] ATP cannot diffuse into the intact cell. Label incorporated into the spectrin component as reported by Palmer and Verpoorte (36). The failure of ATP depleted cells to incorporate label demonstrated the energy dependence for phosphorylation in the intact cell. Incubation with glucose resulted in label incorporation principally into the Band II component of spectrin (in comparison to both Band I and Band II labeling in isolated membrane). Secondly, label also incorporated into the Band III position. The decrease in label in both polypeptides, which occurs in metabolically depleted or inhibited cells, demonstrated a functional phosphorylation-dephosphorylation process in the intact cell which favors phosphorylation under conditions of energy repletion and retention of the biconcave disc, and which favors dephosphorylation with energy depletion and spherocytogenesis. The reduction in label was below levels established during the preincubation and therefore represented a real loss of label rather than a decreased incorporation level due to variation in specific activities of ATP in repleted and depleted cells. The actual kinetic parameters for decay, however, will depend on this factor as well as the competition of the protein kinase and other enzymes for the declining levels of ATP.

The specific function of the substrates of the protein kinase remains an unresolved problem. The effects of phosphorylation on the properties of these proteins are also not known. The spectrin component has been suggested as a structural component of the erythrocyte membrane (37) and it contains a myosin-like Ca++ ATPase (38) which would imply a possible contractile function for this protein. In view of the sensitivity of the phosphorylation of spectrin to conditions which modify cell shape, as reported here, the actual demonstration of the effect of protein modification by phosphorylation would be particularly useful. Jacob, et al. (39) have reported the altered precipitation of membrane protein extracts from HS which may reflect the differing solubility properties of the phosphorylated and unphosphorylated states of the spectrin component. Differential solubility properties for spectrin have been reported by Marchesi et al. (37) and by Clarke (40) and this, too, may reflect the isolation of the protein in a phosphorylated or unphosphorylated state. The deficient phosphorylation of spectrin in HS may effect the organization of this protein at the intracellular face resulting in the reduced deformability and decrease in the biconcave shape. A similar response would result from energy depletion or inhibition of the kinase by sulfhydryl agents.

The phosphorylation defect in the HS membrane warrants further consideration of this reaction in influencing pathophysiological defects in addition to cell shape and deformability. The cell shows an abnormal passive ion permeability (27) which may, of course, be secondary to conformational changes induced in the spectrin molecule. However, the effects of phosphorylation on the Band III polypeptides may be of considerable interest in studies of passive ion permeability, since these polypeptides appear to traverse the membrane interior (41). The potential influence of membrane protein phosphorylation on permeability control has already been noted in synaptic (2) and muscle membrane (6). The HS membrane also shows abnormal agglutination properties (39) which indicates an alteration at the cell surface. Since the modification of the spectrin component can produce transmembrane effects on the distribution of surface charges (42), the defect in spectrin phosphorylation may also be manifested in transmembrane effects on cell surface sites which influence cell agglutinability.

REFERENCES

1. Huijing, F., Lee, E. (Eds.), Protein Phosphorylation in Control Mechanisms, Academic Press, New York, 1973.
2. Maeno, H., Johnson, E., Greengard, P., J. Biol. Chem. 246:134 (1971).
3. Lemaire, S., Pelletier, G., Labrie, F., J. Biol. Chem. 246:7303 (1971).
4. Pannbacker, R. in Kahn, R. and Lands, W. (Eds.), Prostaglandins and Cyclic AMP, Academic Press, New York, 1973.
5. Brown, E., Biochem. Biophys. Res. Comm. 22:406 (1966).
6. Andrews, C., Rosen, A., Alman, R., Appel, S., Science 182:927 (1973).
7. Williams, R., Biochem. Biophys. Res. Comm. 47:671 (1972).
8. Guthrow, C., Allen, J., Rasmussen, H., J. Biol. Chem. 247:8145 (1972).
9. Rubin, C., Erlichman, J., Rosen, O., J. Biol. Chem. 247:6135 (1972).
10. Roses, A. and Appel, S., J. Biol. Chem. 248:1403 (1973).
11. Rubin, C. and Rosen, O., Biochem. Biophys. Res. Comm. 50:421 (1973).
12. Roses, A. and Appel, S., Proc. Nat. Acad. Sci., USA 70:1855 (1973).
13. Greenquist, A.C. and Shohet, S.B., Blood 42:997 (1973).
14. Shohet, S.B. and Greenquist, A.C., Clin. Res. 22:406a (1974).
15. Greenquist, A.C. and Shohet, S.B., FEBS Letters, In Press.
16. Dodge, J., Mitchel, C., Hanahan, D., Arch. Bioc. Biophys. 100:119 (1963).
17. Weber, K. and Osborn, M., J. Biol. Chem. 244:4406 (1967).
18. Fairbanks, G., Steck, T. and Wallack, D., Biochem. 10:2606 (1971).

19. Hokin, L. and Hokin, M., Biochim. Biophys. Acta 84:563 (1964).
20. Watson, E., Vincenzi, F., Davis, P., Biochim. Biophys. Acta 249:606 (1971).
21. Jacob, H., Amsden, T., White, J., Proc. Nat. Acad. Sci. USA 69:471 (1972).
22. Nakao, M., Nakao, T., Yamazoe, S., Nature 187:945 (1960).
23. Weed, R., LaCelle, P., Merril, E., J. Clin. Invest. 48:795 (1969).
24. Shlatz, L. and Marinetti, G., Biochem. Biophys. Res. Comm. 45:51 (1971).
25. Labrie, F., Lemaire, S., Poirier, G., Pelletier, G. and Boucher, R., J. Biol. Chem. 246:7311 (1971).
26. Greenquist, A.C. and Shohet, S.B., Fed. Proc. 33:1532 (1974).
27. Bertles, J.F., J. Clin. Invest 36:816 (1957).
28. Reed, C., Swisher, S., J. Clin. Invest. 45:777 (1966).
29. Weed, R. and Bowdler, A., J. Clin. Invest. 45:1137 (1966).
30. LaCelle, P. and Weed, R., Blood 34:858 (1969).
31. Duffy, M. and Schwarz, V., Biochim. Biophys. Acta 330:294 (1974).
32. Duffy, M. and Schwarz, V., BCSTB5 2:406 (1974).
33. Seeman, P., Chau-Wong, M., Moygen, S., Nature NB 241:22 (1973).
34. Jacob, H.S. and Jandl, J.H., J. Clin. Invest. 41:779 (1962).
35. Petit, F., Roche, T., Reed, L., Biochem. Biophys. Res. Comm. 49:563 (1972).
36. Palmer, R., Verpoorte, J., Can. J. Bioc. 49:337 (1971).
37. Marchesi, S., Steers, E., Marchesi, V., Tillack, T., Biochem. 9:50 (1970).
38. Clarke, M., Griffith, J., Fed. Proc. 31:412 (1972).
39. Jacob, H., Ruby, A., Overland, E., Mazia, D., J. Clin. Invest. 50:1800 (1971).
40. Clarke, M., Biochem. Biophys. Res. Comm. 45:1063 (1971).
41. Bretscher, M., J. Mol. Biol. 59:351 (1971).
42. Nicolson, G.L. and Painter, R.G., J. Cell. Biol. 59:395 (1973).
43. This work has been supported by grants AM-16095 and AM-37237 from the National Institutes of Health, U.S.P.H.S.

DISCUSSION

Dr. Jacob: Our two groups agree on most of what you have presented. I wonder whether you have tried using the protein kinase in red cell membranes to phosphorylate nonendogenous substrates. You have speculated that your results suggest a protein kinase deficiency in spherocytosis. If so, histones and other non membrane substrates might not be expected to be normally phosphorylated.

Dr. Greenquist: No, we haven't looked at the effects of adding exogenous substrates. Certainly it's possible to have a defect in the endogenous membrane protein phosphorylation and not see it with exogenous substrates but we haven't done that.

Dr. Rasmussen: That membrane protein kinase doesn't phosphorylate exogenous substrate very well so if you add histone or casein you get very little phosphorylation.

Dr. Aminoff: Am I to understand from what you're saying that there are some phosphate groups on the red cell surface that are normally present?

Dr. Greenquist: There is phosphate in several polypeptides in the red cell membrane.

Dr. Aminoff: Is there any way of determining what amount there is and to what extent it contributes to the negative charge of the red cell?

Dr. Greenquist: We can estimate how much gets incorporated under our reaction.

Dr. Aminoff: No, that's incorporation. I am talking about how much there is naturally before you artificially incorporate it.

Dr. Greenquist: It could be done but we haven't done it.

Dr. Aminoff: Does anyone know if there is any naturally occuring phosphate on the outside of the membrane that contributes to the overall negative charge of the red cell surface?

Editor's note: No answer from audience.

Dr. Gabuzda: A technical question. I wonder if your membranes from pathologic erythrocytes, such as in hereditary spherocytes, wash as free from Hb as normal erythrocytes do? Do you get them clean?

Dr. Greenquist: They usually have slightly larger amounts of hemoglobin. You can see a trace band on the gel.

Dr. Gabuzda: Would these figures affect your specific activity of phosphorylation?

Dr. Greenquist: Yes, we have corrected for that, but even if we didn't correct for it, it wouldn't produce the deficiency that we have shown. But we have corrected for hemoglobin present.

Dr. Gabuzda: You correct for it? By just deducting it from the optical density of your specific....

Dr. Greenquist: Exactly, by doing hemoglobin determinations by pyridine hemochromagen and determining how much is in the preparations. The effect is small anyway.

Dr. La Celle: Several people have talked about various ATPase activities of membranes, calcium-magnesium dependent which are not the calcium pump. I wonder if your kinase could be related to or the same as those activities?

Dr. Greenquist: We have looked at the effects of ruthenium red on the kinase reaction. That is presumably an inhibitor of the calcium-magnesium ATPase, and it doesn't affect the protein kinase reaction.

DETERMINANTS OF ERYTHROCYTE MEMBRANE ELASTICITY

P. L. La Celle[1,2] and F. H. Kirkpatrick[2]

Depts. Medicine[1] & Radiation Biol. & Biophys.[2]

University of Rochester, Rochester, NY 14642

INTRODUCTION

Three hundred years ago the microscopist van Leeuwenhoek first recognized the remarkable reversible deformation of erythrocytes during capillary flow and modern investigators (Krogh, 1922; Ponder, 1952; Skalak and Brånemark, 1969; Canham, 1969) have re-emphasized the significance of this characteristic. Over the last century fragmentation of red cells has been observed by many investigators and Rous (1917) considered it a mechanism whereby increasing sphericity and resultant loss of deformability of the erythrocyte determines the cells' life span. Krogh noted that in narrow capillaries the erythrocyte may assume a sausage shape and recover the equilibrium biconcave disc shape, indicating its elasticity. By careful measurement of individual erythrocyte dimensions (Canham and Burton, 1968) the minimum cylindrical diameter through which erythrocytes could pass without rupture was predicted to be 3.0 μm. Subsequent studies of aspiration of erythrocytes in glass micropipettes (Rand and Burton, 1964; La Celle, 1969) and filtration through polycarbonate filters (Gregerson *et al.*, 1967) demonstrated that normal human erythrocytes can, in fact, assume a cylindrical shape with minimum diameter 2.7 to 2.8 μm and length 10 to 15 μm and then, presumably by elastic recoil, resume the discocyte configuration.

Early investigators examined the erythrocyte membrane properties by observing behavior at hemolysis (Ponder, 1932) and experiments with swollen erythrocytes (Rand and Burton, 1964), indicated the modulus of elasticity to be 10^7-10^8 dyn/cm^2, similar to that obtained by Katchalsky (Katchalsky *et al.*, 1960). This modulus may correspond to the bulk modulus of the membrane and indicates the two dimensional incompressibility of the membrane material. In studies of fluid shear stress on erythrocytes (Hochmuth and Mohandas, 1972) and analysis of micropipette aspiration of erythrocyte membrane (Evans, 1973a) the elastic constant μ corresponding to the shear modulus is, in contrast to the bulk modulus, very low: approximately 10^{-2} dyn/cm. Katchalsky's analysis suggests that a tension of 1.3×10^6 dyn/cm^2 or greater is required for hemolysis and that the solid viscosity is of the order of 3×10^8 poise, characterizing the erythrocyte membrane as a fairly rigid structure.

Recently evaluation of several models of membrane structure (Bull and Brailsford, 1973) suggests that a protein chain meshwork interacting to provide a skeletal network, with interspersed bimolecular lipid leaflets would provide mechanical properties corresponding to those observed in the erythrocyte membrane. Evans (1973a,b) has proposed a two dimensional elastomer material concept and has demonstrated that this model will accommodate the observed behavior of the erythrocyte membrane undergoing fluid shear which produces the microfilament and tear drop formation; the large strains and fragmentation phenomena observed in micropipette aspiration experiments; and the large strains with elastic recoil typical of capillary flow. A simple statistical thermodynamic calculation to relate the observed elastic shear modulus to the molecular weight of the subchains of the proposed protein network (Evans, 1973a, Evans and La Celle, 1975) suggests that the molecular weight is of the order of 10^5, a magnitude similar to that of spectrin.

Erythrocyte shape affects its deformability, a cell characteristic dependent in part on elasticity (La Celle, 1969). Nakao noted the dependence of the rheologically favorable (elastic, shear compliant) shape on erythrocyte ATP (Nakao *et al.*, 1960a) and correlated cell survival with ATP concentration (Nakao, 1962); and intracellular Ca++ concentration was found to be the important ATP-modulated regulator of cell shape and deformability (Weed *et al.*, 1969). Subsequent studies (Palek *et al.*, 1971a,b) have extended the earlier observations (Wins and Schoffeniels, 1966; Weed *et al.*, 1969) that Ca++ causes "contraction" of erythrocyte ghost membranes. It has been reported that actin- and myosin-like proteins exist in the human erythrocyte membrane (Ohnishi, 1962); such proteins or other contractile membrane proteins may mediate the Ca++-induced discocyte-echinocyte transformation. A variety of amphiphilic agents (Deuticke, 1968) can induce echinocytic or stomatocytic shape changes in erythrocytes. Weed has suggested that such agents may exert their effect by alteration of Ca++ movements and/or pH in the membrane (Weed and Chailley, 1973). It is well known that calcium accumulation in the erythrocyte membrane affects cation permeability (Maizels, 1959; Hoffman, 1962; Palek *et al.*, 1971a; Romero and Whittam, 1971; Porzig, 1973). Many studies of Ca++ binding to erythrocyte membranes have been made; only those studies defining Ca++ binding to the inner membrane surface are useful in understanding Ca++ effects, since these effects on membrane proteins involve proteins at the inner membrane surface. Characterization of Ca binding to isolated proteins (La Celle *et al.*, 1972) indicates significant binding to spectrin, a water soluble protein located on the inner surface; spectrin has a high affinity site with an apparent association constant, $K = 3 \times 10^6$ l/mole.

The experiments described in this paper were undertaken 1) to determine the individual contribution of lipids and proteins to membrane elasticity in an *in vitro* membrane system; 2) to correlate the cellular deformability of normal erythrocyte membranes (resealed ghosts) with intracellular Ca++ concentrations in a Ca EGTA system, where pH is known; and 3) to examine elasticity and its time dependent modification in sickle, thalassemic and hereditary spherocyte cell membranes. The intent is to provide additional insight in the role of membrane proteins in membrane elasticity and also investigate the potential effects of Ca++ on the membrane elastic solid material properties.

METHODS

Preparation of Erythrocytes and Erythrocyte Ghosts

Fresh erythrocytes were obtained from venous blood samples collected with sodium heparin (14 U/ml) as anticoagulant. Cells from hematologically normal donors were utilized for studies of erythrocyte proteins and lipids, for ghost deformability experiments and as controls for cells from four patients having thalassemia major (Th), five having sickle cell disease (SS) and four having hereditary spherocytosis (HS). Erythrocytes separated by centrifugation were washed and resuspended in 2 mM tris-NaCl buffer, pH 7.4, osmolarity = 297 mosm, which contained 0.25% human albumin, except for ghost experiments in which the buffer was modified as noted. Experiments were performed immediately (less than two hours following venesection) or on cells stored up to six hours at $4^{o}C$. Erythrocyte ghosts were made by a one step hypotonic lysis method previously described (Weed *et al.*, 1969) except that the lysis medium contained predetermined Ca EGTA and Ca++ concentrations such that calculated internal [Ca++]i was derived from standard curves obtained from plots of Ca EGTA/EGTA vs. Ca++ at the specified pH. During experiments the reconstituted ghosts were suspended in isotonic 5 mM tris NaCl buffer which contained Ca++ = 1.5 mM; K+ = 4.5 mM; Mg++ = 4 mM.

Isolation of Membrane Proteins

Water soluble proteins were extracted at pH 7.5 in the presence of EDTA by the method of Hoogeveen (Hoogeveen *et al.*, 1970) and the derived protein analyzed by a standard SDS-polyacrylamide gel electrophoresis technique (Fairbanks *et al.*, 1971). Using a high resolution stacking gel system capable of resolving proteins of molecular weight difference of approximately 500 daltons (modified from Neville, 1971) proteins were characterized and compared with chicken skeletal muscle proteins. Ca++ affinity of specific proteins was determined by a flow dialysis method, utilizing ^{45}Ca and known quantities of protein, with Scatchard plot analysis

Estimates of Membrane Elasticity and Cellular Deformability

To assess elasticity small regions of the membrane were stressed in a uniform manner by aspiration into small (0.5 μm) glass micropipette tips in a controlled technique such that force required to aspirate a specified length, D, of membrane could be measured. Figure 1 illustrates such aspiration, indicating the calibrated eyepiece micrometer scale to measure D; D was also measured from a videotape record. The pressure was recorded by means of a calibrated variable reluctance transducer-digital manometer capable of measure-

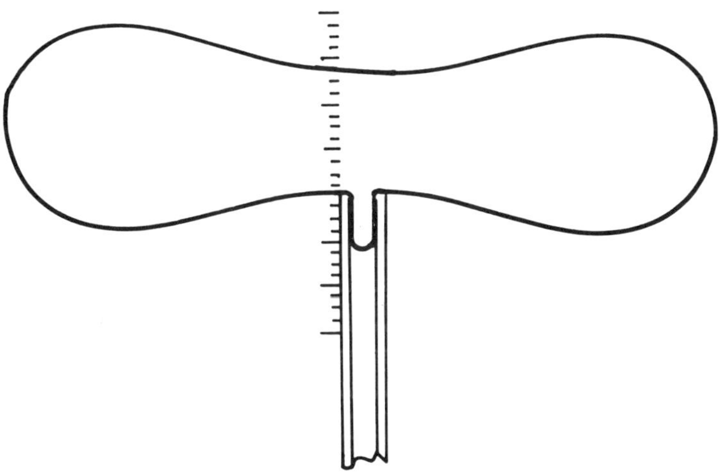

Figure 1. Measurement of membrane extension in a small glass micropipette as a reflection of membrane elasticity. A micrometer scale superimposed allows measurement of D, distance membrane tongue is aspirated into the pipette as a function of force, and the pipette diameter. Use of a small (0.5 μm) pipette avoids induction of tension in the membrane outside the pipette tip, demonstrated by the maintenance of the biconcave shape.

ments to 50 dyn/cm^2. To estimate the loss or modification of elasticity with duration of stress, portions of membrane were held in the extended state for 5, 10, 15 minutes and the permanent membrane strain (length of extension recorded after removal of stress) was measured. Data were recorded as extension ratio λ at the tip of micropipette from the value of D, length of membrane aspirated, and the radius of the micropipette, by the method of Evans (1973b). The strain occurring in the membrane at the micropipette tip is illus-

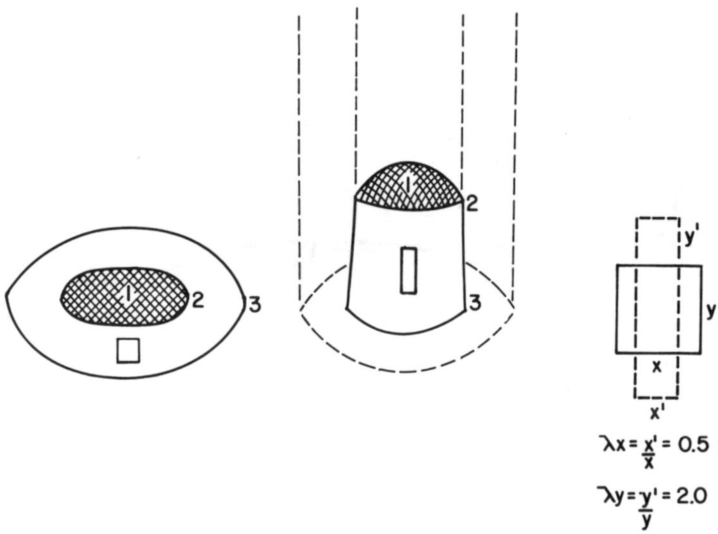

Figure 2. Uniaxial extension of membrane into a micropipette On the left the membrane under the micropipette tip prior to beginning aspiration; in the center diagram membrane strain is indicated by the elongation of the square membrane element and increase in distance 2 to 3 along the axis of the pipette On the right is illustrated the unidirectional extension of a square membrane element with conservation of area by reduction of the second dimension. The extension ratios, λ_x, λ_y, are defined as the ratio of final dimension in the x and y directions to the initial values.

trated in Figure 2 in which a small square element of membrane is shown in the middle diagram to have undergone uniaxial strain in the direction of the micropipette axis, with decrease in the second dimension perpendicular to the axis. λ, the extension ratio, is a function of the ratio of D, length of extension to R_p, pipette radius. No substantial strain occurs in the hemispherical cap of membrane. The strain is confined to the region of the pipette tip and thus the measured force is indicative of the local membrane strain.

Cellular deformability, estimated by recording the force to cause the erythrocyte to enter and transit a 2.7 μm micropipette, reflects membrane characteristics such as elasticity, and the contribution of shape and intracellular contents to the cells' ability to adapt passively to small channel geometry. Force Pt for cellular deformability was measured using the apparatus described above, in limiting diameter (2.7-2.8 μm) glass micropipettes.

Extensibility of Lipid and Lipid-Protein Membranes

To determine the relative contribution of the lipid and protein to membrane elasticity, deformation of lipid membranes was examined by the micropipette method illustrated in Figure 3. On the left, a "black" lipid bilayer formed in a 1 mm aperture in a teflon cup (which in turn is immersed in a Lucite bath) is aspirated into a small (∿0.5 μm) glass micropipette and force recorded as noted above. The solutions on either side of the membrane were the standard solutions noted above, at pH 7.2; to the solution on the side away from the micropipette ("inside") protein extracted from erythrocytes was added to test its effect on the extension ratio λ of the lipid bilayer. Oxidized cholesterol or phospholipid extracts of normal human erythrocytes were used to make bilayers and human erythrocyte spectrin, up to 10 mg/ml was examined for its effect on the lipid membrane. A second approach involved injecting protein into liposomes via a micropipette, illustrated on the right panel of Figure 3, with extension of the membrane recorded prior to and five minutes after this maneuver.

ATPase Activity of Membrane Proteins

ATPase activities of EDTA-extracted proteins, of spectrin purified by isoelectric precipitation, and of ghosts, were measured by extracting $^{32}P_i$ (liberated from γ-^{32}Pi-ATP) with molybdate into isobutanol (Kirkpatrick, *et al.*, unpublished).

RESULTS

Effect of protein on lipid membrane extension in micropipettes

Lipid bilayers rupture when extended approximately the length of the pipette radius as noted in the case of both oxidized cholesterol and phospholipid membranes in Figure 4.

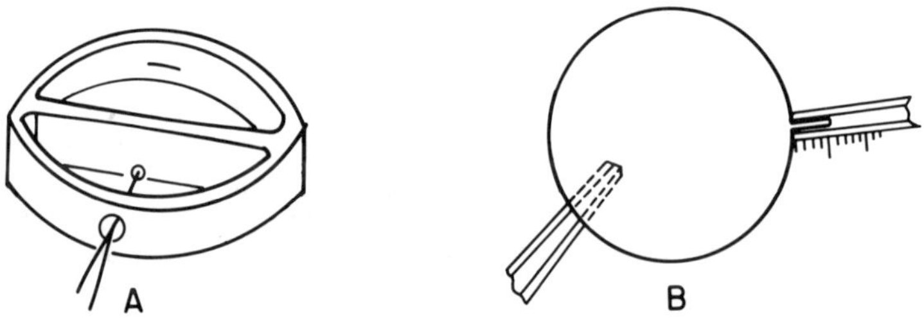

Figure 3. Techniques for determining the effect of absorbed protein (spectrin) on the uniaxial extension of oxidized cholesterol and erythrocyte phospholipid bilayers. On the left the lipid placed over the aperture of the chamber septum is visualized by light microscopy and the extension in a small micropipette recorded. Spectrin is added to the chamber on the opposite side of the membrane. In the illustration on the right liposomes are deformed in a micropipette and effect of protein, injected via a larger pipette, observed.

The cholesterol membranes ruptured at forces 50 to 150 dynes/ cm^2 and the phospholipid bilayers at lesser forces at somewhat greater extension. The force required was the same order of magnitude for extension of normal erythrocyte membranes in the same micropipette. Addition of spectrin 5 μgm/ ml increased the extension of the cholesterol membranes appreciably and rupture occurred at higher forces whereas

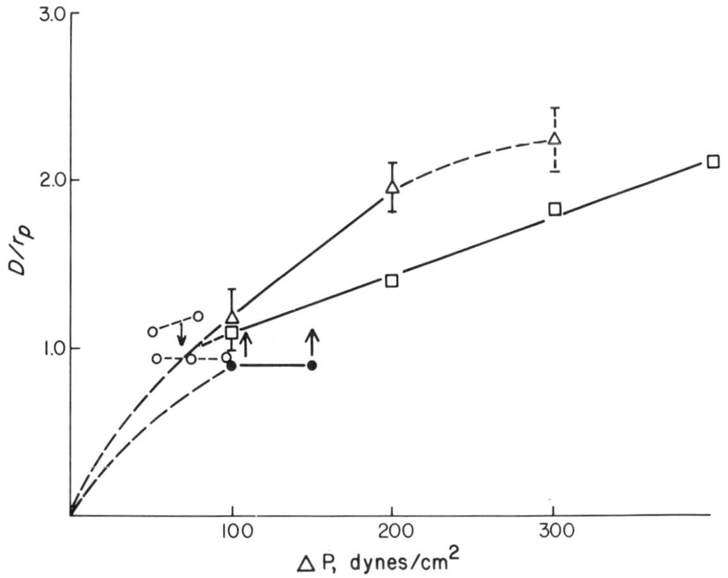

Figure 4. Alteration of extension D/Rp of lipid bilayer membranes by spectrin. Extension D/Rp vs. force: oxidized cholesterol membrane ●—●; oxidized cholesterol + spectrin Δ—Δ; erythrocyte lipids o—o ; erythrocyte lipids + spectrin o---o; normal erythrocyte ghost membranes □-□. ↑ indicates direction of alteration of D/Rp with addition of spectrin.

in the case of phospholipid the extension decreased somewhat and the limited data suggest an increase in force tolerated. Rupture of the simple lipid membranes occurs at approximately the predicted extension (Evans, 1973b) and absorbed protein appears to permit greater extension than expected in the pure lipid bilayers. Rupture of ghost membrane required 50x or greater force than that observed for the lipid bilayers.

Ghost Deformability as a Function of [Ca++]i

Alteration of "cellular" deformability, *ie.*, Pt measurement, in normal erythrocyte ghosts occurred between a calculated 10^{-8} and 10^{-7} M and appeared to reach a plateau at 10^{-6} M, as indicated in Figure 5, which represents a typical experiment. If these calculated data reflect accurately the free [Ca++] in the neighborhood of the inner membrane surface, 10^{-8} M would correspond to the normal deformability and elasticity state of the normal erythrocyte membrane and maximum calcium-related loss of deformability and elasticity would occur at approximately the concentration at which Ca++ begins to induce an increase in K+ permeability (Porzig, 1973). This value is less than that noted by Palek (Palek *et al.*, 1971b) for Ca++-ATPase stimulation and maximal decrease in ghost volume; however, their studies, at pH 7.6 with ATP in the system may not be comparable. It is of interest that the [Ca++] is below 10^{-6} M since our unpublished studies indicate that K+ and Na+ flux is actually decreased in the situation where sphering of ghosts occurs, which would not be anticipated if free [Ca++] were greater than 10^{-6} M, in light of the Porzig studies. These data confirm the small quantities of Ca++ capable of inducing membrane changes and suggest that the free [Ca++] rather than the total membrane related Ca++, as determined by atomic absorption flame spectrophotometry, is the important determinant of membrane dyanamics.

Cellular Deformability of Pathologic Erythrocytes

Table I records cellular deformability of normal, SS, Th and HS erythrocytes and indicates as well the excess rigidity (increased Pt) of poikilocytes from the Th blood

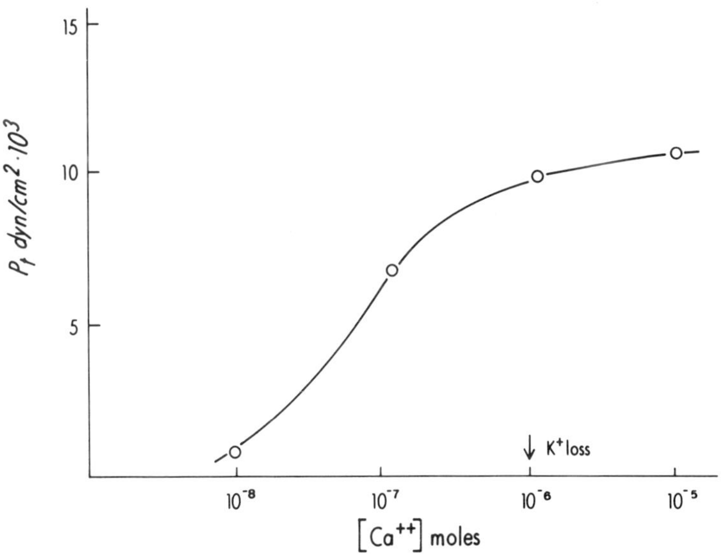

Figure 5. Cellular deformability of normal erythrocyte ghosts as a function of free intraghost Ca++. Free Ca++ concentrations were achieved by use of a Ca EGTA buffer system and Ca++, introduced at the time of hypotonic lysis of erythrocytes to make ghosts by the method of Schatzmann (1973) and Porzig (personal communication). Deformability was measured at temperature 23°C. Each point represents 50 ghost deformability determinations.

samples. In post splenectomy state, Pt was higher, as would be predicted, and in HS, there was not a uniformly strong correlation between relative rigidity of the stomacytic and spherocytic HS cells and life span indicators such as reticulocyte count. HS cells showed a yield stress in a Casson plot of viscosity vs. shear rate, indicating abnormal three dimensional membrane molecular arrangements.

Table 1

Cellular deformability of normal, SS, Th and HS erythrocytes

	Patients	Pt, mm H_2O ± SE	
Control cells		6.1 ± 0.1	
Sickle (SS) RSC	5	6.7 ± 0.4	(deoxy: 20.3±1.8; 9%>100)
ISC	5	2.1 ± 0.1	if minor diameter <dp*
		25 to ∞	if minor diameter <dp
Th	4		
HS presplenectomy	2	28.6 ± 12.4	* dp = pipette diameter
post "	2	109.8 ± 42.7	
all HS	7	37.6 ± 7.4	
Th poikilocytes	1	131.7 ± 30.3	
	1	116.8 ± 33.1	

Elasticity and Residual Deformation

When the extension ratios of SS and Th were obtained SS and Th membranes were found less extensible in 0.5 μm micropipettes than were those of normal erythrocytes. These data are recorded in Figure 6. Figure 6 also shows that irreversibly sickled cells (ISC) are less easily extended than reversibly sickled cells (RSC). ISC are more readily fragmented that RSC if force is applied to relatively narrow portions of the cells. When stress is removed significant residual extension is observed in all cells: SS>Th>normal.

Characteristics of Isolated Membrane Proteins

Spectrin, purified from EDTA extracts by isoelectric precipitation, has an ATPase of low specific activity that is stimulated by Ca++ and Mg++ in a complex pattern which appears to indicate three distinguishable classes of ATPase activity (Kirkpatrick *et al.*). The observed activities co-purify with the 240,000 dalton doublet peptides observed in SDS-gel electrophoresis. The observed turnover number, at

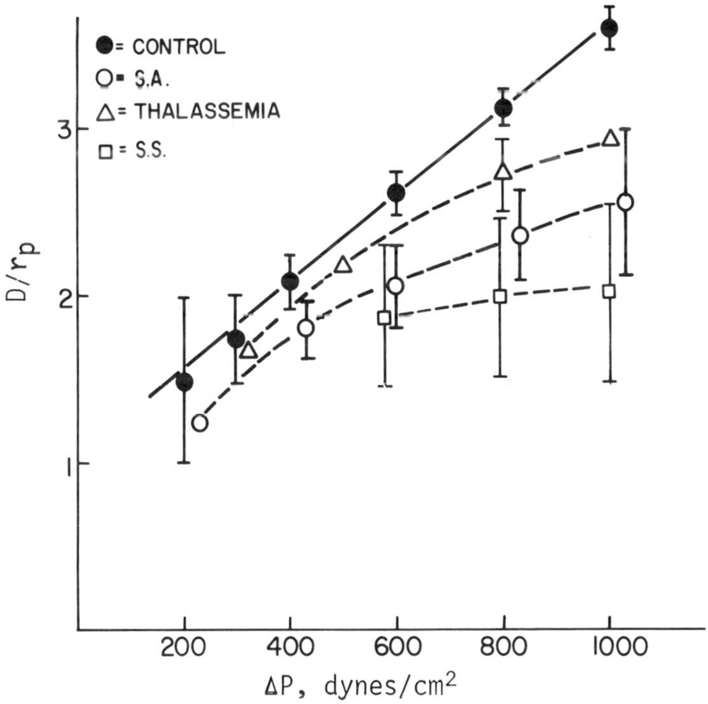

Figure 6. Extension of normal, Th, SS and SA erythrocytes as a function of deforming pressure. Normal =●—●; Th =▲--▲; SA =○--○; SS =□--□. Four different samples of each cell type are recorded; N = 40 cells for each point.

1 mM ATP, 1 mM $CaCl_2$ and 1 mM $MgCl_2$, is of the order of 40 nanomoles Pi/mg protein/hr; this corresponds to one Pi released per spectrin dimer per three minutes.

A low molecular weight protein most widely known as "Band 5" is elicited from erythrocyte membranes at low ionic strength, along with spectrin. It can be separated from "spectrin", the 240,000 dalton doublet, by precipitation of spectrin at pH 5.3, which leaves band 5 in the supernatant. Band 5 was further purified by column chromatography. The molecular weight by polyacrylamide gel electrophoresis in sodium dodecyl sulfate (SDS-PAGE) is about 43,000. Using the high resolution stacking gel system, "Band 5" is found to co-electrophorese with chicken skeletal muscle actin (Brederman and Kirkpatrick, unpublished results). The resolution of the system is sufficient that a molecular weight difference of 500 daltons should have produced observable band splitting. Band 5, thus corresponding to actin in molecular weight does not exhibit ATPase activity.

DISCUSSION

The data indicate that bilipid membranes do not have the potential to confer solid elastic properties on the erythrocyte membrane, rather they behave as liquids with mechanical properties anticipated from interfacial tension. Addition of protein to lipid bilayers, particularly erythrocyte phospholipid tends to modify the liquid behavior toward the solid material elasticity observed in the intact erythrocyte membrane or partially lipid extracted erythrocyte membrane, and supports the predictions inherent in the models of Bull (1973) and Evans (1973) in which protein networks, particularly spectrin dominated structures, account for the solid material properties (Evans, 1973; Evans and La Celle, 1975). This technique may have the potential for elucidation of the role of other protein components and divalent cations on membrane properties.

Clearly very small amounts of free [Ca++] produce major changes in the membrane configuration at the intracellular pH values typical of normal erythrocytes. Evidently the requisite [Ca++] for altered elasticity, as indicated in cellular deformability studies which reflect both the role of shape and membrane elasticity, is smaller than that which the Hoffman (1962) and Porzig (1973) studies suggest causes excess passive K+ permeability. The [Ca++] required for shape and elasticity changes is in the range of that thought important in skeletal muscle contraction. Such an observation suggests some potential similarity between ion requirements of classical contractile systems and the system which accounts for the erythrocyte shape change.

Each hemolytic anemia evaluated in these studies had increase in cellular deformability although only the deoxy

SS and post splenectomy HS cells were remarkably rigid. Of note nine percent of the RSC, normally deformable at high oxygen tension, would not pass the limiting diameter channel when deoxygenated, and the relatively rigid ISC SS cells could pass this restrictive channel only if the minor diameter of the cell was smaller than the channel. Individual Th cells were significantly rigid in postsplenectomy patients; such cells and the poikilocytes examined would have great difficulty surviving, if they behave in a manner similar to that of posttransfusion ACD stored cells having Pt values >100 mmH_2O (La Celle, 1969). The increased yield stress and high mean Pt values in HS cells, particularly in the post-splenectomy state may suggest abnormal three dimensional configuration of membrane proteins to account for abnormal mechanical properties.

The differences in membrane extensibility and greater tendency to permanent deformation following small stresses of several minutes duration may result from excess membrane associated protein in thalassemic cells. In sickle cells both a difference in membrane protein configuration and possibly small amounts of hemoglobin S adherent may cause the abnormality. These alterations may make thalassemic cells more liable to poikilocyte formation and sickle Hb containing to fragmentation at the small forces of the microcirculation.

In light of the elasticity conferred on lipid bilayers by spectrin it is of interest to speculate how spectrin may interact with membrane "actin-like" protein, to modify membrane configuration and elasticity. The ability of spectrin to interact with lipid, and also with itself to form fibers could provide a mechanism for conferring the solid elastic property, especially since the model of Evans (1973b; Evans and La Celle, 1975) does not require crosslinking of the weak elastomer subchains. In such a spectrin system simple addition of Ca++ could cause spectrin aggregation and change of membrane material properties. However, in solution spectrin aggregation requires [Ca++] $\simeq 10^{-3}$ M, whereas ghost experiments showed membrane changes with only 10^{-7} M. Band 2 of spectrin *in vivo* is probably normally phosphorylated (Avruch and Fairbanks, 1975). If dephospho-spectrin can aggregate in the plane of the membrane, while phosphospectrin cannot, then lowering intracellular ATP or increasing Ca++ will increase aggregation and later deformability. If dephosphospectrin also binds more strongly to actin, then even greater changes will be produced. If phosphospectrin can break and remake actin polymers, then the existence of persistent deformations is explained. The ATPase activity of spectrin would be an expression of a protein kinase activity, which might normally regulate spectrin kinase. Alternatively, the *in vivo* function of spectrin ATPase could be to rephosphorylate F-actin ADP to split and remodel actin polymers. Either activity could be decoupled from its normal substrate by solubilization or by calcium.

SUMMARY

Elasticity is conferred on bilayers formed from erythrocyte lipids by absorption of the water soluble erythrocyte protein spectrin, indicated by increased membrane extensibility and reduced fragmentation. In resealed erythrocyte ghosts, membrane extensibility, measured by mechanical experiments with narrow micropipettes, is decreased by free [Ca++] as low as 10^{-7} M. These observations indicate the important role of proteins in determining the solid material properties of the highly deformable erythrocyte membrane, and the sensitive modulation by Ca++.

A water soluble erythrocyte membrane protein having molecular weight similar to skeletal muscle actin has been partially characterized. It is postulated that spectrin, normally in the phospho form aggregates in the plane of the membrane when dephosphorylated as ATP decreases or Ca++ increases; interaction of aggregating spectrin with polymers of this "actin-like" protein may account for "membrane" contraction and loss of elasticity.

Sickle cells, thalassemic cells and hereditary spherocytes differ from normal erythrocytes in elastic properties, indicated by less extensible membranes and decreased cellular deformability, *ie.*, reduced capacity to deform through a minimum capillary channel; both sickle cells and thalassemic cells show greater time dependent permanent deformation than normal cells. Both sickle and hereditary spherocytes fragment more readily than control cells, at forces as low as 2 x 10^3 dynes/cm^2; this contrasts with force ≃ $2x10^7$ dyn/cm^2 for hemolysis.

This work was supported in part by USPHS Research Grant HL 16421-04 and in part by the US Atomic Energy Project at the University of Rochester and has been assigned Publication Number UR 3490-629.

REFERENCES

Avruch, J., Fairbanks, G. (1975). Phosphorylization of endogenous substrates by erythrocyte membrane protein kinases. I. A monovalent cation-stimulated reaction. *Biochem.* in press.

Bull, B.S. and Brailsford, J.D. (1973). The biconcavity of the red cell: an analysis of several hypotheses. *Blood* 41:833.

Canham, P.B. (1969). The difference in geometry of young and old human erythrocytes explained by a filtering mechanism. *Circ. Res.* 25:39.

Canham, P.B. and Burton, A.C. (1968). Distribution of size and shape in populations of normal human red cells. *Circ. Res.* 22:405.

Deuticke, B. (1968). Transformation and restoration of biconcave shape of human erythrocytes induced by amphiphilic agents and changes of ionic environment. *Biochim. Biophys. Acta* 103:494.

Evans, E.A. (1973a). A new material concept for the red cell membrane. *Biophys. J.* 13:926.

Evans, E.A. (1973b). New membrane concept applied to the analysis of fluid shear and micropipette-deformed red blood cells. *Biophys. J.* 13:941.

Evans, E.A. and La Celle, P.L. (1975). Intrinsic material properties of the erythrocyte membrane indicated by mechanical analysis of deformation. *Blood* in press.

Fairbanks, G., Steck, T.L. and Wallach, D.F.H. (1971). Electrophoretic analysis of the major polypeptides of the human erythrocyte membrane. *Biochem.* 10:2606.

Gregerson, M.I., Bryant, C.A., Hammerle, W.E., Usami, S.

and Chien, S. (1967). Flow characteristics of human erythrocytes through polycarbonate sieves. *Science* 157:825.

Hochmuth, R.M. and Mohandas, N. (1972). Uniaxial loading of the red cell membrane. *J. Biomech.* 5:501.

Hoffman, J.F. (1962). Cation transport and structure of the red cell plasma membrane. *Circ.* 26:1201.

Hoogeveen, J.Th., Juliano, R., and Rothstein, A. (1970). Water soluble proteins of the human red cell membrane. *J. Membr. Biol.* 3:156.

Katchalsky, A., Kedem, O., Klibansky, C. and de Vries, A. (1960). Rheological considerations of the haemolysing red blood cell. *Flow Properties of Blood and Other Biological Systems*. London, Pergamon, p. 150.

Krogh, A. (1929). *The Anatomy and Physiology of Capillaries*. New Haven, Yale University Press, p. 8.

La Celle, P.L. (1969). Alteration of deformability of the erythrocyte membrane in stored blood. *Transf.* 9:238.

La Celle, P.L., Kirkpatrick, F.H. and Udkow, M.P. (1972). Relation of altered deformability, ATP, DPG and Ca++ concentrations in senescent erythrocytes. *Erythrocytes, Thrombocytes, Leukocytes, Recent Advances in Membrane and Metabolic Research*. Stuttgart, Georg Thieme, p. 49.

La Celle, P.L., Kirkpatrick, F.H., Udkow, M.P. and Arkin, B. (1973). Membrane fragmentation and Ca++ membrane interaction: potential mechanisms of shape changes in the senescent red cell. *Red Cell Shape*. Heidelberg, Springer, p. 69.

Maizels, M. (1959). Calcium ions and the permeability of human red cells. *Nature* 184:366.

Marchesi, V.T. and Steers, E. (1968). Selective solubilization of a protein component of the red cell membrane. *Science* 159:203.

Nakao, M., Nakao, T. and Yamazoe, S. (1960). Adenosine triphosphate maintenance of shape of the human red cell. *Nature* 187:945.

Nakao, M., Wada, T., and Kamiyama T. (1962). A direct relationship between ATP level and *in vivo* viability of erythrocytes. *Nature* 194:877.

Neville, D.M. (1970). Molecular weight determination of protein-dodecyl sulfate complexes by gel electrophor-

esis in a discontinuous buffer system. *J. Biol. Chem.* 246:6328.
Ohnishi, T. (1962). Extraction of actin and myosin-like proteins from erythrocyte membrane. *J. Biochem. (Tokyo)* 52:307.
Palek, J., Curby, W.A. and Lionetti, F.J. (1971a). Effects of calcium and adenosine triphosphate on the volume of human red cell ghosts. *Am. J. Physiol.* 220:19.
Palek, J., Curby, W.A. and Lionetti, F.J. (1971b). Relation of Ca++-activated ATPase to Ca++-linked shrinkage of human red cell ghosts. *Am. J. Physiol.* 220:1028.
Ponder, E. (1952). *Hemolysis and Related Phenomena.* New York, Grune and Stratton.
Porzig, H. (1970). Calcium efflux from human erythrocyte ghosts. *J. Memb. Biol.* 2:324.
Porzig, H. (1973). Effect of divalent cations on Na and K permeability of human red cell ghosts. *Exper.* 29:747.
Rosenthal, A.S., Kregenow, F.M. and Moses, H.L. (1970). Some characteristics of Ca++-dependent ATPase activity associated with a group of erythrocyte membrane proteins which form fibrils. *Biochim. Biophys. Acta* 196:254.
Rous, P., and Roberston, O.H. (1917). The normal fate of erythrocytes. I. The findings in healthy animals. *J. Exptl. Med.* 25:651.
Schatzmann, H.J. (1973). Dependence on calcium concentration and stoichiometry of the calcium pump on human red cells. *J. Physiol.* 235:551.
Skalak, R. and Brånemark, P.O. (1969). Deformation of red blood cells in capillaries. *Science* 164:717.
Weed, R.I., La Celle, P.L. and Merrill, E.W. (1969). Metabolic dependence of red cell deformability. *J. Clin. Invest.* 48:795.
Weed, R.I. and Chailley, B. (1973). Calcium-pH interactions in the prediction of shape change in the erythrocyte. *Red Cell Shape.* Heidelberg, Springer, p. 55.
Wins, P. and Schoffeniels, E. (1966). ATP and Ca++-linked contraction of red cell ghosts. *Arch. Int. Physiol. Biochem.* 74:812.

DISCUSSION

Dr. Castro: Did you study several patients with hereditary spherocytosis that were not splenectomized?

Dr. La Celle: We have three that are not splenectomized. They are all in their eighties and they say they have done so well that they don't see the point of splenectomy. And we have studied them.

Dr. Castro: What I was referring to is whether you have found some of their red cells to be actually more deformable or actually better suited to circulate than those of splenectomized patients. We've studied RBC's from patients with spherocytosis in the rat model and found uniformly short survival of RBC's from splenectomized patients. In contrast, the RBC's of some non-splenectomized patients had longer survivals than normal human red cells.

Dr. La Celle: Well, I can simply reply that in the three we've seen who subsequently were splenectomized and in whom we've done studies after splenectomy, there has been a uniform worsening of deformability after splenectomy. The spleen is the most restrictive portion of the circulation and when you take it out, then cells that are basically worse in terms of deformability can survive in the circulation. This has been consistent in those three patients. On the other hand, one can't predict what the life span of cells will be simply from deformability *in vitro*. That is to say, one must look at the whole system. I think this is understandable from various studies including one by Wylie which tends to show that there wasn't a terribly good correlation between such simple things as hemolytic rate because one apparently has to look at the spleen, and what's going on there. "Conditioning" may allow some spleens to accept a more rigid cell than others.

Dr. Mizukami: Two questions. With respect to the quantity lambda you have measured, is there any change according to the age of each cell? Second, do you expect this quantity lambda to be the same at any portion of the cell, i.e., will there be any difference of this quantity on the side of the cell from that on the top or bottom of the cell?

Dr. La Celle: The first question relates to age and we don't have any systematic studies of elasticity as a function of age. I think one might predict, though, that since the cell membranes are thicker "if you accept some peoples' work" that elasticity probably will be different. Total cellular deformability decreases with age. In terms of whether there is different elasticity in various portions of the normal biconcave disc, I think I'm on shaky ground. Rand and Burton who looked at the micro-pipettist's technique 10 years ago felt that there was no difference in their hands, but they were using a rather unique situation, basically looking at swollen cells. When we first started we felt that there wasn't any difference, but then at this point, I think, we didn't see any difference because: 1) our equipment wasn't good enough or we weren't good enough, and 2) we used relatively large pipettes which didn't allow us the sensitivity of measurement. Dr. Evans and Lablond in their studies showed, as I recall, rather clear differences in parameters of the cell as the most convex portion of the cell compared to the more flat biconcave or simple region, and this would be expected in terms of any mathematical analysis of what's going on as a function of tension in the membrane. So in answer to your question, I think one should expect to find differences over the surface if he has the technique whereby to measure it with sensitivity.

Dr. Mizukami: Thank you.

Dr. Greenquist: Have you ever looked at the deformability of the hereditary spherocytosis membrane ghost in the presence of EDTA? Is the reduced deformability changed by EDTA?

Dr. La Celle: Well, we didn't do the right experiment. We looked at ghosts with EDTA on the outside and couldn't see any change, but then these were only short term experiments with about an hour's incubation.

Dr. Brewer: Do you have any thoughts on the echinocytic

changes in the membrane such as those induced by calcium for instance? What they're due to and so forth?

Dr. La Celle: Actually, probably the local expert would be Dr. Evans who has thought about this a lot more than I. Would you like to speculate on this Evan?

Dr. Evans: I would speculate that there are aproximately 30 to 50 Ca++ pump sites per erythrocyte, based on the rates we have observed the Ca pump to extrude labelled Ca++, and this happens to correspond to the number of spicules seen in echinocytes. This obviously proves nothing about a correlation between number of pump sites and number and loci of echinocytic spicules but is intriguing to contemplate. I would suggest that echinocytes could result due to alteration of Ca pump function by agents which induce echinocyte formation and that resultant local accumulation of Ca++ could cause a "contraction" phenomenon at the inner membrane surface, involving aggregation of spectrin, with possible intimate participation of an actin-like protein which could thus be the "multiplier" component, with Ca++ the trigger. Reversibility is the result of resumption of the Ca++ pump.

Dr. La Celle: Does that satisfy you, Dr. Brewer? I'm sure I can't add much to it. I guess I'm impressed that a very small amount of calcium ions in the region of the membrane can cause a lot to happen and one almost has to think of a multiplier system intermediate between the calcium and the end result just as one would have to, I think, in the case of Dr. Rasmussen's studies where a very small number of molecules appear to have a very major effect over the membrane. There must be some intermediate which gives you some multiplication of the initial phenomenon.

BLOOD SUBSTITUTES

Chairwoman: N. Meyers

Blood Substitutes: Introductory Comments

N. Meyers

The University of Michigan Medical School

Ann Arbor, Michigan

A precedent is being set today, for this is the first time an international conference on red blood cell metabolism and function has assigned a special session to blood substitutes. Blood substitutes, artificial blood, and breathable liquids appear to have sprung upon the scene, or so it seems, because of the publicity given to the almost science-fiction aspects of some of the experiments. Breathable liquids and blood substitutes are, in fact, two different aspects of an interrelated field.

First, the breathable liquids is an area in which our second speaker, Dr. Leland Clark, is well known. His picture in magazines and on television has been widely published alongside his famous mouse, submerged in a beaker containing a clear breathable fluid. The mouse is bright-eyed and his mouth is wide open to suck in the oxygen containing fluid. After hundreds of such experiments with many different types of media the animals now stay submerged longer and recover to live normally.

Second, blood substitutes, or "life support systems" as Dr. Geyer would like to call them, make use of emulsified fluids which dissolve large amounts of oxygen and carbon dioxide as a substitute for all or part of the whole blood in the animal. This is in contrast to blood extenders which do not dissolve oxygen and must be used with red blood cells. Dr. Geyer, the first speaker, has concentrated on the goal of replacing 100% of an animal's blood and has achieved good results using perfluorochemical emulsions. His rat is usually pictured in a desiccator immediately after such a transfusion, drinking water, washing himself, carrying out all his natural functions, and happily pumping his milk-like substitute blood. All the while he is breathing oxygen-enriched air.

It's natural, however, to recoil at the thought of lungs filled with fluid to breathe, or a colorless blood substitute replacing our own red cells, but we can no longer afford philosophic discussions about whether we should or could accept blood substitutes. Blood must be considered a natural resource, which, like oil and other natural resources, has been used wastefully in the past and is now and in the future in short supply. It has been stated that 90% of the world's population does not have access to blood banks. If blood substitutes were not already here, we would be challenged to invent them. That we already have a good start is due to the invention and synthesis of two kinds of chemicals, which were originally designed for other uses, such as electrical insulation, as cooling agents, detergents, and surfactants. These materials are used to make perfluorochemical emulsions. They are carbon and nitrogen derivatives in which all of the hydrogen has been replaced by fluorine atoms. Most of them are quite inert, but they had one fault: According to the industrial users, some dissolved too much oxygen. However, it was not long before biochemical researchers turned this fault into an asset, screening them at first in organ perfusion experiments. Of the early workers, Dr. H.A. Slovitor and Dr. T. Kamimoto of the University of Pennsylvania, first emulsified a fluorochemical with albumin to perfuse a living brain.

But the perfluorochemicals on their own were not really successful as blood substitutes. They did not have the right flow properties for circulation in the animal body.

Fortunately, about this time, new types of surfactants and emulsifying agents were entering the commercial market.

They were non-toxic; many of them are now used in the food and drug industries. Some of them were found to protect red blood cells in freeze-thaw experiments. These compounds, "the pluronics," are ethylene and propylene oxypolymers. The molecules have hydrophobic and hydrophilic components. They cause the very dense perfluorochemicals to form fine emulsions in the presence of a suitable source of energy such as sonication or homogenizing machines. Dr. Geyer has stated that, "the problems associated with obtaining proper circulation proved to be much more difficult than those related to the capacity of perfluorocompounds to carry oxygen."

Dr. Clark, who is the inventor of the most commonly used heart lung machine, long ago realized the need for a blood-like material to prime the pump. Furthermore, red blood cells rupture easily when continuously circulated and need to be replaced with costly human blood. In a recent magazine article, it was said that Dr. Clark had "accidentally" made the discovery of using a breathable liquid by simply plunging an animal into it. However, he had reasoned that lungs are functional, and are not necessarily violated by nonhydrolizing fluid. If that fluid can deliver oxygen and remove carbon dioxide, it is doing what red blood cells do. At first he used silicone oils which dissolve 20% oxygen, the composition in air, but later turned to the clear perfluorocompounds. I've read also where he is quoted as saying that he expects to try breathing some of these breathable fluids himself in the very near future. We shall anxiously await the results. He also predicts that breathable fluids will be used by deep sea divers. For example, he has decompressed an animal in a breathable substance from a simulated 500 foot depth, in one second. The animal survived because the liquid was noncompressible and no bubbles were formed in his blood. He envisions that breathable liquids could be used in cystic fibrosis to clean up patients' lungs. Clinical testing is yet to be accomplished, but that may not be too far off.

At the April, 1974, Washington conference to discuss the state of the art in this field, some of the most enthusiastic supporters for blood substitute research were the blood bank center representatives themselves, who are certainly in a position to realize its need. At the end of that meeting Dr. Geyer, who made the summarizing speech, gave a list of at least fifteen uses for blood substitutes. Although he has made considerable progress in complete substitution of animal blood, he sees more immediate goals as partial replacement of blood in such situations as:

1) Hemorrhagic emergencies; blood substitutes are imminently suitable because they are easy to store, since most of them do not need refrigeration; they are not antigenic, hence need no blood typing; they can be sterilized, and would not contain such contaminants as serum hepatitis;
2) Replacement of surgical blood losses;
3) The perfusion of organs, especially those awaiting transplantation;
4) In hemolytic anemias;
5) In sickle cell anemia, to help deliver the oxygen as needed and as a possible "oxygen buffer;"
6) Removal of toxins from the blood;
7) Removal of leukemic cells;
8) In veterinary medicine.

In case you are confounded by the black-magic aspect of the subject, may I show samples of first, a fluorochemical liquid, FC 47 (perfluorotributylamine), and second, the pluronic polyol, F 68, a waxy white solid which acts as the emulsifying agent. In a typical preparation, an aqueous 5-10% g/v solution of the F 68 is combined with the 10% v/v of the dense oil perfluorocompound, which forms an oily layer at the bottom of a beaker. When subjected to sonication for about an hour, a milky emulsion is formed which would not excite attention on a laboratory shelf. In the correct particle size range (below 0.2 μ) appropriate pH, buffer, and ion content, it may be used as a blood substitute.

Now, may I present Dr. Robert Geyer.

STUDIES WITH "BLOODLESS" ANIMALS

Robert P. Geyer

Harvard Department of Nutrition

Boston, Massachusetts

Animals without red cells or plasma proteins provide unusual opportunities for conducting many experiments impossible under normal circumstances. Such animals must be provided a means of oxygen and carbon dioxide transport and a way to maintain pH and oncotic and osmotic pressures. Because of the scarcity of artificial materials which can assume the functions of hemoglobin or plasma proteins, there are very few choices when formulating artificial whole blood substitutes. What compounds are available that could possibly be utilized for these purposes must do so while flow properties, viscosity, toxicity, and other related characteristics are kept within relatively narrow limits. Thus, the final preparation to be used must have both the potential to provide essential functions and the intrinsic properties to allow this potential to be realized.

METHODS AND PROCEDURES

The materials utilized in the present studies were Pluronic F-68 (BASF Wyandotte Corp., Wyandotte, Mich.), hydroxyethyl starch (McGaw Laboratories, Glendale, Calif.), perfluorotributylamine (FC-47) and perfluorobutyltetrahydrofuran (FX-80) (3M Co., St. Paul, Minn.), perfluorodecalin (PP-5) and perfluoromethyldecalin (PP-9) (ISC Chemicals, Ltd., Bristol, England), and Freons 1, 2, 3, 4, and 5 of the E

Series (E. I. Du Pont de Nemours & Co., Inc., Wilmington, Del.). The methods of dispersing the perfluorochemicals and other details concerning the preparation of the artificial mixtures have been given (Geyer, 1973; Geyer *et al.*, 1974).

Details of the method of perfusing the rats have been reported (Geyer, 1973; Geyer *et al.*, 1974; Geyer *et al.*, 1968). In brief, the rats are lightly anesthetized with ether:O_2 and perfused through a tail vein while blood is being removed at the same rate from the exterior jugular vein. Approximately 0.5 to 0.7 ml of perfusion fluid per gram body weight is required to remove essentially all red cells and plasma proteins. At the end of the perfusion after the catheters are removed, the animal is allowed to awaken and then kept in 10 to 100% O_2 for 24 hours. The "bloodless: rat regenerates red cells and plasma proteins during the subsequent 8 to 10 days and then continues to grow and develop, living out a normal life span.

Blood volumes were determined by the method of Wang and Hegsted (1949) using one-half the amount of Evan's Blue indicated. Lactic and pyruvic acids were determined by the methods of Horn and Bruns (1956) and Redelzki *et al.* (1956), respectively. Other determinations have been previously described (Geyer, 1973; Geyer *et al.*, 1974; Geyer *et al.*, 1968).

RESULTS AND DISCUSSION

Several different ways of artificially supplying oxygen and carbon dioxide transport are possible (Table I). Direct introduction of microbubbles of oxygen into the bloodstream has been carried out but has not as yet proven practical. Free hemoglobin solutions have always had an appeal because they not only carry oxygen but have oncotic properties as well. Obviously the latter advantage becomes a disadvantage when the concentration of hemoglobin desired for oxygen transport exceeds physiological limits of oncotic pressure. Much progress has been made towards the goal of preparing stable stroma-free hemoglobin solutions, and it is possible suitable preparations will soon be generally available.

Table I. Possible Means of Providing Oxygen to Tissues

I. REVERSIBLE OXYGEN-BINDING CHELATES

A. Heme-Type - Natural

1. Hemoglobin
2. Myoglobin

B. Heme-Type - Synthetic

1. Hemoglobin "heme"
2. Myoglobin "heme"

C. Cobalt Chelates

1. Coboglobin
2. Bis-histidinato complex

II. PHYSICAL SOLVENTS OF OXYGEN

A. Aqueous Solvents Such as Plasma

B. Organic Solvents

1. Lipids
2. Silicones
3. Perfluorochemical liquids

III. OTHER

A. Hyperbaric Chambers

B. Direct Introduction of O_2 Bubbles into Blood

Such solutions of free hemoglobin will be useful chiefly in short term (2 - 4 hours) emergency situations unless modified hemoglobins having a long half-life in circulation are developed, or unless hemoglobin can be used in conjunction with other oxygen carriers. Microencapsulated hemoglobin solutions have proven unsuccessful to date (Chang *et al.*, 1966).

Hemoglobin binds oxygen at fairly low oxygen tensions and serves as a model in the design of artificial iron chelates capable of reversibly binding oxygen. Until recently no such artificial compounds had been synthesized. Baldwin and Huff (1973) prepared an iron chelate which reversibly bound oxygen at temperatures below -40°C. Subsequently Baldwin has reported another chelate displaying reversible oxygen binding at 20°C. These important developments clearly suggest that it is but a matter of time before practical artificial oxygen-binding chelates will be available capable of functioning under normal physiological conditions. Perhaps by suitable modifications they will then also be tailor-made for different applications both *in vivo* and *in vitro*. Oxygen binding chelates of metals other than iron pose problems of heavy metal toxicity. However, because of the fundamental importance of oxygen in biology and medicine, it seems appropriate that the development of a number of different kinds of chelates continue in order to facilitate obtaining fundamental data in this area. Needless to say all such chelates are of importance to an understanding of oxygen chelate chemistry itself.

Another way to transport oxygen in the circulating fluid is by dissolving it. Even though its solubility in water is poor, certain biomedical situations can still make use of the limited amount of oxygen that does dissolve. Thus, where the body temperature can be lowered, the reduced oxygen demand can be met at least for short intervals by using oxygenated saline-albumin solutions. A naturally occurring example of this is the case of the so-called "ice fish". These fish live at the South Pole and have no red cells or hemoglobin in circulation. Instead reliance is on the oxygen which dissolves in their plasma. Their total plasma volume is significantly larger than other fish which have red cells, and, of course, their body temperature is extremely low. A frequently employed *in vitro* analogue of this is the perfusion of isolated organs at low temperature with oxygenated plasma. At more normal physiologic temperatures oxygen requirements cannot be met by such means, and the ice fish, for example, die with a rise in temperature of only a few degrees.

Fortunately there are better solvents for oxygen than water. These are solvents that are non-polar, and even lipids dissolve more of this gas than water does. Liquid silicones and perfluorochemicals are, however, much better solvents, and have received much attention. To date most progress has been made with the perfluorochemicals both in perfusing organs *in vitro* (Sloviter and Kamimoto, 1967; Triner *et al.*, 1970) and in replacing natural blood *in vivo* (Geyer, 1973; Clark *et al.*, 1973; the Green Cross Corp., 1974; Sloviter *et al.*, 1969). Initially in a number of both kinds of studies these compounds were themselves used as the circulating liquids, and generally unsatisfactory results were obtained. In large part the problems centered around the embolic effects of the unemulsified liquids even though they possessed very low surface tensions. Emulsification of the perfluorochemical liquids in an aqueous phase minimized the danger of such adverse reactions. Sloviter and Kamimoto (1967) utilized a bovine albumin stabilized emulsion of the perfluorocyclic ether, FX-80 to successfully perfuse rat brains *in vitro* for several hours. Such dispersions given to rats intravenously resulted in almost immediate death. In experiments in this laboratory dog heart-lung preparations were successfully perfused with dispersions of perfluorotributylamine, FC-47. Living rats were also totally perfused with similar preparations and kept alive for as long as eight hours (Geyer *et al.*, 1968). These and results obtained by a number of other investigators clearly demonstrated that oxygen dissolved in liquid perfluorochemicals was readily available from a biological standpoint.

The results with the totally perfused rats suggested that further improvements might make it possible to obtain total blood replacement in living animals and yet have the animals continue to live in a normal manner. A series of experiments were therefore carried out in which the maximum whole blood replacement with any given artificial substitute was determined. As these studies progressed, it became clear that 95 to 98% of the animal's normal blood could be removed with relatively little difficulty and still allow the animal to live and develop (Geyer, 1970). The reasons for the apparent essentiality of the 2 to 5% residual whole blood was not evident, especially since the substitution of either red cells or serum for the residual blood was effective in preserving the life of the animal. Since all of the evidence indicated that the dispersed fluorocarbon furnished adequate oxygen, attention was directed toward the oncotic pressure and flow characteristics of the preparations.

As with oxygen carriers, there are few suitable agents which can be used to replace the plasma proteins (Table II). The most widely used artificial plasma expander is Dextran, but this material cannot be used in rats at all because of their intolerance to it. The original oncotic agents used in our artificial blood substitute were high molecular weight polyols of the polyoxyethylene polyoxypropylene type. These served also as emulsifying agents for dispersing the liquid fluorocarbons. As one phase of modifying the artificial whole blood substitutes, several other oncotic agents were investigated as components of the final mixture. Of these polyvinylpyrrolidone (PVP) and hydroxyethyl starch (HES) received the most attention. They were used by substtuting them isooncotically for some of the polyols. These various mixtures were tested by the complete replacement technique in rats. No combination involving PVP proved successful. Rats given PVP-containing preparations withstood complete blood exchange and were in excellent condition. However, during the next 24 to 48 hours the animals became lethargic and died. Poor red cell regeneration occurred during this time and may have played a role in the animals' deaths or was itself due to some adverse effects of the procedure. Some degree of lung edema was routinely found.

In contrast to the findings with PVP, mixtures contain-

Table II. Compounds Possessing Colloid Osmotic Pressure Characteristics

I. NATURAL OR MODIFIED NATURAL MATERIALS

A. Albumin
B. Globulins
C. Starch
D. Hydroxyethyl starch
E. Dextrans
F. Gelatin
G. Oxygelatin

II. SYNTHETIC MATERIALS

A. Polyoxyethylene polyoxypropylene compounds
B. Polyvinylpyrrolidone
C. Polypeptides

Table III. Composition of Artificial Substitutes*

COMPONENT		CONCENTRATION (Per 100 ml)
Perfluorotributylamine		12 ml
Polyols		2.8 - 3.5 g
Hydroxyethyl starch		2.5 g
$NaHCO_3$		0.336 g
Na, K, Mg, Ca, PO_4, SO_4, Cl	Equivalent to	0.9 g NaCl
Dextrose		100 mg
Penicillin		10,000 units
Streptomycin		10 mg

* Details are given in a publication by Geyer (1973).

ing HES were well tolerated by the rats (Geyer, 1973). Not only did these animals withstand the complete exchange treatment, but they continued to live, regenerate new blood components, and develop and grow in a normal manner. Because of the superior performance obtained with the use of HES, this oncotic agent was routinely incorporated into the artificial blood substitute preparations. In this way the oncotic pressure requirements were met in part by the polyols and in part by the HES. To date attempts to replace most of the polyols with HES have given unsatisfactory results.

The overall view of the total blood replacement studies is given in Figure 1. The composition of an artificial substitute for whole blood which has been used successfully for total blood replacement is given in Table III.

It is essential that the pH of the circulating artificial blood substitute be kept within normal limits. The liquid perfluorochemicals are very good solvents for carbon dioxide and can function to transport this gas from tissues to lungs. In this manner the perfluorochemicals may be said to aid indirectly at least in pH control. Bicarbonate buffer is an integral part of the artificial system and is present in such a concentration that equilibration with 95% O_2: 5% CO_2 is possible. The completely exchanged rat can maintain the pH of its circulating fluid adequately (Table IV). When the bicarbonate is omitted, the pH cannot be maintained, indicating that although the liquid perfluorochemicals are capable of transporting CO_2, this not sufficient to prevent the pH from drifting downwards. This drift is probably due to the lactic and other similar acids which are formed and which must be buffered by water-soluble compounds. Ordinarily the plasma proteins and hemoglobin play important buffering roles. Since these are absent in the case of bloodless animals, the bicarbonate assumes the sole means of maintaining the pH. It is likely that the introduction of an additional buffering system would be desirable, especially under conditions where excess lactic acid and CO_2 may be encountered. Fortunately additional buffers are not needed when normal living rats are totally exchange perfused with the artificial blood substitutes (Tables IV and V).

Figure 1

OVERALL VIEW OF

TOTAL BLOOD REPLACEMENT EXPERIMENTS

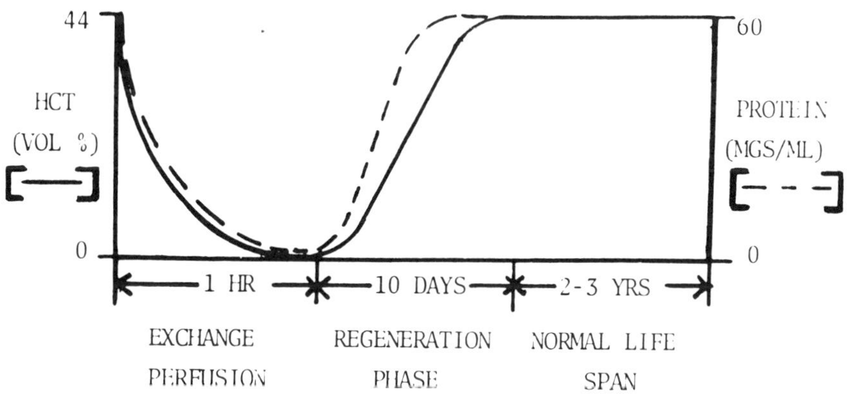

The animals are completely exchange perfused usually during approximately a one hour period. In the subsequent regeneration phase the red cells and plasma proteins are made by the animal and return into circulation. The rats then continue to grow and develop normally.

Table IV. Values of Various Determinations Before and After Complete Perfusion

DETERMINATIONS	PRE-EXCHANGE	POST-EXCHANGE
Blood volume (ml/100 g. body wt.)	6.1 - 6.9	5.8 - 6.7
Hematocrit (vol. %)	41 - 44	Less than 0.2
WBC (cells/mm^3)	8,000 - 13,000	500 - 2,000
Total plasma proteins (mgs/ml)	58 - 65	0.5 - 1.2
Osmolality (mOsm)	284 - 291	286 - 293
pH	7.42 - 7.48	7.35 - 7.43
pO_2 (mm Hg)	46 - 95	280 - 460*
pCO_2 (mm Hg)	38 - 44	36 - 48

* The pO_2 subsequently decreases in the post-exchange period, partly because O_2 is no longer being introduced by vein.

Table V. Lactic and Pyruvic Acid Contents of Circulating Fluid During Total Blood Replacement

VOLUME PERFUSED (ml)	LACTIC ACID CONTENT (mg/100 ml)				PYRUVIC ACID CONTENT (mg/100 ml)			
RAT:	1	2	3	4	1	2	3	4
0	15	13	18	28	2.3	2.2	2.8	2.1
10	16	13	16	26	2.1	2.2	2.2	4.1
20	16	14	18	16	3.4	2.1	2.0	2.3
25	24	11	19	11	3.1	2.2	2.0	2.3

Osmotic pressure control has presented no problems (Table III). The mixture of electrolytes employed was adjusted to 290 mOsm. During the perfusion the osmotic pressure remained close to 290 mOsm, and in the post-perfusion period ranged between 285 to 300 mOsm. When the osmotic pressure of the artificial blood substitute was purposely adjusted downward to 260 or 240 mOsm, the effluent perfusate from the animal always showed an upward shift in osmolality which ranged between 10 to 30 mOsm. Animals totally perfused with such preparations were in excellent condition throughout the perfusion as well as during the early post-perfusion period. Within the subsequent 20 hours the rats began to deteriorate and eventually died. No significant gross abnormalities were found on autopsy. It should be noted that during the perfusion the animals would lose the electrolytes which were responsible for the increase in osmolarity. This would amount to the equivalent of 800 to 1000 mOsm depending upon the volume used for perfusion. In small rats this could be an important drain on their electrolyte pool.

The effect of hyperosmotic preparations on the response of rats to total perfusion was also investigated. In these experiments osmolalities up to 350 mOsm were employed. During the exchange perfusion the osmolality of the effluent showed a downward shift of 20 to 30 mOsm. As the perfusion continued the animals given the hypertonic preparation required much less etherization to maintain them in a light state of anesthesia. After the total exchange had been completed, and the catheters removed the animals required 10 to 20 minutes before they awakened fully. They were then fairly inactive, but survived and continued to grow and develop. Because both high and low deviations from normal osmolality appeared to be detrimental, the routine artificial blood substitutes were always adjusted to 288 $\pm$ 5 mOsm before use and after gassing with 95% O_2:5% CO_2 at the temperature of use.

As stated previously, the perfluorochemical was used to aid in O_2 and CO_2 transport, and in this sense replaced the red cells. The particles of perfluorochemicals obviously do not have the chemical composition, enzymatic capabilities, or physical characteristics of erythrocytes. The fact that rats survive without red cells does not prove the foregoing attributes of red cells are unimportant. There is, in fact, much room for further development in this area in addition to simply introducing new perfluorochemicals.

The leukocyte counts (Table IV) do not show the same degree of decrease as the hematocrit. This may mean that lymphocytes are constantly entering the circulation at a rate faster than that at which red cells are being produced. Thoracic duct cannulation experiments may help clarify this situation. Blood volume is well maintained by the artificial substitute (Table IV). This argues for the efficacy of the osmotic colloid properties of the polyols and HES.

The red cell has many unique properties. One is that, being grossly too large for passage through capillaries, it still manages to do so quite well. By deforming as shown by A in Figure 2 the cell negotiates even the smallest diameter capillary. In so doing its interaction with the capillary wall may have some important physiological or biochemical result. The diameter of the perfluorochemical droplets may be selected such that they need minimum deformation to pass through the capillary as shown in B of Figure 2. This may, however, be prone to create the situation depicted in C (Figure 2) in which the particles in vying to enter the capillary create a jam and thereby occlude the opening. To avoid this, very small particles are resorted to and presumedly pass through the capillary without difficulty (D, Figure 2). A problem may still remain, however, in that fairly unaltered laminar flow might occur even in the small vessels. This may decrease the movement of oxygen from the center to the periphery. If such is the case, it would be more pronounced with preparations of higher viscosity. It would appear that the presence of red cells, even in small numbers, would disturb the laminar flow pattern in the capillaries and perhaps aid in getting the oxygen to the tissue cells.

In addition to the above considerations are the selection of the particular liquid perfluorochemical used and the

Figure 2. Selection of Particle Size Range of Liquid Perfluorochemicals

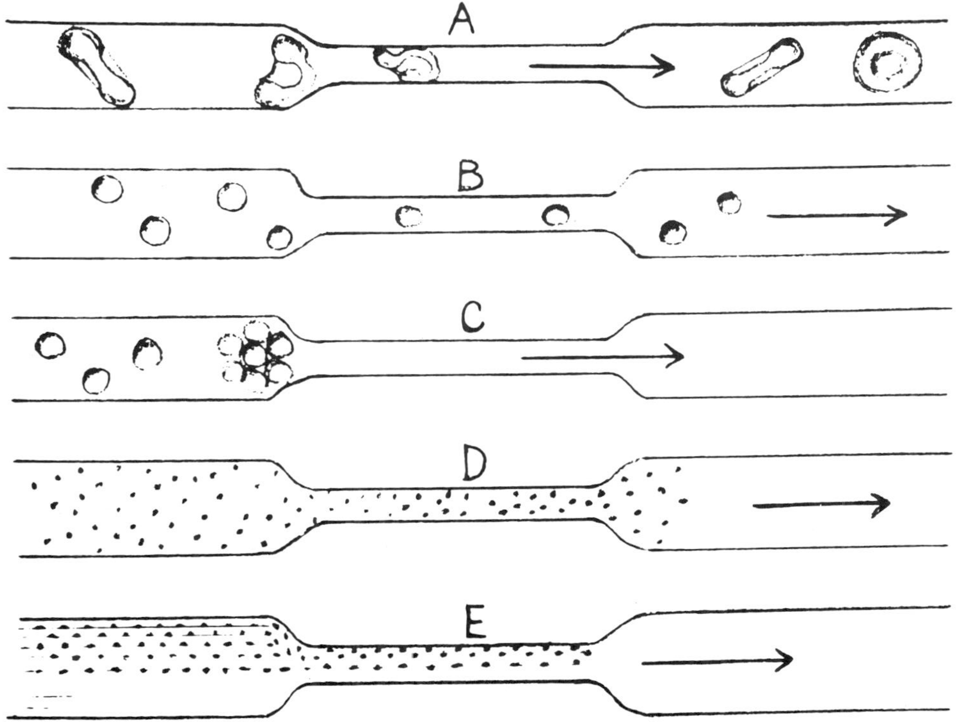

emulsifying agent to aid in dispersing it. It is well recognized that different liquid perfluorochemicals behave in very different ways both during emulsification and in animals (Table VI). We have continued to use FC-47 as the "standard" perfluorochemical for several reasons. First, it forms very stable, finely dispersed preparations. Second, we have associated no ill effects with its use either during complete exchange perfusion or in the subsequent post-exchange period. In earlier studies (Geyer *et al.*, 1968) we found no change from normal in the O_2 consumption of tissue slices from perfused animals, or of normal tissue slices incubated in the presence of the FC-47 emulsions. No gross pathology is seen in the tissues of rats which have undergone complete exchange with FC-47-containing preparations. The exposed tissues seen in Figure 3B are from a rat (Figure 3A) seven months after being completely perfused with 62 ml of a 12% FC-47 mixture. At the time of perfusion the animal weighed 60 grams. Microscopically no pathology is seen except for occasional non-staining very small droplets which are presumedly residual fluorocarbon. Animals allowed to live out their normal life span show no deleterious effects of the total blood exchange procedure or residual FC-47.

The entire question of how materials used in artificial blood substitutes should be tested is unclear. If large excess quantities of red cells or plasma proteins are given, serious consequences can occur. Iron toxicity from multiple transfusions is well recognized. We believe the contemplated use of the material should have a real bearing on the manner of testing. To infuse large quantities of artificial blood substitute into normal animals will expand the blood volume. If the preparation has oncotic properties, the degree of expansion can be very serious indeed. Even when no or little oncotic pressure effect is exerted by the mixture, the volume of perfluorochemical itself would add to the total blood volume while it remained in circulation. There are other responses to the administration of effective artificial blood substitutes which also argue against indiscriminate large dose testing procedures. These arguments will be presented elsewhere.

Table VI. Liquid Perfluorochemicals Used in Total Blood Replacement Studies

DESIGNATION	NAME	EXTENT OF REPLACEMENT*	
		PARTIAL	COMPLETE
FC-47	Perfluorotributylamine	Yes	Yes
FX-80	Perfluorobutyltetrahydrofuran	No	No
PP-5	Perfluorodecalin	Yes	No
PP-9	Perfluoromethyldecalin	Yes	Yes
PP-1	Perfluorohexane	No	No
Freon E Type	$F-(CF(CF_3)CF_2O)_n-CHFCF_3$		
	n = 1 or 2	No	No
	n = 3, 4 or 5	Yes	No

* SUBSEQUENT SURVIVAL WAS ALSO OBTAINED.

Figure 3. Growth and Lack of Liver Damage in Completely Exchange Perfused Rat

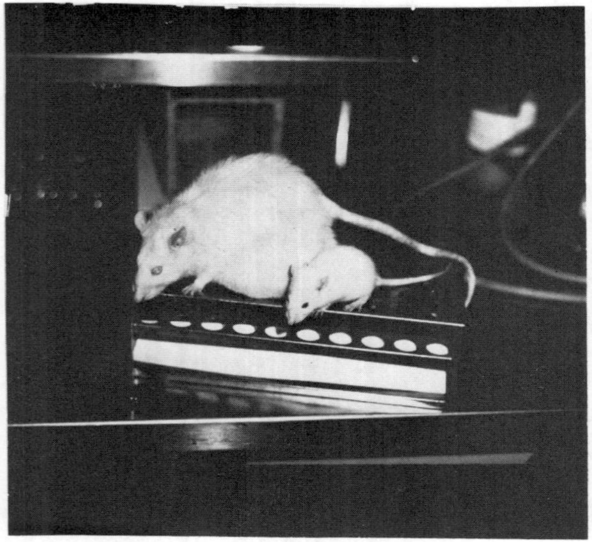

A

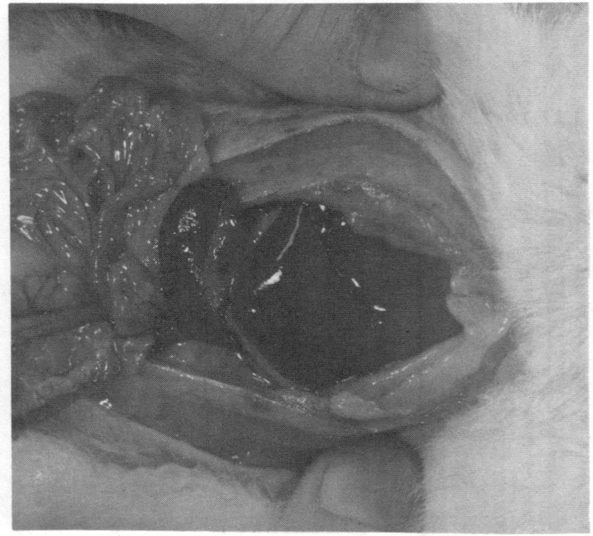

B

The large rat in Figure A (Wt., 360 g) was completely exchange perfused when it was the size of the small rat (wt. 60 g). A laparotomy was performed on the large rat and no abnormal liver or other abdominal organs were found (Figure B). The perfluorochemical used was FC-47.

Although perfluorochemicals such as PP-5 (perfluorodecalin) are very attractive because of their rapid disappearance from tissues (Clark *et al.*, 1973; Green Cross Corp., 1974), they can be difficult to incorporate into stable emulsions of the type used in these complete replacement studies. Finely dispersed emulsions can be prepared but they will deteriorate over a period of days. To date no rat totally perfused with a PP-5-containing preparation has survived (Table VI). Such animals undergo the perfusion satisfactorily, but then die within 12 to 24 hours. No cause of death has been found. It is still possible that PP-5 will be used successfully for this purpose. Studies done by others have involved only partial replacement, which in no way indicates whether total replacement would have been possible with the same preparations.

At present the only commercial source of perfluorochemical dispersions is the Green Cross Corporation in Osaka, Japan (1974). One product recommended for organ perfusion consists of FC-47 dispersed with Pluronic F-68. Another is for blood replacement *in vivo* and is made from perfluorodecalin, egg lecithin, and an adjuvant (not yet disclosed). Testing of these products by a number of investigators remains to be done. It should be pointed out that neither of these mixtures are comparable to those used in the total replacement studies reported in the present paper. Whether they will be efficacious in this regard remains to be determined.

One of the important considerations in evaluating artificial blood substitutes is the fact that the presence of even small concentrations of plasma proteins and/or red cells have very significant effects on the results of the testing. Under the conditions employed here, for example, when the liquid perfluorochemicals were omitted from the preparation, the rats withstood removal of approximately 80% of their own blood. Thus, an hematocrit of 10 is sufficient to furnish adequate oxygen transport. As a consequence of this, more than 90% of the blood should be replaced just to demonstrate that the preparation is indeed fulfilling a vital role in gas transport. The most stringent and reliable test of an artificial substitute is to use it to replace completely the blood of animals. In this way the remaining normal blood is not present to give a falsely optimistic evaluation of the artificial substitute.

It is likely that other artificial mixtures will be developed in the near future which will prove even more efficacious than those now on hand. The full extent to which they will be used *in vivo* and *in vitro* remains to be determined. That there are many possible applications is clear (Geyer, 1974). No doubt many others will be uncovered.

SUMMARY

"Bloodless" animals are living animals having no red cells or plasma proteins. Instead they circulate in their vascular system a completely synthetic mixture capable of fulfilling at least the most critical functions of normal blood. Emulsified liquid perfluorinated chemicals are utilized to transport oxygen and carbon dioxide. This is possible because these gases are quite soluble in the liquid perfluorochemicals. High molecular weight polyols and hydroxyethyl starch furnish the required colloid osmotic pressure. Other components include buffers, glucose, antibiotics, and essential electrolytes. Using such preparations it was possible to replace all of the normal blood of living rats without impairing the life or activities of the animals. In the immediate post-exchange period the "bloodless" rats drank, washed, ate, urinated, and showed other aspects of normal behavior. During the subsequent week to ten days the normal number of red cells and concentrations of proteins returned to circulation. The animals not only survived the episode of complete blood replacement, but continued to grow and develop in the usual manner. The results of these studies show that total whole blood substitution with artificial preparations is possible. Many eventual uses for such preparations and such "bloodless" animals are evident. As additional compounds, including oxygen-binding iron chelates and new oncotic agents become available, artificial blood substitutes designed for specific purposes will be possible.

References to the literature relating to artificial blood substitutes may be found in the following publications: Norman (1968); Clark (1970); Riess (1974) and Geyer *et al.* (1974).

ACKNOWLEDGMENTS

This research has been supported by a grant from the John A. Hartford Foundation, Inc., and a grant (HL15520-02) from the National Institutes of Health. I am indebted to Dr. P. Willard of the 3M Co., St. Paul, Minn., for providing Fluorocarbon FC-47; to Dr. I. Schmolka of BASF Wyandotte, Wyandotte, Mich., for providing Pluronic polyols; to Dr. J. Brake of McGaw Lab., Glendale, Calif., for providing hydroxyethyl starch; to Mr. B. D. Joyner of ISC Chemicals Ltd., Bristol, Engl., for PP-1, PP-5 and PP-9; to Mr. E. C.Coyner of E. I. Du Pont de Nemours & Co., Inc., Wilmington, Del., for providing Freons E1, E2, E3, E4, and E5; and to Mr. Ken Taylor, Mr. Robert Eccles and Mrs. Ethel Duffett for their excellent technical assistance.

REFERENCES

Baldwin, J. E., and Huff, J. (1973). Binding of dioxygen to iron(II). Reversible behavior in solution. *J. Amer. Chem. Soc.* 95: 5757.

Chang, T. M. S., MacIntosh, F. C., and Mason, S. G. (1966). Semipermeable aqueous microcapsules. *Can. J. Physiol. Pharmacol.* 44: 115.

Clark, L. C., Ed. (1970). Symposium on Inert Organic Liquids for Biological Oxygen Transport. *Fed. Proc.* 29:1695.

Clark, L. C., Becattini, F., Kaplan, S., Obrock, V., Cohen, D., and Becker, C. (1973). Perfluorocarbons having a short dwell time in the liver. *Science* 181: 680.

Geyer, R. P. (1970). Studies on acute blood replacement with fluorocarbon-polyol preparations. *Med. u. Ernähr.* 11:256.

Geyer, R. P. (1973). Fluorocarbon-polyol artificial blood substitutes. *New Engl. J. Med.* 289: 1077.

Geyer, R. P. (1974). Potential uses of artificial blood substitutes. (Presented at Workshop on Artificial Blood, April 5-6, 1974, Bethesda, Maryland). To be published in *Fed. Proc.*

Geyer, R. P., Monroe, R. G., and Taylor, K. (1968). Survival of rats totally perfused with a fluorocarbon-detergent preparation. In *Organ Perfusion and Preservation*, 1968, J. C. Norman, Ed., Appleton-Century-Crofts, New York, pp. 85-96.

Geyer, R. P., Sherer, P. B., and Weiler, J. (1974). Workshop on Artificial Blood (April 5-6, 1974, Bethesda, Maryland), to be published in *Fed. Proc.*

Green Cross Croporation, Osaka, Japan (1974). Fluosol-43 for perfusion of isolated organs. Fluosol-DC for circulatory replacement. *Technical Information Ser. No. 1,* (Sept. 11, 1974, RN/ky/yd).

Horn, H. D., and Bruns, F. H. (1956). Quantitative bestimmung ven L(+) milchsare mit milchsauredehydrogenase. *Biochim. Biophys. Acta* 21: 378.

Norman, J., Ed. (1968). *Organ Perfusion and Preservation*, Appleton-Century-Crofts, New York.

Redelzki, H., Bloedorn, H., and Bansi, H. W. (1956). Einfluss of Thioctinsaure auf den Boenztraubensaure and alphaketoglutosaure blutspiegel bei leberkranken. *Klin. Wscher.* 34: 845.

Riess, J. G. (1974) Les fluorocarbones transporteurs de gaz dissous comme substituts du sang. To be published in *An. Franc. Anesth.*

Sloviter, H., and Kamimoto, R. (1967). Erythrocyte substitute for perfusion of brain. *Nature* (London) 216: 458.

Sloviter, H. A., Petkovic, M., Ogoshi, S., and Yamada, H. (1969). Dispersed fluorochemicals as substitutes for erythrocytes in intact animals. *J. Appl. Physiol.* 27: 666.

Triner, L., Verosky, M., Habif, D. V., and Nahas, G. G. (1970). Perfusion of isolated liver with fluorocarbon emulsions. *Fed. Proc.* 29: 1778.

Wang, C. F., and Hegsted, D. M. (1949). Determination of blood and plasma volumes, thiocyanate space, and bromsulfalein clearance in rats. *Am. J. Physiol.* 156: 227.

DISCUSSION

Dr. Fuller: I am a clinical hematologist and a blood banker. I came to this conference with a sharp pencil and notebook to write down all the things I could do for my patients next week, but I must say that I haven't gotten writer's cramp so far! However, the prospect of artificial blood is very exciting for those of us in clinical practice who see some unusual and difficult transfusion problems.

Several years ago, for example, we had a patient who was a Jehovah's Witness who had continued bleeding after delivery. She finally bled down to a hemoglobin of less than 2 grams, survived a hysterectomy at that level and is doing well today. The word got around that we could and would take care of people without giving blood and we have seen a number of similar patients since then but some of them have not done so well.

Several years ago I called Dr. Geyer in regard to a patient with a bleeding peptic ulcer who was also a Jehovah's Witness hoping that his blood substitute might be ready for clinical use. It was not, and the patient steadfastly refused transfusion and died. About six weeks ago we had another patient with underlying leukemia and an associated Coombs positive hemolytic anemia that prevented transfusion. The most compatible blood was tagged with radioactive chromium and showed complete elimination of an aliquot sample in a few hours. When his hemoglobin dropped to about 3 grams I called Dr. Clark and begged for some help since I had heard that his product might be nearly ready for clinical trials. He expressed great interest and was gracious but did not feel that his product could be used without preliminary further animal trials. This patient also died. Many of us do see clinical problems where blood is needed but cannot be given. In such situations a blood substitute might well be the only life saving treatment.

Several other aspects of the problem are of interest. First, your comment about the low white cell yield would be as expected since the white cells are merely transported in the blood and represent a very small fraction of the white cell reserve. Significant numbers cannot be harvested without the use of special techniques such as continuous flow centrifugation. You mentioned that the animals did not bleed with replacement of their total blood volume and I would wonder what studies have been done on the coagulation parameters. Many of the patients that we see with abnormal plasma factor coagulation or abnormal platelets do not bleed without trauma. I do think that this is an important area in which to have more information if blood substitutes are to be used clinically. I am sure that such investigation will be required before approval by the FDA. Finally, you note that the vehicle in which the material is suspended dramatically increases blood flow rates. This is fascinating from the standpoint of whether the vehicle itself might not have--Dr. Clark mentioned this--some clinical application in itself, such as in patients who have sickle cell anemia, other hemolytic problems associated with "rigid red cells" or in those who have DIC or similar conditions.

Thank you very much for your presentation.

Dr. Geyer: Thank you. The clotting aspects of this work are such that in the bloodless animal, one does not have these animals bleeding--they are not going to bleed to death. I think the important part of that would be to do these studies in partially exchanged animals, where you have enough of the clotting factors left to really do suitable tests. In these animals I think the concentrations are extremely low, and we feel that perhaps some of the materials still in the tissues play an important role. In terms of sickle cell anemia, we wondered whether just increasing the oxygen capacity of what would really be the plasma, by the use of some mixture like this, would indeed prevent crises from occuring because you would overcome anoxic conditions. I think for this to work, one needs a preparation that stays in the circulation for a very long time. And we have often joked about the idea that if we could get a prep that never left the circulation, we could always tell the FDA just where it was, and at any time just drain it out, and put back ordinary blood. I think eventually preps like this will become available. I see no stumbling block here.

Unidentified Speaker: Is there any gastrointestinal absorption of this material?

Dr. Geyer: We have not found any. I should also point out that no one to my knowledge has done any work with radioactive perfluorochemicals, unless it's been done very recently. The reason is that the companies which provide these chemicals don't want to provide the funds to make such compounds. We're hoping that through some sort of joint effort we may get them. Then we'll know a lot more about them.

Dr. MacFarlane: What happens to the compound in the circulatory system when the animals replace it with their normal plasma proteins and red cells?

Dr. Geyer: Well, what we have is obviously not an equilibrium; the material that we inject is leaving the circulation. The half life in the circulation for a number of these preparations is approximately three days in our experience.

Dr. MacFarlane: Do you know where it goes?

Dr. Geyer: These very fine preparations go into almost all the tissues. I know that Dr. Clark has given very large amounts of material to dogs and has shown that the liver really shows a lot of changes. In our experiments, doing them the way we're doing them, we don't find any histological problems or growth problems. Material of the type we use--the FC47--will stay in the tissues for a long time, and on electron microscopic examination, even as late as eight months later, you can still see very small places where the fluorocarbon must have been before the processing. But there's no tissue reaction to this. The perfluorodecaline does get out rapidly, and that's what's so intriguing about it. I don't think anyone knows exactly how it does get out.

Dr. MacFarlane: Do you know whether these compounds are metabolized?

Dr. Geyer: We have done some work in looking for fluoride formation. We have not yet looked at bones, which I think would be worth looking at to see if they've trapped fluoride. Our best indication is that it's not touched, it's an inert material, but this still has to be proven.

Dr. McFarlane: Thank you.

Dr. Brewer: I'm rather impressed by the lack of hemorrhage; actually I don't know whether you'd call it hemorrhage if the loss is non red cell containing fluid, but I've always viewed coagulation as a very finely balanced thing, where if the platelets get too low, you have hemorrhage, or if the various coagulation parameters--any one of them--get too low, you have hemorrhage. Yet, these rats don't bleed. Does the material have some sort of property which prevents it, or what?

Dr. Geyer: What we do know is that some preparations definitely will go the other way. And part of the time that we spent in the last 5 or 6 years has been trying to learn what was going on. I don't know why they don't hemorrhage. I did have a series of slides I didn't bring that show the animal with heparin not hemorrhaging either. We then exchanged in the reverse direction with heparinized blood, and it leaked all over. Now, if someone in the audience has a good reason for this, we'd like to know it because I think this is one of the fascinating areas. We have, for instance, done laparotomies on the rats, taken out the spleen and most of the liver, sewed them back up, and they're fine.

Dr. Brewer: Is CO_2 transported by the fluorocarbons, or does it just accidentally end up being normalized under the usual conditions?

Dr. Geyer: No, as a matter of fact, its solubility is much greater than oxygen. We wish it was just the reverse.

PERFLUORODECALIN EMULSION INFUSION IN AN AWAKE RHESUS MONKEY

Leland C. Clark, Jr., Samuel Kaplan, Carolyn Emory, Eugene P. Wesseler
Children's Hospital Research Foundation
Elland and Bethesda Avenues
Cincinnati, Ohio 45229

With the discovery (1) that highly perfluorinated liquids (PFL) could be breathed there emerged the possibility that synthetic organic compounds might serve as gas transporting agents. These liquids, as well as silicone and other oils which are good oxygen solvents, are not soluble in water. At the present time, therefore, the only way they can be used is in the form of emulsions.

Sloviter (2) reported the use of PFL emulsions to perfuse isolated brain and Geyer (3) is pioneering in the use of PFL emulsions in the total replacement of blood. Clark (4,5,6) has described the physiological application of such emulsions. The finding (7) that certain cyclic perfluorocarbon liquids leave the body shortly after administration has increased the possibility that such emulsions may find clinical use as a substitute for whole blood.

In order to meet the oxygen requirement of isolated perfused organs without using whole blood, the temperature must be lowered or the oxygen carrying capacity of the perfusion media must be increased. Addition of stroma-free hemoglobin is one solution and addition of PFL is another.

In this paper I will explore the possible future uses of such emulsions, report some new findings since our last publications (8,9), and try to weigh the merits of various PFL emulsions in perfusion systems.

Materials and Methods

All of the methods used in this research have been previously reported (1,4,5,6,7,9) except those involving the Rhesus (Macaca mulatta) monkey.

The monkey was initially anesthetized with intravenous phencyclidine (2mg/kg) and maintained with sodium amytal (4mg/kg). The inferior vena cava was cannulated via the right femoral vein with a No. 5 French vinyl catheter which was filled with Ringer's solution containing heparin and the animal was allowed to wake up in a special restraining chair. He was hand fed with biscuits, raw peanuts and bananas and, because he refused water, he was fed Gatorade which he drank in copious amounts.

Blood was collected from the cannula with a 12 ml syringe containing heparin. The blood was analyzed for pO_2, pCO_2, pH, hematocrit, "fluorocrit", perfluorodecalin content, GC in the vapor phase, bacteriological culture, complete blood count, including a differential count. Plasma was analyzed as shown in the table by routine methods, including Technicon procedures, in use at the Cincinnati General Hospital.

Samples of breath were taken in glass microliter syringes and analyzed by gas chromatography using nitrogen carrier gas, a ^{63}Ni electron capture detector, and a SE-30 column.

The emulsion consisted of 100 ml of PP5 (ISC Ltd., St. Andrews Rd., Avonmouth, Bristol BS11 9HP, England) which had been purified by spinning band distillation, 225 ml. of 20% Pluronic F68, 322 ml of sterile water, 333 ml of Ringer's solution and 20 ml of 10% Beta-propiolactone. It was homogenized first in a Waring Blendor, then in a Gaulin homogenizer to a final optical density of 0.55. The emulsion was filtered through a Gelman fiberglass filter (Fisher Scientific, Cat. No. 9-730-62). The entire operation was conducted under sterile conditions. Analysis of the final emulsion showed it was 9.7% by volume perfluorodecalin. The emulsion was infused at a dose of 30 ml/kg (total dose=130 ml) into the femoral venous cannula.

Table 1

SAM	TOT PRO	ALB	CA	INO PHO	GLU	BUN	URI ACI	CRE	TOT BIL	PP5
	gm%	gm%	mg%	mg%	mg%	mg%	mg%	mg%	mg%	V%
cont	8.0	5.1	10.4	3.7	140	27.7	0.40	1.3	0.3	0.0
0.5H	5.8	3.6	8.5	3.2	146	25.0	0.32	1.2	0.3	1.3
1H	5.6	3.4	8.3	3.4	110	22.5	0.30	1.1	0.4	2.5
2H	6.4	4.2	9.1	3.3	145	20.3	0.30	1.2	0.3	2.6
18H	6.7	4.2	9.2	3.5	92	10.4	0.23	1.0	0.2	1.6
1D	5.8	3.2	7.8	3.3	120	17.4	0.27	1.1	0.1	1.6
2D	5.9	3.6	8.1	3.3	95	18.4	0.21	1.0	0.1	0.5
3D	5.9	3.6	8.4	2.1	115	22.9	0.51	1.1	0.2	0.1
4D	6.5	3.4	8.7	3.1	94	24.9	0.24	0.9	0.3	0.01
5D	7.1	3.7	9.0	3.3	130	20.8	0.20	0.8	0.3	0.0
6D	6.9	3.5	8.7	3.7	78	19.0	0.13	0.8	0.2	0.0
2W	9.5	4.2	10.5	5.2	113	32.0	0.40	1.0	0.2	0.0
3W	9.8	4.6	10.4	5.8	126	12.5	0.20	1.1	0.1	0.0
4W	8.9	4.4	10.8	4.3	139	26.7	0.21	1.2	0.1	0.0

Blood chemistry of monkey after infusion of PP5 ct emulsion.

Table 2

SAM	ALK PHO	LDH	SGOT	Na	K	Cl	CO_2	Hct	Fct
	U/ml	mU/ml	mU/ml	mEq/L	mEq/L	mEq/L	mEq/L	%	%
cont	488	364	64	163	3.5	114	21	34	0
0.5H	295	287	50	151	3.1	108	28	28	2
1H	295	333	57	156	3.2	109	29	29	4
2H	338	440	67	154	3.0	108	27	33	5
18H	328	405	97	154	4.3	111	25	29	3
1D	315	330	80	152	4.3	110	23	29	2
2D	237	337	57	156	3.7	112	28	25	1
3D	223	352	55	156	4.6	118	21	28	0
4D	328	338	53	157	4.1	118	21	23	0
5D	432	325	45	150	4.2	113	20	27	0
6D	408	310	38	154	4.0	113	25	25	0
2W	>350	405	46	173	6.5	123	9	34	0
3W	472	240	27	160	4.4	109	13	40	0
4W	>350	406	39	159	5.8	115	7	40	0

Blood chemistry of monkey after infusion of PP5 ct emulsion.

Results

The infusion of emulsion was performed with the monkey alert and apparently feeling fine. He appeared to be completely unaware of the fact that blood was being withdrawn and that the emulsion was being infused. His carotid pulse was about 120 and did not change significantly. He was bothered only by the flash on the camera. A total of 73 ml of blood was withdrawn and 130 ml of emulsion was given, about 15 ml of Ringer's solution was used in flushing the cannula. He weighed 4.3 kg on the day of infusion. He has varied in weight between 4.3 and 5.0 kg and one month after the infusion he weighs 4.7 kg. He has remained in good health and appears normal in all respects.

The results of the chemical analysis of the blood are given in tables 1, 2, and 3. Aside from the expected change in perfluorodecalin level there were essentially no effects of the infusion. The venous pO_2 did not increase because the animal was not breathing oxygen. Gas chromatography of breath samples indicated the presence of the fluorocarbon in gradually decreasing amounts over a period of many days. A culture of the emulsion gave a positive test for _Pseudomonas._ A blood sample taken the first day also showed these same rods. One or two later samples, from the cannula were positive for _Staphylococcus aureus_ and _Enterobacter._

Table 3

SAMPLE	INFERIOR VENA CAVA BLOOD		
hour	pO_2	pCO_2	pH
Control	36	41	7.41
0.5	30	38	7.43
1.0	23	46	7.35
2.0	28	46	7.36

Discussion

While this paper deals with the infusion of fluorocarbon emulsion in only one monkey it is being reported here at this time because as a single experiment it is the culmination of a number of years of research. The final goal is the use of such an emulsion in humans. As part of our final preclinical testing we plan to test the perfluorodecalin emulsion in 10 or 15 monkeys.

The oxygen and carbon dioxide transport function of the various fluorochemical liquids are quite predictable and therefore this phase of the problem was not studied here.

This experiment illustrates that after many experiments using thousands of animals to perfect the method of making useful oxygen carrying emulsions, reasonable success has been achieved. In early experiments, a few years ago, it was not uncommon to lose many of the animals tested. Many others were sick for a number of days. We were not sure why some animals survived in good health while others did not.

Careful attention must be paid to each aspect of making an emulsion for intravenous use. Reproducible means of making an emulsion, such as sonicating or shearing to an optical density plateau, must be carefully followed. Apparatus must not only be sterile but clean. There are many other details involved but they will be dealt with elsewhere.

Success in harmlessly replacing part or all of the blood with a fluorocarbon emulsion in an animal paves the way for the use of such substances as artificial blood for clinical use in man and other animals.

The fact that there are no significant changes in serum enzymes, uric acid, creatinine, etc., together with our previous findings that no residual morphological changes can be found in liver probably indicates that no damage has been done to the liver and kidney.

An emulsion which is satisfactory as a substitute for blood in an intact animal, and in this sense perfuses all the organs, may not be satisfactory for perfusion of an isolated organ. Emulsions tend to break down in a system containing a perfusion machine and an isolated organ, more than in an intact animal. Emulsions will probably have to be tailored for each perfusion system.

Emulsions used in intact animals (a closed system) must have vapor pressures within narrow limits while those used to perfuse organs (generally open systems) may safely have higher vapor pressures and volatility.

Summary

A perfluorodecalin-Pluronic F68 emulsion given intravenously to an awake Rhesus monkey caused no measurable physiological, chemical or psychological changes. Approximately 1/3 of his blood volume was withdrawn and replaced with the emulsion. This accomplishment is analyzed in terms of the requirements for artificial blood for clinical use and isolated organ preservation.

Acknowledgements

This research is supported in part by NIH grants HL12419, HL17587, HL17353, the American Heart Association and the Southwestern Ohio Chapter of the American Heart Association. This research is supported by the Children's Hospital Research Foundation. We wish to thank Sara Devine, Lilam Stanley, Mary E. Schneider, Eleanor Brinkmoeller, Dr. Steele F. Mattingly, Dr. J. B. Lal, Frank Knapke, Sidney Hughes, Barbara Libbey, Sandy Hoffman, Robert Moore, Raymond Plevey. Drs. Christ Tamborski and Donald Denson for valuable technical advice.

References

1. Clark, L.C., Jr., and Gollan, F. (1966). Survival of mammals breathing organic liquids equilibrated with oxygen at atmospheric pressure. Science 152, 1755-1756.

2. Sloviter, H.A., and Kamimoto, T. (1967). Erythrocyte substitute for perfusion of brain. Nature (London) 216, 458-460.

3. Geyer, R.P., Monroe, G., and Taylor, K. (1968). Survival of rats having red cells totally replaced with emulsified fluorocarbon. Fed. Proc. 27, 384.

4. Clark, L.C., Jr., Kaplan, S., Becattini, F., and Benzing, G. III (1970). Perfusion of whole animals with fluorocarbon emulsions using the Clark bubble-defoam heart-lung machine. Fed. Proc. 29, 1764-1770.

5. Clark, L.C., Jr., Kaplan, S., and Becattini, F. (1970). The physiology of synthetic blood. J. Thorac. Cardiovasc. Surg. 60, 757-773.

6. Clark, L.C., Jr., Becattini, F., and Kaplan, S. (1972). Can fluorocarbon emulsions be used as artificial blood? Triangle 11, 115-122.

7. Clark, L.C., Jr., Becattini, F., Kaplan, S., Obrock, V., Cohen, D., and Becker, C. (1973). Perfluorocarbons having a short dwell time in the liver. Science 181, 680-682.

8. Clark, L.C., Jr., Wesseler, E.P., Miller, M.L., and Kaplan, S. (1974). Ring versus straight chain perfluorocarbon emulsions for perfusion media. Microvas. Res. 8, 1-21.

9. Clark, L.C., Jr., Wesseler, E.P., Kaplan, S., Miller, M., Becker, C., Emory, C., Stanley, L., Becattini, F., and Obrock, V. (1974). Organic oxygen solvents for artificial blood. Fed. Proc. (in press).

10. Technical information Ser. No. 1. Sept. 11, 1974, RN/ky/yd. The Green Cross Corporation, Osaka, Japan.

DISCUSSION

Dr. Geyer: I was very interested in your monkey results. We had had success going to 75% replacement in Rhesus monkeys. We haven't gone beyond that because it's technically difficult to work with these animals in a high oxygen atmosphere under our limited financial arrangements. We've not found that the albumin is being interfered with at all; it seems to come back very nicely. We simply think that when you observe derangements in the protein synthesis, something is wrong with the preparation and not with the idea. I would like to back up your statements about organ perfusion. We started out with organ perfusion and we're very elated. We went to the whole animals and now we feel that organ perfusion is going to be a tough area because we think most people perfusing organs simply work in the "push it through" principle. I think you just can't do that, you have to have as much care, or more care with organs as you do with the whole animal. I think this is going to be an extremely interesting area in which to work.

Dr. Fuller: Getting back to the question about coagulation, I think that this is a really fascinating aspect. It is inconceivable that there are not major detectable changes in the coagulation system including platelet function and number. Having been involved to a degree in platelet storage evaluation in regard to FDA licensing, there's no question that the FDA will want to have studies in this regard and I think it would be high priority to get this material approved for clinical use.

Dr. Clark: Yes, it is difficult to decide, even at this stage, what blood measurements should be made to satisfy everyone that perfluorodecalin emulsion is safe. I am sure we will find changes in many things, such as platelets, but such changes must be balanced with the need for artificial blood. There are many changes in blood components during open-heart surgery, but sometimes the surgery is essential.

Dr. Woosley: It would seem that these animals would be immuno-suppressed. Have you noticed any increased incidence of infection in any of the animals which you have re-transfused?

Dr. Clark: I am sure that the animals are imuno-suppressed, after all, we are giving particles in a concentration of perhaps 500 million per cm. We can increase the size of the liver manyfold. But we have had no problem with infection in the beagles or the monkey.

Dr. Woosley: One other quick question. I'm not sure about the physiology of the monkey, but I believe that dogs auto-transfuse themselves by splenic contraction when they are phlebotomized. I wonder if monkeys also do this and could this be the reason why their hematocrits didn't fall dramatically in your studies.

Dr. Clark: Yes, that must be the reason. Perhaps this is the time to mention that healthy dogs can survive very low hematocrits, down to 4 or so. We are not sure about the Rhesus yet.

Dr. Kraus: Has anybody looked at erythropoietin in this system?

Dr. Clark: I don't know of anybody; Dr. Geyer do you?

Dr. Geyer: No, I don't. However, we have had about 12 people who would love to look into it. That's an interesting area.

Dr. Button: Dr. Clark, have you had any opportunity to explore any changes in the bone marrow of these transfused animals?

Dr. Clark: We're in the middle of that. What should we look for?

Dr. Button: Changes in the morphology and cell ratios of the marrow after the animals have refilled their blood space with blood.

Dr. Woosley: Since a lot of people who receive emergency transfusions may be surgical candidates, has anyone administered anesthetics, especially gases, to animals after they have been given fluorocarbon blood substitutes to see if they can be anesthetized? I would think that the drugs could possibly be trapped in the circulation and surgical anesthesia could not be obtained.

Dr. Clark: Because of the high solubility of fluorinated anesthetics in fluorocarbon, induction and recovery take a little longer with Halothane, which we use. We have looked for metabolites of the perfluorinated substances we use for emulsions, using electron capture gas chromatography, and have never found any. Even the ones which contain -O- or -N- in the molecule are not metabolized, as judged by GC patterns. We have found no changes in blood or urine fluoride levels.

Dr. Hoekstra: Have you looked for dimers or trimers or higher polymers of these compounds being formed in the body?

Dr. Clark: No, we haven't only in the sense that I just mentioned; the gas chromatograph would change then we would....

Dr. Hoekstra: Perhaps one of the reasons that such compounds are so effective is that they obviate the problem of oxidant damage. In other words, the types of oxygen present may be less damaging or these compounds may scavenge free-radicals and thereby interact to form dimers and trimers which may be stable or may be slowly reconverted to monomers. The oxygen carried in such a system may be a poorer source of damaging species than is the oxygen bound hemoglobin.

Dr. Clark: That's a very interesting comment.

Unidentified Speaker: There is another way you can give oxygen that Dr. Geyer had on his slide. That is to give hydrogen peroxide. It doesn't work but you can....

Dr. Geyer: That's no laughing matter. We have given our bloodless rats hydrogen peroxide, I.V., because they don't have catalase in enough quantity to cause gas bubble formation. You can perfuse hydrogen peroxide this way for a long period. We had at one time hoped we could actually fuel these animals with hydrogen peroxide and maybe apply this to the space program.

TRACE METALS AND THEIR BLOOD CELL EFFECTS

Chairman: A. Prasad

ROLE OF ZINC IN MAN AND ITS DEFICIENCY IN SICKLE CELL DISEASE

Ananda S. Prasad, E. B. Schoomaker, J. Ortega, G. J. Brewer, D. Oberleas and F. J. Oelshlegel, Jr.

From the Department of Medicine, Wayne State University, Detroit General Hospital and Grace Hospital, Detroit; V. A. Hospital, Allen Park; and Department of Human Genetics, University of Michigan, Ann Arbor, Michigan.

INTRODUCTION

Zinc is known to be essential for the growth of micro-organisms, plants, animals and man (Underwood, 1971; Prasad, 1966). Its essentiality for growth of Aspergillus niger was recognized almost one hundred years ago (Raulin, 1869). Forty years later, its role in growth of plants was demonstrated (Bertrand & Javillier, 1911). Todd et al (1934) reported for the first time that zinc was necessary for life in animals and suggested that it was probably an essential nutrient for man also. Nevertheless the ubiquity of zinc made it seem unlikely that alterations in zinc metabolism could lead to significant problems in human nutrition or clinical medicine. For example, in 1962 Underwood (Underwood, 1962) stated that "an uncomplicated dietary deficiency of zinc has never been observed in man". Since then, zinc deficiency has been observed in man, and thus in 1971 Underwood (Underwood, 1971) included man among the species in whom a deficiency syndrome had been demonstrated. This was the result of reports of primary zinc deficiency in Egypt by Prasad et al (1963), and in Iran by Halsted et al (1972).

In addition, Caggiano et al (1969), in the United States, observed zinc deficiency in a patient with hypogammaglobulinemia with nodular lymphoid hyperplasia of the small intestine and bronchiectasis. More recently, also in the United States, Hambidge et al (1972) reported cases of low hair zinc concentration and low taste acuity that were responsive to zinc supplementation.

The clinical manifestations of zinc deficiency in man include growth retardation, delayed onset of puberty and hypogonadism in the males, rough skin, poor appetite and mental lethargy (Prasad et al, 1963). We have observed that some sickle cell anemia (SCA) patients show similar features and inasmuch as zinc is an important constituent of red blood cells, it appeared possible that continued hemolysis for a prolonged period of time in patients with SCA might lead to a zinc deficient state secondarily. Delayed healing of leg ulcers and beneficial effect of zinc therapy on leg ulcers in SCA patients as reported by Sergeant et al (1970) would also appear to be consistent with the above hypothesis.

In this paper we wish to present evidences which support our concept that some patients with SCA are zinc deficient and that therapy with zinc may be beneficial to such subjects.

METHODS

Patients from Detroit General Hospital Sickle Cell Anemia Adult Clinic, were investigated. Eighteen men and 18 women comprised the group. The diagnosis of SCA was established by history, physical examination, and hematological studies which included cellulose acetate hemoglobin electrophoresis and quantitative determination of A_2, F and S hemoglobins*. Hemoglobin electrophoresis revealed S-S pattern, quantitation of A_2 hemoglobin gave normal values and F hemoglobin was less than 20 percent in all our cases. The controls were healthy non-anemic Black males and females with ages ranging from 23 to 57. The ages of SCA patients ranged

* We are grateful to Dr. D. Rucknagel for these determinations

from 15 to 69.

The usual precautions to avoid contamination with zinc during collection of samples were taken throughout the study (Prasad et al, 1965). Zinc was assayed with an atomic absorption spectrophotometer† according to methods published earlier (Prasad et al, 1965). Plasma was diluted (1:4) and assayed directly by using standards made up in 15% glycerol. Undiluted samples of urine were assayed directly by atomic absorption spectrophotometry. Washed red cells were lysed by deionized water and then digested by concentrated HNO_3 prior to assay. Hair samples were washed with hexane and alcohol. These washed samples were dried overnight at 125° and then digested with concentrated HNO_3 prior to assay.

RNase (alkaline) activity in plasma was assayed by a method reported previously (Prasad & Oberleas, 1973). Red cell carbonic anhydrase content was measured by a radioimmunosorbent technique (Magid et al 1973).**

Plasma and red cell zinc were also assayed in other anemic subjects, including patients with megaloblastic anemia, iron deficiency anemia, anemia associated with chronic diseases and in one patient with auto-immune hemolytic anemia.

Seven men and two women with SCA have received zinc sulfate, 660 mg daily for varying lengths of time. The clinical effects of this therapy are summarized in the results section.

RESULTS

Of 18 men with SCA, 13 manifested signs of hypogonadism as evidenced by decreased or absent facial, axillary, chest and pubic hair and delayed onset of puberty. In contrast, only 4 women showed decreased gonadal function as suggested by late onset of menarchy and menstrual abnormalities. This

† Perkin Elmer Corp., Model 303, Norwalk, Conn.
** We are grateful to Dr. R. E. Tashian for this assay.

observation is consistent with the known greater susceptibility of male gonads to a lack of zinc.

The height and weight of the patients with SCA were compared with data obtained by the Ten-State Nutrition Survey conducted by the U.S. Department of Health, Education and Welfare in 1968-70*. Two men with SCA were below the 10th height percentile, 14 were less than the 15th weight percentile and 2 were in the 50th weight percentile for their ages.

The RBC zinc level (mean ± S.E.) was significantly less in 27 SCA patients as compared to the 23 controls (35.2 ± 1.6 vs. 41.7 ± 1.2 μg/g Hb, $p < .01$). Of the 27 SCA patients in which RBC was analyzed for zinc, 6 had very low red cell zinc levels (less than 2 S.D. below the control mean) and 6 older subjects (over 30 years) had normal red cell zinc. RBC zinc correlated with age, r being + 0.58 and $p < .01$, suggesting that older subjects had higher zinc content in the red blood cells. The hair zinc concentration (mean ± S.E.) was also decreased in the 21 SCA patients as compared to the 17 controls (149 ± 10.3, vs. 193 ± 4.3 μg/g, $p < .01$). Mean plasma zinc levels (mean ± S.E.) in 27 SCA patients were significantly less than the 23 controls (102 ± 2.7 vs. 112 ± 2.5 μg%, $p < .025$). The excretion of urinary zinc (mean ± S.E.) in 12 SCA patients was increased as compared to 10 controls (739 ± 60 vs. 495 ± 35 μg/g creatinine, $p < .01$).

The activity of plasma RNase (mean ± S.D.), an enzyme which is inhibited by zinc, showed significantly higher activity in 31 SCA patients as compared to the 16 controls (0.43! ± .011 vs. 0.31 ± .003, ΔOD/min/ml, $p < .001$). The red cell zinc concentration correlated closely with the carbonic anhydrase (a zinc metalloenzyme) content ($r = 0.94$, $p < .001$). A significant negative correlation ($r = -0.71$, $p < 0.05$) between 24 hour urinary zinc excretion and red cell zinc levels in SCA patients was observed.

*Ten-State Nutrition Survey, 1968-1970, U.S. Department of Health, Education & Welfare, III-Clinical, Anthropometry, Dental, D.H.E.W., Publication #72:8131, III-48 & III-54.

Following zinc therapy, one 17 year old male patient gained 5 cm in 49 weeks and another 17 year old male gained 7 cm in 42 weeks. Normally by age 17, the height curve shows a plateau. Except for one female who lost 0.5 Kg during the period of observation, an average of 2.06 Kg weight gain was observed in 8 subjects (observation period 7 to 60 weeks).

Five out of 7 males have shown a positive effect on growth of body hair as a result of zinc therapy. One male has been on zinc for only 4 weeks, rather too soon to show such an effect, and the other has not shown any effect of zinc on body hair growth so far.

Two males and one female in this group have had chronic leg ulcers for many years. In one male subject, the ulcers healed within 6 weeks of zinc therapy and in the cases of the other two, some benefit of zinc therapy on healing of ulcers was noted.

DISCUSSION

Our data show that some SCA patients are zinc deficient although the severity varied considerably from one patient to another in this group. This conclusion is supported by the clinical and biochemical data obtained in this study. The older subjects showed higher red cell zinc levels, the significance of which is not clear at present. It is possible that red cell zinc concentrations may have some prognostic significance but this must await future longitudinal clinical studies in a larger group of subjects. A good correlation between red blood cell zinc and carbonic anhydrase further supports our conclusion that tissue zinc was depleted in our subjects. Activity of RNase is inhibited by zinc and in zinc deficient tissues its activity is increased (Prasad & Oberleas, 1973). Thus an increased RNase activity in plasma of SCA patients may indicate a zinc deficient state.

In spite of tissue zinc depletion in SCA patients, the mean urinary excretion of zinc was higher than in the controls. This may have been directly a result of increased filtration of zinc by the glomeruli due to continued hemolysis, or there may have been a defect in tubular re-absorption of zinc somehow related to SCA. The latter possibility cannot be excluded at present. Continued hyperzincuria may have been responsible for tissue depletion of zinc as suggested by a significant negative correlation between 24 hour urinary zinc excretion and red cell zinc levels. At this stage, however, one cannot rule out additional factors such as predominant dietary use of cereal protein and other nutritional factors which affect zinc availability adversely, thus accounting for zinc deficiency (Prasad, 1966; Prasad and Oberleas, 1970). Further work is warranted for proper elucidation of pathogenesis of zinc deficiency in SCA.

Zinc is known to be a constituent of a number of metalloenzymes. These include: carbonic anhydrase, pancreatic carboxypeptidase, liver and yeast alcohol dehydrogenase, alkaline phosphatase, tryptophan desmolase, malic dehydrogenase, glutamic dehydrogenase, lactic dehydrogenase and probably other pyridine nucleotide-dependent metallo-dehydroxyenzymes. In addition, zinc increases the activity of a number of other enzymes apparently as a "co-factor" in a nonspecific manner. These include arginase, enolase, yeast, aldolase, oxalacetic decarboxylase, lecithinase, histidine deaminase, carnosinase, aminopeptidase, tripeptidase, dehydropeptidase and glycylglycine, glycyl-L-leucine, alanylglycine, and leucylglycine dipeptidases (Vallee, 1959; Prasad, 1966).

One may suggest that the level of zinc in cells may control the physiological processes through the formation of zinc-sensitive enzymes. Our studies of tissue-enzyme changes in zinc deficient animals would support this concept (Prasad et al, 1967, 1969, 1971; Prasad & Oberleas, 1971). The rapidity with which a low-zinc diet under experimental conditions affects the growth, even in the absence of a general depletion of tissue reserves of zinc, suggest that the primary site of action of zinc must be in a component of tissue that suffers an extremely high turnover rate at a site at which this metal is freely exchangeable in the enzyme molecule or other macromolecules for which zinc is essential for normal function. Our recent study has shown that the activity of thymidine kinase, an enzyme regarded as essential for DNA synthesis and cell division, is adversely affected rapidly as a result of zinc deficiency (Prasad & Oberleas, 1974). RNA polymerase (Sandstead and Rinaldi, 1969) also required zinc for their function and zinc is an inhibitor of RNase (Prasad and Oberleas, 1973). Thus zinc has an important role in nucleic acid metabolism and this may account for its profound effect on growth. The precise role of zinc in male gonadal function is not well understood. An impairment of spermatogenesis in zinc deficiency may be a result of an adverse effect of zinc lack on DNA metabolism, however other effects of zinc on hypothalamic or anterior pituitary function cannot be ruled out at present.

Our recent studies have demonstrated a potential beneficial effect of zinc on the sickling process, in vitro, mediated by its effect on the oxygen dissociation curve (Oelshlegel et al, 1973, 1974) and the red cell membrane (Brewer and Oelshlegel, 1974; Brewer et al, 1974). Thus it is suggested that SCA patients may derive potential benefits from zinc therapy in more ways than one. The results of our limited clinical trial with zinc therapy revealed beneficial effects of zinc on growth, development of secondary sexual characteristics in male subjects and healing of chronic leg ulcers. These observations support our biochemical data that deficiency of zinc was a complicating factor in our SCA patients. Zinc therapy in such patients therefore should be considered. In addition to the above, apparent symptomatic improvement, presumably related to the anti-sickling effect of zinc, was also noted in our patients. Double-blind studies however must be done before any conclusion can be reached regarding symptomatic improvement.

We have observed no serious toxic side effects due to zinc administration so far. Occasionally some patients have complained of nausea following zinc intake in a fasting state. In general, zinc administration has been tolerated well by our patients. However, inasmuch as long term effects of zinc administration in doses utilized in this study are not known, one must be cautious in treating SCA patients with zinc on a prolonged basis.

SUMMARY

Delayed onset of puberty, short stature, hypogonadism and delayed healing of chronic leg ulcers are common clinical findings in patients with SCA. Similar clinical problems are also found in zinc deficient human subjects. We have hypothesized that a secondary zinc deficient state may develop in SCA as a result of hyperzincuria secondary to hemolysis inasmuch as red blood cells are rich in zinc.

During the past 2 years we have studied 18 men and 18 women with SCA. Of 18 male patients, 13 manifested signs of hypogonadism as evidenced by decreased or absent facial, axillary, chest and pubic hair, delayed onset of puberty and decreased sexual function. In contrast, only four females showed decreased gonadal function as evidenced by late onset of menarchy and menstrual abnormalities. This observation is consistent with the known greater susceptibility of male gonads due to a zinc lack. Two males and 2 females were below 10th height percentile whereas 16 males and 13 females were below 50th weight percentile for their ages.

The plasma, RBC, and hair zinc were decreased and the urinary zinc excretion increased in SCA patients in comparison to their controls. A significant inverse correlation between RBC zinc and daily urinary zinc excretion in SCA patients ($r = -.63$, $p < 0.001$). RNase activity in the plasma was significantly greater in SCA subjects as compared to the controls. Zinc is known to be an inhibitor of the activity of this enzyme and an increased activity in zinc deficient tissues have been previously reported by one of us.

We have administered zinc sulfate, 660 mg orally daily to 7 men and 2 women with SCA so far. Two 17 year old males have gained 5 cm and 7 cm in height in 49 and 42 weeks of zinc therapy, respectively. Normally at this age the height curve shows a plateau. All patients with the exception of one female who lost 0.5 Kg during the observation period, have gained weight ranging from 0.5 Kg to 4.1 Kg. Five out of 7 males have shown positive effect on growth of pubic, axillary, facial and body hair. One male has been on zinc for only 4 weeks, rather too soon to show such an effect, and the other has not shown any effect on body hair growth so far. Two males and one female in this group had chronic leg ulcers for many years. In one male subject the ulcers healed in 6 weeks on zinc and in the cases of the other two, some benefit of zinc therapy on healing of ulcers was noted.

In addition to the above, apparent symptomatic improvement, presumably related to the anti-sickling effect of zinc, was also noted in our patients. Double-blind studies must be done before any conclusion can be reached regarding symptomatic improvements.

In conclusion, our data suggest that a significant number of SCA patients have zinc deficiency. Supplementation with zinc has been beneficial with respect to growth, development of secondary sexual characteristics and healing of leg ulcers.

Supported by Contract No. I-HB-2-2918 from National Heart and Lung Institute Sickle Cell Disease Branch, N. I. H.

REFERENCES

Bertrand, G., and Javillier, M. (1911). Influence du zinc et du manganese sur la composition minérale de L' aspergillus niger. C. R. Acad. Sci. (Paris) 152:1337.

Brewer, G. J., and Oelshlegel, F. J., Jr. (1974). Anti-sickling effects of zinc. Biochem. Biophys. Res. Commun. 58:854.

Brewer, G. J., Oelshlegel, F. J., Jr., Prasad, A. S., Knutsen, C. A., and Meyers, N. (1974). Antisickling effects of zinc. First National Symposium on Sickle Cell Disease, June 27-29, 1974, N. I. H., Bethesda, Maryland (abstract).

Caggiano, V., Schnitzler, R., Strauss, W., Baker, R. K., Carter, A. C., Josephson, A.S., and Wallach, S. (1969).

Zinc deficiency in a patient with retarded growth, hypogonadism, hypogammaglobulinemia and chronic infection. Amer. J. Med. Sci. 257:305.

Halsted, J. A., Ronaghy, H. A., Abadi, P., Haghshenass, M., Amirhakemi, G. H., Barakat, R. M., and Reinhold, J.G. (1972). Zinc deficiency in man: The Shiraz experiment. Amer. J. Med. 53:277.

Hambidge, K. M., Hambidge, C., Jacobs, M., and Baum, J. D. (1972). Low levels of zinc in hair, anorexia, poor growth, and hypogeusia in children. Pediat. Res. 6:868.

Magid, E., DeSimone, J., and Tashian, R.E. (1973). Genetic variation in the carbonic anhydrase isoenzymes of Macaque monkeys. I. The radio-immunosorbent assay. Biochem. Genetics 8:157.

Oelshlegel, F. J., Jr., Brewer, G. J., Prasad, A. S., Knutsen, C., and Schoomaker, E. B. (1973). Effect of zinc on increasing oxygen affinity of sickle and normal red blood cells. Biochem. Biophys. Res. Commun. 53:560.

Oelshlegel, F. J., Jr., Brewer, G. J., Knutsen, C., Prasad, A. S., and Schoomaker, E. B. (1974). Studies on the interaction of zinc with human hemoglobin. Arch. Biochem Biophys., In Press.

Prasad, A. S., Miale, A., Farid, Z., Schulert, A., and Sandstead, H. H. (1963). Zinc metabolism in normals and patients with the syndrome of iron deficiency anemia, hypogonadism and dwarfism. J. Lab. Clin. Med. 61:537.

Prasad, A.S., Oberleas, D., and Halsted, J. A. (1965). Determination of zinc in biological fluids by atomic absorption spectrophotometry in normal and cirrhotic subjects. J. Lab. Clin. Med. 66:598.

Prasad, A. S. (1966). Zinc Metabolism. Charles C. Thomas, Springfield, Illinois.

Prasad, A. S., Oberleas, D., Wolf, P. L., and Horwitz, J. (1967). Studies on zinc deficiency: Changes in trace elements and enzyme activities in tissues of zinc-deficient rats. J. Clin. Invest. 46:549.

Prasad, A. S., Oberleas, D., Wolf, P., Horwitz, J. P., Miller, E. R., and Luecke, R. W. (1969). Studies on zinc deficiency: changes in trace elements and enzyme activities in tissues of zinc deficient pigs. Am. J. Clin. Nutr. 22:628.

Prasad, A. S., and Oberleas, D. (1970). Zinc: human nutrition and metabolic effects. Annals Int. Med. 73:631.

Prasad, A. S., and Oberleas, D. (1971). Changes in activities of zinc-dependent enzymes in zinc-deficient tissues of rats. J. Appl. Physiol. 31:842.

Prasad, A. S., Oberleas, D., Miller, E. R., and Luecke, R. W. (1971). Biochemical effects of zinc deficiency: changes in activities of zinc-dependent enzymes and ribonucleic acid content of tissues. J. Lab. Clin. Med. 77:144.

Prasad, A. S., and Oberleas, D. (1973). Ribonuclease and deoxyribonuclease activities in zinc-deficient tissues. J. Lab. Clin. Med. 82:461.

Prasad, A. S., and Oberleas, D. (1974). Thymidine kinase activity and incorporation of thymidine into DNA in zinc-deficient tissue. J. Lab. Clin. Med. 83:634.

Raulin, J. (1869). Études cliniques sur la végétation. Ann. Sci. Nat. Botan. Biol. Végétale. 11:93.

Sandstead, H. H., and Rinaldi, R. A. (1969). Impairment of deoxyribonucleic acid synthesis by dietary zinc deficiency in the rat. J. Cell. Physiol. 73:81.

Serjeant, G. R., Galloway, R. E., and Gueri, M. C. (1970).

Oral zinc sulphate in sickle-cell ulcers. Lancet 2:891.

Todd, W. R., Elvehjem, C. A., and Hart, E. B. (1934). Zinc in the nutrition of the rat. Amer. J. Physiol. 107:146.

Underwood, E. J. (1962). Trace Elements in Human and Animal Nutrition, Ed. 2. Academic Press, New York, pp. 157-186.

Underwood, E. J. (1971). Trace Elements in Human and Animal Nutrition, Ed. 3. Academic Press, New York, pp. 208-252.

Vallee, B. L. (1959). Biochemistry, physiology and pathology of zinc. Physiol. Rev. 39:443.

DISCUSSION

Dr. Hines: Do you have any data with respect to nitrogen balance studies in any of these patients? It would appear that you are dealing with total state, at least a marginally negative state in those two males particularly. They showed a marked increase in weight. I just wondered if you had any comments on that?

Dr. Prasad: We have not done any metabolic studies in our sickle cell patients so far. However, Dr. Reinhold from Shiraz, Iran has published a great deal on metabolic balance studies in zinc deficient subjects. High phytate content of cereal diet appears to adversely affect nitrogen balance.

Dr. McCormack: We reported in June at the First National Symposium on Sickle Cell Disease in Washington, the results of some pilot studies on the growth and development of children with sickle cell trait. I wonder whether or not you have looked at possible zinc deficiency in sickle cell trait since we have found that on some anthropometric measures, the sickle cell trait children showed slower rates of development compared to normal black children?

Dr. Prasad: We have not investigated sickle cell trait patients so far. The possibility that in this population marginal deficiency of zinc may be prevalent must be considered. However, more work needs to be done in order to settle this point.

Dr. McCormack: Did you look at the improvement in the skeletal age of your treated sickle cell anemia patients?

Dr. Prasad: Yes. With one year of treatment I think they gained two years of bone age. Is that correct, George?

Dr. Brewer: Yes, with one year of treatment the gain in skeletal maturation was approximately two years or a little more. I might mention that in the last three months there has been additional 3 cm. gain in height in one patient and I think about the same in the other.

Dr. McCormack: Is this effect the same for males and females with sickle cell anemia?

Dr. Prasad: We have not treated our female zinc deficient subjects yet. We have two but they have elected not to be in this program. I am very anxious to get some females into this study. I would suspect that as far as growth is concerned, they would behave just like the males. But with respect to secondary sexual characteristics it will be different.

Dr. Button: Could you tell us anything about the nature of these patients' zinc absorption? Do they have normal thymic shadows, and also how anemic do they become?

Dr. Prasad: Are you referring to the sickle cell patients or zinc deficient dwarfs from the Middle East? With respect to anemia in the Middle East, subjects all were iron deficient because the same factors which affect the availability of zinc also affect the availability of iron. We administered pure iron to some of the dwarfs in the Middle East. Their anemia was corrected but they gained no height, or weight, and no changes in secondary sexual characteristics were noted. The group receiving zinc remained anemic but they grew. Thus, we were able to separate the tissue effects of iron and zinc. In the sickle cell patients here we have a complicated situation, inasmuch as there was hemolysis. We have not looked for thymic shadows per se, but routine chest x-rays have showed no abnormality. The most recent evidence from Dr. Sandstead's laboratory indicates that there is a ligand that is released from the pancreas and this then transports zinc from the gut to the mucosa. It appears that absorption of zinc utilizes a complicated mechanism.

Dr. Perutz: I think superoxide dismutase is another zinc enzyme, but what I really wanted to ask Dr. Prasad is how he first discovered these cases of dwarfism that are due to zinc deficiency?

Dr. Prasad: When I first saw these patients in the Middle East, it was the impression of the local physicians that they were hypopituitary dwarfs. We do know now that the effect of growth hormone and zinc on growth are by separate mechanisms and there was no clear cut evidence for hypopituitarism in those patients. The main reason why I suspected that this may be due to zinc deficiency was the clinical similarity which these patients showed to what was reported in zinc deficient animals. It was already known that animals do not grow properly when they lack zinc. I was also reasonably certain that iron deficiency was not the cause of growth retardation and hypogonadism. These facts led me to look for some other nutritional aspect.

Dr. Orten: In the 1974 National Research Council, so called recommended daily dietary allowances, I noticed for the first time they have included zinc and at the surprising level of 15 mg. Surprisingly this is about the same as the recommended RDA for iron. I just wondered if you would comment on that? Do you think it is justified?

Dr. Prasad: In 1970, I believe the National Research Council had their first meeting concerned with the requirements for zinc. It was more or less arbitrarily determined that 15 to 18 mg. of zinc may be needed in an American diet. I wish to point out, however, that this requirement may be altered greatly by unfavorable dietary conditions and diseased states.

Dr. Maile: Do you have any idea of the relative frequency of zinc deficiency in your sickle cell population and how you identify patients that might be zinc deficient? Do any of the zinc deficient sickle cell patients have co-existent liver disease? In addition, I wasn't clear on the reason they had an increased urinary excretion of zinc with a low plasma zinc.

Dr. Prasad: We have not found any evidence of liver disease so far by the usual routine liver function tests. We have not done any liver biopsies. With respect to why they lose zinc in the urine, we feel that perhaps the destruction of red cells released zinc for increased glomerular filtration. At this point we cannot rule out the possibility that there may be a defect in tubular reabsorption of zinc in sickle cell patients. As I mentioned to you earlier, there seems to be a spectrum of zinc deficiency in our population of sickle cell subjects. Approximately one fourth were markedly zinc deficient by our criteria and a fourth in the elderly age group were normal.

Dr. Maile: How many sickle cell patients were negative as far as their evaluation for zinc? Did you have any that you suspected were zinc deficient and really were not?

Dr. Prasad: None so far in our studies.

Dr. Maile: You did not identify anything in the diet as you had in the Middle Eastern subjects that was particularly unusual?

Dr. Prasad: As I mentioned, this is one area which we should really look into very carefully. It is very difficult to get a good nutritional history by the usual means. The possibility that marginal nutritional deficiency of zinc may be an additional problem must be considered.

Dr. Maile: Was there any improvement in parameters other than growth and development in these children after correction of zinc deficiency?

Dr. Prasad: As you heard from Dr. Brewer, they feel well and some of them have shown symptomatic improvements.

Dr. Moore: Do you find that the same kind of response is made to a given dosage of zinc among members of different races? Is the response to a given dosage of zinc approximately similar in your black patients and the Middle East subjects? Is an approximately equivalent amount of zinc absorbed from a given dosage in the black, Middle East, and white subjects (laboratory personnel studied)?

Dr. Prasad: The response to zinc administration in our Middle Eastern dwarfs was more dramatic as compared to what we find here in the sickle cell patients. This may be because we haven't stopped them from hemolyzing completely such that they are still continuing to lose zinc. Dr. Caggiano's zinc deficient patient in New York was a Puerto Rican. He gained approximately six inches in about 15 months on zinc supplementation at the age of 18.

Dr. Moore: And are there any changes in testosterone levels associated with growth in your patients?

Dr. Prasad: This is one thing which we are evaluating right now in the sickle cell patients. It's our impression that they tend to have low FSH and low testosterone levels. The growth hormone is normal and we have not seen any other abnormal endocrine parameters. We have just begun to stimulate their hypothalamus by giving them hypothalamic releasing factor. I believe the effect of zinc lack is an end organ effect on testes and affects spermatogenesis adversely. Detailed studies in this area are currently being done in our laboratories.

METABOLIC ABNORMALITIES OF VITAMIN B6 AND MAGNESIUM IN ALCOHOL-INDUCED SIDEROBLASTIC ANEMIA

John D. Hines, M.D.

Case Western Reserve University School of
Medicine at Cleveland Metro. General Hospital
3395 Scranton Road, Cleveland, Ohio 44109

ABSTRACT

Chronic and excessive alcohol abuse has been shown to create cellular depletion of folate, pyridoxal phosphate (PLP), potassium and magnesium in a significant number of patients. Studies reported herein document a striking association of hypokalemia, hypomagnesemia and abnormalities of vitamin B6 metabolism frequently resulting in erythroid mitochondrial iron-overloading. Selected well nourished, chronic alcoholic subjects were studied, utilizing metabolic balance studies. Graded amounts of ethanol in the form of 86 proof bar whiskey were isocalorically substituted for carbohydrate and the patients were observed from 40 to 60 days. The results of these investigations revealed the following:

1) a progressive fall in serum and erythrocyte PLP and magnesium concentrations;
2) a state of negative magnesium balance, but not of potassium or calcium;
3) a progressive decrease in erythrocyte pyridoxal phosphokinase concentrations not corrected by administration of magnesium or pulse doses of pyridoxine;

4) the demonstration of a plasma inhibitor of erythrocyte and hepatic pyridoxal phosphokinase in certain of these subjects.

INTRODUCTION

A reversible form of sideroblastic anemia (Figure 1) has been well documented in a significant number of chronic alcoholics admitted to hospitals for acute withdrawal (1-4). A significant number of such patients have been shown to have abnormal vitamin B6 metabolism (3-5), coexistent folate abnormalities and clinical and/or biochemical evidence of liver disease (2, 3, 4, 6, 7). Chronic ethanol abuse has also been associated with hypomagnesemia and to a lesser degree hypokalemia (8-17). In a significant number of these alcoholic subjects a coexisting depletion of intramuscular K^+ and Mg^{++} was demonstrated (11).

The present studies were undertaken to 1) determine the pathogenesis of alcohol-induced erythroid mitochondria iron overload (sideroblastic alterations); 2) define the mechanism of altered vitamin B6 metabolism observed in alcoholic subjects; and 3) evaluation of magnesium and potassium metabolism in well nourished, chronic alcoholic subjects receiving ethanol in conjunction with an otherwise normal diet.

METHODS

Subjects

Two groups of patients were investigated. The first consisted of 65 patients (46 male, 19 female) who were admitted to Cleveland Metropolitan General Hospital for symptoms of acute alcohol withdrawal. Eighty percent of these subjects had clinical and/or biochemical evidence of liver disease. The second group comprising these studies were well nourished, chronic alcoholic subjects who had been hospitalized for a minimum of 12 days and in no instance was there any evidence of liver or renal disease. The criteria for eligibility for investigation have been previously described (3). These subjects were housed on the Metabolic

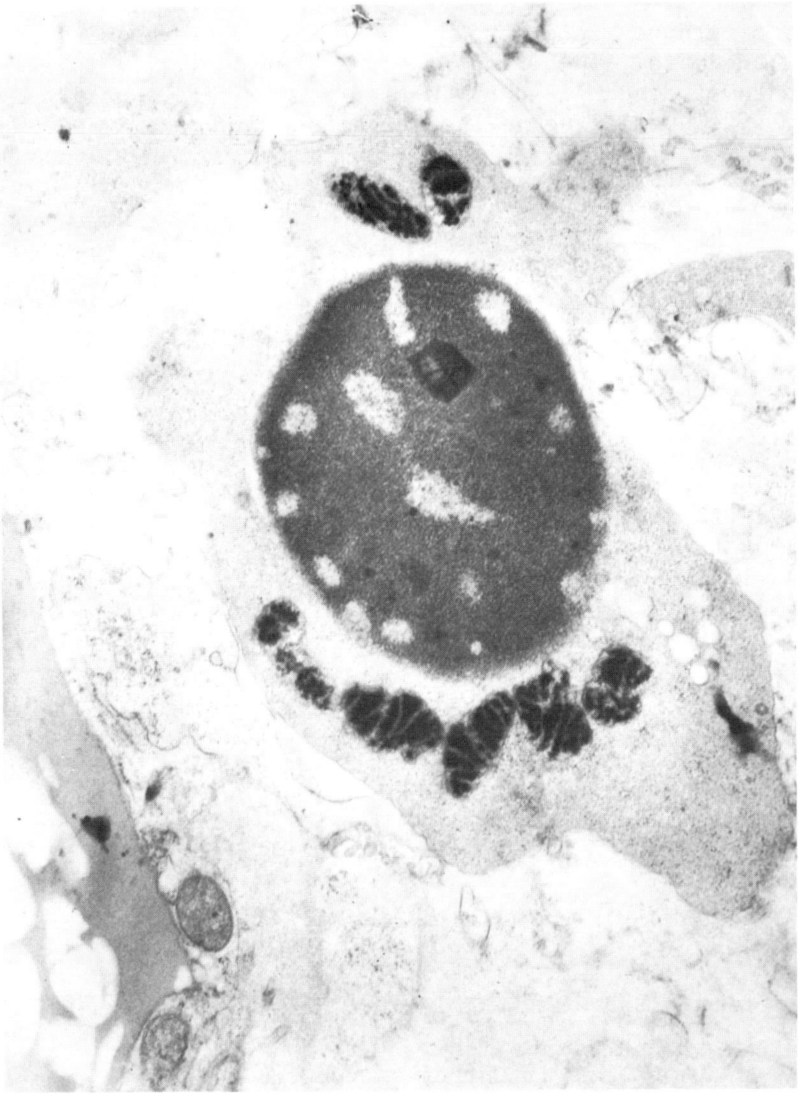

Figure 1. Electron photomicrograph of abnormal iron-laden sideroblast in a patient with alcohol-induced sideroblastic anemia (x 15,000).

Ward and received a standard hospital diet containing approximately 1500 µg of "total" folate and 5-6 mg of pyridoxine per day. Ethanol in the form of 86 proof blended bar whiskey was isocalorically substituted for carbohydrate. Serum levels of ethanol in excess of 250 mg/100 ml were achieved in all subjects. The investigations were performed in accordance with the Helsinki Declaration and were approved by the Hospital Committee on Investigation in Humans.

MATERIALS AND METHODS

Routine hematologic studies were performed according to standard methods (18). Serum and erythrocyte folate levels were assayed by both Lactobacillus casei (19, 20) and the radiochemical method of Kamen and Caston (21) employing partially purified hog kidney folate binder.

Serum, erythrocyte and hepatic concentrations of pyridoxal phosphate (PLP) were determined by the method of Hines and Love (22). Erythrocyte and hepatic pyridoxal phosphokinase estimations were performed according to the method previously described (4). Serum vitamin B12 levels were performed employing the Euglena gracilis (23) and serum iron and total iron binding capacity were measured by the method of Schade and co-workers (24). Estimation of the *in vivo* conversion of intravenous pyridoxine to PLP was performed by the method of Hines and Cowan (3). Serum, urine, erythrocyte and fecal (extracted) potassium and magnesium were determined by atomic absorption spectroscopy. Serum and urine calcium sodium and chloride were determined by autoanalytic method.

RESULTS

Incidence of Hypomagnesemia, Hypokalemia, Subnormal Vitamin Levels, and Marrow Sideroblast Abnormalities in Chronic Alcoholic Subjects

Results from this and other laboratories have illustrated that the majority of chronic alcoholic patients ad-

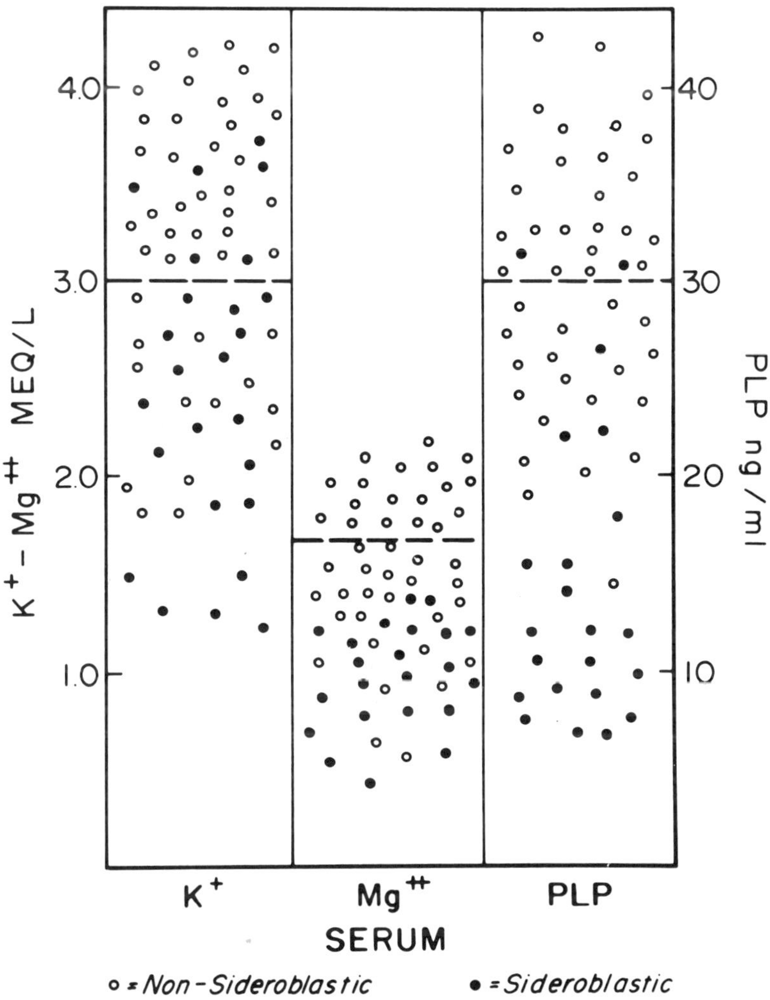

Figure 2. Serum K+, Mg++, and PLP levels in 65 chronic alcoholics admitted for acute withdrawal. Hatched lines are the lower limits of normal values.

mitted for acute withdrawal have subnormal serum folate and PLP levels (1-5). Figure 2 illustrates the admission serum, K+, Mg++, and PLP levels in 65 chronic alcoholic subjects admitted for acute withdrawal manifestations. Sixty-five percent had subnormal serum levels of K+ and Mg++ and 60% were subnormal for serum PLP. Thirty-five percent of the patients had marrow sideroblastic alterations on admission and all of these subjects had subnormal serum Mg++ levels and all but two subnormal PLP concentrations. The mean PLP level for the patients with marrow sideroblastic abnormalities was statistically significant (student T test) at the $P < 0.005$ level.

Figures 3 and 4 illustrate the red cell concentrations of PLP and magnesium respectively in the alcoholic subjects compared to hematologically normal hospital control subjects. There was a statistically significant difference in both Mg++ and PLP in the alcoholic non-sideroblastic and alcoholic sideroblastic subjects, the latter having the lower red cell values.

Sixty-six percent of all these patients had both a subnormal serum folate and morphologic signs of folate deficiency in the marrow specimens. Erythrocyte folate levels were below normal in 58% of patients. There was no significant correlation between subnormal serum or erythrocyte folate and PLP levels.

These studies confirm and extend previous observations that abnormal folate and vitamin B6 metabolism and hypokalemia and hypomagnesemia are significant features in chronic alcoholic subjects admitted to a hospital for acute withdrawal manifestations. In order to further delineate the effects of excessive alcohol ingestion on vitamin B6 metabolism, magnesium and potassium balance, and development of sideroblastic marrow abnormalities, six well nourished, chronic alcoholic volunteer subjects (vida supra) were investigated on the Metabolic Unit. The clinical and hematologic status of these six individuals were normal. All

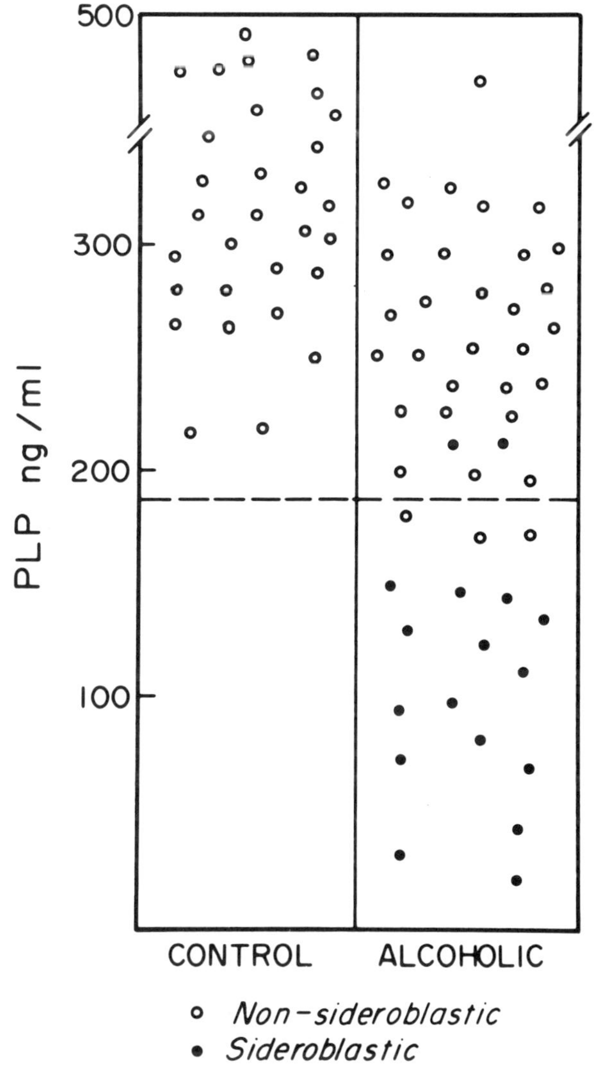

Figure 3. Red cell PLP levels in normal control and alcoholic subjects. Hatched line is lower limit of normal values.

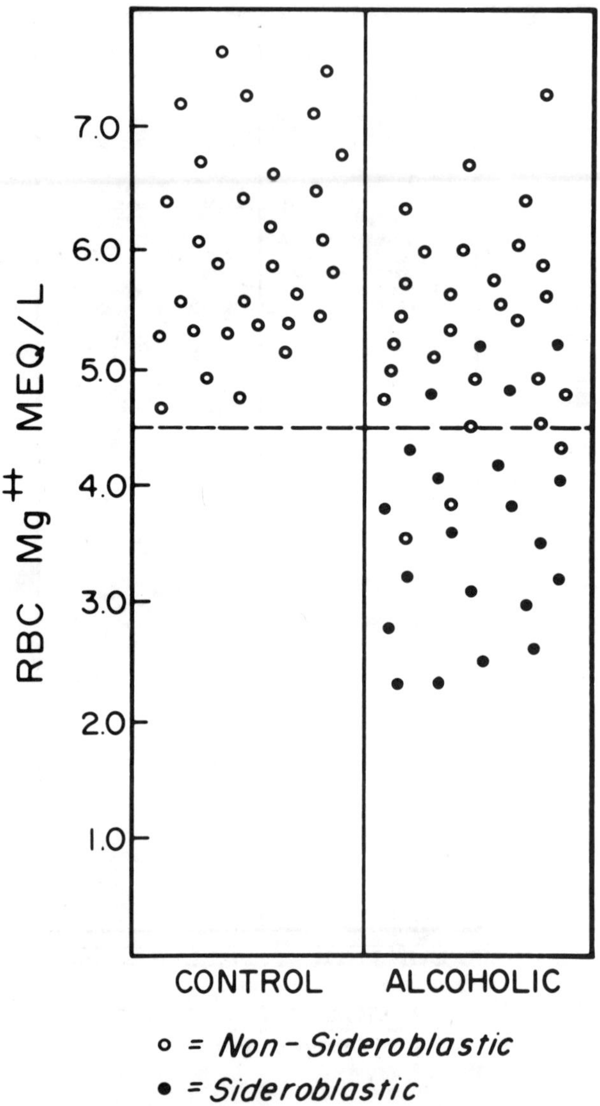

Figure 4. Red cell magnesium levels in normal control and alcoholic subjects. Hatched line is lower limit of normal values.

were caucasian males, age range between 29 and 54 years, and all had ingested a standard hospital diet without ethanol for 3 weeks prior to investigation. Graded amounts of 86 proof ethanol of 900-1100 ml per day were administered with the standard balanced diet (vida supra). The daily dietary content for magnesium varied from 28 to 32 Meq per day and and for potassium approximately 80 Meq per day. After ingesting alcohol for two weeks the in vivo conversion of intravenous pyridoxine to PLP was tested as follows: 20 mg of intravenous pyridoxine was administered to each subject and serum for PLP assay was drawn at 0, 30, and 90 minutes. The net increase in serum PLP represented in vivo pyridoxine conversion to PLP which in man is primarily due to hepatic pyridoxal phosphokinase (PL-kinase) and oxidase enzyme activity. The mean values for PLP were compared to ten age-matched, normal, control subjects. The peak increase in PLP in the six alcoholic subjects was significantly less than controls ($P < 0.001$) indicating defective oxidation and/or phosphorylation of the vitamin. It has been previously demonstrated in this laboratory that this conclusion is indeed valid since intravenous infusion of PLP resulted in a peak increase in serum PLP activity which was not different from normal control subjects (25). The latter observation ruled out the possibility that failure of rise in serum PLP in alcoholic subjects subsequent to receiving I.V. pyridoxine was due to accelerated egress of PLP from the circulation. These observations strongly suggested that chronic, excessive ingestion of alcohol despite an adequate diet impaired the oxidation-phosphorylation of the vitamin.

To test this possibility, assessment of the patients' erythrocyte hemolysate pyridoxal-phosphokinase (PL-kinase) was performed employing the method previously described (4). The results of this study are depicted in Figure 5. It can readily be discerned that after from two to nine weeks of alcohol ingestion there is a precipitous drop in erythrocyte PL-kinase activity. These results prompted speculation as to whether or not chronic, excessive alcohol intake in some fashion generates a circulating inhibitor to PL-kinase. To test this assumption, plasma was obtained from the six subjects from three to six weeks after alcohol ingestion. Ali-

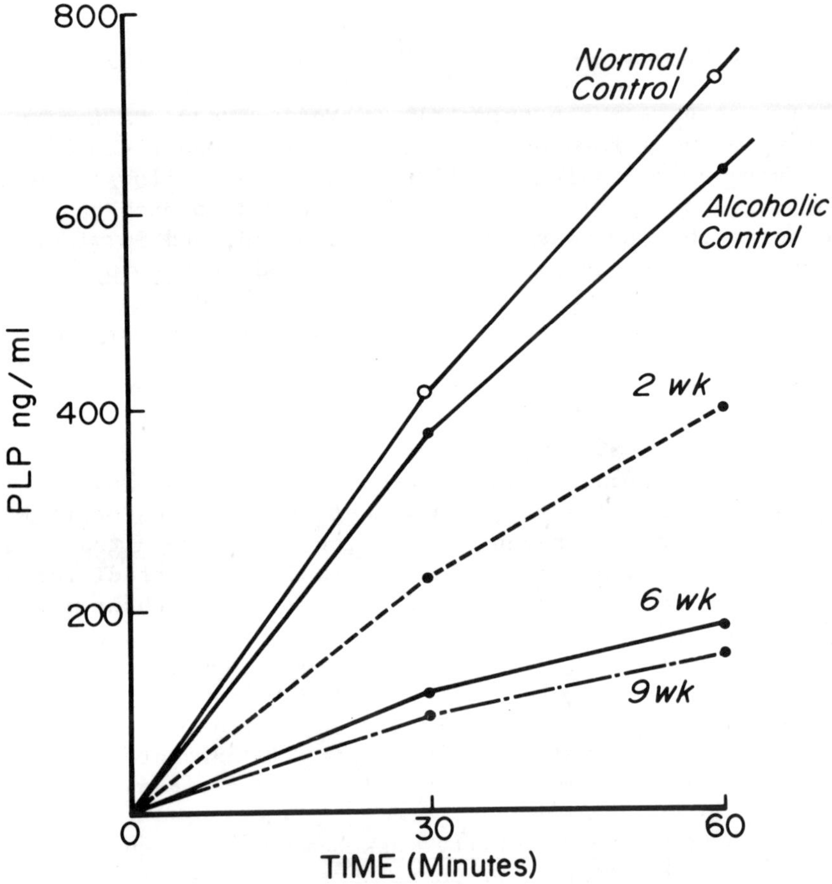

Figure 5. Red cell PL-kinase values in alcoholic subjects before and up to nine weeks of ingestion.

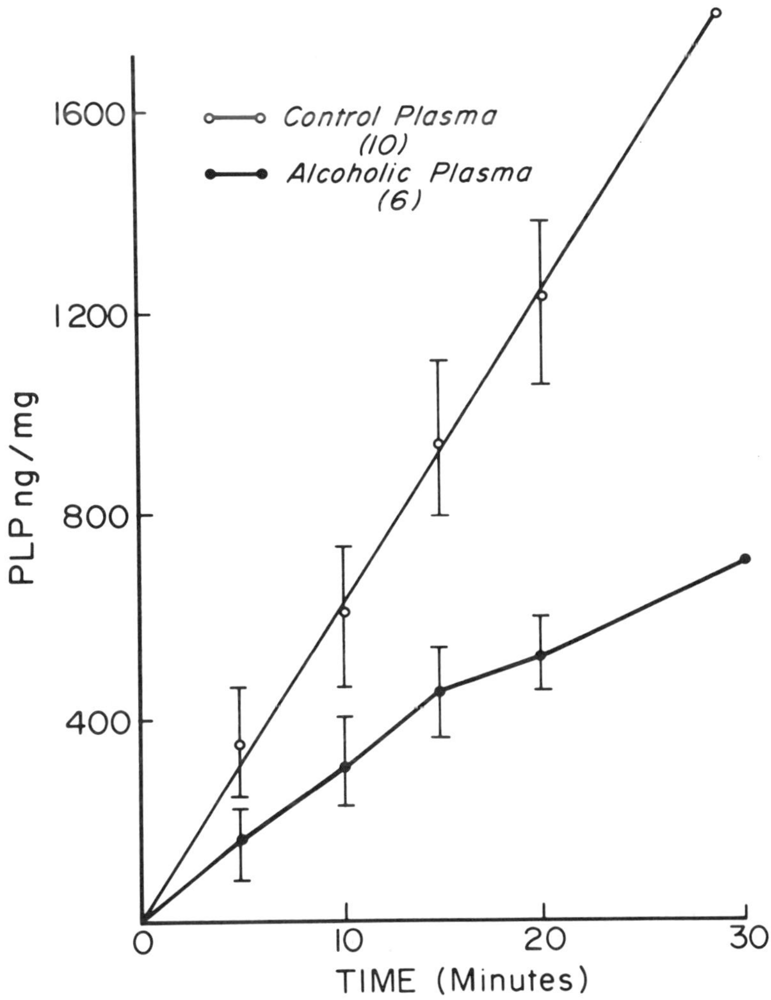

Figure 6. Hepatic PL-kinase in liver slices pre-incubated with control (normal) and alcoholic plasma.

quots of the alcoholic and normal control plasma were preincubated with histologically normal human liver slices (obtained from patients during cholecystectomy) and subsequently, PL-kinase was estimated. The results are illustrated in Figure 6. Preincubation of the liver in alcoholic plasma caused a profound decrease in PL-kinase activity. Further studies in this laboratory have shown that the plasma "inhibitor" is non-dialyzable, heat labile (56°C), and is not lactate, acetaldehyde or orate or phospholipid (25).

Magnesium and Potassium Balance Studies

Complete metabolic balance studies were carried out in six well nourished, chronic alcoholic subjects before, during, and subsequent to excess alcohol intake with an adequte diet (vida supra). Figure 7 illustrates the mean serum magnesium in these subjects. A statistically significant decrease in serum and in erythrocyte magnesium (not illustrated) occurred in these subjects by day 25 and was maintained through day 40 of alcohol ingestion. The decrease in erythrocyte magnesium was most pronounced in the three alcoholic subjects who developed marrow sideroblast abnormalities (from 6.5 to 3.4 Meq/L). Immediately post withdrawal the serum magnesium concentration dropped even further for the first 48 hours similar to the fall observed by Mendelsohn (16).

Fecal magnesium concentration did not change significantly from pre-alcohol control at any time of alcohol ingestion (range 16.3 to 18.5 Meq/day). In striking contrast all patients exhibited a progressive state of negative magnesium balance peaking at 35-50 days (Figure 8). The daily urinary excretion exceeded stool loss after 30 days of alcohol ingestion.

In contrast to the magnesium results, no significant change in serum or urine potassium occurred (Figure 9). The magnesium and potassium studies are summarized in Table I.

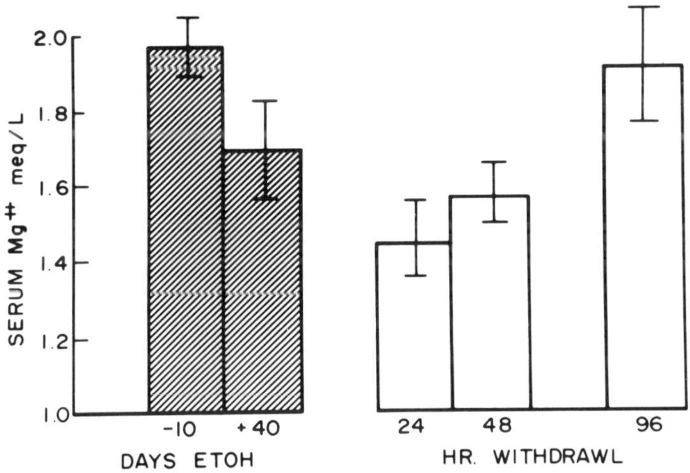

Figure 7. Serum magnesium levels in alcoholic study subjects before, during, and after ingestion.

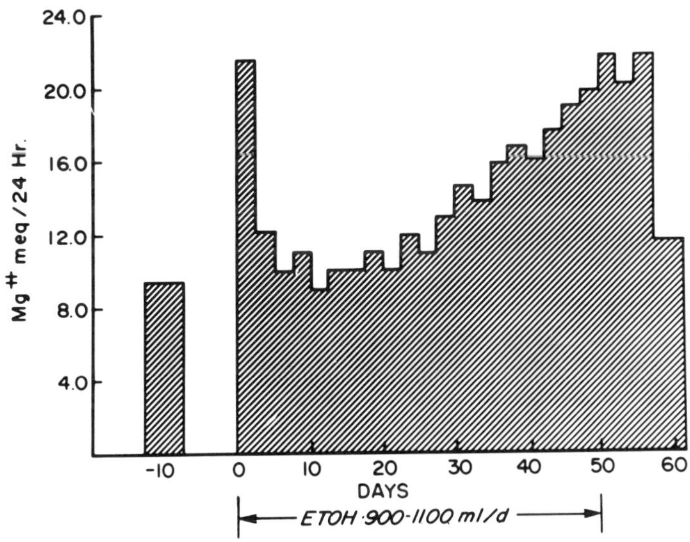

Figure 8. Magnesium balance study illustrating relatively severe hypermagnesuria and negative balance.

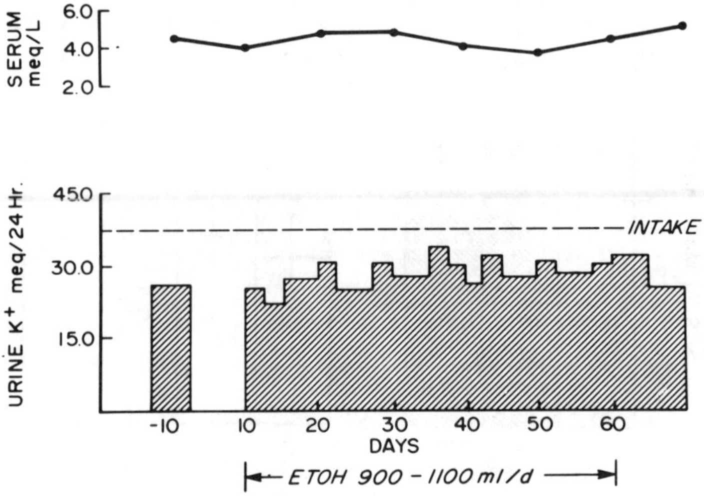

Figure 9. Potassium balance study showing no significant abnormality.

MAGNESIUM:	SERUM meq/L	ERYTHRO -CYTE meq/L	URINE meq/24 hr	FECAL meq/24 hr
NORMAL	*1.98 ±0.55*	*6.32 ±0.84*	*7.94 ±0.96*	*16.08 ±1.78*
SUBJECTS NO. 6				
PRE ALCOHOL -10d	1.92 ±0.16	5.98 ±0.73	7.91 ±0.88	16.09 ±1.70
DURING ALCOHOL	1.68 ±0.22	3.96 ±0.68	16.07 ±1.33	15.97 ±1.91
POST ALCOHOL 14d	1.97 ±0.12	4.84 ±0.71	7.06 ±0.93	16.37 ±1.63

Table I. Summary of magnesium balance study in six subjects before, during, and after alcohol ingestion.

No significant changes occurred in serum or urine concentrations of sodium calcium CO_2 or chloride (not illustrated). Electrocardiograms taken every seventh day remained normal in all six subjects throughout the study as did sequential careful neurologic examinations. No data were obtained with respect to electromyography or peripheral nerve conduction. None of the patients became anemic although three of the six subjects manifested marrow sideroblastic changes by the third week of study and in two subjects this was reversed by 10 mg of PLP intramuscularly every six hours for one day while ethanol consumption continued. In the third subject with sideroblastic marrow alterations, the administration of intravenous magnesium sulfate 2 gm every six hours for one day had no demonstrable effect on marrow sideroblastic changes.

DISCUSSION

Pyridoxal phosphate constitutes the major fraction of vitamin B6 congeners in human serum and concentrations of the coenzyme in serum and erythrocytes are considered to be a reliable indication of vitamin B6 nutritive in man (22, 26). The studies reported herein demonstrate that alteration of vitamin B6 metabolism occurs relatively soon after excessive alcohol ingestion is monitored with a nutritionally adequate diet and in the absence of clinical and/or biochemical evidence of liver disease. Liver biopsy specimens were not obtained in our subjects since the studies of Lieber and Rubin (27, 28) have clearly shown a reversible abnormality in hepatic architecture in normal subjects after several days of alcohol abuse. Although vitamin B6 depletion is associated with altered hepatic histology in rats and monkeys (29, 30), no such causal effect has been demonstrated in man.

The possibility exists that there may be multiple mechanisms operative in the evolution of vitamin B6 metabolic abnormalities occurring in chronic alcoholics. The studies reported herein strongly support one possible mechanism which is the acquired defect in conversion of pyridoxine to

PLP via PL-kinase. Both the *in vitro* and *in vivo* studies support this possibility. An additional possible mechanism has been reported recently by Lumeng and Li (5) who demonstrated that acetaldehyde, and not ethanol, impaired the net total concentration of PLP in erythrocytes. This effect of acetaldehyde was totally abolished by addition of 80 mM Pi ostensibly because of its inhibition of B6-phosphate phosphatase. These authors showed the phosphatase was membrane bound and upon appropriate incubation demonstrated it resulted in accelerated degradation of phosphorylated B6 congeners in erythrocytes. Whether or not this has pathologic significance *in vivo* remains to be tested. Unpublished observations in this laboratory have failed to detect any appreciable decrease in erythrocyte PLP concentration in a hemolysate system when incubated at 37°C with up to 1.0 mM acetaldehyde for up to 30 minutes. The studies reported herein clearly failed to demonstrate any effect of ethanol or acetaldehyde on hepatic PL-kinase concentrations. Regulation of erythrocyte PLP concentration depends upon pyridoxine phosphate oxidase, pyridoxal phosphokinase, and on B6 phosphate phosphatase (5, 31). The major body site for PLP biosynthesis is the liver. Very little is known regarding the possible role of B6 phosphate phosphatase with respect to regulation of hepatic PLP synthesis. The studies reported herein have demonstrated that certain healthy, well nourished, chronic alcoholic subjects, when ingesting excessive alcohol, generate in some way a circulating protein-bound inhibitor for erythrocyte and hepatic PL-kinase. The precise physiochemical nature of this substance remains to be elicited.

Beginning with the studies of Flink and co-workers (8) a number of investigators have documented the strong association between chronic alcohol abuse and hypomagnesemia and/or hypokalemia (9-17). Martin and co-workers (10) in a study of 44 patients entering the hospital with acute alcoholism found hypomagnesemia in 60% and hypokalemia in 30% of the subjects. Muscle biopsy studies have definitely established a cellular depletion of Mg^{++} and K^{+} (11). Studies in this laboratory showed a similar incidence of hypomagnesemia (65%) but a higher incidence of hypokalemia (60%) in 65 chronic alcoholics admitted for acute withdrawal. It has been emphasized that the possibility exists that intracellular K+ depletion in alcoholics may be the resultant of co-existing Mg++ depletion; that restoration of intracellular K+ may be more efficiently accomplished clinically if Mg++ repletion is concurrently instituted (32-35). Observation of hypermagnesuria following ingestion of alcohol has been implicated as one of the modes of depleting Mg++ in alcoholic subjects (13-15). Studies in this laboratory on six well nourished, healthy, chronic alcoholic volunteer subjects, receiving chronic daily excessive alcohol intake with an adequate diet clearly show an evolution of hypomagnesemia closely paralleling hypermagnesuria with no change in fecal excretion. Subsequently, a significant diminution in erythrocyte Mg++ ensued, more marked in the patients who developed marrow sideroblastic abnormalities. Surprisingly, no significant change in potassium balance was detected in any of the six subjects.

Studies in experimental magnesium deficiency have indicated that increased aldosterone secretion apparently accompanies this disorder (36, 37). Unfortunately, no assessment of aldosterone status was made in these subjects. The fact that no significant serum or urine Na+ or K+ alterations occurred in these subjects on alcohol lends indirect support against major changes in aldosterone secretion as it might affect Mg++ balance. Certainly it does not rule out a more subtle effect of aldosterone and magnesium balance.

Supported by Grants AA-00225-07 and 5 RO1 AM00745-20 of National Institutes of Health.

REFERENCES

1. Hines, J. D. Reversible megaloblastic and sideroblastic marrow abnormalities in alcoholic patients. Brit. J. Haem., 16:87, 1969.
2. Eichner, E. R., and Hillman, R. S. The evolution of anemia in alcoholic patients. Am. J. Med., 50:218, 1971.
3. Hines, J. D., and Cowan, D. H. Studies on the pathogneesis of alcohol-induced sideroblastic bone marrow abnormalities. N. E. J. M., 283:441, 1970.
4. Hines, J. D., and Cowan, D. H. Anemia in alcoholism. IN: Drugs and Hematologic Reactions. Dimitrov, N. V., and Nodine, J. H., eds. Grune and Stratton. The Twenty-ninth Hahnemann Symposium, 1974, p. 148.
5. Lumeng, L., and Li, T. K. Vitamin B6 metabolism in chronic alcohol abuse. J. Clin. Invest., 53:693, 1974.
6. Sullivan, L. W., and Herbert, V. Suppression of hematopoiesis by ethanol. J. Clin. Invest., 43:2048, 1964.
7. Sullivan, L. W., and Herbert, V. Mechaniam of hematosuppression by ethanol. Am. J. Clin. Nutr., 14:238, 1964.
8. Flink, E. B., Stutzman, F. L., Anderson, A. R., et al. Magnesium deficiency after prolonged parenteral fluid administration and after chronic alcoholism complicated by delirium tremens. J. Lab. Clin. Med., 43:169, 1954.
9. Flink, E. B. Magnesium deficiency syndrome in man. J. Am. Med. Assoc., 160:1406, 1956.
10. Martin, H. E., McCuskey Jr., C., and Tupikowa, N. Electrolyte disturbance in acute alcoholism. Am. J. Clin. Nutr., 7:191, 1959.
11. Jones, J. E., Shane, S. R., Jacobs, W. H., et al. Magnesium balance studies in chronic alcoholism. Ann. N. Y. Acad. Sci., 162:935, 1969.
12. Welt, L. G., Hollander Jr., W., and Blythe, W. B. The consequences of potassium deficiency. J. Chron. Dis., 11:213, 1960.
13. Heaton, F. W., Pyrah, L. N., Beresford, C. C., et al. Hypomagnesemia in chronic alcoholism. Lancet, 2:802, 1962.
14. Kalbfleisch, J. M., Lindeman, R. D., Ginn, H. E., et al.

Effects of ethanol administration on urinary excretion of magnesium and other electrolytes in alcoholic and normal subjects. J. Clin. Invest., 42:1471, 1963.
15. Dick, M., Evans, R. A., and Watson, L. Effect of ethanol on magnesium excretion. J. Clin. Path., 22:152, 1969.
16. Mendelsohn, J. H., Ogata, M., and Mello, M. K. Effects of alcohol ingestion and withdrawal on magnesium states of alcoholics: clinical and experimental findings. Ann. N. Y. Acad. Sci., 162:918, 1969.
17. Mendelsohn, J. H. Biologic concomitants of alcoholism. N. E. J. M., 283:71, 1970.
18. A Syllabus of Laboratory Examinations in Clinical Diagnosis. Edited by L. B. Page, P. J. Culver. Cambridge, Harvard University Press, 1960.
19. Herbert, V. Aseptic addition method for Lactobacillus casei assay of folate activity in human serum. J. Clin. Pathol., 19:12, 1966.
20. Hoffbrand, A. V., Newcombe, B. F. A., and Mollin, D. L. Method of assay of red cell folate activity in the value of the assay as a test for folate deficiency. J. Clin. Pathol., 19:17, 1966.
21. Kamen, B., and Caston, D. Direct radio chemical assay for serum folate: competition between folic acid and 5-methyl tetrahydrafolate for a folate binder. J. Lab. Clin. Med., 83:1964, 1974.
22. Hines, J. D., and Love, D. S. Determination of serum and blood pyridoxal phosphate concentrations with purified rabbit skeletal muscle phosphorylast b. J. Lab. Clin. Med., 73:343, 1969.
23. Anderson, B. B. Investigations into the Euglena methods for the assay of vitamin B12 in serum. J. Clin. Pathol., 17:14, 1964.
24. Schade, A. L., Oyama, J., Reinhart, R. W., et al. Bound iron and unsaturated iron-binding capacity of serum: rapid and reliable quantitative determination. Proc. Soc. Exp. Biol. Med., 87:443, 1954.
25. Hines, J. D. Hematologic abnormalities involving vitamin B6 and folate metabolism in alcoholic subjects. Ann. N. Y. Acad. Med., IN PRESS.
26. Sauberlich, H. E., Canham, E. M., Bauer, N., et al.

Biochemical assessment of the nutritional status of vitamin B6 in the human. Am. J. Clin. Nutr., 25:629, 1972.

27. Lieber, C. S., and Rubin, E. Alcoholic fatty liver in man on a high protein and low fat diet. Am. J. Med., 44:200, 1968.
28. Rubin, E., and Lieber, C. S. Alcohol-induced hepatic injury in non-alcoholic volunteers. N. E. J. M., 278: 869, 1968.
29. Okoda, M., and Ochi, A. The effect of diet protein level on transaminase activities and fat deposition in the vitamin B6-depleted rat. J. Biochem. (Tokyo), 70: 581, 1971.
30. Greenberg, L. D. Arteriosclerotic dental and hepatic lesions in pyridoxine deficient monkeys. Vit. Horm., 22:677, 1964.
31. Anderson, B. B., Fulford-Jones, C. E., Child, J. A., et al. Conversion of vitamin B6 compounds to active forms in the red blood cell. J. Clin. Invest., 50: 1901, 1971.
32. Shills, M. E. Experimental human magnesium depletion. Clinical observations and blood chemistry alterations. Amer. J. Clin. Nutr., 15:133, 1964.
33. Shills, M. E. Experimental human magnesium depletion. Medicine (Balt.), 48:61, 1969.
34. Whang, R., et al. The influence of sustained magnesium deficiency on muscle potassium repletion. J. Lab. Clin. Med., 70:895, 1967.
35. Ryan, M. P., and Hingerty, D. Effects of magnesium deficiency on restoration of potassium and sodium levels in potassium depleted muscle. Irish J. Med. Sci., 2: 137, 1969.
36. Ginn, H. E., et al. Aldosterone secretion in magnesium deficient rats. Endocrin., 80L969, 1967.
37. Cantin, M. Relationship of juxtaglomerular apparatus and adrenal cortex to biochemical and extracellular fluid volume changes in magnesium deficiency. Lab. Invest., 22:558, 1970.

DISCUSSION

Dr. Brewer: We've been interested in whether plasma magnesium might have an influence on red cell glycolysis. Has anybody measured DPG or ATP in the red cells of these hypomagnesemic patients?

Dr. Hines: The only data I'm aware of were in patients who had a high retic count and they were hypomagnesemic. The DPG's were elevated and they were appropriately elevated to the reticulocyte index.

Dr. L. G. Moore: I noticed that the drop in red cell magnesium was far greater than the decreases in serum, fecal, or urinary magnesium levels observed among the alcoholics relative to the normal subjects. Would you comment on the apparent greater susceptibility of the red cells to magnesium loss?

Dr. Hines: All we can surmise is that they're leaking magnesium from the erythrocyte at a rate that again cannot be accounted for by red cell turnover in terms of developing cells being deficient. I think it has been shown before by some other investigators that the red cells will leak magnesium.

Dr. Embury: As you know, we've studied some idopathic sideroblastic patients and found that in addition to synthesizing heme and globin slowly, they've had some nucleic acid metabolism abnormalities. To my knowledge, nobody has done this in alcoholics. Have you done this, John, or do you know if anybody has?

Dr. Hines: I don't think anybody has. It is obviously the next step that one would like to do, and in light of your mentioning to me the success you've had in getting normoblasts separated from marrow, I think this is a real four plus for us. We've been struggling with reticulocytes which are horrible to work with, and we would like a cellular component to work with with respect to looking at the PLP content of the mitchondria. Have you had any opportunity to do oxidative phosphorylation experiments in your marrow preps? Do they look normal?

Dr. Embury: We haven't done the experiments. We've just been concentrating on nucleic acids in view of the globin synthesis which is depressed.

Dr. Hines: John Light and Alli in London showed in the sideroblastics they studied that there was definitely a defect in globin synthesis. You might comment on this. This is not alcoholic, but refractory sideroblastic. It seemed to me they couldn't relate definitely that there was an effect on heme synthesis that was affecting the globin in the feedback mechanism.

Dr. Embury: We don't know which is cause and which is effect or how they are interrelated. We just noticed both.

Dr. Hines: That is an interesting observation.

THE ROLE OF COPPER IN THE BIOSYNTHESIS OF HEME

James M. Orten, Aline Underhill Orten,
Vishwanath M. Sardesai, and Linda C. Cheng
Departments of Biochemistry, Medicine, and Surgery
Wayne State Univesity School of Medicine
Detroit, Michigan 48201

INTRODUCTION

The essentiality of copper for the biosynthesis of hemoglobin in the animal organism was demonstrated first in 1928 (Hart, Steenbock, Waddell, and Elvehjem, 1928) in rats fed a whole cow's milk diet supplemented with iron as a highly purified ferric salt. Despite the addition of the supplemental iron, the rats became severely anemic and died usually within 10 to 12 weeks. The addition of small amounts of copper (25 to 50 micrograms per day) as purified cupric sulfate was rapidly effective both in preventing and in curing this type of "nutritional anemia", the hemoglobin levels returning to normal values in 4 to 6 weeks. This now classical work was soon confirmed (Underhill, Orten, and Lewis, 1931) and extended to other species including rabbits, chicks, and pigs (Elvehjem and Hart, 1932). Copper was shown to be unique in its hemopoietic effect, some twelve other inorganic elements, including purified salts of antimony, arsenic, cadmium, chromium, cobalt, germanium, lead, manganese, mercury, nickel, tin and zinc, being completely ineffective at different dosage levels. (Waddell, Steenbock, and Hart, 1929; Underhill, Orten, and Lewis, 1931). The foregoing *in vivo* hematopoietic effect of copper appeared to be that of a catalyst or cofactor since it could not be detected as a constituent of hemoglobin or heme (Elvehjem, Steenbock, and Hart, 1929).

Subsequent investigations have amply confirmed and extended the above classical in vivo studies, some in human subjects. Recent work using radioactive iron has shown that the effect of copper is due to its enhancement of the release of iron from the duodenal mucosa, the hepatic parenchymal cell, and the reticuloendothelial system (Lee, et al., 1968) and its transfer into the plasma where it would become available for hemoglobin synthesis in the bone marrow. Other recent studies (Osaki, Johnson, and Frieden, 1971) indicate that copper is active as a plasma copper enzyme, ferroxidase ("ceruloplasmin"), which mobilizes ferrous iron from the intestinal mucosa and other tissues and enhances its incorporation as Fe (III) into transferrin. Iron is thus made available for transport and for the formation of heme and hemoglobin in the bone marrow.

There is some evidence that copper may also be involved in hemopoiesis in another way. Preliminary studies of Iodice et al. (1958) suggested that copper may be a constituent of the enzyme, delta-aminolevulinic acid dehydratase (ALAD), which is involved in the biosynthesis of heme. However, these investigators subsequently reported that all of the copper from the ALAD preparations could be removed without loss of enzyme activity (Wilson et al., 1959). Other studies (Anderson and Tove, 1958), however, indicated that the rate of incorporation of glycine into heme was reduced in erythrocytes from copper-deficient chicks and that the rate increased upon the addition of copper in vitro. These investigators subsequently were unable to reproduce these results consistently (Anderson, 1959). More recent studies (Komai and Nielands, 1969) appear to support the original claim, at least in fungi, however, showing that copper is essential for the action of ALAD in U. sphaerogena. Preliminary studies in the author's laboratory also indicate some role of copper in the activity of ALAD (Chen, Weissman, and Orten, 1973). Lee and co-workers (1968), on the other hand, have been unable to demonstrate any defect in heme synthesis in copper-deficient swine. They conclude that copper is essential for the normal utilization of iron or possibly for the synthesis of globin. The former possibility is in accord with the data of Osaki et al. (1971) described previously.

The trace element, cobalt, likewise is well-known to be implicated in hemopoiesis. A small amount of this element administered daily to rats in the presence of sufficient amounts of iron and copper produces a striking polycythemia (Orten, et al., 1932). The polycythemic effect of cobalt may result from an increased formation of the hemopoietic hormone, erythropoietin (Goldwasser, et al., 1958; Smith, Ignarro, and Fisher, 1974). Erythropoietin, in turn, appears to stimulate the formation of increased amounts of the regulatory enzyme of heme biosynthesis, ALA-synthetase, and thus produce an increase in heme-hemoglobin levels and a polycythemia (Bottomly and Smithee, 1969).

There is some evidence that other trace elements may affect hemopoiesis. Several of these, as will be described, were included in the present study, partly also as controls. An anemia due primarily to a deficiency of zinc has been demonstrated in man (Prasad, 1967). A small amount of manganese appears to be necessary for hemopoiesis in rats (Orten, et al., 1932; Wachtel, et al., 1943). This effect of manganese has been shown to increase still further with the inclusion of arsenic in the diet (Skinner and McHargue, 1932). Molybdenum, as ammonium molybdate, has been alleged to increase reticulocytes and erythrocytes in rats with an experimental anemia induced by an exclusive milk diet plus bleeding (Biryukova, 1967). Still other trace elements, including uranium, thorium, beryllium, increase porphyrin excretion in the urine (Goldberg, 1962) although this effect may result from inhibition of certain steps in heme synthesis rather than from increased synthesis.

The foregoing in vivo studies thus are indicative of roles of copper, cobalt, and possibly other trace elements in heme-hemoglobin formation. The present investigation was designed to determine whether certain of these elements when added to in vitro porphyrin-heme synthesizing systems exert any direct effect on the biosynthesis of heme. Two such systems were employed, avian erythrocytes and a bovine liver "acetone powder" preparation. The former system is capable of forming porphyrins and heme from the primary precursors, glycine and succinate or acetate. The latter system's primary activity is from delta-aminolevulinic acid (ALA) to protoporphyrin (Sardesai, Melcer, and Orten, 1973). The experiments with the two systems were planned with these facts in mind since it made possible an evaluation of any direct in vitro effect of copper and other inorganic ions studied on the complete spectrum of porphyrin-heme biosynthesis. The alleged relation of copper to heme synthesis via an effect on the activity and/or composition of ALAD was also investigated.

METHODS

A. In Vitro Incubation Studies

Avian erythrocytes. Pooled blood from 10-12 freshly killed white Plymouth Rock chickens was collected in a flask containing 40 mg. heparin, 10 mg. streptomycin, and 10 mg. penicillin dissolved in a minimal amount of 0.9 percent sodium chloride. Erythrocytes were sedimented and washed as described previously (Sardesai, Doehr, and Orten, 1965). Twenty ml. of the packed, washed erythrocytes were suspended in an incubation medium (Krebs-Ringer phosphate, pH 7.4) containing glucose 333 μmoles, adenosine 100 μmoles, glycine 600 μmoles, sodium acetate trihydrate 770 μmoles, penicillin 5 mg. and dihydrostreptomycin 5 mg. The following additions of inorganic ions were made singly to incubation flasks. The amounts used were approximately the same as those used by other investigators in in vivo studies, based on their uniform distribution in total body water. The additions are ferrous iron, 1.0 mg., as $Fe(NH_4)_2(SO_4)_2 \cdot 6H_2O$ (low level) or 25 mg. (high level); EDTA, as the sodium salt, 2.3 mg. or 114 mg.; copper, 5.0 mg as $CuCl_2 \cdot 2H_2O$; cobalt, 5.0 mg as $CoCl_2$, zinc, 5.0 mg. as $ZnSO_4 \cdot H_2O$, molybdenum, 8.1 mg as $(NH_4)_6Mo_7)_{24} \cdot 4\ H_2O$.

The incubation mixtures were gently shaken at 37° for 20 hours. Control flasks without added precursors were similarly prepared.

The total porphyrins and heme formed were isolated at the end of the incubation period by exhaustive extraction with an ethyl acetate-glacial acetic acid mixture, 4:1 ratio. The porphyrins were extracted quantitatively with 3 N hydrochloric acid and separated chromatographically as their methyl esters as described previously (Sardesai, Doehr, and Orten; 1965). The amounts of uro- copro-, proto- and total porphyrins were determined spectrophotometrically.

The residual heme in the above ethyl acetate-acetic acid layer was prepared by evaporating to dryness and crystalized. The heme was then converted to protoporphryin and its methyl ester which was isolated by chromatographing on a silica gel column and the total heme content was estimated (Sardesai, Doehr, and Orten, 1965).

The quantitative effectiveness of the above method was checked by the recovery of pure porphyrin methyl esters and heme (hemin) from avian erythrocytes. Recoveries of 80 to 90 percent were obtained.

Bovine liver acetone powder. 250 mg. of bovine liver acetone powder (General Biochemicals, Chagrin Falls, Ohio) and 8 mg. of neutralized ALA hydrochloride, as the precursor, were used in each incubation flask. Other additions included 20 mg. glucose, 8 mg. adenosine, 3 mg. penicillin, 3 mg. streptomycin and the amounts of inorganic ions given in Tables I and II. The resultant mixture was incubated for 6 hours at 37°. The copro- and protoporphyrins were extracted and determined fluorometrically by procedures previously described (Sardesai, et al., 1965).

B. Determination of Hepatic ALAD Activity and Copper Content

ALAD preparation. Mouse (Swiss Webster) liver ALA dehydratase was purified by the procedure described by Doyle and Schimke (1969). All samples were passed through a Sephadex G-200 column. The material resulting from the G-200 step of purification was 85-95% pure ALA dehydratase by polyacrylamide disc electrophoresis at pH 8.9 and pH 7.6 (Cheng, Weissman, and Orten, 1973). The resulting enzyme preparations had a specific activity in the range of 5.5-6.5 units per mg of protein.

ALAD assay. ALA dehydratase activity was assayed by a modification of the method of Russell and Coleman (1963). The enzyme solution was preincubated with 40 μmoles of potassium phosphate buffer, pH 6.5, and 10 μmoles of GSH, adjusted to pH 6.5, in a final volume of 0.6 ml. After 30 minutes of incubation in 37^{0}C water bath, 15 μmoles of ALA, pH 7.0, in a volume of 0.15 ml was added. The tubes were then incubated for one more hour at 37°C. The formation of porphobilinogen was terminated by adding 1.5 ml of 10% TCA containing 0.1 M $HgCl_2$. After centrifugation, 0.5 ml of aliquot was then added 1.0 ml of 5% TCA solution plus 1.5 ml of modified Ehrlich's reagent. After 5 minutes the optical density of the solution was read at 553 nm. One unit of enzyme activity is defined as that amount of protein necessary to form one μmole of PBG per hour at 37^{0}C. Assays of aliquots of enzyme solutions were usually run in duplicate or triplicate and the values were averaged.

Protein determination. Protein concentrations were determined by a phenol reagent procedure (Lowry et al 1951). Bovine serum albumin was used as a standard.

Metal-ion analyses. 1. Atomic absorption spectrophotometry -- Metal-ion analyses were performed by atomic absorption spectrophotometry on a Perkin-Elmer 303 Atomic Absorption Spectrophotometer, equipped with a model SRL recorder. Prior to analyses, the enzyme preparations were dialyzed against 0.0005 M phosphate buffer, pH 6.5, for 24 hours. The dialysis fluid was used as a blank. The following wavelengths (nm) were used for determinations: zinc, 214; copper, 325; iron, 248; magnesium, 285; and manganese, 279.

2. Determination of copper -- Copper was determined by a procedure modified after that described by Poillon and Dawson (1963). BCS reagent were mixed with enzyme (0.7-1.2 mg) for 30 minutes. The solution was then titrated with 0.2 N NaOH and diluted to 5.0 ml total volume with phosphate

buffer, pH 7.0 The optical density of the solution was then measured at 480 nm in a Perkin-Elmer Spectrophotometer, and the result was corrected for the blank.

3. Electron paramagnetic resonance (EPR) -- These studies were performed with a Varian V-4502 EPR spectrometer to detect the presence of copper (as Cu^{++}) in purified enzyme preparations. The enzyme preparation under liquid nitrogen was divided into 16 small spheres (5 µl/sphere). The experiments were performed at 77°K. Ultramarine (diphenyl-picryl-hydrozyl mixture) was employed as a standard g-value (g = 2.003) to calculate the g-value of the enzyme.

Table I

Effect of Certain Inorganic Ions and of EDTA on Porphyrin-Heme Biosynthesis in Nucleated Erythrocytes

Substance Added @	Porphyrins* Uro	Copro	Proto	Total	Heme*
None	42 ± 5	44 ± 6	409 ± 43	495 ± 59	253 ± 29
Fe (low)	28 ± 4	66 ± 10	239 ± 29	333 ± 41	1698 ± 204
Fe (high)	114 ± 14	34 ± 6	153 ± 18	301 ± 39	566 ± 62
EDTA	37 ± 5	20 ± 4	369 ± 38	426 ± 49	195 ± 26
Cu	18 ± 3	31 ± 5	110 ± 16	159 ± 23	606 ± 73
Co	14 ± 3	20 ± 3	149 ± 19	183 ± 25	**
Zn	14 ± 4	37 ± 5	405 ± 45	456 ± 56	229 ± 28
Mo	**	38 + 4	390 + 43	428 + 48	**

* Amounts are expressed as mumoles of porphyrin or heme formed per incubate. Values given are averages for at least 8 experiments, with standard deviations.

** Value omitted was not determined.

@ Amounts are given in the text

RESULTS

A. Incubation Studies

The results obtained in the in vitro incubation experiments using avian erythrocytes are summarized in Table I. The amounts of uro-, copro-, and proto- prophyrins and of heme given are averages of 8 to 12 separate experiments which agreed within 5 to 10 percent. Standard deviations are shown in the table. It should be noted that the values obtained following the addition of either iron (both levels), EDTA, copper and cobalt do not overlap with those of the controls. Thus, the differences are highly significant (p 0.005). The values obtained following the addition of either zinc or molybdenum, on the other hand, overlap and their differences are not significant.

As might be expected, the addition of ferrous ammonium sulfate, to the medium resulted primarily in a marked increase in heme production with little consistent change in the amounts of uro-, and coproporphyrins (and their respective porphyrinogens), but a decrease in protoporphyrin. The latter is undoubtedly due to an enhanced coversion of protoporphyrin to heme in the presence of added iron. Since only small amounts of uro- and copro- porphyrins (and porphyrinogens) accumulate in avian erythrocytes during the incubation procedure, accurate determination is difficult and hence their amounts are variable and of questionable significance. With the higher level of iron (25.0 mg.) problems of tonicity of the erythrocytes were encountered resulting in marked alterations in their morphology. Nevertheless, the amount of heme formed per incubate was slightly more than double that of the controls.

The addition of EDTA at the lower level (2.3 mg.), an amount theoretically sufficient to chelate all of the iron present in the medium, produced the expected slight decrease in heme in the medium. Uro-, copro- and protoporphyrins (with their respective porphyrinogens) were all decreased somewhat. Similar results were obtained with the higher level of EDTA (data not included in Table I).

The data obtained following the addition of copper to the incubates (Table I) show an increase in heme with a decrease in uro-, copro- and protoporphyrins. These results indicate that the added copper enhances the conversion of protoporphyrin to heme.

The results obtained with cobalt show a lowering of the individual and total porphyrins below control values. Unsatisfactory determinations of heme were obtained in the experiments with cobalt; hence the values are omitted from the table. Added zinc and molybdenum had no consistent effect on either the porphyrin or heme (in the case of zinc) content of the incubated erythrocytes.

Bovine Liver Acetone Powder. The effect of adding several "trace elements" or porphyrin levels in the second *in vitro* system was also studied. Table II shows the average results obtained with standard deviations. It is evident from the data obtained that there is no significant difference between the copro- and protoporphyrin (and their corresponding porphyrinogens) levels in the samples incubated either with added arsenic, molybdenum, uranium or zinc and those of untreated controls. However, in the samples to which either copper or cobalt were added, significantly less copro- and protoporphyrin than in controls were found.

B. Relation of Copper to ALAD Activity and Composition

It has been postulated that ALAD does not require added organic or inorganic cofactors for its activity in mammalian systems (Granick and Mauzerall, 1958). However, the possible participation of tightly bound metal ions involved in the enzymatic catalysis reaction cannot be excluded. In order to test this hypothesis, the purified enzyme was incubated with a series of metal chelating agents and varying degrees of its inhibition were observed.

Effect of EDTA and Other Non-specific Chelating Agents on ALA-dehydratase Activity. It has been reported that all mammalian ALAD preparations are inhibited by EDTA with the

Table II

Effect of Certain Inorganic Ions on Poryphyrin Biosythesis in Bovine Liver Acetone Powder

Substance Added*	Porphyrins formed ***	
	Copro	Proto
None (Control)	27.09 $\pm$ 4.14	65.22 $\pm$ 9.06
Copper (as Chloride)	0.22 $\pm$ 0.16 p 0.0001	0.24 $\pm$ 0.18 p 0.0002
Cobalt (as Acetate)	4.18 $\pm$ 0.96 p 0.0005	38.28 $\pm$ 4.98 p 0.005
Zinc (as Sulfate)	28.98 $\pm$ 3.08	68.25 $\pm$ 0.96
Uranium (as Acetate)	29.08 $\pm$ 4.18	66.98 $\pm$ 9.22
Arsenic (as Sodium arsenite)	28.14 $\pm$ 3.18	69.25 $\pm$ 8.18
Molybdenum ** (as Ammonium molybdate)	26.18 $\pm$ 2.96	63.89 $\pm$ 8.22

* 10 mg. of the inorganic salt added per incubate.

** 16.2 mg. of ammonium molybdate added per incubate.

*** Amounts are expressed as ug. of porphyrin formed per incubate. Values are averages of 12 experiments with standard deviations.

exception of that from mice (Gurba, et al., 1972). As shown by the data in Table III, using highly purified enzyme preparations, EDTA was found to be a powerful enzyme inhibitor in concentrations as low as 0.08 mM. Similarly, 1,10-phenanthroline was strongly inhibitory, whereas 2,2-bipyridine, 8-hydroxyquinoline, and potassium cyanide were only weakly inhibitory. This was true whether the chelating agents were preincubated with the enzyme preparation at 37°C for 30 minutes or whether the chelating agent and substrate were added simultaneously. However, the data indicate that the substrate does protect the enzyme from inhibition by the chelating agents to some extent. The inhibitory effects of EDTA and the limited protective effect of substrate are evident for periods varying from 30 to 90 minutes of incubation.

Table III

Inhibition of Mouse Liver ALA Dehydratase By

Certain Chelating Reagents

Reagents	Concentration (mM)	Inhibition (%) Preincubation[a]	Directly added[b]
	0.34	100	70
EDTA	0.27	98	--
	0.08	80	--
	0.34	100	90
1,10-phenanthroline	0.08	85	--
	0.34	50	20
2,2-bipyridine	0.27	34	--
8-hydroxyquinoline	0.34	20	0
Potassium cyanide	0.34	10	0

a. Chelating agents incubated with enzyme preparation at 37°C for 30 minutes prior to the addition of substrate. Incubation was then continued for 60 minutes.

b. Chelating agent and substrate added simultaneously.

Effect of Specific Copper-binding Chelating Agents on ALA-dehydratase Activity. Since ALAD from *U. spehaerogena* appears to be inhibited by copper-binding chelating agents (Komai and Nielands, 1969), a study of the effect of certain copper-specific binding agents on highly purified preparations of ALAD from mouse liver was made. Bathocuproine disulfonate (BCS) and neocuproine, Cu^{+}-specific agents, and diethyldithiocarbamate, cuprizone, and disulfiram, Cu^{++}-specific agents, were selected for this purpose. Table IV shows that both BCS and neocuproine inhibit enzyme activity. Enzyme preincubation with BCS and neocuproine have stronger inhibition than that observed when the chelating agent and substrate are added simultaneously. The Cu^{++}-binding agents on the other hand, show no inhibition at all with or without preincubation. These data thus demonstrate that inhibitory power is confined to the Cu^{+}-specific agents.

Table IV

Inhibition of Mouse Liver ALA Dehydratase by Copper-Binding Reagents

Reagents	Concentration (mM)	Inhibition (%)* Preincubation[a]	Directly added[b]
	0.34	100	--
Bathocuproine-disulfonate	0.27	99	--
	0.08	85	72
	0.34	84	--
Neocuproine	0.27	80	--
	0.08	52	30
	0.34	0	--
Diethyldithio-carbamate	0.27	0	--
	0.08		0
	0.34	0	--
Cuprizone	0.27	0	--
	0.08	0	0
Disulfiram	0.08	0	0

* Average of 2-4 determinations

a. Chelating agent incubated with the enzyme preparation at 37°C for 30 minutes prior to the addition of substrate.

b. Chelating agent and substrate added simultaneously.

Reversal of Inhibition of ALA-dehydratase with BCS or 1,10-phenanthroline by Cu^{++}. The inhibition of enzyme by BCS can be reversed partially at least when Cu^{++} are added (Table V). With concentrations of BCS greater than 0.01 mM, and Cu^{++} ion addition, little or no restoration of enzyme activity is observed. Lower concentrations (0.001 and 0.0001 mM) of BCS-treated enzyme, however, show 80-91% activity, when low concentrations of Cu^{++} ions (0.001 - 1.0 mm) are added.

Further similar studies demonstrated that concentrations of 1,10-phenanthroline from 0.1 to 1 mM likewise prevent the reversal of enzyme activity by Cu^{++} ions (data not included). However, Cu^{++} ions can reverse the inhibition in the 0.01 and 0.001 mM 1,10-phenanthroline-treated enzyme at a lower concentration (1×10^{-7}M).

Table V

Reversal of Bathocuproine Inhibition by Copper Ion (% Activity)

BCS (mM) \ Cu^{2+} (mM)	0	0.001	0.1	1.0	10.0
1.0	0	0	0	0	0
0.1	4	4	5	2	2
0.01	22	35	29	25	12
0.001	64	88	--	80	44
0.0001	80	--	91	--	47

Metal-Ion Analyses. From metal chelating studies, it has been shown that the purified ALAD may require cuprous copper for its enzymatic activity. In order to determine the copper content of the enzyme, three different methods were employed as follows:

1. Determination of copper content by BCS reagent. It is evident from Table VI that during the process of ALAD purification, there is an increase in activity proportional to the increase in copper content. The most highly purified fraction (5.7 units specific activity per mg) contained 3.23 atoms copper per mole of enzyme.

Table VI

Copper Content by BCS Reagent of ALA Dehydratase At Various Stages of Purification

Purification Stage	Specific Activity (units/mg)	Cu (ug/mg of protein)	Cu/protein[a]
Heat	0.14	0.021	0.082
$(NH_4)_2SO_4$	0.45	0.16	0.629
DEAE Cellulose I	2.7	0.48	1.89
Sephadex G200	5.7	0.82	3.23

a - The copper-protein ratio has been calculated as the atoms of copper per mole of ALA-dehydratase.

2. <u>Determination of copper and other metal ions content by atomic absorption spectrophotometry</u>. Since it was found that the increase in specific activity during purification paralleled that of the copper content as determined by the BCS reagent, the values for copper and certain other metallic ions were determined by atomic absorption on four separate purified ALAD samples. The data are compiled in Table VII. The major metallic constituent, Cu, varies from 0.698 to 0.89 μg per mg of protein corresponding to 2.7 to 3.5 g-atoms per mole of protein, based on a molecular weight of 250,000, with average of 3.0975 ± 0.27. Of the other metal ion contents examined, only the copper content shows a correlation with enzyme activity. These data thus further indicate that Cu is involved in the activity of ALAD.

Table VII

Metal Content* of ALA Dehydratase at Various Stages of Purification

Purification Stage	Specific Activity (units/mg)	Cu[b]	Cu/protein[a]	Other metals[b] Zn	Fe	Other metals Mg	Mn	Ca
DEAE Cellulose I	2.0	0.50	2.0	0.65	-	-	0.07	0.21
DEAE Cellulose II	4.8	0.60	2.36	0.46	1.89	0.32	0	0.62
Sephadex G200	6.0	0.78	3.09	0.23	1.12	0.09	0	0.18
Sephadex G200	5.8	0.698	2.7	-	1.12	0.08	0	0.15
Sephadex G200	6.3	0.89	3.5	0.35	0.63	0.11	0	0.11
Sephadex G200	6.5	0.83	3.1	0.44	0.80	-	-	-

a-The copper-protein ratio has been calculated as atoms of copper per mole of ALA-dehydratase.

b-Metal content is given in microgm. per mg. protein.

*By atomic absorption spectrophotometry. Data are averages of values obtained on <u>four</u> separate purified ALAD preparations.

3. <u>EPR Studies</u>. Analysis of the valence of copper in the highly purified preparations show no Cu^{++} content in the enzyme by EPR studies. It therefore appears that the copper found to be present by the preceding two methods must be in the *cuprous* state.

DISCUSSION

A. Incubation Studies

From the data presented in Tables I and II it is clear that four of the trace elements studied, arsenic, molybdenum, uranium and zinc as their common water-soluble salts, have no direct effect demonstratable by the present *in vitro* incubation technique on porphyrin heme levels when added to bovine liver acetone powder or to avian erythrocytes. Their alleged effect when administered *in vivo*, as described earlier, must therefore involve factors or mechanisms having some *indirect* relation to heme-porphyrin biosynthesis. Further studies will be required to clarify this question.

The addition of either copper or cobalt salts in increaing amounts, on the other hand, to liver preparations are associated with progressive decreases in the total copro- and protoporphyrin contents. Data not included indicate that this effect is due to the *inhibitory* action of excessive amounts cupric and cobaltous ions on porphyrin formation in hepatic tissue. A similar conclusion was reached by Granick using duck erythrocytes (1958) and others. However, it is possible although unlikely, that these ions increase the formation of heme from protoporphyrin thus "drawing off" cellular porphyrin intermediates, resulting in their observed decrease in tissue concentration. Since heme synthesis is considerably less in the adult liver than in nucleated erythrocytes (Sardesar, Doehr, and Orten, 1965) such an explanation appears extremely questionable.

The situation appears to be somewhat different in avian nucleated erythrocytes, however, a type of tissue in which heme synthesis is extremely active, even in the adult. In this case, while both copper and cobalt decreased the amount of porphyrin in the incubated erythrocytes, copper at least increased the amount of heme present. Several explanations of these results appear possible. As indicated earlier (Osaki, et al., 1971), copper appears to enhance the utilization of tissue iron possibly by acting as a ferroxidase. This could have occurred in the present studies, resulting in the observed increase in heme formation. Pertinent also may be the fact that little copper is normally present in erythrocytes, especially after washing as in the present experiments, in contrast to liver which stores relatively significant amounts. Thus added copper might be expected to show different effects in the two systems.

One further point should be mentioned. With the exception of the experiments using iron with EDTA, the possible effects of the trace element ions initially present in avian erythrocytes or in the bovine liver preparations are not evaluated. However, in avian erythrocytes, at least, their possible effects should have been minimized by the washing procedure, unless of course, they are firmly bound to some cellular constituent. Further experiments involving the addition of specific non-toxic cation inhibitors to the *in vitro* system should be helpful in answering this question.

Thus the present studies employing *in vitro* systems further indicate the important roles of the trace elements copper and indirectly cobalt in the biosynthesis of the heme moiety of hemoglobin. The probable role of copper in the biosynthesis of heme as suggested by current experimental evidence is summarized diagrammatically in Figure 1.

Figure I. ROLE OF COPPER IN HEME AND HEMOGLOBIN BIOSYNTHESIS

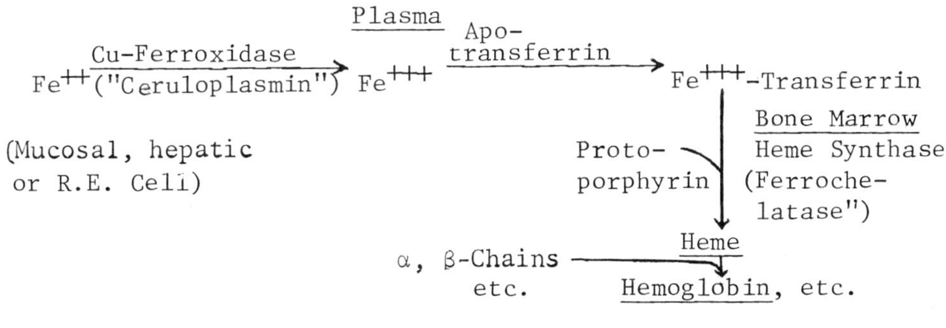

B. Relation of Copper to ALAD Activity and Composition

Evidence in the literature indicates that certain metal ions are involved in the activity of ALAD. Observations on enzyme preparations from mammalian liver and from mammalian and avian erythrocytes indicate that ALAD activities are inhibited by EDTA. Komai and Neilands (1969) have reported that Cu^{+} may be bound tightly to ALAD from U. sphaerogena. In addition, it has been reported that one zinc atom is present per one molecule of ALAD from bovine liver (Gurba, et al., 1972). Shemin (1970) suggested that all ALA-dehydratases contain a metal ion. In certain cases, as ALAD of R. spheroides, the metal ion either is bound tightly or is buried in the molecule and thus cannot chelate with EDTA.

The data obtained in the present studies strongly indicate that the enzymatic activity of highly purified ALAD from mouse liver is dependent upon the presence of cuprous copper. The inhibition with such non-specific chelating agents as EDTA and 1,10-phenanthroline and the specific cuprous copper binding agent, BCS and neocuprine, but not with cupric-copper binding agents (cuprizone, diethyldiothiocarbamate, and disulfiram) constitute definite support for this postulation. Likewise, the quantitative determination of copper by both the bathocuproine and atomic absorption spectrophotometric methods showing the copper content increasing with specific activity while other metal ions decrease (i.e. Zn^{++} or Fe^{++}) or diminished to zero (i.e., Ca^{++}, Mg^{++}, Mn^{++}) gives additional evidence for a role of copper in the activity of ALAD prepared from mouse liver. Further support is also provided by the experiments in which partial restoration of enzymatic activity was achieved by the addition of copper ions to enzyme preparations inactivated by bathocuproine.

The amount of copper in highly purified ALAD was found to be approximately 3 atoms of copper per one mole of enzyme and present in the cuprous state in vitro. This finding is consistent with that reported on U. sphaerogena by Komai and Neilands (1969). It also is in general agreement with the report that purified rat liver ALAD contains 0.1% copper (Wilson, et al., 1959). The finding of the reversal of ALAD inhibition by very low concentrations of BCS or 1,10-phenanthroline could be accomplished by addition of low, but not higher concentrations of Cu^{++} (or possibly Zn^{++} ions), also implies that a relationship exists between this ion and the activity of the functional groups of the enzyme.

It appears possible that copper may be involved in the maintaining the polymeric structure of ALAD which may be necessary for enzymatic activity. To confirm this postulate, further studies on the mechanism action of this metal ion in mouse liver ALAD remain to be performed.

SUMMARY

The possible effects of copper and several other "trace" elements (arsenic, cobalt, molybdenum, uranium, and zinc), alleged to have hemopoietic properties in *in vivo* studies, were investigated in two *in vitro* porphyrin-heme synthesizing sythems, avian (nucleated) erythrocytes and bovine liver "acetone powder".

No direct effect of arsenic, cobalt, molybdenum, uranium or zinc were observed in either system. Therefore, their alleged *in vivo* effects apparently involve factors or mechanisms having some indirect relation to porphyrin-heme formation as has been found true of cobalt.

In contrast, copper increased the formation of heme in avian erythrocytes at the expense of porphyrin intermediates. As to be expected, copper was ineffective in the hepatic acetone-powder system.

Studies in mouse liver preparations of highly purified delta-aminolevulinic acid dehydratase demonstrated that this enzyme is inhibited by specific copper-binding agents, partially reversible by copper ion addition. Copper is present in the enzyme preparations, the amount increasing with purification and activity.

The present results are thus compatible with the concepts that copper increases the biosynthesis of heme by increasing the utilization of iron and that copper may play a related role in increasing the activity of hepatic delta-aminolevulinic acid dehydratase and, in turn, the formation of heme.

REFERENCES

Anderson, R.L. (1959). Role of copper in the formation of heme. M.S. Thesis. North Carolina State College.

Anderson, R.L. and Tove, S.B. (1958). Effect of copper deficiency the synthesis of harm. Nature, 182: 315.

Biryukova, I.V. (1967). Molybdenum in experimental anemia. Tr. Voronezh. Gos. Med. Inst., 58: 104.

Bottomley, S. and Smithee, G.A. (1969). Effect of erythropoietin on bone marrow delta-aminolevulinic acid synthetase and heme synthetase. J. Lab. and Clin. Med., 74: 445.

Cheng, L.C., Weissman, E.B., and Orten, J.M. (1973). Some biochemical characteristics of delta-aminolevulinic acid dehydratrase. Proc. IX Int. Congress Biochem. Stockholm, Sweden, pg. 27.

Doyle, D. and Schimke, R.T. (1969). Genetic and developmental regulation of hepatic delta-aminolevulinic acid dehydratase in mice. J. Biol. Chem., 244: 5449.

Elvehjem, C.A. and Hart, E.B. (1932). The necessity of copper as a supplement to iron for hemoglobin formation in the pig. J. Biol. Chem., 95: 363.

Elvehjem, C.A., Steenbock, H., and Hart, E.B. (1929). Is copper a constituent of the hemoglobin molecule. Distribution of copper in blood. J. Biol. Chem., 83: 21.

Evans, J. L. and Abraham, P. A. (1973). Anemia, iron storage and ceruloplasmin in copper nutrition in the growing rat. J. Nutrition, 103: 196.

Goldwasser, E., Jacobson, L.O., Fried, W., and Plzak, L.F. (1958). Studies on erythropoiesis. V. The effect of cobalt on the production erythropoietin. Blood, 13: 55.

Granick, S. (1958). Porphyrin biosynthesis in erythrocytes. I. Formation of delta-aminolevulinic acid. J. Biol. Chem. 232: 1101.

Granick, S. and Mauzerall, D. (1958). Porphyrin biosynthesis in erythrocytes. II. Enzyme coverting delta-aminolevulinic acid to coproporphyrinogen. J. Biol. Chem., 232: 1119.

Gurba, P.E., Sennett, R.E., and Kobes, R.D. (1972). Studies on the mechanism of action of delta-aminolevulinate dehydratase from bovine and rat liver. Arch. Biochem. Biophys., 150: 130.

Hart, E.B., Steenbock, H., Waddell, J., and Elvehjem (1928). Iron in nutrition. VII. Copper as a supplement to iron for hemoglobin building in the rat. J. Biol. Chem., 77: 797.

Iodice, A.A., Richert, D.A., and Schulman, M.P. (1958). Copper content of purified delta-aminolevulinic acid dehydrase. Fed. Proc., 17: 248.

Komai, K. and Nielands, J.B. (1969). The metalloprotein nature of Ustilago sphaerogena delta-aminolevulinic acid dehydratase. Biochem. Biophys. Acta, 171: 311.

Lee, G.R., Cartwright, G.E., and Wintrobe, M.M. (1968). Heme biosynthesis in copper deficient swine. Proc. Soc. Exp. Biol. and Med., 127: 977.

Lee, G.R., Nacht, S., Lukens, J.N., and Cartwright, G.E. (1968). Iron metabolism in copper-deficient swine. J. Clin. Invest., 47: 2058.

Lowry, O.H., Rosenbrough, N.J., Farr, L., and Randall, R. (1951). Protein measurement with the Folin phenol reagent. J. Biol. Chem., 193: 265.

O'Dell, B.L. (1974). The biochemistry and physiology of copper. In Prasad, A.S., Ed.: Trace elements in human disease: An international symposium. Academic Press, New York, In press.

Orten, J.M., Underhill, F.A., Mugrage, E.R., and Lewis, R.C. (1932). Polycythemia in the rat on a milk-iron-copper diet supplemented by cobalt. J. Biol. Chem., 96: 11.

Osaki, S., Johnson, D.A., and Frieden, E. (1966). The possible significance of the ferrous oxidase activity of ceruloplasmin in normal human serum. J. Biol. Chem., 241: 2746.

Poillon, W.N. and Dawson, C.R. (1963). On the nature of copper in ascorbate oxidase. Biochem. Biophys. Acta., 77: 27.

Prasad, A.S. (1974). Zinc deficiency in man and its toxicity. In Prasad, A.S., Ed.: Trace Elements in human disease. Academic Press, Inc., New York, In press.

Russell, R.L., and Coleman, D.L. (1963). Genetic control of hepatic delta-aminolevulinic acid dehydratase in mice. Genetics, 48: 1033.

Sardesai, V.M., Doehr, S.A., and Orten, J.M. (1965). The subcellular sites of porphyrin biosynthesis in nucleated erythrocytes. Am. J. Physiol., 208: 1270.

Sardesai, V.M., Melcer, I., and Orten, J.M. (1973). The effect of certain inorganic ions on in vitro porphyrin - heme formation. Biochem. Med., 7: 405.

Shemin, D. (1970). On the synthesis of heme. Naturwissen-schaften, 57: 185.

Skinner, J.T. and McHargue, J.S. (1946). Supplementory effects of arsenic and manganese on copper in the synthesis of hemoglobin. Am. J. Physiol., 145: 500.

Smith, R., Ignarro, L.J., and Fisher, J.W. (1974). Lysosomal enzyme release: a possible mechanism of action of cobalt as an erythropoietic stimulant. Proc. Soc. Exp. Biol. Med., 146: 781.

Underhill, F.A., Orten, J.M., and Lewis, R.C. (1931). The inability of metals other than copper to supplement iron in curing the nutritional anemia of rats. J. Biol. Chem., 91: 13.

Wachtel, L.W., Elvehjem, C.A., and Hart, E.B. (1943). Studies on the physiology of manganese in the rat. Am. J. Physiol., 140: 72.

Waddell, J., Steenbock, H., and Hart, E.B. (1929). Iron in nutrition. X. The specificity of copper as a supplement to iron in the cure of nutritional anemia. J. Biol. Chem., 84: 115.

Wilson, M.L., Iodice, A.A., Schulman, M.P., and Richert, D.A. (1959). Studies on liver delta-aminolevulinic acid dehydratase. Fed. Proc., 18: 352.

Supported by National Institutes of Health Research Grant No. HE-10519, the McGregor Fund of Michigan, and the Michigan Heart Association

DISCUSSION

Dr. Hultquist: Do you know the molecular weight of dehydratase and how many subunits you might have in it?

Dr. Orten: Yes, from some work we have done, also Colemen, Doyle et. al. in the literature, the molecular weight of highly purified ALA-dehydratase is about 250,000 daltons. It is composed of six subunits, as far as we have gone, the molecular weight of each being a little over 40,000; each has one binding site for the substrate, ALA. Our own work would suggest, although I think it needs to be verified and extended, that there might be one copper for each two subunits, or possibly one zinc for three subunits, perhaps binding the six subunits--we don't know. This is current work in progress.

SIGNIFICANCE OF SELENIUM AS A COMPONENT OF GLUTATHIONE PEROXIDASE IN RED CELL METABOLISM

William G. Hoekstra

Departments of Biochemistry and Nutritional Sciences, College of Agricultural and Life Sciences, University of Wisconsin-Madison, Madison, Wisconsin 53706

The enzyme, glutathione peroxidase (GSH:H_2O_2 oxido-reductase, EC 1.11.1.9) was discovered by Mills (1957) in red blood cells. This enzyme functions in catalyzing the reaction between 2 GSH (reduced glutathione) and H_2O_2 to produce $2H_2O$ and GSSG (oxidized glutathione) or the reaction between 2 GSH and any of many organic hydroperoxides (ROOH) to produce H_2O + GSSG + the corresponding organic hydroxide (ROH). By catalyzing the reduction of H_2O_2 and of organic hydroperoxides such as lipid hydroperoxides, glutathione peroxidase aids in protecting the oxidant sensitive components of the cell such as the membranes from lipid peroxidation and proteins from oxidative denaturation (for review see Flohe, 1971; Ganther et al., 1975).

Studies on hemolytic anemias of humans, particularly the so-called drug-induced hemolytic anemias (Beutler, 1972), laid the framework for our research which culminated in the discovery that glutathione peroxidase is a selenium-containing enzyme. Such studies demonstrated that genetic defects in enzymes, such as glucose-6-phosphate dehydrogenase, which play a role in providing reduced glutathione (GSH) to the erythrocyte, either by promoting the reduction of oxidized glutathione (GSSG) or by biosynthesis of GSH, caused an increased sensitivity of the erythrocyte to hemolysis in response to "oxidant" drugs. The protective mechanism of GSH in the erythrocyte was shown to relate, at least in part, to its role as the hydrogen-donating substrate in the glutathione peroxidase catalyzed reduction of H_2O_2 and organic hydroperoxides. For this series of reactions to continue requires the continued provision of reducing equivalents to convert GSSG to GSH by the enzyme glutathione reductase. In the case of red blood cells, this means providing glucose whose metabolism by the hexose monophosphate shunt, generates the NADPH necessary for this conversion. Our early discovery (Rotruck et al., 1971, 1972) that the protective effect of vitamin E against erythrocyte hemolysis in vitro did not require the continued presence of glucose in the medium while the protective effect of dietary selenium against such hemolysis did require glucose, suggested a close involvement of selenium, but not of vitamin E, in the GSH-related protection of the cell. Further pursuit of this finding demonstrated that glutathione peroxidase is a selenoenzyme and that activity of this enzyme in tissue is greatly dependent on dietary selenium intake (Rotruck et al, 1973; Oh et al., 1974; Hoekstra, 1974).

The pioneering work on human red blood cell metabolism in relation to hemolytic anemias contributed heavily to this discovery of selenium function. The question may now be asked, "does selenium status of human subjects have a significant bearing on hematological disease of humans?" My primary purpose in this paper is to pose this question. In this regard I will briefly (1) review the nature and extent of erythrocyte defect caused by selenium deficiency in experimental animals which became apparent as we delineated step by step the significance of selenium to oxidant damage in erythrocytes, (2) summarize the now convincing evidence that glutathione peroxidase is in fact a selenoenzyme, (3) discuss the magnitude of the response of erythrocyte glutathione peroxidase to dietary selenium intake in comparison to the response of some other tissues and (4) suggest that selenium status of human subjects be evaluated in relation to certain specific hematological diseases.

ERYTHROCYTE DEFECTS CAUSED BY SELENIUM DEFICIENCY

The erythrocyte is not a primary target for pathological defects resulting from selenium deficiency in animals such as the rat; however, red cells served as a model system and alterations were observed when the red blood cells were studied *in vitro*. These defects are summarized in Table I. In order to observe the protective effect of dietary selenium against hemolysis, it was necessary to have glucose in the incubation medium and for the rats to be deficient as well in vitamin E, but the other effects, such as those on hemoglobin oxidation and glutathione were observed in the presence of adequate dietary vitamin E.

Table I. A Summary of the Metabolic Defects in Selenium-Deficient Rat Erythrocytes

Nature of Erythrocyte Defect	Reference
↑ Sensitivity to hemolysis *in vitro*, both with or without addition of an oxidant stressor such as ascorbate	Rotruck *et al.*, 1971; Rotruck *et al.*, 1972
↑ Formation of methemoglobin *in vitro* upon addition of an oxidant stressor such as ascorbate	Rotruck *et al.*, 1972
↑ Formation of choleglobin *in vitro* upon addition of ascorbate	Rotruck et al., 1972; Rotruck et al., 1973
↑ Formation of Heinz bodies *in vitro* upon addition of an oxidant stressor such as ascorbate	Rotruck et al., 1972
↑ GSH concentration *in vivo*, but little or no change of the rate of GSH disappearance upon incubation with ascorbate *in vitro*	Rotruck et al., 1972
↓ Rate of GSH disappearance in hemolyzates incubated with H_2O_2 (i.e., low glutathione peroxidase activity)	Hafeman et al., 1974

The relationship of selenium to vitamin E has been reviewed recently (Hoekstra, 1974, 1975). Each of the erythrocyte defects was ultimately explained by the much lower activity of glutathione peroxidase in the erythrocytes of selenium-deficient rats. Despite these alterations, hematological parameters *in vivo* in the selenium-deficient rat have remained normal and no evidence of a compensated hemolytic anemia has been found. However, studies to evaluate whether the selenium-deficient rat is more sensitive than the normal rat to a variety of hemolytic agents, particularly those which act as oxidants, remain to be conducted.

GLUTATHIONE PEROXIDASE AS A SELENOENZYME

The evidence that glutathione peroxidase is a selenoenzyme is convincing. Three independent research groups have reported the presence of selenium in homogeneous (Oh *et al.*, 1974; Nakamura *et al.*, 1974) or crystalline (Flohe *et al.*, 1973) preparations of the enzyme as summarized in Table II. The sources of glutathione peroxidase have included erythrocytes (ovine and bovine) and rat liver.

Table II. Characteristics of Some Purified Glutathione Peroxidases

Characteristic	Reference: Oh *et al.* (1974)	Flohe *et al.* (1973)	Nakamura *et al.* (1974)
Source	Ovine erythrocytes	Bovine erythrocytes	Rat liver
Molecular weight (daltons)	88,000	84,000	76,000
Subunit molecular weight	22,000	21,000	19,000
% Selenium	0.34	0.38	0.42
No. Se atoms/mole	3.8	4.0	4.1
Calculated no. Se atoms/subunit	1	1	1

Although some difference in molecular weight of glutathione peroxidase from the three sources is apparent, particularly for rat liver, the enzyme from each of the sources contains four selenium atoms per mole, an average of one selenium atom per enzyme subunit. The fact that purified glutathione peroxidase invariably contains four selenium atoms per mole implies that the selenium is bound rather tightly, but in a still unknown manner. Upon long-term storage of solutions of the purified enzyme at pH values near neutrality, a substantial part of the enzyme precipitates as a selenium-free, inactive protein releasing the selenium in a form which does not react as inorganic selenite or selenate. This still uncharacterized selenium moiety appears to be a low-molecular-weight organic form of selenium, apparently distinct from the known selenium-containing amino acids. Thus, the selenium moiety appears to be bound to the enzyme by non-covalent bonding. Characterization of the nature of the selenium moiety and its biosynthesis from the large variety of biologically active selenium compounds, both inorganic and organic, as well as assessment of the role of the selenium moiety in the biosynthesis of the holoenzyme are prime goals of current research, as is the detailed chemical role of selenium in the enzyme's catalytic role.

RESPONSE OF ERYTHROCYTE GLUTATHIONE PEROXIDASE TO DIETARY SELENIUM INTAKE

It is well documented that dietary selenium intake profoundly affects tissue activities of glutathione peroxidase (Hoekstra, 1974; Hafeman et al., 1974; Lawrence et al., 1974; Noguchi et al., 1973; Chow and Tappel, 1974; Omaye and Tappel, 1974; Reddy and Tappel, 1974; Smith et al., 1974). This subject recently received extensive review (Ganther et al., 1975) and in this paper only brief reference will be made to the magnitude of effect on the erythrocyte as illustrated in Table III. Diets based on Torula yeast as the protein source and containing about 0.01 μg selenium per g which depress the glutathione peroxidase activity in rat liver to an undetectable level, have depressed erythrocyte glutathione peroxidase activity only to about 20-25% of the activity for selenium-adequate controls (usually about 0.1 μg selenium per g diet). This is the case even when the deficiency is very long-term in

Table III. Examples of the Effect of Selenium Deficiency in Weanling Rats on the Decrease in Glutathione Peroxidase Activity of Erythrocytes in Comparison to Liver

Duration of Se-deficiency	Glutathione peroxidase activity as % of Se-adequate control		Reference
	Erythrocytes	Liver	
17 days	59	5	Hafeman *et al.*, 1974
66 days	24	0	
> 6 months	27	0	Lawrence et al., 1974
42 days	22	14	Reddy and Tappel, 1974

relation to red cell life span. In other words, some tissues or cells appear to be protected in some way from glutathione peroxidase depletion more than other tissues or cells. In long-term selenium deficiency, the body components in which glutathione peroxidase is most extensively depleted (as a % of control) due to selenium deficiency include blood plasma, liver, heart, lungs, stomach mucosa, skeletal muscle and eye lens; those showing moderate decreases include kidney, adrenal glands and erythrocytes; and those least subject to depletion are testes and brain (Ganther *et al.*, 1975). Rate of depletion of glutathione peroxidase in different tissues also differs greatly. For example, lens glutathione peroxidase is little affected by short-term selenium deficiency such as 8 weeks, but in long-term deficiency (> 6 months) activity is less than 15% of that of controls (Lawrence *et al.*, 1974). Erythrocytes are depleted in relation to their life span and repletion upon supplementing selenium-deficient animals with selenite is related to the rate at which new cells enter the circulatory system following erythropoiesis in the bone marrow to replace the old, selenium-deficient and glutathione peroxidase-deficient cells (Hafeman et al., 1974). It is interesting that erythrocyte glutathione peroxidase activity does not plateau with increasing dietary intake of selenium as one satisfies the requirement, but continues to increase even to chronically toxic levels of selenium. The increase is in approximate relation to the logarithm of the dietary selenium concentration. This rather surprising observation suggests that excess selenium induces "supernormal" amounts of glutathione peroxidase in the erythrocyte, perhaps because of a "pro-oxidant" effect of excess selenium (Hafeman _et al._, 1974). This aspect has been discussed more fully elsewhere (Hoekstra, 1975; Ganther _et al._, 1975).

POSSIBLE SIGNIFICANCE OF SELENIUM STATUS OF HUMAN SUBJECTS TO HEMATOLOGICAL DISEASE

The discovery that glutathione peroxidase is a seleno-enzyme immediately suggests that the dietary selenium status of humans may determine, in part, the glutathione peroxidase activities of the tissues including the erythrocytes. The obvious question, then, is whether or not nutritional selenium status is likely to differ substantially for different subjects. Allaway _et al._ (1968) studied selenium levels of 210 samples of blood from blood banks in several cities across the United States and found a range of 0.10 to 0.34 μg Se per ml whole blood with a substantial relationship of geochemical selenium status of the area to the mean selenium content of blood from that area. Red blood cells contain nearly twice as much selenium per ml as does plasma so that the red cell selenium must also have differed to about the same extent. If our data on experimental animals such as the sheep (Oh, S. H., Pope, A. L., and Hoekstra, W. G., unpublished) can be extrapolated to humans, the glutathione peroxidase activity of erythrocytes should reflect a similar range of activity as does the total selenium content. This suggests from the study of a very limited number of individuals that the range in glutathione peroxidase activity of human red blood cells as determined by selenium status should be at least 3-fold and possibly much greater.

Selenium deficiency has not been demonstrated in humans, but little attempt has been made to date to exclude the possibility of its occurrence. Such deficiency would not be expected in the geochemically high-selenium areas, but in the low-selenium areas it is a possibility because such areas are very extensive (Kubota _et al_., 1967). It is not possible to estimate selenium intakes from the food items selected because of the great dependence of selenium content to area of origin of that food. Certain food items such as fish, especially ocean fish, are invariably high in selenium, as are foods such as U.S. wheat which is mostly grown in the high-selenium area. Therefore, in the low-selenium areas, many of the human subjects will undoubtedly not be selenium-deficient because of their consumption of such food items. But, do all subjects in these areas consume sufficient of these high-selenium foods? Clearly investigations of selenium status in relation to glutathione peroxidase status of human subjects should be initiated.

Are the cases of low erythrocyte glutathione peroxidase in human subjects (Necheles _et al_., 1970; see Ganther _et al_., 1975 for additional references and discussion) related to genetic causes as is presently assumed, or is nutritional selenium status sometimes the important variable? A parallel to this suggestion is the realization that low glutathione reductase activity of red blood cells, once considered to be of genetic origin, is in fact largely explained by low intakes of riboflavin (Beutler, 1972). Use of selenium-deficient but vitamin E-adequate animals as a model for human deficiency of glutathione peroxidase, whether or not it is shown to depend on nutritional intake of selenium, should be considered. Of course, there may be other still uncharacterized, functioning forms of selenium in animals which might complicate such a model, but other significant forms with respect to red cell metabolism seem less likely, since glutathione peroxidase is estimated to account for 75% of red blood cell selenium of sheep fed natural diets (Oh _et al_., 1974). A further possibility for truly genetically related deficiencies of glutathione peroxidase is that some step in selenium metabolism to form the active moiety of glutathione peroxidase is defective rather than a mutation directly related to the enzyme.

Another condition in humans which should be scrutinized with respect to selenium status is the vitamin E responsive anemia of premature infants (Hassan et al., 1966; Oski and Barnes, 1967; Ritchie et al., 1968; Melhorn and Gross, 1971). Where this condition has been reported it commonly affects premature infants, but apparently in other hospitals, such as the University of Wisconsin Hospital, such anemia is seldom if ever observed. Is this anemia prevalent only in low-selenium areas? Erythrocyte glutathione peroxidase activity has usually, but not invariably, been reported to be lower in newborn infants than in adults (see Ganther et al., 1975 for references and discussion) but overall selenium status has not been investigated. Conditions of low glutathione peroxidase in blood constituents other than erythrocytes, such as platelets (Karpatkin and Weiss, 1972) and leukocytes (Holmes et al., 1970) should also be investigated with respect to selenium metabolism.

SUMMARY

The defects in erythrocytes of selenium-deficient animals represent an increased sensitivity to oxidative damage of membranes and oxidant sensitive proteins such as hemoglobin. Such defects result from glutathione peroxidase deficiency and active glutathione peroxidase has been shown to contain four g atoms of selenium per mole or one selenium per enzyme subunit. Prolonged selenium deficiency decreased erythrocyte glutathione peroxidase to 20-25% of the level for selenium-adequate controls, which is a smaller decrease than for some body components as liver, plasma, heart and lens but a larger decrease than for brain and testes. Furthermore, an excessive selenium intake causes a "supernormal" level of erythrocyte glutathione peroxidase. The suggestion is made that certain hematological diseases of humans such as erythrocyte, platelet and leukocyte glutathione peroxidase deficiencies and the vitamin E responsive anemia of premature infants be investigated with respect to selenium metabolism and dietary selenium intake. A more comprehensive review of selenium and glutathione peroxidase in health and disease is in press (Ganther et al., 1975).

ACKNOWLEDGEMENTS

This research was supported by the College of Agricultural and Life Sciences, University of Wisconsin-Madison, and by United States Public Health Service Program Grant No. AM 14881.

REFERENCES

Allaway, W. H., Kubota, J., Losee, F., and Roth, M. (1968). Selenium, molybdenum, and vanadium in human blood. Arch. Environ. Health 16:342.

Beutler, E. (1972). Drug-induced anemia. Fed. Proc. 31:141.

Chow, C. K., and Tappel, A. L. (1974). Response of glutathione peroxidase to dietary selenium in rats. J. Nutr. 104:444.

Flohe, L. (1971). Die glutathionperoxidase: Enzymologie und biologische aspekte. Klin. Wochenschrift 49:669.

Flohe, L., Gunzler, W. A., and Schock, H. H. (1973). Glutathione peroxidase: A selenoenzyme. FEBS Letters 32:132.

Ganther, H. E., Hafeman, D. G., Lawrence, R. A., Serfass, R. E., and Hoekstra, W. G. (1975). Selenium and glutathione peroxidase in health and disease: A review. In Proceedings of a Symposium on Trace Elements and Human Disease, Wayne State Univ., July 10-12, 1974. To be published as a monograph by The Nutrition Foundation, Inc., New York, Ed. by Prasad, A. S., and Chichester, C. O.

Hafeman, D. G., Sunde, R. A., and Hoekstra, W. G. (1974). Effect of dietary selenium on erythrocyte and liver glutathione peroxidase in the rat. J. Nutr. 104:580.

Hassan, H., Hashim, S. A., Van Itallie, T., and Sebrell, W. H. (1966). Syndrome in premature infants associated with low plasma vitamin E levels and high polyunsaturated fatty acid diet. Am. J. Clin. Nutr. 19:147.

Hoekstra, W. G. (1974). Biochemical role of selenium. In Trace Element Metabolism in Animals-2. Ed. by Hoekstra, W. G., Suttie, J. W., Ganther, H. E., and Mertz, W. University Park Press, Baltimore, p. 61.

Hoekstra, W. G. (1975). Biochemical function of selenium and its relation to vitamin E. Fed. Proc. (in press).
Holmes, B., Park, B. H., Malawista, S. E., Quie, P. G., Nelson, D. L., and Good, R. A. (1970). Chronic granulomatous disease in females. New England J. Med. 283:217.
Karpatkin, S., and Weiss, H. J. (1972). Deficiency of glutathione peroxidase associated with high levels of reduced glutathione in Glanzmann's thrombasthenia. New England J. Med. 287:1062.
Kubota, J., Allaway, W. H., Carter, D. L., Cary, E. E., and Lazar, V. A. (1967). Selenium in crops in the United States in relation to the selenium-responsive diseases of livestock. J. Agr. Food Chem. 15, 448.
Lawrence, R. A., Sunde, R. A., Schwartz, G. L., and Hoekstra, W. G. (1974). Glutathione peroxidase activity in rat lens and other tissues in relation to dietary selenium intake. Expt. Eye Res. 18:563.
Melhorn, D. K., and Gross, R. T. (1971). Vitamin E dependent anemia in premature infants. 1. Effect of large doses of medicinal iron. J. Pediat. 79:581.
Mills, G. C. (1957). Hemoglobin catabolism, Part I. Glutathione peroxidase; an erythrocyte enzyme which protects hemoglobin from oxidative breakdown. J. Biol. Chem. 229:189.
Nakamura, W. Hosoda, S., and Hayashi, K. (1974). Purification and properties of rat liver glutathione peroxidase. Biochim. Biophys. Acta 358:251.
Necheles, T. F., Stimberg, M. H., and Cameron, D. (1970). Erythrocyte glutathione peroxidase deficiency. Brit. J. Haematol. 19:605.
Noguchi, T., Cantor, A. H., and Scott, M. L. (1973). Mode of action of selenium and vitamin E in prevention of exudative diathesis in chicks. J. Nutr. 103:1502.
Oh, S. H., Ganther, H. E., and Hoekstra, W. G. (1974). Selenium as a component of glutathione peroxidase isolated from ovine erythrocytes. Biochemistry 13:1825.
Omaye, S. T., and Tappel, A. L. (1974). Effect of dietary selenium on glutathione peroxidase in the chick. J. Nutr. 104:747.

Oski, F. A., and Barnes, L. A. (1967). Vitamin E deficiency: A previously unrecognized cause of hemolytic anemia in the premature infant. J. Pediat. 70:211.

Reddy, K., and Tappel, A. L. (1974). Effect of dietary selenium and autoxidized lipids on the glutathione peroxidase system of gastrointestinal tract and other tissues in the rat. J. Nutr. 104:1069.

Ritchie, J. H., Mathews, B. F., McMasters, V., and Grossman, M. (1968). Edema and hemolytic anemia in premature infants: A vitamin E deficiency syndrome. New England J. Med. 270:1185.

Rotruck, J. T., Hoekstra, W. G., and Pope, A. L. (1971). Glucose-dependent protection by dietary selenium against haemolysis of rat erythrocytes *in vitro*. Nature New Biol. 231:223.

Rotruck, J. T., Pope, A. L., Ganther, H. E., and Hoekstra, W. G. (1972). Prevention of oxidative damage to rat erythrocytes by dietary selenium. J. Nutr. 102:689.

Rotruck, J. T., Pope, A. L., Ganther, H. E., Swanson, A. B., Hafeman, D. G., and Hoekstra, W. G. (1973). Selenium: Biochemical role as a component of glutathione peroxidase. Science 179:588.

Smith, P. J., Tappel, A. L., and Chow, K. (1974). Glutathione peroxidase activity as a function of dietary selenomethionine. Nature 247:392.

DISCUSSION

Dr. Jacob: Your results are very intriguing and lead to speculation regarding the paradox of acatalasia in humans in which two syndromes are observed. I was privileged to study one acatalasic family in Switzerland who were totally acatalasic--had no catalase in their red cells and other tissues--and had absolutely no difficulties. Yet, as you know, in Japan the original acatalasic patients all had severe, gangrenous mouth ulcerations. It intrigued us as to what sensitized the Japanese to tissue destruction. If selenium deficiency coexisted, an explanation would be forthcoming. Do you know the selenium content of the typical Japanese diet; is it likely to be deficient? You've mentioned that fish is high in selenium, but what if one ate nothing but rice, and so on?

Dr. Hoekstra: I've seen no data on the selenium or glutathione peroxidase status of subjects in Japan. My guess would be that they are not deficient, in fact, they may be taking in amounts of selenium which I postulated may be in the "peroxidant" range. There is an interesting model, the acatalasic mouse. It would be interesting to determine whether selenium deficiency in such mice would cause expecially serious consequences. Glutathione peroxidase has the additional role that catalase does not have, of catalysing the decomposition of organic hydroperoxides such as lipid hydroperoxides. This is an important difference.

Dr. Jacob: May I ask another question? You mentioned that the lens glutathione peroxidase declines by 85% or more in selenium deficient animals. This is of great interest, since cataract formation is frequently due to oxidative denaturation of lens crystallin. Is there any evidence of cataract formation in selenium deficient animals?

Dr. Hoekstra: There are certainly very interesting corollaries between the red cell and the lens in terms of aging phenomena. The spleen is able to sift out the aged red cells, but nothing can sift out the oxidative damage in the lens, so it is more or less permanent marker of such effects. It has been reported from Oregon State that prolonged selenium deficiency in rats produces congenital cataracts. We have observed about a 20 percent incidence of cataracts in the second litter from females raised from weaning on a low-selenium diet.

Dr. Glader: I'm confused. There's a problem we have that you may be able to help us with. We are interested in neonatal red cells, which have probably about 40% of the adult levels of glutathione peroxidase activity, and certainly neonatal red cells are more susceptible to oxidant damage. It's logical to try and equate the two phenomena. We have, in the past, incubated neonatal red cells that have lower activity, with low dose hydrogen peroxide in the Cohen-Hochstein type of system. Under these conditions we see that the rate of glutathione degradation is identical in the two cell types, and the rate of hexose monophosphate shunt stimulation is also identical. We also know, as does anyone who works with glutathione peroxidase, that in vitro there is a significant amount of non-enzymatic oxidation of glutathione with peroxide. I'm raising the old question--how important physiologically is this? I don't doubt your data. You are showing that the enzyme activity does increase, but does it matter physiologically? You demonstrate also that the rate of glutathione degradation in your selenium deficient and sufficient animals were more or less identical--perhaps I'm wrong about that. Did you look at hexose monophosphate shunt stimulation and was there really a difference? And, lastly, could selenium actually be doing something else--could it actually be protecting hemoglobin some other way?

Dr. Hoekstra: It does appear that there may be an excess of the glutathione peroxidase system in the red blood cell, and even when challenged in the ways mentioned, a critical situation does not seem to arise. I think it is critical in certain tissues. For example, if their diet is deficient in vitamin E and selenium, rats will die of liver necrosis at about 5 weeks when glutathione peroxidase has essentially disappeared from the liver. If vitamin E is adequate, the rats will live, but growth is slower, the males can't reproduce and the offspring of the females show marked defects.

I think that the nonenzymic reaction between GSH and H_2O_2 may be important. When the glutathione peroxidase level in liver is essentially zero, one can prevent or at least greatly delay the liver degeneration by providing a higher intake of sulphur-containing amino acids which are precursors of glutathione. It appears that if you have a high enough level of glutathione, it can protect even though the enzyme is at a very low level. That's about all I can comment at this time.

Dr. Brain: I don't want to get into technicalitics, but are there reltively simple methods for measuring selenium in the range of concentrations?

Dr. Hoekstra: Yes, there are. We use a fluorometric procedure (see Biochem. 13: 1825 (1974)). It is also commonly measured by neutron activation analysis.

BIOLOGICAL OXIDATION AND BLOOD CELLS

Chairman: Gerald Cohen

UNUSUAL DEFENSE MECHANISMS AGAINST H_2O_2 CYTOTOXICITY IN ERYTHOCYTES DEFICIENT IN GLUCOSE-6-PHOSPHATE DEHYDROGENASE OR TOCOPHEROL

Gerald Cohen
Department of Neurology
Mount Sinai School of Medicine
New York, N.Y. 10029

This paper deals with two types of red blood cells (RBC's) which undergo oxidative damage during exposure to relatively small amounts of hydrogen peroxide (H_2O_2). Human erythrocytes deficient in glucose-6-phosphate dehydrogenase (G-6-PD) respond *in vitro* to sustained low levels of H_2O_2 with the following changes: 1) disappearance of reduced glutathione (GSH) (Cohen and Hochstein, 1961), 2) accumulation of methemoglobin and 3) depression of the glycolytic pathway (see ahead). Additionally, G-6-PD deficient RBC's undergo oxidative damage and hemolysis *in vivo* when exposed to a number of drugs (Beutler, 1966; Hochstein, 1971). The intracellular generation of H_2O_2 by some of these drugs has been observed both *in vitro* and *in vivo* (Cohen and Hochstein, 1964, 1965). G-6-PD deficient RBC's contain normal catalase levels. The sensitivity to H_2O_2 derives primarily from the disappearance of GSH: As the GSH concentration falls, so does the activity of GSH peroxidase, the enzyme which is primarily responsible for scavenging low levels of H_2O_2 within RBC's (Cohen and Hochstein, 1963; Nicholls, 1972).

The second cell type is the tocopherol (vitamin E)-deficient RBC. Tocopherol is a free radical scavenger and a major biologic lipid antioxidant (Tappel, 1962). The sensitivity of this cell type to H_2O_2 is manifest as hemolysis accompanied by extensive peroxidation of lipids.

Vitamin E-deficient RBC's possess essentially normal levels of GSH, GSH peroxidase and catalase. These cells are sensitive to hemolysis *in vivo* upon exposure to a number of agents, including dialuric acid and alloxan. Generation of H_2O_2 has been reported for dialuric acid *in vitro* (Deamer et al., 1971) and for alloxan *in vivo* (Heikkila, Barden, Cohen, 1974).

Although the research efforts in the study of G-6-PD deficiency and vitamin E-deficiency have undergone different historical developments, there is an area of confluence in the intrinsic sensitivity to H_2O_2. Additionally, there is at least one agent, menadione, to which both G-6-PD deficient RBC's and E-deficient RBC's respond *in vivo* with hemolysis. It has been shown that menadione generates H_2O_2 within RBC's *in vivo* (Cohen and Hochstein, 1965).

STUDIES WITH G-6-PD DEFICIENT ERYTHROCYTES

Washed RBC's from G-6-PD deficient subjects and from normal subjects were suspended in isotonic saline buffered with phosphate at pH 7.4. The RBC's were exposed to H_2O_2 vapor in a closed two-compartment system (Warburg flask or equivalent; see Cohen and Hochstein, 1961; 1963). The RBC suspension was in the outer chamber and a small amount of concentrated H_2O_2 was placed in the center well. During shaking at 37°C, the H_2O_2 vaporized and was transferred by gaseous diffusion to the cells in the main compartment. The rate of addition of H_2O_2 to the cell suspension in these studies was 4.0 - 4.5 μmoles per hour.

It was previously shown (Cohen and Hochstein, 1961) that in the H_2O_2 diffusion system, G-6-PD deficient RBC's sustain a major loss in cellular GSH. The loss can be attributed to a failure to regenerate GSH from its oxidized form (GSSG). The reason is that in RBC's, the hexose monophosphate shunt pathway (which includes G-6-PD) is the sole source for NADPH, the obligatory cofactor for the action of GSSG reductase.

In the current experiments, G-6-PD deficient and normal erythrocytes were exposed to H_2O_2 vapor in the presence of glucose (2 mg per ml) and penicillin G (Squibb, 250 units per ml), which was added as a bacteriostatic agent. The enzyme deficient cells possessed less than 10% of the normal range of G-6-PD activity. At the end of 10 hours, methemoglobin was measured with a standard method (Evelyn and Malloy, 1938). Results are shown in Table 1.

There was significant accumulation of methemoglobin in G-6-PD deficient RBC's from nine separate subjects while negligible methemoglobin levels were observed in RBC's from 19 normal subjects ($p < 0.001$). A likely interpretation of these data is as follows: In G-6-PD deficient RBC's, there is a decline in GSH and, hence, in GSH peroxidase activity. Since catalase cannot adequately remove low levels of H_2O_2 (Keilin and Hartree, 1945; Cohen and Hochstein, 1963) other cellular constituents such as hemoglobin become targets for oxidation. In model studies with both normal RBC's and catalase-deficient RBC's exposed to H_2O_2 in the absence of glucose (to limit hexose monophosphate shunt activity), methemoglobin was observed only after the protective GSH had disappeared (Cohen and Hochstein, 1963; cf. also Aebi and Suter, 1974).

In other experiments, the effect of H_2O_2 on glycolytic capacity was studied. Six ml aliquots of cell suspension (12.5% hematocrit) were exposed to H_2O_2 vapor; control samples for each blood specimen were incubated without H_2O_2. After 16 hours, duplicate samples were pooled, the cells were isolated by centrifugation and they were washed with 0.9% saline. The pH of the cells was adjusted to pH 8.1 (the optimum for glycolysis) by the method of Chapman et al. (1962). The cells were then mixed with one volume of 0.9% saline and two volumes of 0.03 M phosphate buffer (pH 8.1) and incubated for three hours at 37°C to study the rate of disappearance of glucose (rate of glycolysis). Samples were removed at zero time and at the end of the 3 hour incubation period; glucose was measured with a standard glucose oxidase method. In some experiments, ethanol 2 mg/ml was incorporated into the medium during the exposure

TABLE 1. METHEMOGLOBIN FORMATION IN G-6-PD DEFICIENT HUMAN ERYTHROCYTES EXPOSED TO HYDROGEN PEROXIDE VAPOR.

H_2O_2 was added at the rate of 4.5 μmoles per hour to 4 ml of a 1:10 suspension of erythrocytes. Glucose, 2 mg/ml; exposure time 10 hours. The number of blood samples (N) is shown in parentheses.

Sample	MetHb. as % total Hb Mean ± S.D.
Normal cells (N=19)	2.5 ± 1.2
G-6-PD deficient cells (N=9)	25.3 ± 5.9

TABLE 2. PROTECTION BY ETHANOL OF GLYCOLYTIC CAPACITY IN G-6-PD DEFICIENT ERYTHROCYTES EXPOSED TO HYDROGEN PEROXIDE VAPOR.

Exposure time, 16 hours; glucose, 2 mg/ml.

Sample	% Change in Glycolysis Compared to Control (Mean ± S.E.M.)
Normal cells (N=5)	(-) 2.92 ± 3.93
G-6-PD deficient cells (N=8)	(-) 51.88 ± 6.49
G-6-PD deficient cells + ethanol (2mg/ml) (N=8)	(-) 4.88 ± 9.72

to H_2O_2 vapor. Results are shown in Table 2.

It would appear that suppression of glycolysis is illustrative of a more general cytotoxic action resulting from elevated H_2O_2 levels within the RBC's. Some enzymes in the glycolytic chain, such as glyceraldehyde-3-phosphate dehydrogenase, are SH-dependent. These enzymes are sensitive to inactivation by H_2O_2 or by H_2O_2-generating agents. That catalase had not been completely destroyed during exposure to the H_2O_2 vapor was evident from a simple test: Direct addition of concentrated H_2O_2 to the cells produced intense foaming (O_2 generation) without intense darkening (oxidation of hemoglobin). This indicated the presence of high concentrations of intracellular catalase. It should be noted that catalase-deficient cells do not show foaming and the hemoglobin is completely oxidized under the same conditions.

There are at least two possible mechanisms for protection by ethanol. Ethanol is a substrate for the peroxidatic activity of catalase (ethanol + H_2O_2 yields acetaldehyde + $2H_2O$); therefore, ethanol may remove the low levels of H_2O_2 which escape destruction by the catalatic route ($2H_2O_2$ yields oxygen + $2H_2O$). A second possibility is that H_2O_2 is decomposed, in part, to hydroxyl radicals within RBC's (see ahead). Since ethanol is an excellent hydroxyl radical trap, it may serve to detoxify this highly reactive species.

STUDIES WITH VITAMIN E-DEFICIENT ERYTHROCYTES

Vitamin E-deficient RBC's were obtained from rats raised on a tocopherol-deficient diet and from human subjects with abetalipoproteinemia. In the latter disorder, there is a defect in the absorption of fats and,hence, of fat soluble vitamins from the gut. In experiments with RBC's from rats, the cells were first tested by exposure to dialuric acid (Rose and Gyorgy, 1952; Tsen and Collier, 1960). These cells underwent lysis accompanied by formation of lipid peroxides; this indicated that the cells were, in fact, tocopherol-deficient.

Rose and Gyorgy (1952), the originators of the dialuric

acid hemolysis test, considered the possibility that H_2O_2 derived from the autoxidation of dialurate (10^{-3}M) was an important hemolytic component. They tested H_2O_2 *in vitro* and found that it was hemolytic. But, very high concentrations (0.4M) were required and, under the conditions of their test, even RBC's from normal animals exhibited considerable lysis. They concluded that H_2O_2 *per se* could not be the hemolytic agent. However, H_2O_2 added directly is almost instantly decomposed by the high concentrations of catalase found in RBC's. Hence, the direct addition of H_2O_2 cannot be considered comparable to the continuous stress of H_2O_2 generated in smaller amount during the incubation period with dialurate.

When E-deficient rat RBC's were exposed to H_2O_2 vapor for three hours, there was almost total lysis and marked accumulation of lipid peroxides (Table 3). Lipid peroxides were measured with the 2-thiobarbituric acid (2-TBA) test (Cf. Bunyan et al., 1960).

The rate of addition of H_2O_2 to the 10% suspension of RBC's in buffered saline (which contained glucose 2 mg/ml) was equivalent to 16 μmoles H_2O_2 per hour per ml of packed RBC's. This was one thousandth of the amount added in the direct addition test of Rose and Gyorgy. The amount of H_2O_2 added by diffusion can be generated during the cyclic oxidation and reduction of 40 μmoles dialurate per ml of packed RBC's. The results of Table 3 support the point of view that H_2O_2 generated during the autoxidation of dialuric acid plays a critical role in the peroxidative hemolysis of E-deficient RBC's.

During the exposure to H_2O_2 vapor, there was disappearance of polyunsaturated fatty acids from human and rat E-deficient RBC's (Dodge et al., 1967). Furthermore, the accumulation of lipid peroxides tended to precede lysis. This latter point, which is critical to an understanding of the mechanism of cell lysis, can be more clearly demonstrated in another experimental system: Azide (5mM) was first added to inhibit RBC catalase and, then, a relatively small quantity of H_2O_2 was added directly to the erythrocyte

TABLE 3. HEMOLYSIS AND LIPID PEROXIDATION IN VITAMIN E-DEFICIENT RAT ERYTHROCYTES EXPOSED TO HYDROGEN PEROXIDE VAPOR.

Data are the mean ± standard deviation for the number of animals (N) shown in parentheses. Exposure time was 3 hrs.

Diet	H_2O_2 Vapor	Lysis	2-TBA Test (O.D. 532 nm)
Normal (N=9)	Yes	12.7 ± 10.9	0.04 ± 0.01
E-Def. (N=22)	Yes	87.0 ± 11.1	0.48 ± 0.08
E-Def. (N=23)	No	23.1 ± 17.5	0.13 ± 0.08
E-Def. + oral tocoph. suppl. (N=6)	Yes	16.7 ± 6.1	0.08 ± 0.04

TABLE 4. PEROXIDATIVE HEMOLYSIS IN VITAMIN E-DEFICIENT HUMAN ERYTHROCYTES EXPOSED TO HYDROGEN PEROXIDE VAPOR.

Data are the averages for three experiments with two subjects (Cf. Dodge, Cohen, Kayden and Phillips, 1967). Exposure time was five hours.

Additions	H_2O_2 Vapor	Lysis	2-TBA Test*
None	No	1.5	1.6
None	Yes	87.0	13.9
$NaNO_2$ (0.3 mg/ml)	Yes	1.5	1.4
CO (10% in atmposphere)	Yes	5.0	4.8
Glucose (2 mg/ml)	Yes	1.5	1.6
α-Tocopherol (2 μg/ml)	Yes	1.5	1.4

* moles x 10^{-8} malonaldehyde per ml RBC

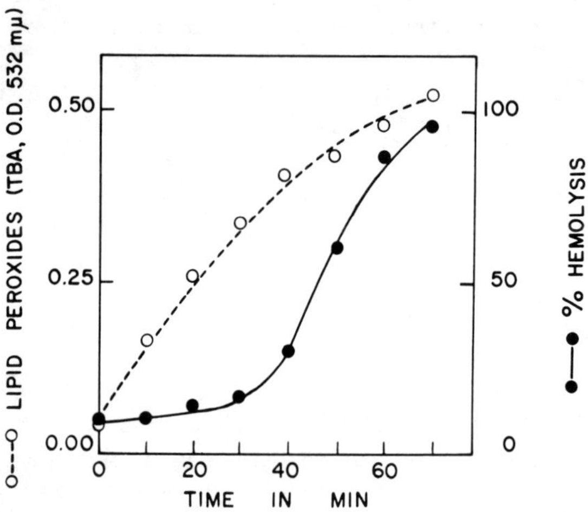

FIGURE 1. LIPID PEROXIDATION AND LYSIS AFTER DIRECT ADDITION OF HYDROGEN PEROXIDE IN A MODIFIED SYSTEM. 10% suspension of RBC's, 5 mM sodium azide, 8 μmoles of H_2O_2 added per ml. of packed RBC's, room temperature.

suspension (8 µmoles H_2O_2 per ml packed RBC's). This amount of H_2O_2 was sufficient to oxidize all of the cellular GSH. The H_2O_2-stressed cell suspension was incubated at ambient temperature and aliquots were removed sequentially for determination of lysis and lipid peroxidation. Results of a typical experiment (Figure 1) showed a steady accumulation of 2-TBA positive material (lipid peroxides). Lysis was not evident until considerable peroxidation had occurred. Lysis, once it began, was a remarkably rapid process. These data support the point of view that peroxidation of membrane lipids is a forerunner of hemolysis in E-deficient cells.

The protective actions of carbon monoxide and sodium nitrite are shown in Table 4 for human E-deficient RBC's. The protective effect of carbon monoxide in E-deficient rat RBC's had been reported previously by Bunyan et al. (1960). Glucose and alpha-tocopherol were also protective. One role for glucose may be to support reduction of GSSG to GSH in these cells; this would maintain GSH peroxidase activity as a defense against H_2O_2. Additionally, glucose can act as a hydroxyl radical trap (Cohen and Heikkila, 1974). Results similar to Table 4 were obtained with E-deficient rat RBC's. However, rat RBC's were much more sensitive and they developed lipid peroxides and underwent lysis in the presence of glucose (see Table 3).

The rationale for testing nitrite (Table 4) was that it might aid in the detoxification of H_2O_2 by acting as substrate for the peroxidatic activity of catalase. This seems unlikely, however, as neither ethanol nor methanol was protective (data not shown), although both are known substrates for catalase. On the other hand, nitrite made the cells methemoglobinemic. Therefore, an alternative and more likely explanation is that nitrite acted similarly to carbon monoxide, namely by decreasing the intracellular concentrations of oxyhemoglobin and/or deoxyhemoglobin.

The importance of hemoglobin in the hemolytic system can be seen from the following experiments with isolated stroma from vitamin E-deficient RBC's. The stroma were washed several times in either distilled water or in dilute

(0.1% w/v) saline. The latter treatment removed trace quantities of hemoglobin. The stromal hemoglobin in water-washed preparations was visible as a pink color. The data of Table 5 show that isolated stroma underwent peroxidation on exposure to H_2O_2 vapor. Although not shown, both nitrite and carbon monoxide diminished peroxidation in this system. When hemoglobin was removed, there was no peroxidation (Table 5). The peroxidation in the presence of hemoglobin required erythrocyte membranes and was not observed in stroma-free lysates (Cf. Bunyan et al., 1960).

DISCUSSION

Both G-6-PD deficient and E-deficient RBC's are sensitive to small amounts of H_2O_2, but through different molecular mechanisms. With G-6-PD deficient cells, there is limited generation of NADPH due to impaired hexose shunt activity; this leads to failure to recycle the oxidized form of glutathione and to resultant impairment of GSH peroxidase activity. As GSH peroxidase activity falls off, the intracellular levels of H_2O_2 rise (Liebowitz and Cohen, 1968). The result is oxidative damage, such as that exemplified by oxidation of hemoglobin or oxidation of SH-dependent enzymes. With diminution of glycolytic capacity, which is the major metabolic route in RBC's for energy production, there should be still further increased susceptibility to oxidant stress. An early demise through either intravascular hemolysis or removal of damaged RBC's by the reticulo-endothelial system would be anticipated.

Oxidation reactions that proceed via one-electron transfers to oxygen to form H_2O_2 generate superoxide radicals as intermediates. Superoxide radicals have been observed during autoxidation of dialuric acid (Cohen and Heikkila, 1974; Fee and Teitelbaum, 1972). Additionally, hydroxyl radicals (Cohen and Heikkila, 1974) are generated from H_2O_2 either by decomposition in the presence of iron catalysts (e.g., Fenton's reagent) or by reaction with superoxide radicals (Haber-Weiss reaction). Hydroxyl radicals can also interact directly with H_2O_2 to form superoxide radicals. The levels of superoxide dismutase (erythrocuprein) in G-6-PD deficient or E-deficient RBC's do not appear to have been studied.

TABLE 5. LIPID PEROXIDATION OF VITAMIN E-DEFICIENT RAT STROMA EXPOSED TO HYDROGEN PEROXIDE VAPOR.

Sample	H_2O_2 Vapor	2-TBA Test (O.D. 532 nm)
Whole lysate	No	0.03
Whole lysate	Yes	0.21
Stroma-free lysate	Yes	0.01
Stroma (water washed)	Yes	0.15
Hemoglobin-free stroma	Yes	0.02

The protective action of ethanol on G-6-PD deficient cells can be rationalized in two possible ways: Either ethanol acted as a hydroxyl radical scavenger or as substrate for the peroxidatic activity of catalase. There was no detectable lipid peroxidation in G-6-PD deficient cells (unpublished observation) and, therefore, cell damage did not appear to proceed via peroxidation of membrane unsaturated fatty acids.

Vitamin E-deficient cells were not protected by ethanol. The mechanism of cell damage in E-deficient cells is best summarized by Figure 2. The E-deficient membrane is extremely susceptible to oxidation of unsaturated fatty acid components. Peroxidation should lead to changes in membrane structure and function, with resultant leakage of cellular components (hemolysis). The protective action of carbon monoxide and sodium nitrite, as well as the requirement for hemoglobin in the peroxidation of isolated stroma, implies that either oxyhemoglobin or deoxyhemoglobin is acting as a catalyst. Catalysis could take the form of the reaction exemplified by Fenton's reagent, in which ferrous iron acts to generate hydroxyl radicals from H_2O_2. Hydroxyl radicals may play a critical role in initiating lipid peroxidation. Although the failure of ethanol to protect cells is inconsistent with this idea, it may be that the extreme lability of lipids in E-deficient membranes and the intimate

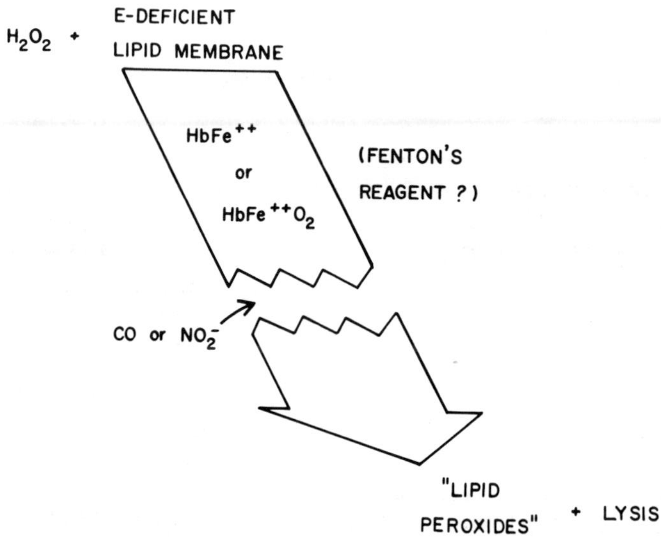

FIGURE 2. MECHANISM OF CELL DAMAGE BY HYDROGEN PEROXIDE IN VITAMIN E-DEFICIENT RED BLOOD CELLS.

association of hemoglobin with the membrane may preclude any strong protective action by ethanol. Additionally, ethanol may exert a detrimental solvent effect on the E-deficient membrane.

There is other evidence that may favor a role for hydroxyl radicals in dialurate (or H_2O_2)-induced hemolysis. In a recent study (Heikkila, Barden and Cohen, 1974), it was observed that ethanol prevented the diabetogenic action of alloxan. Alloxan is the oxidized form (quinone) of dialurate. Both alloxan and dialurate are hemolytic _in vivo_ with E-deficient animals, and both produce experimental diabetes in normal mice or rats via destruction of the beta-cells of the pancreas. An implication of the protective action of ethanol against alloxan-induced diabetes is that the causative agent could well be the hydroxyl radical. After alloxan was administered to normal mice, elevated levels of H_2O_2 were detected within the RBC's (Heikkila, Barden and Cohen, 1974). Thus, the presumptive hemolytic intermediate (H_2O_2 or an oxygen radical) is present within RBC's in vivo during peroxidative hemolysis.

SUMMARY

The preceding experiments constitute strong evidence that H_2O_2 (either directly, or indirectly via derived radical species) is a cytotoxic intermediate in the reaction of hemolytic agents with both G-6-PD deficient RBC's and tocopherol-deficient RBC's. In G-6-PD deficiency, hemoglobin is both a target of the oxidative process (formation of methemoglobin and subsequent breakdown products) and also a constituent of the system for generating H_2O_2 (coupled oxidation with drugs). In vitamin E-deficiency, hemoglobin plays a special role as a catalyst in the oxidative process.

In G-6-PD deficiency, there is impaired capacity to detoxify H_2O_2 and oxidative damage takes several forms, including inhibition of glucose metabolism. In E-deficiency, the detoxification of H_2O_2 may be normal, but there is marked lability of the erythrocyte membrane to peroxidation (a free radical chain process). G-6-PD deficient cells are protected in vitro by ethanol. E-deficient cells are protected by agents such as carbon monoxide or sodium nitrite that interact with the hemoglobin catalyst, but not by ethanol. Although the molecular mechanisms for response of G-6-PD deficient RBC's, E-deficient RBC's and normal beta-pancreatic cells to H_2O_2-producing drugs such as dialurate, alloxan, menadione, primaquine, phenylhydrazine, etc., may differ in detail (site and sequence of oxidative damage), the rapid demise of each of these cell types may involve factors in common, most prominent among which are the generation of reactive free radicals which initiate damage to membranes and SH-dependent enzymes.

REFERENCES

H. Aebi and H. Suter (1974), in "Glutathione", Eds., L. Flohe, H.Ch. Benohr, H. Sies, H.D. Waller and A. Wendel, Georg Thieme Publishers, Stuttgart, p. 192.

E. Beutler (1966), in "The Metabolic Basis of Inherited Disease", Ed. by J.B. Stanbury, J.B. Wyngaarden and D.S. Fredrickson, McGraw-Hill, New York, p. 1060.

J. Bunyan, J. Green, E.E. Edwin and A.T. Diplock (1960), Biochem. J. 77, 47.

R.G. Chapman, M.A. Hennessey, A.M. Waltersdorph, F.M. Huennekens and B.W. Gabrio (1962), J. Clin. Invest. 41, 1249.

G. Cohen and R.E. Heikkila (1974), J. Biol. Chem. 249, 2447.

G. Cohen and P. Hochstein (1961), Science 134, 1756.

G. Cohen and P. Hochstein (1963), Biochemistry 2, 1420.

G. Cohen and P. Hochstein (1964), Biochemistry 3, 895.

G. Cohen and P. Hochstein (1965), J. Pharmacol. Exp. Therap. 147, 139

D.W. Deamer, R.E. Heikkila, R.V. Panganamala, G. Cohen and D.G. Cornwell (1971), Physiol. Chem. Phys. 3, 426.

J.T. Dodge, G. Cohen, H.J. Kayden and G.B. Phillips (1967), J. Clin. Invest. 46, 357.

K.A. Evelyn and H.T. Malloy (1938), J. Biol. Chem. 126, 655.

J.A. Fee and H.D. Teitelbaum (1972), Biochem. Biophys. Res. Commun. 49, 150.

R.E. Heikkila, H. Barden and G. Cohen (1974), J. Pharmacol. Exp. Therap. 190, 501.

P. Hochstein (1971), Exp. Eye Res. 11, 389.

D. Keilin and E.F. Hartree (1945), Biochem. J. 39, 293.

J. Liebowitz and G. Cohen (1968), Biochem. Pharmacol. 17, 983.

P. Nicholls (1972), Biochim. Biophys. Acta 279, 306.

C.S. Rose and P. Gyorgy (1952), Amer. J. Physiol. 168, 414.

A.L. Tappel (1962), Vitamins and Hormones 20, 493.

C.C. Tsen and H.B. Collier (1960), Can. J. Biochem. Physiol. 38, 957.

FORMAL DISCUSSION

ON THE MECHANISM OF THE OXYGEN/DIALURIC ACID INDUCED HEMOLYSIS OF VITAMIN E DEFICIENT RAT RED BLOOD CELLS AND THE PROTECTIVE ROLES OF CATALASE AND SUPEROXIDE DISMUTASE

James A. Fee‡, Robert Bergamini and Robert G. Briggs
Department of Chemistry, Rensselaer Polytechnic Institute, Troy, NY 12181 ‡Present address: Biophysics Research Division, University of Michigan, Ann Arbor, Michigan 48105

Since a detailed description of this work has been submitted for publication elsewhere we will only present the major experimental findings which support our conclusions.

Dialuric acid has been known to induce the hemolysis of vitamin-E deficient red blood cells for some time. The pioneering work of Rose and György (1, 2) left us with the conclusions that neither hydrogen peroxide alone nor alloxan was responsible for the hemolytic effect but some intermediate substance formed during the reaction between dialurate and oxygen. In our preliminary communication (3) on this subject we surmised that superoxide anion may be the intermediate suggested by Rose and György. This has not proven to be true on further investigation.

STUDIES CONCERNED WITH THE AUTOXIDATION OF DIALURIC ACID

Observations:

(a) Dialuric acid reacts with oxygen to form one mole of alloxan and one mole of H_2O_2 (4).
(b) With air saturation at pH 7.8 the time course of the reaction is sigmoidal and half complete at $\sim$30 sec.
(c) It is non-reproducibly inhibited (by as much as a factor of two) by micromolar concentration of superoxide dismutase.

(d) No free radicals were detected by EPR spectroscopy. The concentration of free radicals at any time during the reaction must have been less than 0.1 μmolar.

(e) The maximum concentration of O_2^- generated during the reaction as determined by cytochrome c^{III} reduction, was less than 0.1 μmolar.

Conclusion:

The autoxidation of dialuric acid does not involve the build up of an appreciable concentration of any free radical species, particularly O_2^-.

STUDIES CONCERNED WITH THE HEMOLYSIS OF RED BLOOD CELLS

Observations:

(a) The additions of 1 mM dialuric acid to a washed suspension of vitamin-E deficient rat erythrocytes induces a hemolysis which occurs many minutes after the autoxidation reaction is complete (Fig. 1).

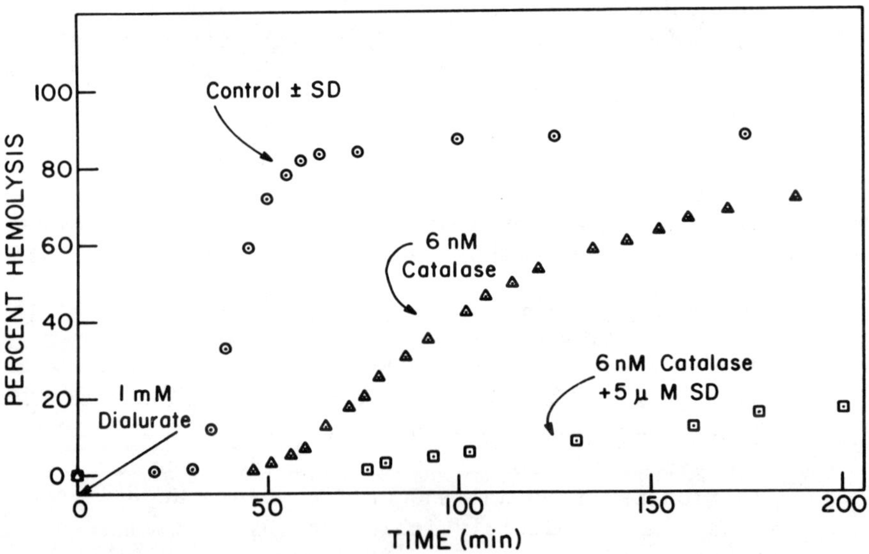

Fig. 1

(b) Superoxide dismutase, even at high concentrations, does not inhibit hemolysis.
(c) Catalase at low concentrations has a partial protective effect while at higher concentrations it will give complete protection (1, 2).
(d) Superoxide dismutase at high concentration potentiates the protective effect of catalase at low concentration.
(e) Addition of the enzymes two minutes after dialuric acid has no influence on hemolysis; removal of the enzymes two minutes after addition of dialuric acid by washing does not alter their protective effect.
(f) No free radicals could be observed by EPR spectroscopy on treatment of red cells with dialuric acid, even with whole blood suspensions. The free radical concentration must be less than 0.1 µmolar.
(g) The following systems do not induce hemolysis: 1-10 mM H_2O_2, 100 mM xanthine with 6-670 nmolar xanthine oxidase, 1 mM hydroquinone, 1 mM alloxan, or 0.1 mM pulse of O_2^- (5).
(h) Lipid peroxidation precedes hemolysis. This and several of the above observations are demonstrated in Fig. 2.

Conclusions:

(a) The modification of the red blood cell which leads to hemolysis is made during the reaction between dialurate and O_2.
(b) Lipid peroxidation is initiated by this modification, and does not depend on the presence of H_2O_2, O_2^- or alloxan and it is not inhibited by externally added catalase or superoxide dismutase.
(c) Neither O_2^-, H_2O_2 nor a mixture of these inflicts the initial lesion on the red blood cell.

Speculation

We believe that dialuric acid reacts with oxygen to form an oxygenated intermediate which is highly reactive toward cellular components.

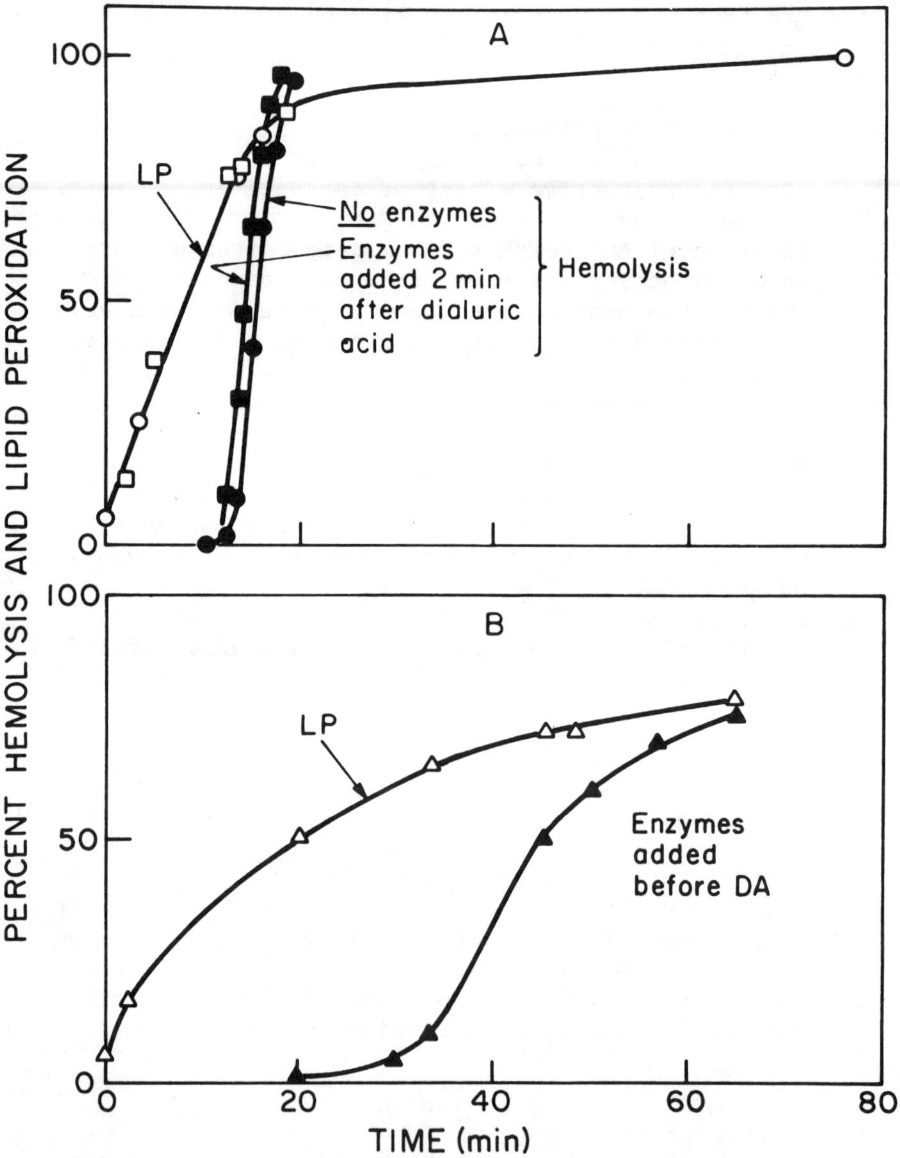
A
B
LP
No enzymes
Enzymes added 2 min after dialuric acid
Hemolysis
LP
Enzymes added before DA
PERCENT HEMOLYSIS AND LIPID PEROXIDATION
100
50
0
100
50
0
0
20
40
60
80
TIME (min)

Fig. 2

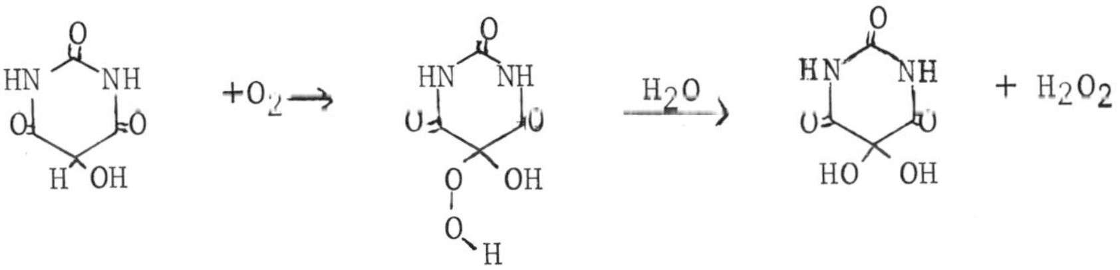

dialuric acid — peroxy intermediate — alloxan

Catalase probably protects by reacting with the intermediate.

Acknowledgements:

This work was supported by a grant from USPHS GM 18869. JAF acknowledges helpful discussions with Dr. Peter Hemmerich concerning the chemistry of dialuric acid.

References:

1. C. S. Rose and P. György, Blood 5, 1062 (1950).

2. C. S. Rose and P. György, Am. J. Physiol. 168, 414 (1952).

3. J. A. Fee and H. D. Teitelbaum, Biochem. Biophys. Res. Comm. 49, 150 (1972).

4. D. W. Deamer, R. E. Heikkila, R. V. Panganamala, G. Cohen and D. G. Cornwell, Physiol. Chem. and Physics 3, 426 (1971).

5. J. A. Fee and P. G. Hildenbrand, FEBS Letters 39, 79 (1974).

DISCUSSION

<u>Dr. Brewer</u>: Would John Eaton like to comment on whether the work he reported at the last conference, on catalase complex II and the effect of ethanol on activating that complex, might be involved with some of the ethanol protection Dr. Cohen is seeing?

<u>Dr. Eaton</u>: We think probably not.

<u>Dr. Cohen</u>: Perhaps Dr. Eaton is being too strong. We have discussed it a bit. Diminishing the catalase level of the cell may play some role, but I don't think it can be the all important role simply because if the catalase level falls off 50%, that may simply be the normal level for another individual, since there are a range of catalase levels. A 50% decline due to accumulation of complex II can't be the overriding factor, but it may contribute.

<u>Dr. Eaton</u>: I would like to ask what you'd anticipate in terms of alloxan sensitivity in acatalasemic vs. normal mice? Have you considered doing this?

<u>Dr. Cohen</u>: No. We haven't considered doing it, and I would not expect oxidant damage to acatalasemic mice. Acatalasemic individuals are not sensitive to acetylphenylhydrazine or primaquine. However, this may depend on how you do the experiment and on how quickly dialurate generates peroxide. If the intracellular peroxide level gets up too high, then the absence of catalase could be important. Also, Dr. Fee has been pointing out to me that catalase may have other functions, for example, the handling of free radicals and perhaps organic peroxides. If so, the absence of catalase could be important.

<u>Dr. Babior</u>: I wonder what Dr. Fee's explanation would be for the effects of catalase and of catalase plus dismutase on hemolysis.

<u>Dr. Fee</u>: I think the catalase entraps an oxygenated intermediate. Catalase is known to react with organic peroxides

such as ethyl peroxides, and so on. Now, the protective effect of the dismutase is more difficult to rationalize. I don't believe that in this system the dismutase was protecting the red cell. It may be, in fact, protecting the catalase, since there are two things that could happen. On interacting with the oxygenated intermediate I propose, the catalase may become inactive, and the dismutase can then regenerate the catalase somehow. That seems a little farfetched. The other point is that superoxide ion is known to react with resting catalase to produce inactive compound III. The effect of the dismutase would be to protect against the formation of compound III, so it's simply protecting the catalase.

Dr. Hoekstra: Dr. Fee, do you know if the dialurate hydroperoxide is a substrate for glutathione peroxidase? If so, wouldn't it be degraded very rapidly, at least inside of the cell?

Dr. Fee: After hearing your talk I planned to test that, but I have not. I agree, the organic peroxide compound should work very well with the glutathione peroxidase.

Dr. Hoekstra: Have you any ideas on singlet oxygen in your studies? Lipid peroxidation can be induced by a free-radical, or it can be induced, with no evidence of free radicals, by singlet oxygen. The singlet oxygen, according to my understanding, reacts directly to produce lipid hydroperoxide, which then initiates peroxidation.

Dr. Fee: There are so many controversies, and singlet oxygen is one I promised to stay out of. I think Bernard Babior, who has looked at this in a good deal more detail than I have could better answer your question. I have deliberately stayed out of the discussion of singlet oxygen. It's a very complicated system.

Dr. Hoekstra: I understand that. Dr. Cohen, I'm not sure I understand the effect of nitrite. I believe that you showed that nitrite interacts with hemoglobin to produce a stoichiometric but small amount of hydrogen peroxide?

Dr. Cohen: Yes, that's right.

Dr. Hoekstra: Then why is it protecting in your current studies?

Dr. Cohen: Well, in the experiments we published some years ago where we showed peroxide formation from nitrite, we also pointed out the difficulty of demonstrating it (Cohen, Martinez, and Hochstein, Biochemistry, 3, 901, 1964). The difficulty relates to why we used nitrite in the first place. Nitrite is a peroxidatic substrate for catalase. If you have a very high concentration of nitrite present, it's very difficult to detect the peroxide generated during the conversion of oxyhemoglobin to methemoglobin. Our positive results were obtained in a very narrow concentration range for nitrite where we were lucky enough to be able to detect the peroxide despite its removal by nitrite and catalase. In the current experiments with vitamin E-deficient cells, we were looking to see if a peroxidatic substrate for catalase would provide protection. But the carbon monoxide experiment took us away from that type of interpretation, and the failure of ethanol to substitute for nitrite also took us away from that interpretation in the E deficient cell. A more likely interpretation relates to hemoglobin as a catalyst.

Dr. Hoekstra: So your idea is that the nitroso- or carbonmonoxy-hemoglobin prevents generation of damaging species. Is that correct?

Dr. Cohen: That's the assumption, yes.

Dr. Hoekstra: And the damaging species are what?

Dr. Cohen: Hydroxyl radical for the time being, O.K.?

Dr. Hoekstra: O.K.

Dr. Dawson: I'm particularly interested in the hemoglobin requirement for oxidative hemolysis. I have this interest because of having published the mechanism for heme-iron absorption in Blood in 1970. The requirement in that reaction was for xanthine oxidase, presumably in a coupled oxidation with the alpha methane bridge converting hemoglobin to choleglobin. Therefore, I wonder what you propose as the mechanism for hemoglobin's participation in oxidant hemolysis?

Dr. Cohen: I've drawn a distinction between oxidant and peroxidant hemolysis. The hemoglobin story--the carbon monoxide and the nitrite--seem relevant to vitamin E deficiency with its peroxidation of the membrane. I don't know about its relevance to so-called oxidant hemolysis, which is generally taken as the G-6-PD type of model. Have I understood your question properly? Have I avoided the answer?

Dr. Dawson: You have avoided the answer, and perhaps the question wasn't terribly clear. I guess the question should be: Does the hemoglobin requirement for oxidant hemolysis have anything to do with oxidation of the protoporphyrin ring at the alpha methane bridge, which would participate in the peroxidation reaction in my system?

Dr. Cohen: In the E deficiency story, I know nothing about the details other than the peripheral evidence you've seen that two agents which bind to hemoglobin in special ways--carbon monoxide and nitrite--are protective. But I cannot give you a detailed answer.

Dr. Dawson: Thank you.

Dr. Hultquist: I'd like to ask for a bit of caution in assuming that when one sees ghosts that are pink it is hemoglobin that is giving the pink color. Depending on the method of lysis there can be an appreciable amount of the hemeprotein that has been referred to as S-protein and we've called hemeprotein 559. This hemeprotein does bind carbon monoxide. It may very well react with nitrite.

Dr. Cohen: Thank you.

Dr. Hoekstra: I'd like to mention some recent unpublished results of Dr. Paul McCay on washed liver microsomal preparations. He is interested in lipid peroxidation in the microsomes. When he exposes microsomes to the xanthine-xanthine oxidase system to generate superoxide anion, he does not get lipid peroxidation. If he adds a small amount of ADP-chelated ferric iron, lipid peroxidation ensues. If he adds a hydroxyl radical scavenger such as mannitol or ethanol, he dramatically reduces the lipid peroxidation. If he adds a singlet oxygen scavenger, it also reduces to some extent the formation of malonic dialdehyde. His implication was that in his system, the hydroxyl radical was the most important in initiating lipid peroxidation but there was also some effect from singlet oxygen.

Dr. Cohen: Thank you. That would be consistent then with the idea that hydroxyl radicals play a role in peroxidative hemolysis. I'd like to direct a comment or question to Dr. Fee or at least indicate my disagreement with one of the conclusions on your slide. The disagreement concerns your conclusion that peroxide itself was not or could not be the initiating species for producing peroxidative hemolysis of an E deficient cell. I think that point of view is difficult to sustain in the face of experiments with peroxide itself as the agent which is added--the experiments I presented here. I think perhaps your conclusion was too strong.

Dr. Fee: I only wanted to make the conclusion with respect to the system that I had studied. In other words, in the experiments I did, I showed that you get one millimolar peroxide formed when one millimolar dialuric acid reacts with oxygen. That means that if it reacts in one minute, the red cell gets a pulse of one millimolar peroxide. By injecting one millimolar peroxide, I felt I was simulating the reaction with the Hamilton syringe. I don't say that the hydrogen peroxide cannot initiate this lesion. I think that Dr. Cohen's results demonstrate that quite clearly. But the two systems are quite different and we don't understand what those differences are.

Dr. McCord: With regard to the alloxan diabetes in mice, I'd like to add for the record that we tried very hard to prevent the development of alloxan diabetes in rats by injection of superoxide dismutase along with, before or after the alloxan, and were totally unsuccessful. So, if ethanol is acting as an hydroxyl radical scavenger, I would suggest that the radical is probably not being produced by reaction of superoxide with hydroxyl radical scavenger, I would suggest that the radical is probably not being produced by reaction of superoxide with hydrogen peroxide in the interstitial fluid. Otherwise, I think we would have seen protection with superoxide dismutase.

Dr. Cohen: If you limit the comment to the interstitial fluid and not to the beta cell of the pancreas whose level of superoxide dismutase we do not know, we can be in agreement.

Dr. McCord: We do not know the level in the beta cell, but we suspect that we have a good idea about it.

SUPEROXIDE AND G-6-PD-TYPE HEMOLYSIS

R. M. Leipzig, G.J. Brewer, and W. C. Kruckeberg

Department of Human Genetics, University of Michigan Medical School, Ann Arbor, Michigan

INTRODUCTION

Glucose-6-phosphate dehydrogenase (G-6-PD) deficiency is an X-linked enzyme deficiency seen in one out of every 10 black American males. The exposure of these individuals to certain agents results in a self-limited hemolytic anemia (Carson et al, 1956). The classical agents producing this anemia are drugs such as the 8-aminoquinoline, acetylphenylhydrazine (APH), and menadione, but fever, infection (Mengel et al, 1967), and acidosis (Gant and Winhster, 1961) have also been implicated in precipitating the hemolytic reaction. The G-6-PD deficient red cells, when exposed to such agents *in vivo*, undergo large decreases in their reduced glutathione (GSH) levels, and Heinz bodies are formed within the cells. Clinically, marked anemia, jaundice, dark urine, and reticulocytosis are seen in such a patient.

The exact biochemical mechanism by which G-6-PD deficiency leads to hemolysis in the presence of these various agents is uncertain. Cells which are G-6-PD deficient generate decreased amounts of NADPH, the cofactor necessary for the reduction of oxidized glutathione by glutathione reductase. The G-6-PD deficient red cells have a lower than normal content of GSH (Beutler et al, 1955) and this decreases even further upon *in vivo* exposure to the various hemolytic agents

(Flanagan et al, 1958). Several explanations have been proposed relating the lowered GSH level to hemolysis. Reduced glutathione constitutes the major source of free sulfhydryl groups in red cells, and it is possibly important in protecting sulfhydryl dependent enzymes, hemoglobin, and other cellular constituents from oxidative damage. It has been suggested that the diminution in the content of GSH in G-6-PD deficient red cells during administration of a hemolytic agent may result in the inactivation of one or more sulfhydryl dependent glycolytic enzymes, leading to a decreased production of energy and subsequent lysis of the cell (Mohler and Williams, 1961). It has also been suggested that membrane oxidation might result due to the lack of NADPH or GSH; or that glutathione might cross-link to the membrane, making it less deformable and therefore more subject to the action of the reticulo-endothelial system. Cohen and Hochstein (1964) have shown that several of the hemolytic drugs produce hydrogen peroxide (H_2O_2). Hydrogen peroxide, spontaneously and in a reaction catalyzed by glutathione peroxidase, oxidizes GSH, and therefore might be an agent responsible for hemolysis. Although several possibilities have been suggested, the actual mechanism of hemolysis remains unclear.

We have begun to examine the possibility that an oxygen free radical, superoxide ($O_2^{\cdot-}$), might be a common intermediate through which the various hemolytic agents cause oxidative damage to G-6-PD deficient erythrocytes (Leipzig et al, 1974) Superoxide spontaneously forms H_2O_2 and singlet oxygen (O_2^1) (Khan, 1970), a high energy form of molecular oxygen capable of effecting lipid peroxidations and nucleic acid oxidations, among other activities (Figure 1). The enzyme superoxide dismutase (SOD) catalyzes the dismutation of superoxide to H_2O_2 and molecular oxygen. The H_2O_2 thus produced either spontaneously or enzymatically can interact with $O_2^{\cdot-}$ as in the Haber-Weiss reaction, forming hydroxyl free radicals ($OH^{\cdot}$) which have also been implicated in lipid peroxidation. The production of $O_2^{\cdot-}$ by hemolytic agents could therefore result in the formation of other potent oxidants such as H_2O_2, O_2^1, and $OH^{\cdot}$, all of which are capable of damaging cellular constituents.

$$1.\quad O_2^{\overline{\cdot}} + O_2^{\overline{\cdot}} + 2H^+ \rightleftharpoons H_2O_2 + {}^1O_2$$

$$2.\quad O_2^{\overline{\cdot}} + O_2^{\overline{\cdot}} + 2H^+ \xrightleftharpoons{SOD} H_2O_2 + O_2$$

$$3.\quad O_2^{\overline{\cdot}} + H_2O_2 \rightleftharpoons OH^{\cdot} + OH^- + O_2$$

Figure 1. Selected oxidant producing reactions of $O_2^{\overline{\cdot}}$. The first reaction depicts the spontaneous dismutation of $O_2^{\overline{\cdot}}$. The second reaction is that catalyzed by SOD. The Haber-Weiss reaction, which results in the production of $OH^{\cdot}$, is shown last.

We hypothesize that $O_2^{\cdot}$ is produced by various hemolytic agents and that directly, and/or indirectly through its conversion to these other oxidants, it is involved in the mechanism of G-6-PD type hemolysis. To test this, we have performed three types of studies. First, we generated $O_2^{\cdot}$ outside whole normal and G-6-PD deficient cells and then measured the effect of this on GSH levels within the cells. Second, we measured the interaction of $O_2^{\cdot}$ with two of the critical reducing components of the cell,NADPH and NADH. Third, we assayed two hemolytic drugs,APH and menadione, for $O_2^{\cdot}$ production.

MATERIALS AND METHODS

The conversion of xanthine (X) to uric acid by xanthine oxidase (XO), a reaction known to produce $O_2^{\cdot}$, is the basis of our $O_2^{\cdot}$ generating system. To measure the effect of $O_2^{\cdot}$ produced outside whole cells on GSH levels within these cells we generated $O_2^{\cdot}$ in a 1.30 ml solution containing 1.0 ml whole blood, 0.584 mM X, and 0.0216 units XO. (All chemicals and enzymes mentioned, unless otherwise stated, were obtained from Sigma Chemical Co., St. Louis, Mo.) Incubation was carried out under mineral oil for 2 hours at 37°C. To test if any observed effects could be inhibited, 0.1 ml SOD [obtained through the generosity of Dr. Donald Hultquist (Reed et al, 1970)], 200 units catalase, or 20 mM benzoate was added to the reaction mixture. GSH was assayed according to the method of Prins and Loos (1969).

A comparable $O_2^{\cdot}$ generating system was used to study the effect of $O_2^{\cdot}$ on NADPH and NADH. 27.5 mM X, 0.0162 units XO, and 0.121 mM NADPH (or 0.121 mM NADH) were contained in a 3.1 ml final volume 0.1 M phosphate buffer, pH 7.4. The change in absorbance at 340 nm was recorded over 35 minutes at 30°C on a Gilford Model 2400-S Recording Spectrophotometer The amount of inhibition of NADPH (or NADH) oxidation by SOD was measured by substituting 0.1 ml SOD for 0.1 ml buffer.

The effect of varying concentrations of H_2O_2 on NADPH was studied in solutions of 0.5 M Tris, pH 7.2, containing final concentrations of 0.74 mM NADPH and 1.4 M H_2O_2, 0.14 M

H_2O_2, 0.014 M H_2O_2, or 0.14 mM H_2O_2. These solutions were incubated for 30 minutes at 25°C after which the absorbance at 340 nm was recorded.

Estimates of $O_2^{\cdot-}$ production by candidate drugs in the presence of red cells were based on modification of the cytochrome c assay of McCord and Fridovich (1969). Superoxide production was estimated by comparing cytochrome c reduction in the absence and presence of SOD. Fresh whole blood was washed three times in a Krebs-Ringer phosphate buffer, pH 7.4, and the cells were resuspended in buffer to simulate a hematocrit of 40. Reduction of cytochrome c in the absence of SOD was measured in a 1.35 ml solution containing, in final concentration, .034 mM cytochrome c (type III), 10 mM EDTA, 1.0 ml resuspended red cell, 0.1 ml buffer, and 1.0 mM drug. Reduction of cytochrome c in the presence of SOD was measured by replacing the 0.1 ml buffer in the above reaction mixture with 0.1 ml SOD. After incubation under mineral oil for 30 minutes at 37°C each tube was spun and an aliquot of the supernatant diluted 1:1 in buffer. Reduced cytochrome c was determined by absorbance at 550 nm.

RESULTS

We have examined the effect of a $O_2^{\cdot-}$ generating system on GSH levels in normal and G-6-PD deficient blood, since one of the common denominators among those agents which precipitate G-6-PD type hemolytic anemia is the ability to decrease red cell GSH levels in deficient but not in normal red cells. Superoxide generated outside G-6-PD deficient cells causes the GSH levels within these cells to decrease about 24%, whereas no significant difference in GSH levels is seen when $O_2^{\cdot-}$ is generated outside normal cells (Figure 2). To see what was mediating this decrease, various scavengers were added to the reaction mixture. The dismutation of $O_2^{\cdot-}$ to H_2O_2 by SOD appears to have no effect on protecting against GSH oxidation. Benzoate, added to scavenge OH· formed from the interaction of $O_2^{\cdot-}$ with H_2O_2, also appears to be ineffective in preventing GSH oxidation. The effects seen upon the addition of catalase, which catalyzes the formation

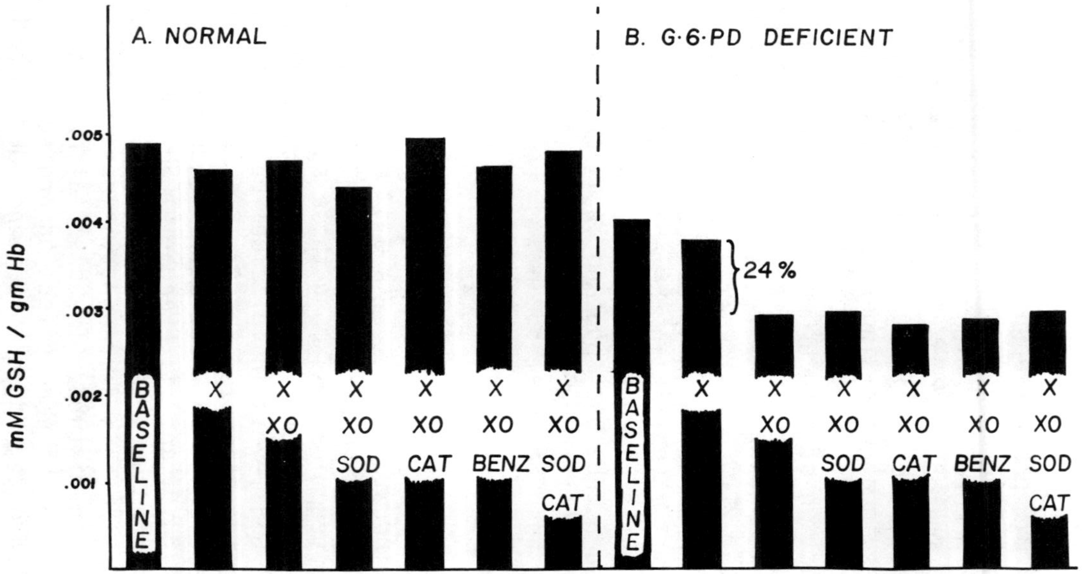

Figure 2. This figure shows the effect of $O_2^{\overline{\cdot}}$ generated outside red cells on GSH levels in normal (A) and G-6-PD deficient cells (B). This figure depicts the averages of three experiments. Key: Baseline is an incubated control with no additions; Benz. refers to the addition of benzoate; cat. refers to the addition of catalase. All other abbreviations are explained in the text.

of H_2O_2 and O_2 from H_2O_2, have been varied. The addition of 200 units of catalase did not effect GSH oxidation in the presence of the $O_2^{\cdot-}$ generating system. Other experiments, however, have at times showed partial protection, and in at least one instance complete protection, of GSH oxidation in the presence of differing amounts of catalase. These results have thus far been inconsistent, and we are currently working on isolating the mechanism of the GSH decrease seen in G-6-PD deficient cells in the presence of a superoxide generating system.

We have found that both NADPH and NADH can be directly oxidized by $O_2^{\cdot-}$ generated in a buffer system (Figure 3). The potential for $O_2^{\cdot-}$ generation in this system is 567 nmoles per 35 minutes (based on the activity of XO). Under these conditions, 6.3 nmoles of NADPH were oxidized, and this was 92% inhibited in the presence of SOD. Four nmoles of NADH were oxidized under these same conditions, and this reaction was totally inhibited in the presence of SOD.

Since the production of $O_2^{\cdot-}$ is always accompanied by the production of H_2O_2, we examined the effect of comparable amounts of H_2O_2 on NADPH oxidation. Figure 4 demonstrates that H_2O_2 is capable of oxidizing NADPH; however, amounts of H_2O_2 comparable to those of $O_2^{\cdot-}$ generated previously (Figure 3), are unable to detectably oxidize NADPH.

Menadione and APH were added to washed red cell suspensions and $O_2^{\cdot-}$ production measured as a function of the inhibition of cytochrome c reduction seen in the presence of SOD. Cytochrome c reduction by menadione was decreased approximately 20% in the presence of SOD (Figure 5). To assure that this decreased reduction was actually due to the activity of SOD, SOD boiled for 15 minutes was added to a reaction mixture. Some inhibition of cytochrome c reduction was still seen in the presence of boiled SOD. This indicates that either boiling the enzyme for 15 minutes does not destroy all the enzymatic activity, or that the decrease in cytochrome c reduction seen in the presence of SOD is not totally due to the enzymatic dismutation of superoxide. Nonetheless, it appears that at least 10-15% of the cytochrome c reduction seen is due to superoxide production by menadione.

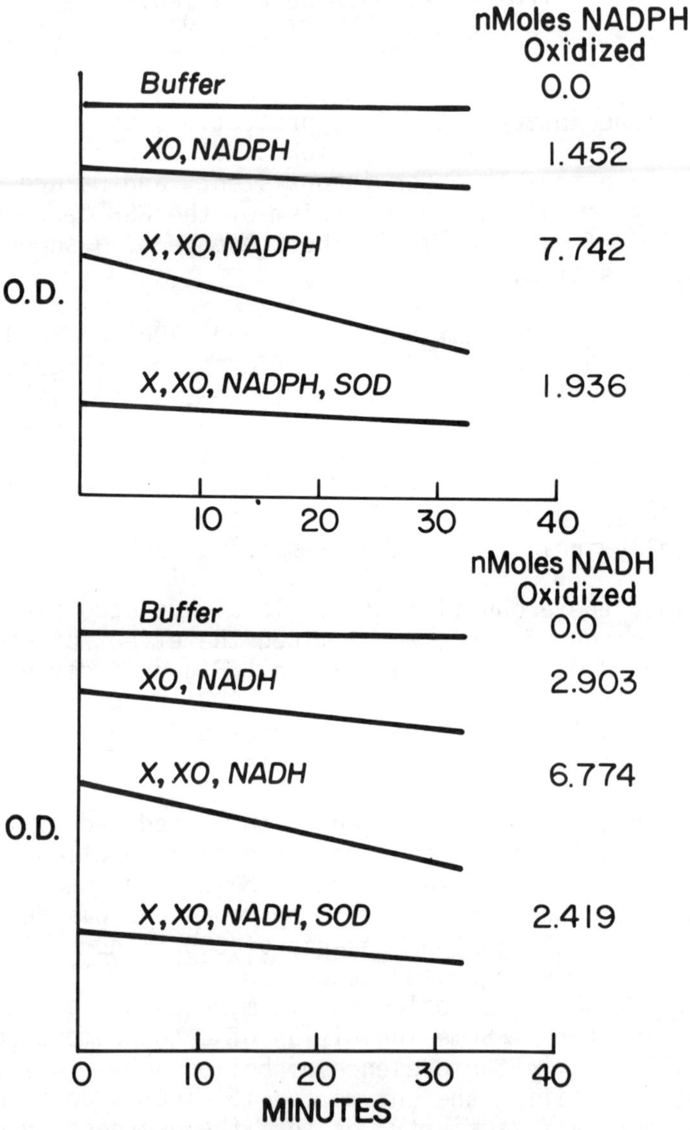

Figure 3. This figure shows NADPH and NADH oxidation by $O_2^{\cdot-}$ over 35 minutes. Details of the system are given in the text

n Moles H_2O_2 Used	n Moles NADPH Oxidized
4,890,000	19.7
489,000	9.2
48,900	2.3
489	0.0

Figure 4. This figure shows the oxidation of NADPH by various concentrations of H_2O_2.

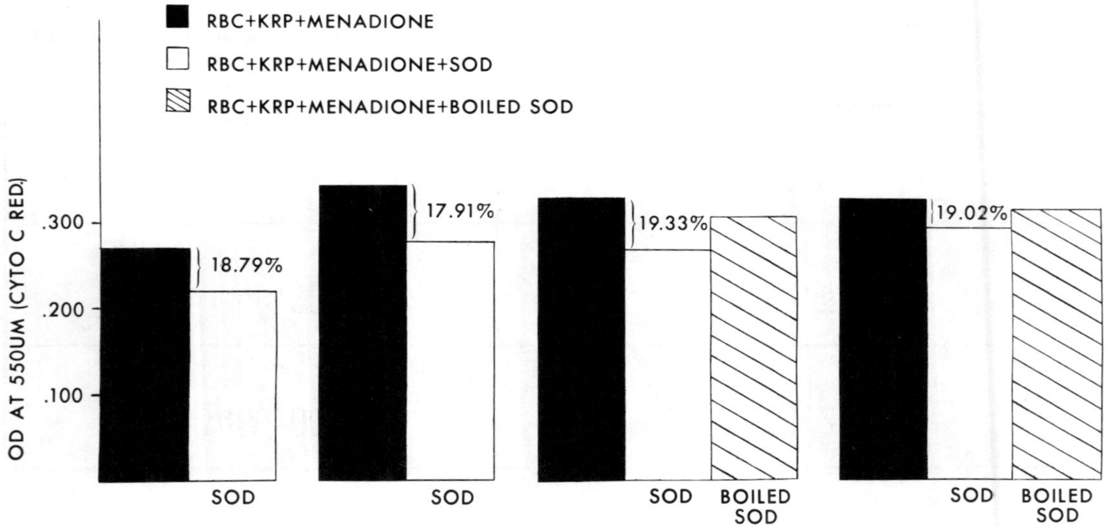

Figure 5. Reduction of cytochrome c by menadione in washed normal RBC's. This figure shows the production of $O_2^{\cdot-}$ by menadione incubated with washed red cells. The effect of boiled SOD in this system is shown in the third and fourth experiments. All blood samples were from non-G-6-PD deficient individuals.

Cytochrome c reduction by APH was decreased 40-60% in the presence of SOD (Figure 6). Boiled SOD, again used as a control, showed less inhibition of cytochrome c reduction than active, unboiled SOD. Taking into account the inhibition seen in the presence of boiled SOD, it appears that at least 15-30% of the cytochrome c reduction seen in the presence of APH is due to its production of $O_2^{\bar{\cdot}}$.

DISCUSSION

The ability of the red cell to maintain adequate levels of NADPH, and therefore GSH, is based on the activity of G-6-PD. Erythrocytes deficient for G-6-PD activity are less able to withstand oxidant stress, and undergo hemolysis during exposure to certain drugs or pathophysiological states. The nature of the oxidant stress, and the mechanisms by which hemolysis occurs in the presence of this stress is uncertain. In this paper, we have examined the possibility that $O_2^{\bar{\cdot}}$ is produced by hemolytic drugs and that $O_2^{\bar{\cdot}}$, or one of the oxidants produced from it, interacts deleteriously with NADPH, NADH, and GSH, compounds known to be important in maintaining red cell integrity.

Our work has shown that NADPH and NADH are directly oxidized by $O_2^{\bar{\cdot}}$. Since $O_2^{\bar{\cdot}}$ spontaneously and enzymatically forms H_2O_2, it is possible that H_2O_2 is the actual agent effecting the oxidation. However, H_2O_2 is produced by SOD, and SOD inhibits the oxidation. It thus appears that $O_2^{\bar{\cdot}}$ is more capable of directly oxidizing NADPH than H_2O_2. To test this hypothesis, we measured NADPH oxidation by H_2O_2 and $O_2^{\bar{\cdot}}$. 567 n moles of $O_2^{\bar{\cdot}}$ oxidized 6.3 n moles NADPH, whereas 489 n moles of H_2O_2 caused no detectable oxidation. Superoxide, therefore, appears to cause greater NADPH oxidation than comparable amounts of H_2O_2.

Many hemolytic drugs, _in vivo_, cause a decrease in GSH levels in G-6-PD deficient but not in normal cells. We found that the generation of $O_2^{\bar{\cdot}}$ outside intact whole cells results in this response. We are currently determining whether the agent mediating the GSH decrease is $O_2^{\bar{\cdot}}$ itself or another

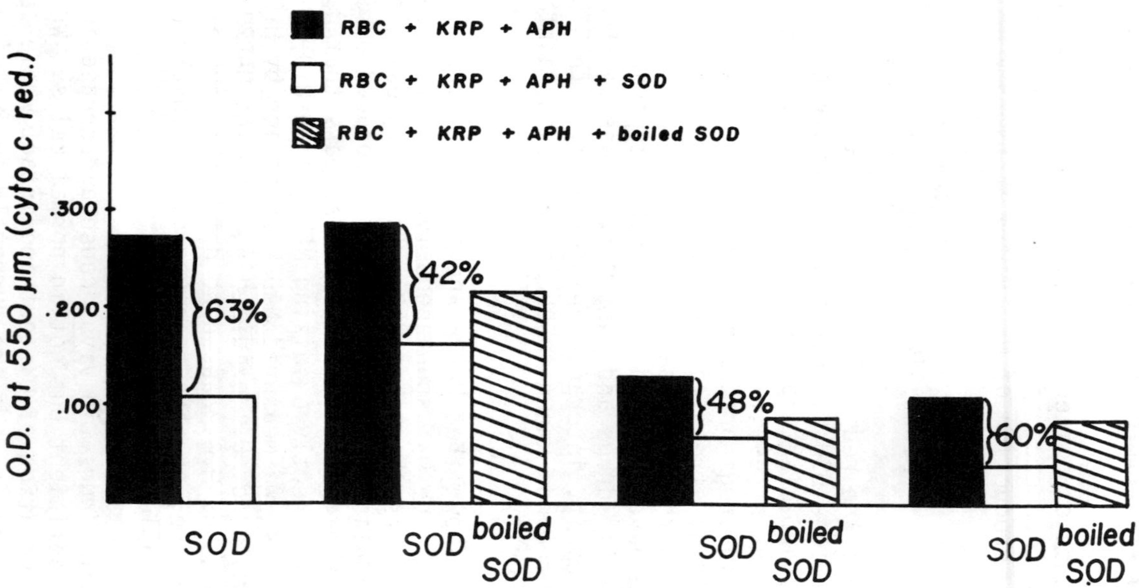

Figure 6. Reduction of cytochrome c by APH in washed, normal RBC's. This figure shows the production of $O_2^{\overline{\cdot}}$ by APH incubated with washed red cells. The concentration of cytochrome c in the first two experiments is double that in the last two experiments. All blood samples were from non-G-6-PD deficient individuals.

of the oxidants it produces. Hopefully this will give us more insight as to the nature of the oxidant stress seen in G-6-PD deficient hemolytic anemia.

Our hypothesis that $O_2^{\overline{\cdot}}$ generation is one of the initiating mechanisms for G-6-PD type hemolysis is supported by our findings that APH and menadione produce $O_2^{\overline{\cdot}}$. Menadione, as well as several other hemolytic drugs, have previously been found to produce H_2O_2 in vitro (Cohen and Hochstein, 1964). We speculate that some of this H_2O_2 production arises from the dismutation of $O_2^{\overline{\cdot}}$ produced by these drugs. We have found that the hemolytic drugs APH and menadione are capable of producing $O_2^{\overline{\cdot}}$ in the presence of suspended washed red cells, leading us to speculate that a common feature of the G-6-PD type hemolytic agents may be $O_2^{\overline{\cdot}}$ production. We would like to emphasize that we are not suggesting that $O_2^{\overline{\cdot}}$ is the only molecule causing damage, or even that it is the most important toxic molecule; we are suggesting that production of $O_2^{\overline{\cdot}}$ in the body may be a common route for initiating the hemolytic mechanism in G-6-PD deficiency. Besides the hemolytic drugs, fever, acidosis, and infection should also be examined for the possible production of $O_2^{\overline{\cdot}}$. It has recently been reported that $O_2^{\overline{\cdot}}$ is produced by phagocytizing polymorphonuclear leukocytes (Babior et al, 1973). This may be the source of the H_2O_2 these cells are also known to produce. The precipitation of G-6-PD type hemolytic anemia during infection, therefore, might be related to the release of $O_2^{\overline{\cdot}}$ or H_2O_2 by these leukocytes.

The possible effects of $O_2^{\overline{\cdot}}$ production on G-6-PD deficient red cell metabolism are shown in Figure 7. The production of $O_2^{\overline{\cdot}}$ by hemolytic agents could lead to a number of reactions making the cell more susceptible to hemolysis. The production of $O_2^{\overline{\cdot}}$ can cause loss of GSH by directly oxidizing NADPH, thereby decreasing the cofactor required for GSH reductase and decreasing the cell's ability to reduce oxidized glutathione. Superoxide, through its spontaneous or enzymatic conversion to H_2O_2 could also oxidize NADPH, resulting in the same consequences for GSH. Hydrogen peroxide is also capable of oxidizing GSH through glutathione peroxidase. A further drain on the cell's NADPH supply occurs

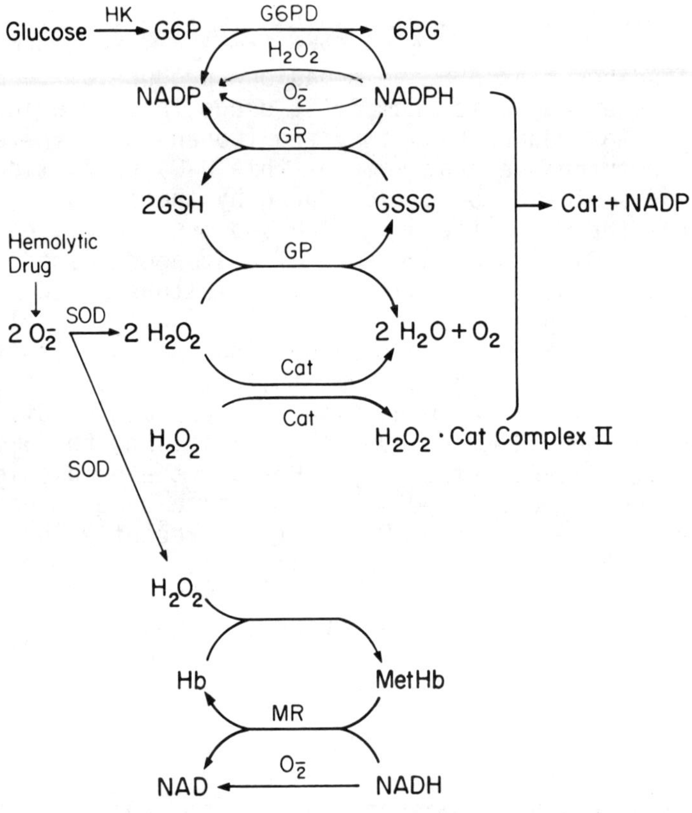

Figure 7. This figure summarizes the possible interactions of $O_2^{\dot{-}}$ with normal red cell metabolism. Key: GR is glutathione reductase; GP is glutathione peroxidase; cat. is catalase; MR is methemoglobin reductase; and HK is hexokinase. All other abbreviations are explained in the text.

when H_2O_2 reacts with catalase forming an inactive $H_2O_2\cdot$ catalase complex II. This complex requires NADPH oxidation for its dissolution. Hydrogen peroxide can oxidize hemoglobin to methemoglobin, and $O_2^{\cdot}$ can interfere with the reduction of methemoglobin by oxidizing NADH.

It thus appears that the production of $O_2^{\cdot}$ could interfere with red cell metabolism. Other investigators have recently shown that O_2^1 and $OH\cdot$, which are produced from $O_2^{\cdot}$ and its interactions with H_2O_2, are capable of oxidizing membrane lipids. These membrane alterations could make the cell more susceptible to lysis or to the action of the reticuloendothelial system. Thus we have at least four candidate molecules, $O_2^{\cdot}$, H_2O_2, O_2^1, and $OH\cdot$, acting alone or in concert, which may produce the hemolysis characteristic of G-6-PD deficiency.

ACKNOWLEDGEMENTS

This work was supported by NIH Training Grant 5-T01-GM-71.

REFERENCES

Babior, B.M., Kipnes, R.S., and Curnette, J.T. (1973)., J. Clin. Invest. 52:741
Beutler, E., Dern, R.J., Flanagan, C.L., and Alving, A.S. (1955)., J. Lab. Clin. Med. 45:286
Carson, P.E., Flanagan, C.L., Ickes, C.E., and Alving, A.S. (1956)., Science 124:484
Cohen, G., and Hochstein, P. (1964)., Biochemistry 3:895
Flanagan, C.L., Schrier, S.L., Carson, P.E., and Alving, A.S. (1958)., J. Lab. Clin. Med. 51:600
Gant, F.L., and Winhster, G.F. (1961)., Clinical Research 9:27
Khan, A.V. (1970)., Science 168:476
Leipzig, R.M., Brewer, G.J., and Oelshlegel, F.J. (1974)., Clinical Research 22:397A
McCord, J.M., and Fridovich, I. (1969)., J. Biol. Chem. 244:6049

Mengel, C.D., Metz, E., and Yancy, W.S. (1967)., Arch. Intern. Med. 119:287

Prins, H.K., and Loos, J.A. (1969) in Biochemical Methods in Red Cell Genetics (J.J. Yunis, ed.) Academic Press, p. 127

Reed, D.W., Passon, P.G., and Hultquist, D.E. (1970)., J. Biol. Chem. 245:2954

DISCUSSION

Dr. McCord: I may have missed this but did catalase have any inhibitory effects on NADH oxidation by superoxide generated by xanthine oxidase and xanthine or was that experiment done?

Ms. Leipzig: That experiment wasn't done.

Dr. McCord: That is a good experiment because it may well be hydroxyl radical generated by reaction of superoxide with hydrogen peroxide that's the actual oxidant. Dr. Bielski has reported fairly recently that superoxide will oxidize NADH bound to lactate dehydrogenase and I believe he could not see very much reaction with free NADH, although I don't know what sort of rate constants we're talking about. Maybe there was some oxidation of free NADH but the enzyme bound·NADH was oxidized much faster, I believe.

Dr. Cohen: I wondered if you looked at some of the other hemolytic agents? I have in mind the difficulty we had in working with primaquine added directly to erythrocytes and even in intact animals as we were fussing around trying to look for peroxide. I wonder if you experienced some of the same difficulties in your system.

Ms. Leipzig: We haven't used primaquine in this system, but prior to using the cytochrome c assay we assayed for $O_2^{\cdot}$ by adding NBT to whole blood. A large increase in reduced NBT was normally seen upon incubation of whole blood with NBT, but when we added primaquine to this system we found no reduction of NBT at all. We became concerned about the cellular permeability of NBT and its possible perturbations of cellular metabolism, and we therefore switched to a detection system which didn't enter the cell, that is, cytochrome c.

Dr. Brewer: There is a problem with primaquine in that it may require degradation in the animal or in the human to obtain an active metabolite. We have stayed away from it because of the difficulties in knowing what the actual molecule is that causes the hemolysis.

Dr. McCord: It might be a good idea to assay your boiled SOD because it is not impossible that it is still partly active. Depending upon the ionic strength, it can survive boiling. It is a very tough enzyme.

Ms. Leipzig: We're planning to do that. We have found that with increased boiling time we are getting a decreased inhibition.

Dr. Cohen: I would add an "Amen" to that because we had a lot of difficulty at first by assuming that if we boil the enzyme for a few minutes that we were doing something biological to it. It is quite resistant, at least under our conditions. What is the direction of effect with ionic strength?

Dr. McCord: At low ionic strength the enzyme is more stable to boiling.

Dr. Hoekstra: I'd like to emphasize Dr. McCay's point once more because I think it could be extremely important. According to his observations, iron in a chelated form in a system at the site where these reactions are going on is extremely important. McCay uses ADP-ferric iron; ATP-ferric iron is not as good. The longer he stores the ADP-iron, the more effective it becomes. The nature of this chelated iron is not well understood, but it is clearly very important. Where you don't get these effects outside the cell and you do inside, it may be caused by differences in chelated iron, such as hemoglobin, etc. McCay implied to me that ordinary phosphate buffer usually has sufficient iron to cause this catalysis, which he regards primarily as the production of hydroxyl radicals. Sucrose containing media also usually have sufficient iron impurity to cause such catalysis, but a number of other buffer systems do not. I think that differences in chelated iron may be very important in determining the results of experiments such as yours.

Dr. Eaton: Apropos of ways of inhibiting superoxide dismutase, I might mention that we've recently found that incubation of the enzyme with very high concentrations of penicillamine may be a good way of inhibiting it, perhaps more effective than boiling.

Dr. Cohen: That is very exciting. But it seems very strange. Penicillamine is given in such large doses in patients who have Wilson's disease.

Dr. Eaton: That is right, but I doubt if these doses even approach those we've used in vitro.

Dr. Cohen: It is also an inhibitor of glutathione peroxidase; partially an inhibitor. I have one more comment. I guess I wasn't surprised when I saw the data that catalase added to the outside of red blood cells was ineffective in stopping whatever was being generated by xanthine oxidase from producing damage on the inside. The reason I'm not surprised is that there is so much catalase on the inside as well. You can destroy a good part of a high level of peroxide with catalase but it is that steady state level that escapes the external catalase that can still penetrate and escape the internal catalase and still continue to produce loss of glutathione through the reaction of glutathione peroxidase. I don't mean to exclude other possibilities such as hydroxyl radicals, but I think the data are still consistent with some simplistic thoughts about its just being peroxide.

Dr. Geyer: Does a high Vitamin C dose given orally cause trouble in these patients?

Dr. Brewer: Years ago we gave Vitamin C in high doses to G6PD deficient subjects and saw a slight shortening of the chromium 51 survival, but it was relatively insignificant.

Dr. Geyer: What happens if you give intravenous Vitamin C and some iron at the same time? What I'm getting at is iron-Vitamin C capable of doing this or have you tried it in your system in vitro?

Dr. Brewer: We haven't, but it might be interesting.

Dr. Geyer: In work we reported years ago, Vitamin C and ferrous iron were able to tear saturated fatty acids apart starting at the carboxyl end, and if you had various types of SH compounds present you got all sorts of different results in keeping with what I think Dr. Hoekstra is saying. This is an extremely potent agent and hydrogen peroxide with iron or any of the other combinations we tried would not do this.

FREE RADICALS AND INFLAMMATION: STUDIES ON SUPEROXIDE-MEDIATED NBT REDUCTION BY LEUKOCYTES

Joe M. McCord and Marvin L. Salin

Departments of Biochemistry and Medicine
Duke University Medical Center, Durham, N.C.

Superoxide dismutases are present in all oxygen-metabolizing organisms. They serve to scavenge the superoxide radical, a reactive and potentially detrimental free radical intermediate and by-product of oxygen reduction, by catalyzing its dismutation:

$$O_2^-\cdot \;+\; O_2^-\cdot \;+\; 2H^+ \longrightarrow H_2O_2 \;+\; O_2 \;.$$

The enzyme appears to be vital for oxygen-metabolizing organisms. Strict anaerobes, organisms which die upon exposure to air, lack the enzyme (McCord et al., 1971). A temperature sensitive mutant of *Escherichia coli* deficient in superoxide dismutase when grown at 43°C was also unable to tolerate the presence of oxygen at the elevated temperature, and became functionally a strict anaerobe (McCord et al., 1973). Mammalian tissues contain two distinct types of superoxide dismutases. One is cytosolic, containing two atoms of copper and two atoms of zinc per molecule (McCord and Fridovich, 1969). It is composed of two identical subunits and has a molecular weight of 31,400. The other

---

This work was supported by USPHS Research Grant AM 17091 and by a USPHS Postdoctoral Research Fellowship NS 01322 to Dr. Salin.

enzyme is located in the mitochondria and is a tetrameric molecule with a molecular weight of approximately 80,000. It contains two moles of manganese per mole of enzyme (Weisiger and Fridovich, 1973). Together, these superoxide dismutases are very effective scavengers of any superoxide generated within the cell. It may be calculated from their reactivities with the superoxide radical and from their concentrations in liver, for example, that the average lifetime of $O_2^{-}\cdot$ in the cell is decreased by about six orders of magnitude by their presence. Mammalian extracellular fluids, however, contain only very small amounts of superoxide dismutase activity. Table I compares the concentrations of superoxide dismutase in several extracellular fluids with those of two representative tissues: liver and erythrocytes. Other tissues examined have activities within this range. The extracellular fluids contain concentrations of the enzyme two to three orders of magnitude lower than intracellular levels. These concentrations are not negligible, but they can not completely scavenge the superoxide that might be generated in such fluids. Thus, although the interior contents of cells are well protected against superoxide-induced damage, the extracellular components and the exterior surfaces of cells bathed by the various extracellular fluids

TABLE I. Superoxide Dismutase Concentrations in Various Tissues and Fluids

	mg/l
Erythrocytes	100
Liver	500
Blood plasma	0.7
Synovial fluid	1.0
Cerebrospinal fluid	0.35
Aqueous humor	0.9

enjoy, at best, only partial protection against any superoxide that may be generated in these fluids (McCord, 1974). We might infer from the relative lack of extracellular superoxide dismutase that extracellular sources of superoxide are not sufficiently large under normal physiological conditions to cause much of a problem. We might suppose, however, that if under abnormal conditions a sizable amount of superoxide were to be generated extracellularly, damage to extracellular components or to exterior cell surfaces might result. The work of Dr. Babior and coworkers has provided insight into one such source of superoxide production in extracellular spaces-- the metabolically activated, phagocytosing polymorphonuclear leukocyte (PMN) (Babior et al., 1973). It was originally suggested that superoxide was produced by the phagocytosing PMN as a bactericidal agent. A considerable body of evidence now supports that hypothesis (Johnston et al., 1973; Yost and Fridovich, 1974; Curnutte et al., 1974). The important feature for the present consideration, however, is that a substantial fraction of the superoxide which is generated by the PMN escapes into the extracellular medium. In an inflamed or infected tissue, the interstitial space may be heavily infiltrated with activated, perhaps phagocytosing, PMN. If these cells are exposing the surrounding tissue to a flux of superoxide, this free radical is a likely candidate as a chemical mediator of inflammation.

The experiments described in the following were designed to shed some light on the possible role of superoxide in cell-mediated inflammation.

MATERIALS AND METHODS

Isolation of cells. All procedures employed plastic or siliconized glass containers. Venous blood was drawn from human volunteers into heparinized syringes. The blood was diluted fourfold with 0.9% saline and, following the procedure of Boyum (1967), the monocytes and lymphocytes were isolated in a Ficoll-Hypaque gradient. The pellet containing the erythrocytes and PMN was brought to the original volume with 0.9% saline, then an equal volume of 3% dextran (Sigma Chemical Co., St. Louis, Mo., average mol wt 500,000) in 0.9% saline was added. After 20 min of sedimentation under gravity, the supernate was withdrawn and centrifuged at 120 g for 10 min. The pellet containing PMN was freed of contaminating erythrocytes by suspension in 10 ml of 0.2% saline followed 30 sec later by the addition of 10 ml of 1.6% saline and centrifugation at 120 g. This hypotonic lysis of erythrocytes was repeated until the pellet was visibly free of erythrocytes. The leukocyte pellet was then suspended in 0.5 ml of Ringer-phosphate buffer, pH 7.4, and microscopically examined. Cell viability, as judged by ability to exclude trypan blue, was greater than 98%. The cells were greater than 98% PMN with less than one platelet per four PMN.

Alternately, a mixed population of leukocytes containing greater than 80% PMN could be isolated by omission of the Ficoll-Hypaque gradient.

Polyacrylamide disc gel electrophoresis. The procedure of Davis (1964) was used with 10% acrylamide resolving gels. The activity staining procedure described by Beauchamp and Fridovich (1971) was modified as follows: gels were soaked in individual tubes in the dark for 40 min in a single solution containing 50 mM potassium phosphate, pH 7.8, 1 mM EDTA, 0.25 mM nitroblue tetrazolium (NBT), 20 mM tetramethylethylenediamine, and 0.03 mM riboflavin. Where indicated, the staining solution also contained 1 mM potassium cyanide. The solution was prepared in subdued light immediately before use. After the soaking period, the gels were removed from the solution and exposed to an incandescent desk lamp for about 20 min. The photogenerated $O_2^-\cdot$ reduced the NBT to the insoluble purple formazan, except at the areas where superoxide dismutase scavenged the radical, resulting in achromatic bands. Human liver, electrophoresed for comparison to leukocytes, was obtained from autopsy at Duke University Medical Center. Approximately 2 g of tissue was homogenized at 4°C in 40 ml of Ringer-phosphate buffer and centrifuged at 5,000 g for 10 min. The supernate was used for electrophoresis.

Quantitative NBT test. The quantitative NBT test was performed in 10 x 75 mm siliconized test tubes, containing a total volume of 1.0 ml of Ringer-phosphate buffer with 5% autologous plasma. The incubation mixture contained 1.0 mM NBT and approximately 5 x 10^6 leukocytes. Where indicated, the leukocytes were stimulated by the addition of 10^8 *E. coli* cells which had been washed in deionized water and stored frozen. Superoxide dismutase was also added where indicated. Tubes were incubated in a water bath at 37°C and at intervals, aliquots were removed and 200 to 300 cells were microscopically counted. Cells containing the dark blue formazan particles were scored as NBT-positive. Results are expressed as percent NBT-positive cells. The extraction of the formazan by pyridine and its spectrophotometric determination were performed by the method of Baehner and Nathan (1968). The superoxide dismutase used was prepared from human erythrocytes or from bovine liver by the method of McCord and Fridovich (1969), or was obtained from Diagnostic Data, Inc., Mountain View, California. Endotoxin from *Salmonella typhosa* was obtained from Difco Laboratories, Detroit, Michigan. A lymphokine preparation was kindly provided by Mr. Linville Meadows.

RESULTS

The results of activity-stained disc gel electrophoresis of a sonicated preparation of human PMN are shown in Fig. 1, with supernate from homogenized human liver for comparison. The two preparations show identical cyanide-sensitive and cyanide-insensitive bands of superoxide dismutase activity. Identical results were also obtained with other human tissues. We conclude that PMN contain intracellular superoxide dismutases which are apparently identical to the cytoplasmic copper-zinc (cyanide-sensitive) enzyme and the mitochondrial manganese (cyanide-insensitive) enzyme found in other tissues which have been examined (Fridovich, 1974).

It is a well-known and clinically useful fact that activated leukocytes reduce NBT (Baehner and Nathan, 1968). Since PMN have been shown to produce superoxide (Babior et

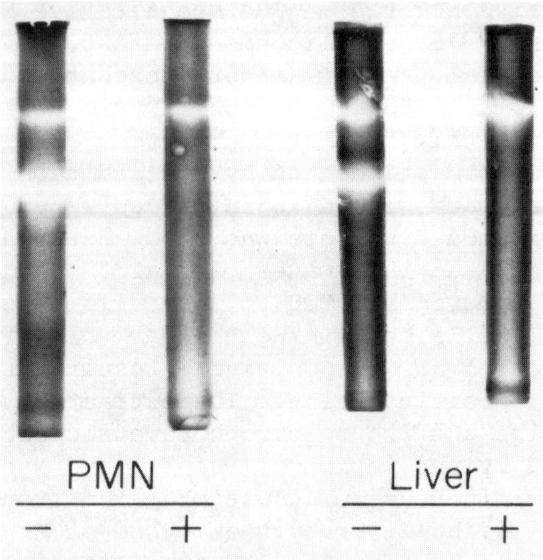

Figure 1. Results of polyacrylamide gel electrophoresis stained for superoxide dismutase activity. Gels labeled PMN received 30 µl of a sonicated suspension of human polymorphonuclear leukocytes containing 10^8 cells/ml. Gels labeled Liver received 5 µl of the human liver preparation described under METHODS. The gels designated + were stained in the presence of 1 mM potassium cyanide.

al., 1973), and since superoxide has been shown to be an efficient reductant of NBT (Beauchamp and Fridovich, 1971), it follows that at least part of the NBT reduction by leukocytes may be due to superoxide released in the medium. The susceptibility of NBT reduction by phagocytosing PMN to inhibition by the addition of exogenous superoxide dismutase is shown in Fig. 2. A considerable baseline of NBT reduction exists in resting cells which shows little or no response to the addition of superoxide dismutase to the medium. This is probably due to a variety of intracellular dehydrogenases which are capable of reducing NBT directly. If the cells are phagocytosing *E. coli*, however, the rate of formation of NBT-positive cells is increased from two- to four-fold for a time. This

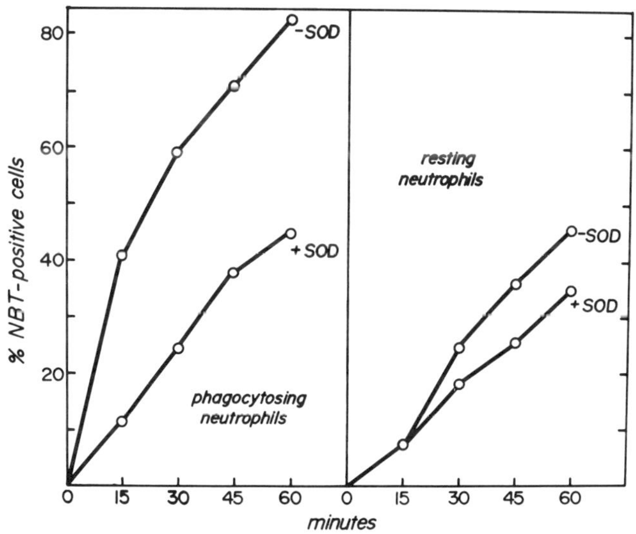

Figure 2. Effect of superoxide dismutase on NBT reduction by phagocytosing and resting PMN. Incubations contained 5 x 10^6 leukocytes, with (phagocytosing) or without (resting) E. coli as described under METHODS. Those labeled + SOD contained 500 µg of superoxide dismutase.

phagocytosis-induced enhancement of NBT reduction can be almost completely inhibited by the addition of superoxide dismutase. The response of the phagocytosis-induced component of NBT reduction to increasing amounts of superoxide dismutase in the medium is shown in Fig. 3. Since superoxide dismutase and NBT are in direct competition for $O_2^-\cdot$, the point at which 50% inhibition is obtained is a function of the relative concentrations of the two scavengers. The concentration of NBT used in the experiment described in Fig. 3 was 1 mM, which essentially saturated the rate of phagocytosis-induced NBT reduction in the absence of added superoxide dismutase.

On occasion, NBT reduction was quantitatively determined by pyridine extraction of the incubation mixtures, in addition

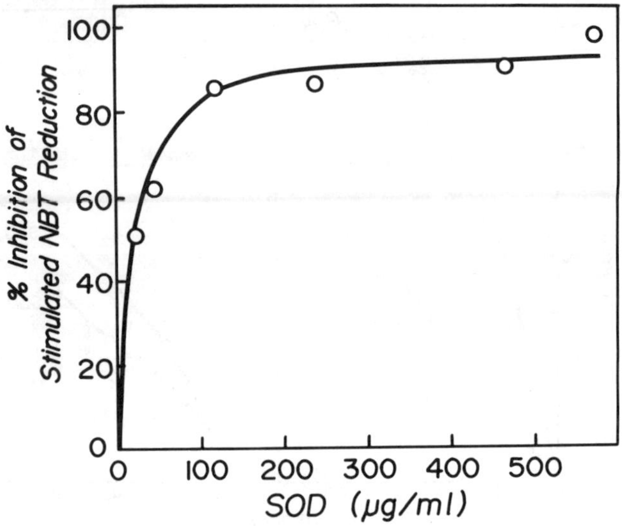

Figure 3. Inhibition of phagocytosis-induced NBT reduction by superoxide dismutase. Incubations were performed as described under METHODS, in the presence of E. coli and with the indicated amounts of superoxide dismutase. Complete inhibition indicates stimulated and resting NBT scores are identical.

to microscopic counting of NBT-positive cells. These two methods were in excellent agreement in all experiments involving PMN.

It is known that a variety of stimuli can cause increased rates of NBT reduction by PMN, and that particles to phagocytose are not an absolute requirement. Since there are two components to NBT reduction by PMN (a baseline rate not inhibited by superoxide dismutase, and a stimulated rate which is totally due to superoxide liberated from the cells), it seemed important to determine how each of these two components is affected by various other stimuli. Fig. 4 illustrates the effects of two soluble factors, endotoxin and lymphokine, on NBT reduction by isolated PMN. The endotoxin is a soluble

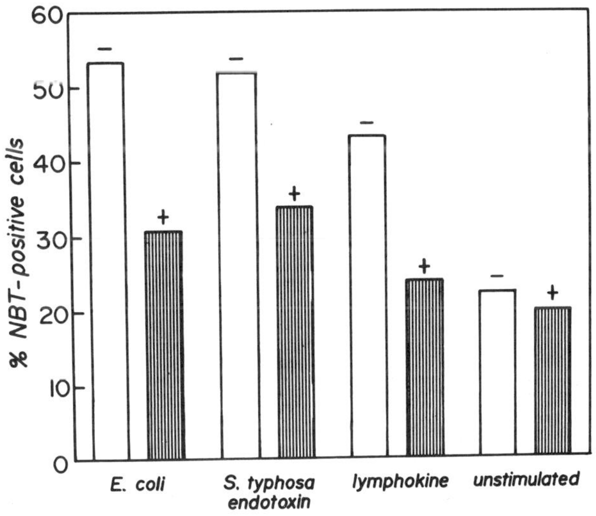

Figure 4. Effects of several stimulants on superoxide production by PMN. Incubations were performed as described under METHODS, with the following additions: E. coli, 10^8 cells; S. typhosa endotoxin, 400 µg; lymphokine, a ten-fold dilution of supernate from 10^6 concanavalin A-stimulated lymphocytes per ml. Superoxide dismutase was present where indicated (+) at 450 µg/ml.

lipopolysaccharide preparation from S. typhosa. Lymphokine represents one or more soluble mediators of inflammation released from lymphocytes which are incubated with a non-specific mitogen (such as concanavalin A) or with an antigen to which they have been sensitized (Snyderman and Altman, 1973). Lymphokine is a chemotactic factor for other leukocytes. While the baseline or uninhibitible NBT reduction showed a modest increase in the presence of all three stimuli, the superoxide mediated NBT reduction showed a dramatic increase in each case. We conclude that phagocytosis of particles is not the only circumstance which "turns on" superoxide production by PMN.

The data presented above have dealt with superoxide production by PMN. Can other phagocytic leukocytes such as monocytes produce superoxide? A mixed population of monocytes and lymphocytes was isolated using a Ficoll-Hypaque gradient. A differential count of Wright stained cells revealed approximately 11% monocytes and 89% lymphocytes. The cell preparation was tested for its ability to reduce NBT under the same conditions used for PMN. Cell density in the incubation mixtures was 2.5×10^6 cells/ml. When the cells were microscopically examined, essentially none showed the characteristic inclusion of purple formazan particles. A visual inspection of the incubation mixtures, however, showed that the tube containing stimulated cells without superoxide dismutase was distinctly more purple than the mixture containing stimulated cells plus superoxide dismutase. This was confirmed by a pyridine extraction of the formazan in the mixtures, and the results are shown in Table II. It appears that phagocytosing monocytes release superoxide which reduces NBT in the medium, but that they do not phagocytose the formazan particles as readily as do PMN.

TABLE II.

NBT Reduction by a Population of Monocytes and Lymphocytes

	$O.D._{515}$
Stimulated leukocytes	
- superoxide dismutase	0.692
+ superoxide dismutase	0.450
Nonstimulated leukocytes	
- superoxide dismutase	0.463
+ superoxide dismutase	0.455

DISCUSSION

Reports appeared in the literature at approximately the same time that PMN were lacking a cytoplasmic superoxide dismutase (Beckman et al., 1973) and that PMN, when phagocytosing, liberated significant amounts of superoxide into the medium (Babior et al., 1973). These two observations seemed to fit together quite well. The most logical explanation seemed to be that cytoplasmic metabolism should be stimulated by the events of phagocytosis, leading to increased production of superoxide in the cytoplasm. With no superoxide dismutase there to scavenge it, a large part of the superoxide would diffuse out of the cell and into the medium. Perhaps it could diffuse into the phagocytic vacuole to participate in bactericidal action. Our finding of both cytoplasmic and mitochondrial superoxide dismutases in PMN, which has been described elsewhere in greater detail (Salin and McCord, 1974), calls for a revision of the above hypothesis. The amount of cytoplasmic superoxide dismutase present in the PMN eliminates the possibility of cytoplasmic generation of the radical and diffusion out of the cell. Rather, it seems more plausible that superoxide is generated on the outer surface of the cell membrane. It is this surface, of course, that invaginates to line the phagocytic vacuole. If superoxide is generated intentionally by the cell for a bactericidal purpose, the cell might ideally prefer to generate the radical only on that portion of the outer membrane which is actually used to line the vacuole. If this could be accomplished, no superoxide would escape into the medium, as it would have to diffuse through cytoplasm which contains superoxide dismutase on its way out of the cell. Apparently, though, the radical is generated on membrane surface still in contact with the external medium, and much of the superoxide escapes its intended purpose of bombardment of a captive bacterium and instead may merely serve to provide chemical insult to surrounding healthy tissue. What explanation can we offer for the phagocyte's less than optimal control over this potentially detrimental chemical weapon? Perhaps it is a reflection of the relative evolutionary newness of the immune response system that a more sophisticated set of controls does not exist. If our understanding of the cell's reason for generating superoxide is correct, other inappropriate responses of the system are demonstrated by the results shown in Fig. 4. Here we see that superoxide production may be triggered by stimuli which do not directly or even necessarily involve bacteria. Thus, one might suspect that any stimulus which "turns on" a leukocyte in any way may result in turning on superoxide production. One might further suspect that any tissue which experiences an infiltration of leukocytes also experiences a perhaps purposeless bombardment by superoxide radicals. In rheumatoid arthritis, for example, huge numbers of activated PMN invade the synovial fluid of an affected joint. In vitro studies have shown that superoxide, via secondary reaction with hydrogen peroxide to generate the hydroxyl radical, is capable of causing depolymerization of purified hyaluronic acid or of whole synovial fluid, a characteristic of rheumatoid arthritis (McCord, 1974). It may be calculated from the numbers of PMN commonly found in diseased joints, and from the amounts of superoxide such cells can produce in vitro, that superoxide-mediated depolymerization is quantitatively feasible as the in vivo mechanism for synovial fluid degradation. The possible role of superoxide in various disease states is expanded by the realization that PMN are not alone in their ability to produce the radical. Our mixed preparation of monocytes and lymphocytes liberated a considerable amount of superoxide into the medium when given E. coli and serum, presumably due to the phagocytic monocytes. Karnovsky (1974) has reported that phagocytosing mouse macrophages liberate amounts of superoxide comparable to PMN. Obviously, a great deal remains to be discovered regarding the specific mechanism of superoxide production by leukocytes and the specific roles the radical may play as a chemical mediator of inflammation. One obvious implication remains to be made. If superoxide is a mediator of inflammation, superoxide dismutase might be expected to display anti-inflammatory activity under certain conditions. Several reports to this effect have already appeared (Lund-Olesen and Menander, 1974; Autor, 1974; Davies and Davies, 1974).

The clinical usefulness of the unstimulated NBT test for diagnosis of bacterial infection has been greatly weakened by the recognition that a great many conditions other than bacterial infections can cause false positive tests (Bittner et al., 1973). In view of the response of the superoxide-producing mechanism to such stimuli as lymphokine, for example, it is not difficult to understand such false positives. It is also possible, however, that some of the false positive conditions result from an increased "baseline" rate of NBT reduction, which would not be inhibited by exogenous superoxide dismutase. It might therefore be worthwhile to re-examine such conditions, performing the NBT test in the presence and absence of exogenous superoxide dismutase. Perhaps this added dimension would render the test more meaningful.

SUMMARY

Reduction of nitroblue tetrazolium (NBT) by leukocytes is a process which appears to consist of two components. Resting cells reduce NBT in a manner which cannot be inhibited by exogenous superoxide dismutase. Cells which are metabolically stimulated by incubation with E. coli, endotoxin, or lymphokine reduce the dye at rates two to four times the unstimulated or resting rate. All of the stimulated enhancement of NBT reduction is susceptible to inhibition by superoxide dismutase in the medium. We propose that activated leukocytes produce $O_2^{-}\cdot$ on the outer surface of their cell membrane and that much of the superoxide escapes its intended bactericidal purpose, becoming instead a chemical mediator of inflammation.

REFERENCES

Autor, A. P. (1974) Reduction of paraquat toxicity by superoxide dismutase. Life Science 14: 1309.

Babior, B., Kipnes, R., and Curnutte, J. (1973) Biological defense mechanisms: The production by leukocytes of superoxide, a potential bactericidal agent. J. Clin. Invest. 52: 741.

Baehner, R. L., and Nathan, D. G. (1968) Quantitative nitroblue tetrazolium test in chronic granulomatous disease. New Engl. J. Med. 278: 971.

Beauchamp, C. O., and Fridovich, I. (1971) Superoxide dismutase Improved assays and an assay applicable to acrylamide gels. Analyt. Biochem. 44: 276.

Beckman, G., Lundgren, E., and Tarnvik, A. (1973) Superoxide dismutase isozymes in different human tissues, their genetic control and intracellular localization. Human Heredity 23: 338.

Bittner, S., Kieff, E., Windhorst, D., and Meier, P. (1973) The use of the unstimulated nitroblue tetrazolium test as a routine screening test for bacterial infection in an adult population: A reassessment. Am. J. Clin. Pathol. 60: 843.

Boyum, A. (1967) Isolation of mononuclear cells and granulocytes from human blood. Scand. J. Clin. Lab. Invest. 21 (suppl. 97): 77.

Curnutte, J., Whitten, D., and Babior, B. (1974) Defective superoxide production by granulocytes from patients with chronic granulomatous disease. New Engl. J. Med. 290: 593.

Davies, D. S., and Davies, D. L. (1974) Effect of D-propanolol and superoxide dismutase on paraquat reduction and adrenochrome formation by rat liver microsomes. Fed. Proc. 33: 228 (Abstract).

Davis, B. (1964) Disc electrophoresis II. Method and application to human serum proteins. Ann. N. Y. Acad. Sci. 121: 404.

Fridovich, I. (1974) Superoxide dismutases, in A. Meister (ed.) Advances in Enzymology, John Wiley & Sons, New York, vol. 41, pp 35-97.

Johnston, R., Jr., Keele, B., Webb, L., Kessler, D., and Rajagopalan, K. V. (1973) Inhibition of phagocytic bactericidal activity by superoxide dismutase: A possible role for superoxide anion in the killing of phagocytized bacteria. J. Clin. Invest. 52: 44a (Abstract).

Karnovsky, M. L. (1974) Biochemical aspects of the functions of polymorphonuclear and mononuclear leukocytes, in J. Bellanti and D. H. Dayton (eds.), Conference on the Phagocytic Cell in Host Resistance. Raven Press, New York.

Lund-Olesen, K., and Menander, K. (1974) Orgotein: A new anti-inflammatory metalloprotein drug: Preliminary evaluation of clinical efficacy and safety in degenerative joint disease. Curr. Therap. Res. 16: 706.

McCord, J. M., and Fridovich, I. (1969) Superoxide dismutase: An enzymic function for erythrocuprein (hemocuprein). J. Biol. Chem. 244: 6049.

McCord, J. M., Keele, B., and Fridovich, I. (1971) An enzyme-based theory of obligate anaerobiosis: The physiological function of superoxide dismutase. Proc. Natl. Acad. Sci. USA 68: 1024.

McCord, J. M., Beauchamp, C., Goscin, S., Misra, H., and Fridovich, I. (1973) Superoxide and superoxide dismutase, in T. E. King, H. S. Mason, and M. Morrison (eds.), Oxidases and Related Redox Systems. University Park Press, Baltimore, vol. 1, pp 51-76.

McCord, J. M. (1974) Free radicals and inflammation: Protection of synovial fluid by superoxide dismutase. Science 185: 529.

Salin, M. L., and McCord, J. M. (1974) Superoxide dismutases in polymorphonuclear leukocytes. J. Clin. Invest. 54: 1005.

Snyderman, R., and Altman, L. (1973) Mediators of delayed hypersensitivity, in C. A. Frazier (ed.), Annual Review of Allergy. Med. Exam. Publ. Co., Flushing, New York, p. 377.

Weisiger, R. A., and Fridovich, I. (1973) Superoxide dismutase Organelle specificity. J. Biol. Chem. 248: 3582.

Yost, F. J., Jr., and Fridovich, I. (1974) Superoxide radicals and phagocytosis. Arch. Biochem. Biophys. 161: 395.

DISCUSSION

Dr. Babior: I was wondering if you could tell me what the relative quantity of SOD in white cells is compared with, say, red cells or liver.

Dr. McCord: It's less. The concentration in the cytoplasm is probably about a tenth as much as red cells. That is low, in fact lower than any other tissue we've looked at.

Dr. Perutz: Listening to talks about the superoxide dismutase at the International Congress of Chemistry in Stockholm last summer, I understood people to say that these white cells actually liberate H_2O_2 rather than superoxide itself.

Dr. McCord: They do liberate H_2O_2 and it's not clear if that is produced secondarily from the dismutation of superoxide or if it is generated directly. Probably it is generated by the dismutation of superoxide. Probably the oxygen is first reduced univalently and then enzymatically or spontaneously dismutates.

Dr. Perutz: I'm afraid I may have missed something but I didn't quite get what is the enzyme responsible for the actual production of the superoxide itself in those cells?

Dr. McCord: That is a very intriguing question and I think I'll leave that for Dr. Babior since he will have some things to say about it. There is an O_2 consumption burst that is associated with the activation of white cells and it's NADH dependent or NADPH dependent, so presumably there is an NADH or an NADPH oxidase that is making the superoxide.

Dr. Perutz: From what?

Dr. McCord: From molecular oxygen. I would propose that this enzyme is located on the membrane surface of the leukocytes. I propose that because I don't think cytoplasmically generated superoxide could get past the cytoplasmic SOD to escape from the cell. If the oxidase is located on the membrane surface, this invaginates to line the phagocytic vacuole. I think the cell can't discriminate between that portion of the membrane which is going to line the vacuole and that which is still covering the outside of the cell. So I envision the activated white cell as making superoxide on most, if not all, of its outer membrane surface, parts of which will invaginate to make vacuoles.

Dr. Perutz: I was most intrigued by this superoxide story. In my student days and later I attended D. Keilin's lectures on heme enzymes because every year he would tell us something interesting and new. He always lectured about catalase, but was embarrased when you asked him what catalase was for. At that time there was no reason to suppose that any H_2O_2 was actually produced in vivo, so why would all cells need catalase? It was only now, many many years later, that we realized why white cells must have catalase. They need it to mop up the H_2O_2 that is produced by the superoxide dismutase.

Dr. McCord: A lot of hydrogen peroxide is produced directly. It can come from enzymes and from oxidations that do not go via superoxide intermediate.

Dr. Eaton: The dogma has been that peroxide was central in the killing of bacteria. Yet it now appears that superoxide itself is quite significant. Would you care to comment on this?

Dr. McCord: Again, I think I'll let Dr. Babior do that. He is more qualified to discuss that aspect than I am. I would like to state that I think there are a number of bactericidal mechanisms in the white cell and that superoxide may play a major role in one of these mechanisms, but by no means accounts for the killing of every bacterium that is encountered.

Dr. Fee: Did you, in your system, ever see any inhibition of phagocytic activity by added dismutase?

Dr. McCord: We did not look at that but others have and did not. I believe that is Johnston and coworkers. I don't know if that's in print or not but SOD apparently does not inhibit phagocytosis.

Dr. Fee: If the chairman will allow me, I would like to take about one minute to make a comment toward something that Joe McCord has presented and also directed toward something that Dr. Hoekstra has told us. This deals with the Haber-Weiss reaction. Now Joe and I have had a long-standing argument; Joe has put his argument on paper and I have not. The Haber-Weiss reaction was postulated in 1934 (F. Haber and J. Weiss, Proc. Roy. Soc. A. 147, 332 (1934)) to account for the fact that iron salts added to peroxide would actually decompose more peroxide than could be stoichiometrically accounted for. Therefore, a chain reaction was postulated. The reaction that was postulated is the so-called Haber Weiss reaction between peroxide and superoxide,

$$O_2^{\dot{-}} + H_2O_2 + H^+ \rightarrow {}^{\bullet}OH + H_2O + O_2$$

Today, many biochemists treat the Haber-Weiss reaction as if it were a fact. This has its roots in some sort of logic and the basic points of that logic are first of all that it is now generally accepted, if not stated, that superoxide ion itself is not a very strong or potentially dangerous cytotoxin. Therefore, secondly, it is assumed to be the progenitor of something which is cytotoxic. The Haber-Weiss reaction was a convenient mechanism for that because it produced the well-known hydroxyl radical, the extreme reactivity of which is well documented in the chemical literature. The third point of logic is that in these myriad effects of superoxide dismutase and catalase one often finds cases where both enzymes are affecting the reaction or observation. Therefore one argues that catalase takes care of peroxide, superoxide dismutase takes care of superoxide and the production of toxic ${}^{\bullet}OH$ via the Haber-Weiss reaction is wiped out. The fourth point is that there is an absolute specificity assumed for these enzymes. I think even Joe will admit that a study of the specificity of the dismutases has never been done. So, if one assumes that the Haber-Weiss reaction goes then a vehicle has been provided for preserving the status quo of the superoxide toxicity.

However, a search of the chemical literature reveals that the Haber-Weiss reaction has never been observed. An attempt to observe the reaction was made in 1938 (Bray, J. Am. Chem. Soc., 60, 82 (1938)), and it was concluded that it did not go. In a very careful study by Philip George, (Disc. Faraday Soc. 2, 196, 219 (1947)), he also concluded that it did not go. Finally, radiation chemists have never observed any effects attributible to a reaction between $O_2^{\cdot-}$ and hydrogen peroxide (e.g., J. Rabini and S.O. Nielsen, J. Phys. Chem. 73, 3736 (1969)). The point I wish to make is that if we're going to discuss the effects observed in these systems, we should consider something that has a basis in physical reality. Can someone test, seriously test, the Haber-Weiss reaction? I think that the chemical results which have been published will stand. We're going to have to look for something else.

Dr. McCord: Let me respond first to the last point. The laboratory of Dr. Irwin Fridovich will have data forthcoming which I hope will put some of this to rest. To one of your first comments I'd like to respond that we don't treat the Haber-Weiss reaction as fact. I treat it as a hypothetical reaction with which much of our data is consistent and for which you cannot provide me a reasonable alternative, even on paper. If you provide a reaction that is equally as consistent with our data and will give me a compound X that will replace the hydroxyl radical, I'd be very happy. Many phenomena have been observed that are inhibited by both superoxide dismutase and by catalase and by scavengers of the hydroxyl radical like ethanol, benzoate and some others. All of this is perfectly consistent with that very simple little reaction. As far as the inability of radiation chemists to document it, according to my conversations with Dr. Bielski, no one has ever really looked to document it. No one has tried to test it. He too had some intuitive dislike for that reaction, but he couldn't really answer why. I, for one, am very open to accepting a substitute for that reaction, but I think you're going to have to propose a substitute because we can't just say that this phenomenon is inhibited by SOD, by catalase, and by benzoate, and we don't know what the heck is going on. I think the Haber-

Weiss reaction nicely fills the bill and if something comes along that is obviously better, we'll accept it. But until then, I think we have to grab for whatever hypothetical reaction works.

Dr. Cohen: The comment was that these were the effects of trace metals?

Dr. Fee: Yes. I think the results of McCay are extremely important here because what you're talking about is a reaction that proceeds as you write it. Now if your system contains a bunch of iron, then the hypothetical reaction of H_2O_2 with the $O_2^{\dot{-}}$ will be replaced by the known reaction between the H_2O_2 and Fe^{++}. O.K., that's my answer to that.

Dr. McCord: But are you saying that Fe^{++} will, for example, make ethylene from methional or depolymerize hyaluronic acid? Because it won't.

Dr. Fee: I think it will, yes. In the presence of hydrogen peroxide, very definitely.

Dr. McCord: In the presence of hydrogen peroxide by making hydroxyl radical?

Dr. Fee: Yes.

Dr. McCord: Well, that is essentially the same reaction.

Dr. Fee: It is?

Dr. McCord: You're simply saying that it's iron catalyzed. I wouldn't find that at all objectionable. I see no reason for including iron in the reaction scheme, however, until we have data that suggest such a role. The reaction we propose is the simplest one consistent with our data.

Dr. Fee: The fact is that Fe^{++} can do it and $O_2^{\dot{-}}$ cannot do it.

Dr. Hoekstra: I'm strickly a second-hand expert, but McCay's idea is that the $O_2^{\cdot}$ dismutates to form hydrogen peroxide and oxygen, the $O_2^{\cdot}$ also reacts with ADP-complexed ferric iron to produce ferrous iron complex, and the ferrous iron complex then reacts with hydrogen peroxide to produce hydroxyl radical. In this way the iron complex catalyses or causes the production of $^{\cdot}OH$ from $O_2^{\cdot}$.

Dr. Fee: That is the Fenton reaction.

Dr. Cohen: I'd like to invite the participants in this debate to remain on and continue the debate after the last speaker, but I think the audience should have the opportunity to hear Dr. Babior if that's what they have come for. You're welcome to remain on afterwards.

SUPEROXIDE AND THE OXYGEN-REQUIRING BACTERICIDAL PROCESSES OF GRANULOCYTES

Bernard M. Babior

Tufts New England Medical Center
171 Harrison Avenue
Boston, Massachusetts

Certain oxidative processes are of great importance in granulocytes, because they provide agents that are used to destroy invading microorganisms. In these processes, oxygen is reduced to yield compounds which are themselves bactericidal, and which undergo secondary reactions to form substances with even greater antibacterial potency. In the present review these processes are discussed, emphasis being placed on the generation and function of superoxide (O_2^-) in these cells.

Attention was first directed to the special role of oxygen in granulocyte function by Sbarra and Karnovsky (1), who showed that uptake of particles by these cells, a process which occurred efficiently under anerobic conditions, nonetheless resulted in two- to threefold increase in the rate of cellular oxygen consumption. Shortly thereafter, an increase in H_2O_2 production was reported to occur under the same conditions (2,3), accompanied by a tenfold rise in glucose oxidation via the hexosemonophosphate shunt (4). It was apparent that special metabolic events were taking place in the stimulated granulocyte.

The purpose behind this metabolic activity became clear with the discovery that cells from patients with chronic granulomatous disease, a condition in which the granulocytes are unable to kill certain species of bacteria, failed to show the characteristic changes in oxidative metabolism displayed by normal cells (5), and the finding that myeloperoxidase, an enzyme present in very large quantities in granulocytes (6), catalyzed the formation of a highly bactericidal agent from H_2O_2 and halide ion (7,8). These observations suggested that the special metabolic events which occurred in stimulated granulocytes were part of a mechanism used by these cells to kill ingested bacteria. Partial correction of the killing defect in chronic granulomatous disease by the introduction into the granulocyte of an H_2O_2-generating system provided further evidence that these events were important in the bactericidal activity of the cell (9).

The foregoing observations, plus much additional evidence not cited here, indicate strongly the existence of a granulocytic bactericidal mechanism involving an interaction between myeloperoxidase, halide ion and the H_2O_2 generated by oxidative metabolism. It was therefore of great interest to learn of a family, some of whose members have no detectible myeloperoxidase in their granulocytes but who nonetheless are troubled very little by infections (10). If the H_2O_2-halide-myeloperoxidase mechanism were the only oxygen-dependent bactericidal mechanism in the granulocyte, myeloperoxidase-deficient patients would be expected to have as much difficulty with infections as patients with chronic granulomatous disease. The fact that they are largely free of bacterial infections implies that the granulocyte possesses other oxygen-dependent bactericidal mechanisms besides the one involving myeloperoxidase.

The clue to a possible alternative mechanism was provided by the discovery by McCord and Fridovich (11, 12) of superoxide dismutase, an enzyme catalyzing the dismutation of superoxide to hydrogen peroxide and oxygen:

$$O_2^- + O_2^- + 2H^+ \longrightarrow O_2 + H_2O_2$$

O_2^- is the compound formed by the one-electron reduction of oxygen. In terms of granulocyte metabolism, the discovery of superoxide dismutase was important for two reasons: it implied that biological systems had to be protected from O_2^- (otherwise, why would the enzyme have evolved?), and it provided a means by which the production of O_2^- in such systems could be detected. With the aid of this enzyme, we began to investigate the possibility that O_2^- was involved in the oxygen-dependent bactericidal processes of granulocytes.

The Production of O_2^- by Granulocytes

The first experiments performed in this investigation were designed to answer the least differentiated question of all: do granulocytes produce O_2^-? To detect O_2^- production, granulocytes were incubated with ferricytochrome c, an electron acceptor dye which is reduced by O_2^- to form ferrocytochrome c:

$$O_2^- + \text{Cyt } \underline{c}\ (Fe^{3+}) \longrightarrow O_2 + \text{Cyt } \underline{c}\ (Fe^{2+})$$

Incubations were conducted in the presence and absence of superoxide dismutase, and the difference between ferricytochrome c reduction under these two conditions was taken to represent O_2^- production by cells. The results are shown in Table 1.

Table 1. O_2^- production by granulocytes

Additions	O_2^--dependent cyt c reduction (nmoles/3 x 10^6 cells/30 min)
None	3.7
Serum	9.2
Bacteria	6.7
Serum & Bacteria	30.3

It is apparent that granulocytes manufacture O_2^-, and that its rate of production is augmented by serum and bacteria (13, 14).

The next series of experiments concerned the relationship between O_2^- production and the changes in oxygen metabolism occurring in stimulated granulocytes. The augmentation in O_2^- production on exposure of granulocytes to serum plus bacteria suggested already that, like oxygen uptake, O_2^- production was "turned on" by stimulation of the cells. Several additional lines of evidence have confirmed this notion. The course of O_2^- production following the exposure of granulocytes to a stimulus (Fig. 1) is very similar to the course of the changes in oxygen uptake observed under the same conditions (14); both processes

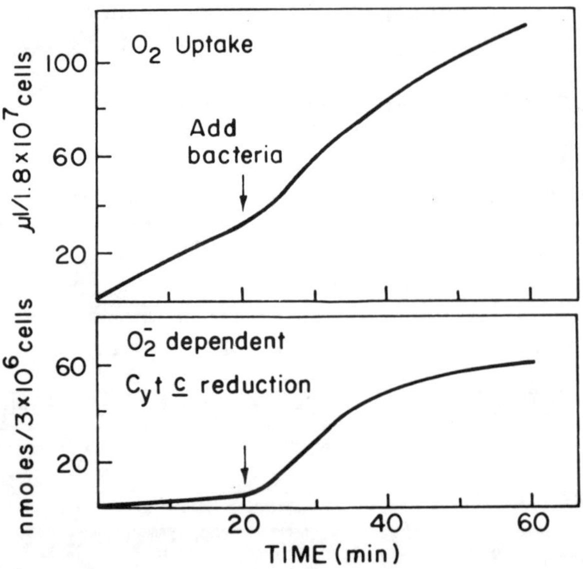

Fig. 1. Comparison between O_2^- production and oxygen uptake in stimulated granulocytes

increase in rate over 5-10 minutes to a maximum, then after another 20-30 minutes subside once again to the resting level. (The magnitude of the changes relative to the resting level, however, are very different for the two processes. Oxygen uptake typically increases by a factor of 2 or 3, while the maximum rate of O_2^- production exceeds its resting level by a factor of 10 or more. At its peak, O_2^- production accounted for 25% of the incremental increase in oxygen consumption in stimulated cells; this is a minimum value, since it represents only that fraction of manufactured O_2^- which escaped from the cells into the surrounding medium). Both processes are similarly affected by metabolic inhibitors, being unchanged by heme enzyme poisons and an uncoupler of oxidative phosphorylation but greatly impaired by sulfhydryl reagents (1) (Table 2).

Table 2. The effect of metabolic inhibitors on O_2^- production and stimulated oxygen uptake in granulocytes

Agent	Rate (% of control)	
	Stimulated oxygen uptake*	O_2^- production**
Cyanide	59	92
Antimycin A	103	93
2,4-Dinitrophenol	80	105
Sulfhydryl reagents***	16	7

* Adapted from reference 1
** Curnutte and Babior, submitted for publication
*** Iodoacetate, iodoacetamide, p-hydroxy-mercuribenzoate

Table 3. O_2^- production by granulocytes from patients with chronic granulomatous disease (CGD)

Subjects	O_2^- production (nmoles/3 x 10^6 cells/30 min)	
	Resting cells	Stimulated cells
Normal adults	12.4	29.7
Children without CGD	10.9	26.1
Children with CGD		
1	0.3	0.9
2	0.2	0.9

Neither process occurs in cells from patients with chronic granulomatous disease (5,15) (Table 3). All these findings confirm that a substantial increase in the rate of O_2^- production is one of the changes in oxygen metabolism that takes place when the granulocyte is stimulated.

O_2^- and Bacterial Killing

The chemical reactivity of O_2^-, the previously discussed findings indicating that it is produced in large quantities by stimulated granulocytes, and the presence of superoxide dismutase in aerotolerant microorganisms, but not in obligate anerobes (16), all suggested that O_2^- is a bactericidal agent used by granulocytes for the destruction of ingested microorganisms. Notwithstanding these considerations, data available so far fail to support a direct bactericidal effect of O_2^-. What they appear to indicate is that certain products formed in secondary reactions involving O_2^- are the agents that destroy bacteria.

O_2^-, once formed, rapidly undergoes a series of reactions leading to the production of singlet oxygen, H_2O_2

and possibly hydroxyl radical (·OH) (12, 17, 18).

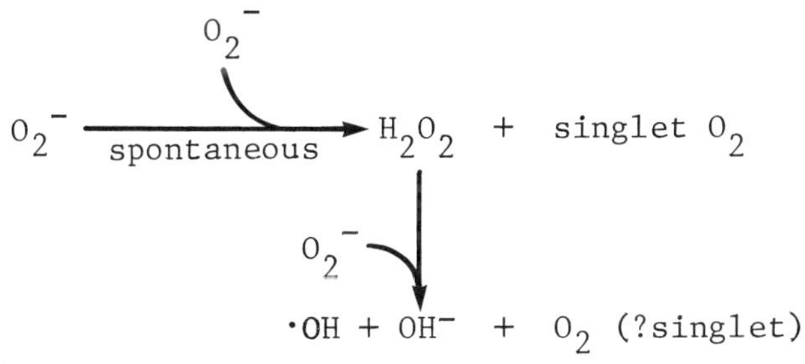

The formation of other reactive oxygen derivatives by reactions unknown at present cannot be excluded, and in fact seems likely considering the reactivity of the compounds listed above.

Any of these compounds may be considered as a candidate antibacterial agent. Of those definitely known to arise by reactions involving O_2^-, two have been shown to have antibacterial activity: H_2O_2, and a compound (·OH?) formed in a reaction between H_2O_2 and O_2^-.

The participation of H_2O_2 in the bactericidal mechanisms of granulocytes has been documented largely by the work of Klebanoff (7,8). In high concentrations, H_2O_2 is by itself bactericidal. Its antibacterial potency is greatly increased in the presence of myeloperoxidase and a halide ion, under which circumstances it is able to destroy bacteria at remarkably low concentrations. H_2O_2 is effective in this system whether added directly or generated in situ by the spontaneous or enzyme-catalyzed dismutation of O_2^- arising from the xanthine oxidase-catalyzed conversion of xanthine to uric acid (19). One manner in which O_2^- is involved in the bactericidal activity of granulocytes, therefore, is as a precursor of the H_2O_2 used in the peroxide-halide-myeloperoxidase system.

There are several observations, however, indicating that the participation of O_2^- in bacterial killing may involve more than merely the generation of H_2O_2. The evidence for this conclusion rests largely on the finding that killing of bacteria in certain systems is abolished by superoxide dismutase, an enzyme which catalyzes the formation of H_2O_2 during the course of its activity. Reports from Fridovich's laboratory have indicated that the killing by an O_2^--generating system of two species of microorganism--*L. plantarum*, and a strain of *E. coli* which was grown on an iron-deficient medium to deplete the organism of its periplasmic superoxide dismutase--was greatly reduced when superoxide dismutase was added to the system (20, 21). The former organism was also protected by catalase; the effect of catalase on the killing of the dismutase-deficient *E. coli* was not tested. Our own observations have supported Fridovich's findings. We studied the killing of *E. coli* and *S. epidermidis* by an O_2^--generating system (purine plus xanthine oxidase) (22). Both organisms were killed by this system (Table 4). *E. coli* was protected by catalase, but not by superoxide dismutase (this strain of *E. coli* was a wild-type strain obtained from ATCC, and presumably possessed a full complement of its own periplasmic dismutase), while *S. epidermidis* was protected both by

Table 4. Killing of microorganisms by a purine-xanthine oxidase system

Addition	Colonies (% of control)	
	E. coli	*S. epidermidis*
Superoxide dismutase		
Active	21	73
Autoclaved	15	18
Catalase		
Active	91	133
Boiled	6	0

catalase and by superoxide dismutase. Thus, in this system E. coli appeared to be killed by H_2O_2 alone, while the killing of S. epidermidis required the product of a reaction between H_2O_2 and O_2^-, since it was prevented by both catalase and superoxide dismutase.

For killing to occur, xanthine oxidase had to be present in high concentrations. E. coli survival was affected in a conventional way by changes in the concentration of the enzyme, falling smoothly as the xanthine oxidase concentration rose. In contrast, the survival of S. epidermidis showed a very sharp dependence on xanthine oxidase concentration, falling from almost complete survival to no survival at all over less than a threefold increase in the concentration of enzyme (Fig. 2). This finding suggests a high order dependence of killing on O_2^- concentration, consistent with a mechanism requiring the participation of several O_2^- molecules (three, in the simplest formulation) in the formation of the bactericidal agent.

The identity of the agent responsible for the killing of S. epidermidis in this system is not known. Although ·OH, possibly formed as noted above in a reaction between

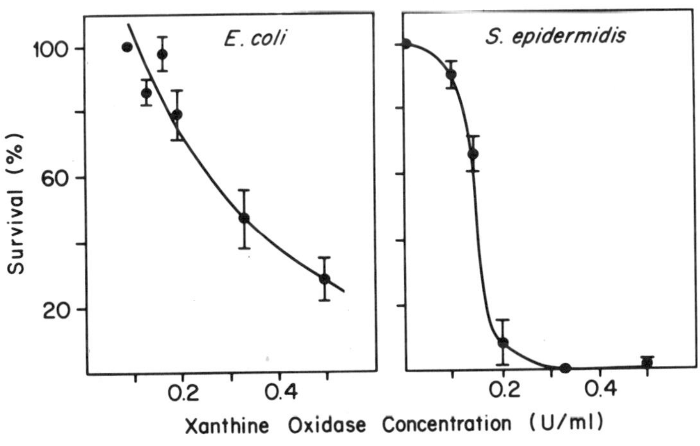

Fig. 2. Survival of bacteria in a purine-xanthine oxidase O_2^--generating system as a function of xanthine oxidase concentration

O_2^- and H_2O_2, is an obvious candidate, evidence for its participation in this process is inconclusive.

Does O_2^- participate in bacterial killing in granulocytes as anything other than a precursor of H_2O_2? A preliminary report published by Johnston et al (23) suggests that it does. These workers found that the killing of E. coli and S. aureus by granulocytes was inhibited when either superoxide dismutase or catalase was present in the incubation medium. The effect of these enzymes was greatly augmented in the presence of latex particles, which appeared to facilitate entry of the enzymes from the incubation medium into the phagocyte. If these data are confirmed, they will provide conclusive evidence for the participation of O_2^- in a bacterial killing mechanism independent of the peroxide-halide-myeloperoxidase system.

O_2^- Metabolism in Granulocyte Homogenates

Most of the studies of O_2^- metabolism in granulocyte homogenates have dealt with the occurrence of superoxide dismutase in these preparations. Eukaryotic cells ordinarily contain two types of dismutase--a manganese-containing enzyme in the mitochondria and an enzyme containing copper and zinc in the cell sap--and evidence has been reported for the presence of both types of enzyme in human granulocytes (24-26). Presumably these dismutases, while protecting the cell against the small quantities of O_2^- produced in the resting state, are present at concentrations too low to deal with the amounts of O_2^- generated by the stimulated cell.

Of more relevance to the oxygen-dependent bactericidal mechanism per se would be an investigation of the O_2^--forming apparatus of the granulocyte in a cell free system. We have recently undertaken such an investigation. Using as an assay a modification of the method described by Misra and Fridovich involving the O_2^--mediated oxidation of epinephrine to adrenochrome, we were able to demonstrate O_2^- production by a homogenate of human granulocytes. Repeated failures to demonstrate a requirement for a reducing agent led us to conclude that epinephrine itself is the reducing agent in this system. With an assay based on the O_2^--dependent reduction of nitro blue tetrazolium to the corresponding formazan, however, we were able to obtain preliminary evidence that granulocyte homogenates catalyze O_2^- formation using a reduced pyridine nucleotide as electron donor.

SUMMARY

O_2^-, formed when oxygen is reduced by one electron, is produced by granulocytes. Augmentation of its rate of production is one of the changes in oxidative metabolism which occur when granulocytes are stimulated. O_2^- appears to be involved in the antimicrobial activity of granulocytes, both as a precursor of H_2O_2 used in the peroxide-halide-myeloperoxidase system and as a reactant which in combination with H_2O_2 generates an antimicrobial agent which acts independently of myeloperoxidase. Preliminary evidence suggests that O_2^- is formed in the granulocyte by the pyridine nucleotide dependent reduction of oxygen. In addition to an O_2^--generating apparatus, granulocytes contain superoxide dismutase, an enzyme which converts O_2^- to oxygen and H_2O_2, to protect themselves against the deleterious effects of O_2^-.

REFERENCES

1. Sbarra, A.J. and Karnovsky, M.L. (1959). The biochemical basis of phagocytosis. I. Metabolic changes during the ingestion of particles by polymorphonuclear leukocytes. J. Biol. Chem. 234, 1355.

2. Iyer, G.Y.N., Islam, M.F., and Quastel, J.H. (1961). Biochemical aspects of phagocytosis. Nature Lond. 192, 535.

3. Paul, B. and Sbarra, A.J. (1968). The role of the phagocytes in host-parasite interactions. XII. The direct quantitative estimation of H_2O_2 in phagocytizing cells. Biochim. Biophys. Acta 156, 168.

4. Baehner, R.L., Gilman, N., and Karnovsky, M.L. (1970). Respiration and glucose oxidation in human and guinea pig leukocytes: comparative studies. J. Clin. Invest. 49, 692.

5. Holmes, B., Page, A.R., and Good, R.A. (1967). Studies of the metabolic activity of leukocytes from patients with a genetic abnormality of phagocytic function. J. Clin. Invest. 46, 1422.

6. Schultz, J. and Kaminker, K. (1962). Myeloperoxidase of the leukocytes of normal human blood. I. Content and localization. Arch. Biochem. Biophys. 96, 465.

7. Klebanoff, S.J. (1967). Iodination of bacteria: a bactericidal mechanism. J. Exp. Med. 126, 1063.

8. Klebanoff, S.J. and Hamon, C.B. (1972). Role of myeloperoxidase-mediated antimicrobial systems in intact leukocytes. J. Reticuloendothel Soc. 12, 170.

9. Baehner, R.L., Nathan, D.G., and Karnovsky, M.L. (1970). Correction of metabolic deficiencies in the leukocytes of patients with chronic granulomatous disease. J. Clin. Invest. 49, 865.

10. Lehrer, R.I. and Cline, M.J. (1969). Leukocyte myeloperoxidase deficiency and disseminated candidiasis: the role of myeloperoxidase in resistance to Candida infection. J. Clin. Invest. 48, 1478.

11. McCord, J.M. and Fridovich, I. (1969). Superoxide dismutase. An enzymic function for erythrocuprein (hemocuprein). J. Biol. Chem. 244, 6049.

12. Fridovich, I. (1972). Superoxide radical and superoxide dismutase. Account Chem. Res. 5, 321.

13. Babior, B.M., Kipnes, R.S., and Curnutte, J.T. (1973). Biological defense mechanisms: the production by leukocytes of superoxide, a potential bactericidal agent. J. Clin. Invest. 52, 741.

14. Curnutte, J.T. and Babior, B.M. (1974). Biological defense mechanisms. The effect of bacteria and serum on superoxide production by granulocytes. J. Clin. Invest. 53, 1662.

15. Curnutte, J.T., Whitten, D.M., and Babior, B.M. (1974). Defective superoxide production by granulocytes from patients with chronic granulomatous disease. New Engl. J. Med. 290, 593.

16. McCord, J.M., Keele, B.B., Jr., and Fridovich, I. (1971). An enzyme-based theory of obligate anaerobiosis: the physiological function of superoxide dismutase. Proc. Nat. Acad. Sci. USA 68, 1024.

17. Khan, A.U. (1970). Singlet molecular oxygen from superoxide anion and sensitized fluorescence of organic molecules. Science 168, 476.

18. Haber, F. and Weiss, J. (1934). The catalytic decomposition of hydrogen peroxide by iron. Proc. Roy. Soc. A 147, 332.

19. Klebanoff, S.J. (1974). Role of the superoxide anion in the myeloperoxidase-mediated antimicrobial system. J. Biol. Chem. 249, 3724.

20. Gregory, E.M., Yost, F.J., Jr., and Fridovich, I. (1973). Superoxide dismutases of Escherichia coli: intracellular localization and functions. J. Bacteriol. 115, 987.

21. Gregory, E.M. and Fridovich, I. (1974). Oxygen metabolism in Lactobacillus plantarum. J. Bacteriol. 117, 166.

22. Babior, B.M., Curnutte, J.T., and Kipnes, R.S. (1974). Biological defense mechanisms. Evidence for the participation of superoxide in bacterial killing by xanthine oxidase. J. Lab. Clin. Med., in press.

23. Johnston, R.B., Jr., Keele, B., Webb, L., Kessler, D., and Rajagopalan, K.V. (1973). Inhibition of phagocytic bactericidal activity by superoxide dismutase: a possible role for superoxide anion in the killing of phagocytized bacteria. J. Clin. Invest. 52, 44a.

24. Beckman, G., Lundgren, E., and Tarnvik, A. (1973). Superoxide dismutase isoenzymes in different human tissues: their genetic control and intracellular localization. Hum. Hered. 23, 338.

25. DeChatelet, L.R., McCall, C.E., McPhail, L.C., and Johnston, R.B., Jr. (1974). Superoxide dismutase activity in leukocytes. J. Clin. Invest. 53, 1197.

26. Johnston, R.B., Jr. and DeChatelet, L.R. (1974). Protection against superoxide anion. New Engl. J. Med. 290, 1383.

DISCUSSION

Dr. McCord: *E. coli* contain two SOD's, one is a manganese enzyme in the cytoplasm and one is an iron enzyme in the periplasmic space, which is between the cell membrane and the cell wall. I believe that Yost and Fridovich have shown that SOD will protect *E. Coli* which are iron deficient against superoxide generated by xanthine oxidase. It seems to me to be a reasonable point that *E. coli* and similar microorganisms that grow in nature, and not in a rich culture medium, might be iron deficient. I don't know how much iron there is available to bugs that are growing in a systemic infection, for example. A naturally occuring *E. coli* might be iron deficient, relative to one that we grow in a rich medium.

Dr. Brewer: Do you have any idea what the serum factor might be which is involved in the stimulation?

Dr. Babior: I can tell you some things that it isn't. We are obviously looking for what it is. It is not complement, at least from C_3 on, because serum heated at 56° for 45 minutes is just as effective as unheated serum. That's point one. Point two is that whatever it is, after it is activated, it is heat labile because when you boil the serum you destroy the activity. Point three is that we looked at serum from a patient who was tentatively diagnosed as having Fletcher factor deficiency, which is a deficiency of circulating prekallikrein. We tried that serum and in addition tried some purified kallikrein that Bob Colman in Philadelphia was kind enough to send us. These experiments showed that kallikrein was not it. It is not any of the conventional opsonins or anything like that. I think it is going to be very interesting to find out what it is. And, believe me, we're working on it.

Dr. Eaton: It's been shown that a chemotactic factor exists in the supernatant of E. coli cultures. Might your factor be something like this?

Dr. Babior: One problem with that suggestion is that

microorganisms don't have the effect of serum that has been previously exposed to microorganisms. Now you could argue, of course, that the serum has released endotoxin from the microorganisms and now the white cell is able to see the bottom side of the endotoxin and the lipid A is doing the activation while the side of the endotoxin that the white cell sees when the microorganism is coated with it.... obviously, that is certainly a possibility that can't be excluded.

Unidentified speaker: I don't see how you make the distinction between something in serum that has been activated by the microorganism versus something in the microorganism that has been activated by something in the serum, and subsequently released. Isn't it just a symmetrical problem?

Dr. Babior: Yes, that's right, it could be.

Dr. Geyer: What happens to the white cell during this time? What is protecting it from the damage and why are bacteria much more susceptible apparently?

Dr. Babior: Let me say first of all that this is something that we have to look at. We have to do trypan blue exclusion and things like that to determine if the white cell is surviving. On the other hand, even if the white cell dies in the sense that it is going to disintegrate in an hour or two it may be in a sense clinically dead--it is hanging together sufficiently to keep the microorganism in a phagocytic vacuole and generate O_2^- into it. It could be like the snake that bites you after it is dead. Even if the cell itself is sufficiently destroyed so that it can't exclude trypan blue, which I'm not sure is the case, actually.

Dr. Geyer: What is the mechanism of the killing action itself, do you know or can you postulate?

Dr. Babior: I wouldn't be surprised if it has something to do with the membrane in the cell. There are other killing mechanisms that may do other things but I suspect that the O_2^- dependent killing mechanism is going to involve the surface of the microorganism in some respect. I don't think anyone has looked at this question as yet. Maybe Joe McCord, because I know he has been interested in what O_2^- does to biological macromolecules, but nobody else has to my knowledge.

Dr. Geyer: I would think that if Dr. McCord's idea is right that this is generated in the membrane, the concentration in the membrane must be terribly high compared to anything that is any distance from the cell and with all the various lipids present in those membranes, I certainly would think it would not only effectively damage the cell but I would think lipids would be a scavenger for these oxygen radicals.

Dr. Babior: I'm not sure whether or not it is made in the membrane. I think your point is well taken, I just think that nobody really knows at this moment about the effects of the agent on the white cell itself, which I gather is the question you were asking.

Dr. McCord: I think the self destruction of white cells plays a considerable role in inflammation. I like to think of white cells as little Kamikaze pilots and I think that is a fairly good analogy. After they have done their job on whatever it is they have ingested and killed, they go on to lyse and dump all sorts of contents, hydrolytic proteases and all sorts of digestive enzymes into the interstitial fluid in whatever tissue they happen to have invaded. I think that subsequent reactions of these lysosomal enzymes can be a big factor in the side effects of this process which we see as inflammation.

Dr. Babior: I think this is the general view but I am not sure that the white cells will put lysosomal enzymes into the medium without necessarily dying. The work of Weissman and Peter Henson and others have indicated that. I think that the evidence that the white cells really are dead an hour after they see microorganisms is not certain. I really haven't seen anyone who has studied that specific question although I certainly may have missed an article.

Dr. McCord: I have some preliminary data that have not been published that show that extracellular SOD does inhibit release of lysosomal enzymes from activated white cells--acid phosphatase, for example.

INDEX